NONINVASIVE INSTRUMENTATION AND MEASUREMENT IN MEDICAL DIAGNOSIS

Biomedical Engineering Series

Edited by Michael R. Neuman

Published Titles

Electromagnetic Analysis and Design in Magnetic Resonance Imaging, Jianming Jin

Endogenous and Exogenous Regulation and Control of Physiological Systems, Robert B. Northrop

Artificial Neural Networks in Cancer Diagnosis, Prognosis, and Treatment, Raouf N.G. Naguib and Gajanan V. Sherbet

Medical Image Registration, Joseph V. Hajnal, Derek Hill, and David J. Hawkes

Introduction to Dynamic Modeling of Neuro-Sensory Systems, Robert B. Northrop

Noninvasive Instrumentation and Measurement in Medical Diagnosis, Robert B. Northrop

Forthcoming Titles

Handbook of Neuroprosthetic Methods, Warren E. Finn and Peter G. LoPresti

The BIOMEDICAL ENGINEERING Series
Series Editor: Michael R. Neuman

NONINVASIVE INSTRUMENTATION AND MEASUREMENT IN MEDICAL DIAGNOSIS

Robert B. Northrop

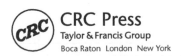

CRC Press
Taylor & Francis Group
Boca Raton London New York

CRC Press is an imprint of the
Taylor & Francis Group, an **informa** business

CRC Press
Taylor & Francis Group
6000 Broken Sound Parkway NW, Suite 300
Boca Raton, FL 33487-2742

First issued in paperback 2019

© 2002 by Taylor & Francis Group, LLC
CRC Press is an imprint of Taylor & Francis Group, an Informa business

No claim to original U.S. Government works

ISBN-13: 978-0-8493-0961-8 (hbk)
ISBN-13: 978-0-367-39693-0 (pbk)

Visit the Taylor & Francis Web site at
http://www.taylorandfrancis.com

and the CRC Press Web site at
http://www.crcpress.com

Library of Congress Cataloging-in-Publication Data

Northrop, Robert B.
    Noninvasive instrumentation and measurement in medical diagnosis / Robert B. Northrop.
        p. ; cm.--(The biomedical engineering series)
    Includes bibliographical references and index.
    ISBN 0-8493-0961-1 (alk. paper)
    1. Diagnosis, Noninvasive--Instruments. I. Title. II. Biomedical engineering series
(Boca Raton, Fla.)
    [DNLM: 1. Diagnostic Techniques and Procedures--instrumentation. 2. Laboratory
    Techniques and Procedures--instrumentation. WB 141 N877n 2001]
    RC71.6 .N67 2001
    616.07′5—dc21   20001037312

Library of Congress Card Number 20001037312

Preface

This text is about the instruments, and sometimes the procedures, that are used for noninvasive medical diagnosis. Why stress "noninvasive"? Noninvasive medical diagnosis (NIMD) is preferred whenever possible to avoid the risks and expense attendant to surgically opening the body surface, e.g., infection; adverse systemic reactions to anesthesia, dye injection, antibiotics and other medications; and surgical error. In many instances, NIMD is less expensive than equivalent invasive procedures, in other cases (e.g., imaging), it is the *only* practical means of diagnosis, but, in some cases (e.g., imaging), it is the most expensive diagnostic modality because of the complex technology involved.

This text was written based on both the author's experience in teaching EE 370, Biomedical Instrumentation I, for more than 25 years in the Electrical and Computer Engineering Department at the University of Connecticut, and on his personal research on certain prototype noninvasive medical instrumentation systems. The contents of EE 370 have evolved with instrumentation technology and our knowledge of human diseases, physiology, biochemistry, and cell biology.

Because NIMD is a rapidly growing interdisciplinary field, a number of the systems described in this text are prototypes that are currently in the research phase of their development. In the author's opinion, these systems will probably be effective, and we will eventually see their general acceptance by the medical community. I expect photonics and photonic means of measurement to play an increasingly important role in future NIMD instrument development. As the reader will see, the photon is here to stay.

This text is intended for use in an introductory classroom course on Noninvasive Medical Instrumentation and Measurements, which is taken by juniors, seniors and graduate students in biomedical engineering. It will also serve as a reference book for medical students and other health professionals interested in the topic. Practicing physicians and nurses interested in learning the state of the art in this important field will also find this text valuable. Physicists, biophysicists and physiologists working in the biomedical field will also find it of interest.

Readers are assumed to have had introductory core courses in human (medical) physiology, biomedical engineering, engineering systems analysis, and electronic circuits. Their mathematical skills should include an introductory course on differential equations, as well as college-level algebra and calculus. Having taken these courses, the readers should be skilled in understanding systems block diagrams, simple electronic circuits, the concepts of frequency response and transfer functions, and ordinary differential equations. It is also important to have an understanding of how the physiological parameters being measured figure in human health. Much of the material in this text is descriptive, but many systems are analyzed in detail. The teacher who considers adopting this text for classroom use should be advised that there are no chapter home problems.

In writing this text, I have been amazed at the depth, breadth and quality of the information available on the topic of NIMD and all its modalities on the World Wide Web. I can perhaps be criticized for using and citing Internet sources because they are ephemeral in the purest sense. Those readers who wish to pursue some of my Web references for additional details on a topic ought to act fast. I estimate the half-life of a Web resource as being 1.5 years. Web resources offer a window on cutting-edge technologies, however. Sometimes, the view begins with university press releases on new research. A good search engine, such as google.com, is invaluable. I have also relied on standard texts and references in my writing.

Noninvasive Instrumentation and Measurements in Medical Diagnosis is organized into 17 chapters, including an Index and an extensive Bibliography and References section. Below, I summarize the chapter contents:

Chapter 1, Introduction, defines what is meant by noninvasive measurements and gives many examples. (Some persons might argue that use of a colonoscope or a bronchoscope is, in fact, an invasive procedure; we classify their use as minimally invasive.) Also provided is an overview and history of the use of simple, noninvasive procedures to diagnose disease as practiced in the 19th century and earlier, and I explain their importance in modern medicine

Chapter 2, Visual Inspection of Tissues with Endoscopes and Other Optical Devices, describes the simple, modern optical instruments that allow the medical practitioner to directly inspect tissues for foreign objects, infections, tumors, etc. Attention is given to the use of ophthalmoscopes and slit lamps to inspect the retina, the cornea and internal structures of the eye. Various types of endoscopes are described that allow direct inspection of a variety of tissues and organs accessible from without the body (e.g., the lungs, colon, stomach, urethra, bladder, and renal pelvis). Modern, coherent fiber-optic bundles are used in some applications with miniature high-resolution CCD TV cameras.

Chapter 3, Sounds from Within the Body, treats the medically important sounds arising from within the body (the heart, lungs, joints, blood vessel bruits, and otoacoustic emissions, as well as the fetal heart). Basic instrumentation is described, including the stethoscope, microphones, filters, and the use of FFT frequency analysis. The growing importance of time-frequency spectrograms in the description of sounds, and in NIMD, is stressed.

Chapter 4, Measurement of Electrical Potentials from the Body Surface, first describes the sources of skin-surface electrical potential from electrically active internal organs (heart, brain, muscles, retina, cochlea, nerves). The signal-coupling properties of various bioelectrodes are treated, followed by sections on the medical significance of each of the potentials (ECG, EMG, EEG, ERG, EOG, ECoG). Differential and medical isolation amplifiers are covered in detail, as are low-noise amplifier analysis and design. The SQUID, and biomagnetic measurements with SQUID arrays, are also described.

In Chapter 5, NI Measurements of Blood Pressure, the use of the sphygmomanometer is described (manual and automatic) in measuring systolic and diastolic blood pressure. Blood pressure estimates can also be made from finger plethysmographs.

Chapter 6, Body Temperature Measurements, considers the basic thermometer, (mercury and electronic) and its importance in detecting fever or hypothermia. Basic heat flow relations are used to describe thermometer response time. The design and physics of the no-touch, LIR thermometer, which reads body temperature from the eardrum, is elaborated..

Chapter 7, Noninvasive Blood Gas Sensing with Electrodes, describes the use of electrochemical electrodes on heated skin used to sense tissue pCO_2 and tissue pO_2.

Chapter 8, Tests on Naturally Voided Body Fluids, reviews a number of analytical instrumental techniques that can be used on body fluids (urine, saliva and breath) to measure the concentrations of certain ions, glucose, urea, drugs, etc. Various analytical instruments used in laboratory medicine are described, including dispersive and non-dispersive spectroscopy, surface plasmon resonance, ion-selective electrodes, flame photometers, gas chromatography, and mass spectrometry. It then goes on to review what can be found of diagnostic significance in urine, feces, saliva and breath.

Chapter 9, Plethysmography, describes the applications of plethysmography in quantifying body volume changes due to breathing, muscle contraction, blood flow, etc. Volume changes can be measured by water displacement, pneumatically, or electronically.

Chapter 10, Pulmonary Function Tests, first describes the volume displacement spirometer, then the use of turbines and pneumotachs to electronically measure respiratory flow and volumes. Spirometers are used to quantify mechanical respiratory functions with such parameters as lung tidal volume, forced expiratory volumes, etc. Their use is critical in detecting obstructive lung diseases and plotting their progress. Also covered is the use of inhaled inert gases in the measurement of respiratory function.

The Measurement of Basal Metabolism is described in Chapter 11. The physiology behind the measurement protocol is explained, and the apparatus and protocol are given. Basal metabolism measurement is a basic NI means of assessing thyroid function.

Chapter 12, Ocular Tonometry, discusses the importance to vision of monitoring the intraocular pressure. The designs of various tonometers, including the no-touch air-puff applanation system are described.

Chapter 13, NI Tests Involving the Input of Audible Sound Energy, treats measurements in which low-frequency acoustic energy (generally 2 to 2000 Hz) is used to characterize the respiratory system or the ear canal and eardrum. It first describes the concepts of acoustic resistance, capacitance, and inertance (inductance), and shows how complex acoustic impedance can be simply measured.

The RAIMS system is described for the measurement of the acoustic Z of the lungs and bronchial tree. Acoustic Z is also shown to be useful in characterizing the compliance of the eardrum and the tympanal reflex. Finally, a means of measuring the acoustic transfer function of the chest cavity and lungs with transmitted white noise is described. The measurement and acoustic Z of the lungs have application in detecting and quantifying obstructive lung disease.

Chapter 14, NI Tests Using Ultrasound (Excluding Imaging), begins by describing the physics and mathematics associated with the Doppler effect. Next covered is the use of CW and pulsed Doppler ultrasound to measure blood velocity, and its diagnostic utility. Another application is the use of air-coupled ultrasound to measure the ocular pulse. The closed-loop, constant phase, NOTOPM system of Northrop and Nilakhe is described, and the uses of the ocular pulse in diagnosis are detailed. A significant improvement on the NOTOPM ocular pulse system, the constant-phase, closed-loop, type 1 ranging system (CPRS) is presented and its possible future applications in the quantitative measurement of aneurisms, heart motion, and the shape of internal organs are described. (The CPRS system gives a simultaneous output of distance and velocity.)

Chapter 15, NI Applications of Photon Radiation (Excluding Imaging), covers a wide spectrum of topics (pun intended): X-ray bone densitometry by the DEXA method; tissue fluorescence spectroscopy; optical interferometric measurement of nanometer tissue displacements; laser Doppler velocimetry — percutaneous IR spectroscopy; glucose measurement in the aqueous humor of the eye by polarimetry (the rotation of linearly polarized light); pulse oximetry — applications of Raman spectroscopy in detecting cancer and dissolved glucose are described.

Chapter 16, A Survey of Medical Imaging Systems, first considers the input modalities of coherent light, X-rays, ultrasound, and γ-rays from radioisotopes. The mathematical means for tomographic imaging are described, including the Radon transform and deblurring techniques. The production of X-rays and their use in flat imaging and CT scanners is treated. Also covered are magnetic resonance imaging (MRI), positron emission tomography (PET) imaging, radionuclide (isotope) imaging (SPECT), ultrasonic imaging, and passive LIR thermal imaging in diagnosis. The present and future imaging capabilities of the emerging field of optical coherence tomography (OCT) are described. Also explored is the new use of coherent X-ray diffraction imaging in high-resolution mammography — all you need is a synchrotron ....

In Chapter 17, Future Trends in NI Measurements and Diagnosis, we consider possible modalities whereby medical professionals can noninvasively examine DNA for mutations, expediting the diagnosis of cancer and research on genetically caused diseases. The DNA microarray, or "gene chip" and the means of reading out probe hits on target molecules are described. The use of fluorescence tagging and laser scanning to read out gene chips, as well as electrical readouts, is described. Biochips are also being designed that can test for specific antibodies to bacteria and viruses, as well as the pathogen coat proteins themselves. The detection of other, non-DNA molecules found in urine and saliva that may be associated with cancer growth is described.

Robert B. Northrop
Chaplin, CT
13 April 2001

The Author

Robert B. Northrop was born in White Plains, NY. He majored in electrical engineering at MIT, graduating with a bachelor's degree. At the University of Connecticut, he received a master's degree in control engineering, and, led by a long-standing interest in physiology, he received his Ph.D. from UCONN in physiology, doing research on the neuromuscular physiology of molluscan catch muscles.

He rejoined the UCONN EE Department as a lecturer, and later as an assistant professor of EE. In collaboration with his Ph.D. advisor, Dr. Edward G. Boettiger, he secured a 5-year training grant from NIGMS (NIH), and started one of the first interdisciplinary biomedical engineering graduate training programs in New England. UCONN awards M.S. and Ph.D. degrees in this field of study.

Throughout his career, Dr. Northrop's areas of research have been broad and interdisciplinary, and have been centered around biomedical engineering. He has done sponsored research on the neurophysiology of insect vision and theoretical models for visual neural signal processing. He also did sponsored research on electrofishing and developed, in collaboration with Northeast Utilities, effective, working systems for fish guidance and control in hydro-electric plant waterways using underwater electric fields.

Still another area of sponsored research has been in the design and simulation of nonlinear, adaptive, digital controllers to regulate *in vivo* drug concentrations or physiological parameters, such as pain, blood pressure or blood glucose in diabetics. An outgrowth of this research led to his development of mathematical models for the dynamics of the human immune system that have been used to investigate theoretical therapies for autoimmune diseases, cancer and HIV infection.

Biomedical instrumentation has also been an active research area: An NIH grant supported studies on the use of the ocular pulse to detect obstructions in the carotid arteries. Minute pulsations of the cornea from arterial circulation in the eyeball were sensed using a no-touch ultrasound technique. Ocular pulse waveforms were shown to be related to cerebral blood flow in rabbits and humans.

Most recently, Dr. Northrop has been addressing the problem of noninvasive blood glucose measurement for diabetics. Starting with a Phase I SBIR grant, he has been developing a means of estimating blood glucose by reflecting a beam of polarized light off the front surface of the lens of the eye, and measuring the very small optical rotation resulting from glucose in the aqueous humor, which, in turn, is proportional to blood glucose. As an offshoot of techniques developed in micropolarimetry, he developed a sample chamber for glucose measurement in biotechnology applications. Another approach being developed will use percutaneous long-wave IR light in a nondispersive spectrometer to noninvasively measure blood glucose.

Dr. Northrop has written four textbooks: one on analog electronic circuits, one on instrumentation and measurements, another on physiological control systems, and the last on neural modeling.

Dr. Northrop was a member of the Electrical & Computer Engineering faculty at UCONN until his retirement in June, 1997. Throughout this time, he was program director of the Biomedical Engineering Graduate Program. As emeritus professor, he now teaches courses in biomedical engineering, writes texts, sails, and travels. He lives in Chaplin, CT, with his wife and two cats.

13 April 2001

Table of Contents

1 Introduction to Noninvasive Measurements

1.1 DEFINITION OF NONINVASIVE MEASUREMENTS, MINIMALLY INVASIVE MEASUREMENTS, AND INVASIVE MEASUREMENTS

A truly noninvasive medical measurement is any measurement system that does not physically breach the skin or enter the body deeply through an external orifice. Thus, the measurement of body temperature with a thermometer in the mouth, rectum, or ear canal is considered noninvasive, as is the use of an otoscope to examine the outer surface of the eardrum. Similarly, the opthalmoscope and the slit lamp, which shine light in the eyes to examine the retina and the cornea and lens, respectively, are considered noninvasive procedures. The transduction of sounds from the body surface (heart, breath, otoacoustic emissions, etc.) is truly noninvasive, as is the recording of electric potentials from the heart (ECG), muscles (EMG), brain (EEG), etc. Medical imaging techniques such as X-ray, X-ray tomography (CAT scan), ultrasound, MRI, PET, etc., are noninvasive; they do involve the input of energetic radiation into the body, however, which generally carries low risk when proper energy levels and doses are observed.

Much can be learned from blood samples; i.e., ion concentrations, red and white blood cell densities, the concentrations of certain hormones, antibodies, cholesterol, drug concentrations, DNA type, etc. The drawing of blood from a superficial vein is a *minimally invasive procedure,* requiring sterile technique.

Endoscopy is a technique for visualizing tissues deep within the body, yet topologically on the outer surface of the body. An example is bronchosopy, where a bronchoscope is inserted through the mouth and larynx into the trachea and bronchial tubes of the lungs to permit visualization of their surfaces and the surfaces inside larger alveoli. Another endoscope is the cystoscope, which is inserted into the urethra to inspect the ureter and the inside of bladder. Many other types exist (see section 2.3). As a rule, endoscopes require sterile technique, and, in some cases, local or general anesthesia; I consider them to be *minimally invasive instruments.*

Some endoscopes, such as laparoscopes, which are inserted into the abdomen through a small incision in the wall of the abdomen or back are used *invasively.* They are used to observe the outsides of the internal organs (intestines, liver, spleen, uterus, bladder, etc.), looking for tumors, infection, damage from trauma, etc. Another invasive procedure is cardiac catheterization, e.g., viewing heart valves with a fiber optic endoscope. One can argue that there are fuzzy classification boundaries separating invasive, minimally invasive, and invasive diagnostic procedures. Anyone who has undergone proctoscopy might be quick to declare that it is a more invasive than minimally invasive diagnostic procedure, considering the preparation, medication, and discomfort involved.

This book is about the instruments and measurement systems used in making modern, noninvasive (NI) medical diagnoses. Some of the instruments and systems described are well established FDA-approved systems; others are prototype systems that eventually may prove affordable and medically effective. It is important for the reader to know where the field of noninvasive diagnostic instrumentation is headed, as well as its present status. Its evolution is rapid, fueled by the advances in information processing and storage, as well as in fields including photonics, molecular biology and medical physics.

Throughout the history of medicine, up to the end of the 19th century, medical diagnosis was necessarily noninvasive. Physicians used their eyes to observe skin lesions or inflammation in the nose, throat and ears. Tactile senses in the hands were used to feel skin temperature, edema, swelling due to infection, lumps under the skin, etc. The ear was used to listen to breath, bowel and heart sounds. The odor of infection was sensed by the physician's nose. Exploratory surgery was seldom done because of the risk of shock due to pain and blood loss, and of infection.

Today, emphasis is on the use of NI diagnosis in health maintenance and emergency medicine. Most of it can be carried out on an outpatient basis, and has little risk of infection or complications that would add to the cost. On the other hand, certain NI instruments, such as the various medical imaging systems, are very expensive to build and maintain and their use fee is commensurately large. Indeed, NI diagnostic procedures, including imaging systems, have been accused of driving up the cost of health maintenance and care (Breindel, 1998). Use of effective but simple NI instruments such as the electrocardiograph, the spirometer and the slit lamp certainly are not culprits in this respect. The advantage of being able to see tumors in the middle of soft tissues such as the brain, lungs, liver, spleen and breasts will continue to drive the need to improve the resolution of expensive imaging systems, and to ensure their use, where indicated.

1.2 MODALITIES OF NI INSTRUMENTATION

Noninvasive medical instruments can be broadly classified between those passive systems that put no energy into the body, and those that input some form of radiation energy (e.g., microwaves, IR, visible and UV light, X-rays, γ-rays, sound and ultrasound), and measure the energy that is either reflected or transmitted. Among the purely passive systems are the well known electrical measurements based on active nerve or muscle membranes. These include potentials recorded via the skin surface from the heart (ECG), brain (EEG), muscles (EMG), ears (ECocG), and eyes (EOG). Sounds from the body's interior, including sounds from the heart valves, pericardium, blood vessels, lungs, bronchial system, pleural cavity, eardrums (spontaneous otoacoustic emissions), joints, etc, can also be recorded from the skin's surface. Body temperature can be sensed from the infrared radiation from the eardrum, or by physically measuring the temperature of the saliva under the tongue or the temperature in the rectum by a liquid-in-glass thermometer, or a thermometer based on a thermistor or platinum resistance element. Tissue pO_2 and pCO_2 can be measured transcutaneously with special chemical electrodes. The only energy put in by endoscopes is white light required to visualize or photograph the tissue being inspected. Blood pressure can be measured noninvasively by Korotkoff sounds emitted by the brachial artery as the pneumatic pressure in a sphygmomanometer cuff is slowly reduced.

Just about every other medical modality that can be measured noninvasively requires some small input of energy. An important class of NI imaging systems uses pulsed ultrasonic energy. The energy level of the input ultrasound is made low enough to avoid tissue-destroying cavitation or heating. Other NI non-imaging diagnostic systems that use continuous-wave (CW) ultrasound include Doppler blood velocity probes and Doppler probes used to sense the fetal heartbeat or detect aneurisms.

Electromagnetic radiation includes radio waves — infrared (IR), visible, and ultraviolet — as well as X-rays and γ-rays (see Figure 1.1). The photons from UV radiation and X- and γ-rays have sufficient energy to knock atomic electrons out of their inner orbits and rupture certain molecular bonds, causing DNA mutations, etc.; UVB, X- and γ-rays are called *ionizing radiations* because of the potential destruction they can cause to biomolecules as the result of ionization of water and other molecules. Thus, the use of NI instruments that emit ionizing radiation is not without some small risk. UVB photons do not penetrate the skin deeply, hence UV damage to skin can include reddening and the creation of various types of skin cancers. The corneas and lenses of eyes given excessive UVB radiation can develop cataracts. X- and γ-ray photons on the other hand, can penetrate the body deeply, causing cell damage in the organs. A high-energy X-ray photon can directly damage a DNA molecule, leading to a cellular mutation if not internally repaired by the cell. If a photon-dislodged electron strikes a water molecule, it can create a *free radical*. The estimated lifetime of a free radical is c. 10 μs, which means it can drift and encounter a DNA molecule, producing indirect damage as stable molecular configurations are restored. Note that we are mostly concerned with electromagnetic ionizing radiations in this text. Certain radioisotopes used in medical imaging and in cancer therapy emit energetic *alpha particles* (He nuclei), *beta particles* (electrons) or *neutrons*. These energetic particles can also generate free radicals and cause DNA damage and cell death.

X-ray machines of all sorts, bone densitometers, and CAT and PET scanners thus carry a small risk of inducing cancer, including leukemia, in the patient. However, most healthy persons absorb far more ionizing radiation in the form of 5.5 MeV alpha particles from the radioactive breakdown of inhaled naturally occurring *radon gas* than they do from X-rays.

Other NI instrumentation systems, such as impedance plethysmographs, pass low levels of ac current (in the microamp range) in the range from 25 to 100 kHz through the tissue being studied. The input of this current is apparently without risk; it is way below the level that will affect the heart, and there is no heating effect on the deep tissues.

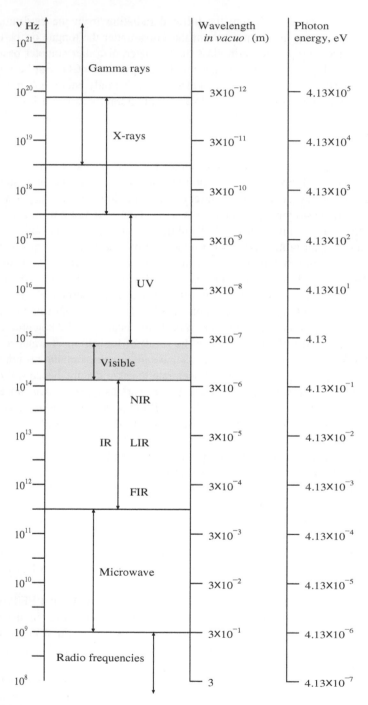

FIGURE 1.1 The electromagnetic spectrum range that finds application in medical diagnosis. Photon energies in electron Volts at a given wavelength are given in the right-hand column.

1.3 SUMMARY

This introductory chapter has made the distinction between truly noninvasive, minimally invasive, and invasive diagnostic instruments and procedures. NI instruments and procedures are important because most can be done on an outpatient basis in a doctor's office or clinic. There are generally few side effects, and minimum risk from infection or other complications.

The following 16 chapters are about the design and application of the instruments used in NI medical diagnosis. Certain signal processing algorithms, such as time-frequency analysis, are also described because of their importance in helping diagnosticians do their job. The final chapter indulges in speculation about where the field of NI diagnosis is heading, considering the on-going contributions from genetics, immunology, molecular biology, and biophotonics. Enjoy.

2 Visual Inspection of Tissues Using Endoscopes and Other Optical Devices

2. 1 INTRODUCTION

The oldest form of medical diagnosis is the direct visual observation of the patient's skin, tongue, eyes and mucous membranes. Health care providers in the millennia before antibiotics were adept at diagnosing local infections, such as those that might have resulted from cuts, abrasions, contusions (bruises), etc., as well as bacterial skin infections such as furuncles and carbuncles. Swelling, skin color, and local heat are external signs of subcutaneous inflammation, which can be caused by bacterial infection, insect bites, or allergy. A fulminating tissue infection can be fatal if the pathogen spreads and attacks organs such as the heart, lungs, kidneys, or brain. A localized or compartmented infection can produce pus, and, in extreme cases, if the pathogen is anaerobic, gas (H_2, N_2).

Malignant melanoma skin lesions are identified by size, color and texture. Touching the skin allows the examiner to detect edema (pitting or non-pitting), and evaluate the general health of the peripheral circulation by the speed of capillary refill (return of skin color on removal of local pressure). Changes in skin color (pallor, yellowing of jaundice) are also diagnostic signs. Eye whites become yellowish in jaundice. The color of the skin on the palms of the hands is also a sign of liver condition. Elevated skin temperature (as sensed by the examiner's hand) can indicate a fever; if the skin is cold and wet (diaphoretic), it may indicate shock.

General aspects of certain tissues are also diagnostic: A baggy face and puffy eyelids, indicative of non-pitting edema, can be the result of extreme hypothyroidism; the same swollen face can be caused by the systemic administration of steroids such as prednisone to control implant tissue rejection. Bulging eyes (exophthalmic condition) can be the result of hyperthyroidism, or severe meningitis. An abdomen swollen with fluid (ascites) can be a sign of congestive heart failure, or a severe blood protein imbalance (low serum oncotic pressure caused by hypoalbuminemia, and high portal venous pressure) due to liver damage (e.g., from alcoholic cirrhosis, or hepatitis). The color of the lips, gums, and tissues around the eyeballs, if pale, can indicate anemia; if blue, cyanosis; if deep red, CO poisoning. The same applies for the tissue under the fingernails.

Fortunately, a given medical condition is accompanied by several symptoms, the non-intersection of which can often lead to a fairly certain diagnosis. Perhaps today, many physicians pay less attention to outward signs than they do to blood and urine chemo-analyses and various imaging readouts to make diagnoses. Still, direct observation is the place to begin any diagnosis. The following sections describe many instrumental enhancements for direct observation of various tissues. Note that certain endoscopic procedures are moderately invasive, and require sterile technique.

2. 2 OPHTHALMOSCOPES, SLIT LAMPS AND OTOSCOPES

2. 2.1 OPHTHALMOSCOPES

The ophthalmoscope is an optical instrument that permits the noninvasive visualization of the front surface of the eye's retina (also known as the fundus), showing blood vessels, general color, surface smoothness, any tears or detachments, and the condition of the macula, etc.

These features are normally viewed by the eye of the examining ophthalmologist, and in modern instruments can also be photographed or recorded as digital color images.

The progenitor of the modern hand-held ophthalmoscope was invented in 1850 by Herrmann von Helmholtz, who appreciated the need for the viewer's line of sight to be collinear with the illuminating beam from the light source. He made a primitive half-silvered mirror from four thin glass microscope slides stacked together. This design allowed the illumination source to be at right angles to the gaze axis of the examiner and patient's eyes (see Figure 2.1) (Eyenet, 2000). Within a year, in order to avoid the intensity losses inherent in partially reflective mirrors, a fully silvered mirror with a hole in it was used to direct the illumination source through the cornea and lens to the retina. The hole allowed the clinician an unobstructed view of the illuminated fundus. An accessory lens was placed in the viewer's sight path to bring the fundus into clear focus, regardless of the combined optical power of the eye's lens and cornea.

A modern ophthalmoscope uses a high-intensity halogen lamp as a light source; often certain colored filters are used over the illumination source to enhance the visibility of features of the fundus. The accessory viewing lens is selected by a turret or wheel. For example, the Neitz model BXa ophthalmoscope has lenses with corrective powers ranging from +36 to −36 diopters, in 1 D steps; two lens wheels are used. In one inexpensive "pocket" ophthalmoscope (Welch-Allyn Model 129), the collimating lens is built into the miniature halogen lamp, and instead of having a hole in the mirror, the sight line to the eye is over the flat top of the mirror. A small imaging lens wheel contains lenses of −15, −8, −5, −3, −1, 0, +1, +3, +5, +8, +12 and +20 diopters. Because of the small size of the lenses, the W-A 129 ophthalmoscope is only marginally effective at resolving retinal details.

Although the optics of the ophthalmoscope are relatively simple, its design has been steadily improved since its invention 150 years ago. The current state of the art is the binocular ophthalmoscope, in which the observer uses both eyes to visualize

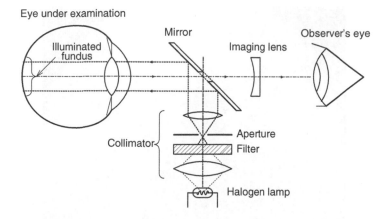

FIGURE 2.1 Schematic of the optical design of an ophthalmoscope. Housing not shown.

the fundus. The scanning laser ophthalmoscope (SLO) and the confocal SLO (CSLO) eliminate the need for direct human observation of the fundus. By rapidly scanning a finely focused low-power laser beam over the retina in a precise pattern and collecting the back-scattered light with a photosensor, it is possible to electronically image the fundus in good detail that is limited only by the optics of the eye under study (cornea, lens and vitreous humor). In CSLO, a pinhole lens is placed in front of the photodiode on a conjugate plane to the retina. Light reflected from different focal planes in the retina is selected by moving the pinhole, allowing tomographic (slice) images of the retina to be constructed over small areas. Using a 785 nm wavelength diode laser source and a novel, double-Gaussian fitting algorithm, it was possible to resolve 32 slices of the retina, 100 μm thick (Vieira, 2000). Very detailed, albeit monochrome, 3-D pictures of the optic disk in normal patients and those with macular edema were obtained. True color was sacrificed for fine textural detail. The use of NIR light minimizes scatter in cloudy media, and lenses with beginning cataracts. SLO and CSLO make it possible to detect the signs of early age-related macular degeneration (ARMD), choroidal neoplasms, and retinas damaged by glaucoma (Kelley et al., 1997).

One of the visible signs of ARMD is the presence of drusen in the retina. According to Cavallerano et al., 1997: "Drusen are yellow to yellowish white nodular deposits found in the deeper layers of the retina. Along with pigmentary abnormalities, drusen are often the earliest ophthalmoscopic signs of aging in the retina. Visual acuity may be normal at this stage. Drusen alone are not enough to satisfy the definition of AMD when vision is normal. Several types of drusen have been described. The lesions are categorized by size, confluence, uniformity and sharpness of borders. Some form of drusen are found in the macular area in 50–95 percent of persons over age 70. Among persons with drusen, 10–15 percent may eventually develop exudative manefestations of ARMD."

Figure 2.2 illustrates a typical fundus showing macular drusen bodies. About 15% of the cases of ARMD are of the "wet" type, in which there is abnormal proliferation of leaky retinal blood vessels. These leaky vessels damage the macula

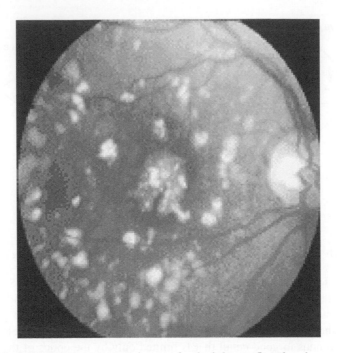

FIGURE 2.2 Ophthalmoscope camera image of retinal drusen. In color, drusen appear yellowish against the red retinal background. The fovea, containing drusen, is at the center of the image. The optic nerve entry is the light area on the right. (This image in color and many other interesting fundus images are available at the Washington Academy of Eye Physicians and Surgeons website: www.wa-eyemd. org.)

and fovea (responsible for central high-resolution color vision), and are responsible for 90% of ARMD vision loss (Rowell, 2000).

The reader will appreciate the tremendous diversity in the vascular anatomy of the fundus. Indeed, the unique "retinal print" has been used for biometric identification of individuals in security applications. (The retinal print has now been largely replaced by the use of the random patterns inherent in the iris for biometric identification purposes. The iris pattern is easier to acquire optically.) Thus, the use of the ophthalmoscope to detect retinal pathologies is not as simple as examining a chest X-ray for a broken rib. There is randomness and order in each fundus, and the challenge is to find features that are signs of disease in the image. Accordingly, there are many "fundus atlases" in print and on-line to guide diagnosis by example.

The modern fixed-base office ophthalmoscope allows the examining optometrist or ophthalmologist to inspect a fundus with binocular vision using a variety of light source wavelengths. The same instrument also allows the capture of color digital images, or color positive film images for archival purposes.

2.2.2 SLIT LAMPS

We have seen that the ophthalmoscope permits visualization of the features of the inner surface of the retina, including signs of ARMD, damage from diabetes, and mechanical damage from trauma. The slit lamp, on the other hand, allows examination of the optical structures of the eye for pathologies, damage and foreign objects, including the cornea, the lens, the iris, and the vitreous body. The components of a slit lamp consist of a long-working-distance binocular microscope, normally directed at the eye under study in the horizontal plane. The microscope can be of the zoom type, giving magnification in the range of 5x to c. 50x. The (azimuth) angle of the microscope axis with respect to the eye's gaze axis can be varied in the horizontal plane. The slit lamp also has a flexible light source based on a high-intensity halogen lamp. The lamp filament is projected onto a slit (adjustable in width, height and angle with the vertical). The slit's image is, in turn, directed to the desired part of the eye by a focusing lens. A cobalt-blue filter can be inserted into the slit beam (pass peak at c. 400 nm) to selectively excite the 550 nm green fluorescence of the stain, fluorescein sodium. Fluorescein is used to identify corneal abrasions, cuts, etc., where it selectively concentrates. A long-wave pass filter is used over the microscope objective to cut the blue light and improve contrast of the fluorescent images.

The microscope and slit illuminator systems of a slit lamp are coupled around a common center of rotation so that the microscope will always be focused where the slit beam is projected. The slit source and microscope can also be independently directed for applications such as viewing sclerotic scatter in the cornea. The slit lamp must also have a head and chin rest to restrain the patient's head (and eyes) from moving during observation. Some slit lamps allow the slit source beam to be moved out of the horizontal plane, i. e., be directed at the eye from above or below the horizontal plane. To see a comprehensive summary of diagnostic procedures that can be done with a slit lamp, visit the Riley 1996 web site. Figure 2.3 schematically illustrates a top view of the basic components of a slit lamp.

2.2.3 OTOSCOPES

The otoscope allows the examining physician to observe the condition of the outer surface of the eardrum and the lining of the external auditory canal. Like the basic ophthalmoscope, it is a hand-held instrument viewed by one eye of the clinician. Figure 2.4 (A) shows a cross-sectional view of a conventional otoscope. A miniature high-intensity halogen lamp with a built-in lens is used as the source, and a convex (magnifying) lens is used by the operator to enlarge the view of the eardrum. The earpieces are disposable, and come in various sizes to fit the patient's ear canal diameter. Figure 2.4 (B) shows an otoscope with coaxial illumination (analogous to an ophthalmoscope); the rays from the halogen lamp are collected by a concave mirror and focused on the eardrum by lens L_1. L_1 and L_2 form a microscope, enlarging the normally illuminated object. Such a coaxial illumination system is used in the Hotchkiss™ otoscope, as described on the Preferred Product website: www.preferred product.com/prod01.html.

The otoscope can be used to locate impacted cerumen (earwax) in the ear canal, as well as foreign objects (insects, Q-tip heads, beans, etc.). The otoscope is also useful in diagnosing middle-ear infection through eardrum color. Convexity can mean fluid pressure in the middle ear, and, of course, tears and perforations can signify trauma or infection. The coaxial design of the Hotchkiss™ otoscope is

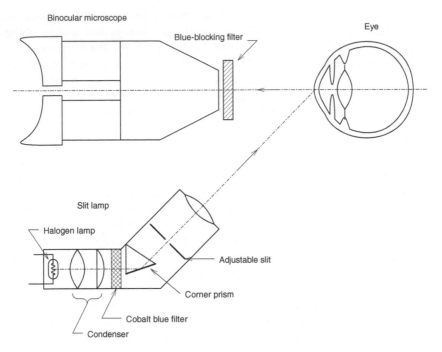

FIGURE 2.3 Schematic top view of the optics of a slit lamp.

particularly well suited for observation of ear canal procedures as they are done (e.g., removing cerumen or foreign objects).

Many otoscopes are easily converted to ophthalmoscopes. The handle holds the batteries, switch and rheostat to control the lamp brightness, and has a universal bayonet-type fitting that enables either a conventional otoscope head or an ophthalmoscope to be powered.

2.3   ENDOSCOPES

An endoscope is an optical instrument that allows a physician to visually inspect the surfaces of certain body organs, internal cavities and tubes, or the surfaces of joints. Endoscopy is a minimally invasive (or invasive) procedure that generally requires sterile technique, and, in most cases, local or general anesthesia.

There are two major categories of endoscope: the rigid (straight tube) and the flexible (fiber optic bundle) type. The following "*scopys" are common to modern medical practice:

- **Arthroscopy**: examination of the surface of joints for diagnosis and treatment.
- **Bronchoscopy**: examination of the trachea and bronchial tubes of the lungs to reveal foreign objects, lesions, infections, cancer, tuberculosis, alveolitis, etc. Guides the taking of biopsy samples.

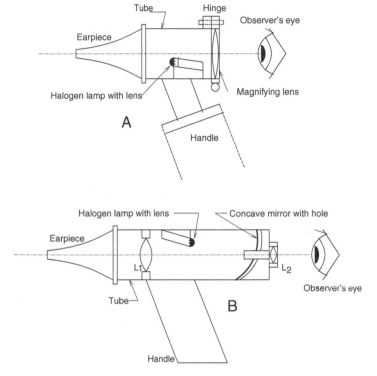

FIGURE 2.4(A) Cut-away side view of a conventional otoscope. **(B)** Cut-away side view of a direct-view otoscope of the Hotchkiss type.

- **Colonoscopy**: examination of the interior of the large intestine to reveal polyps, diverticula, cancer, lesions, etc. Also guides the taking of biopsy samples.
- **Colposcopy**: visualization of the lining of the vagina and the cervix to detect infection, lesions, cancer, etc., also biopsies.
- **Cystoscopy**: the endoscope is inserted through the urethra to examine the urethra, bladder, and, in men, the prostate, for lesions, infection, and cancer.
- **Endoscopic retrograde cholangio-pancreatography** (ERCP): highly invasive procedure used to examine the liver's bilary tree, the gallbladder, the pancreatic duct, etc., to check for stones, lesions, cancer, etc.
- **Esophogealgastroduodenoscopy** aka gastroscopy (EGD): examination of the upper GI tract; the esophagus, stomach, and pyloric valve to reveal ulcers, hemorrhage, hiatal hernia, duodenal ulcers, cancers, etc.
- **Laparoscopy**: visualization of the exterior of abdominal organs such as the uterus, ovaries, bladder, intestines, pancreas, liver, etc. The laparascope is inserted through a small incision in the abdomen; the abdomen is inflated with sterile CO_2 gas for better visualization. (Perhaps helium would be a better gas to use for abdominal inflation because it is absorbed rapidly and is chemically inert (Northrop, 1994).)

- **Laryngoscopy**: examination of the larynx.
- **Proctoscopy**: examination of the rectum and sigmoid colon (see colonoscopy).
- **Thorascopy**: a flexible fiber optic (FO) endoscope is inserted between the ribs to view the pleural cavity between the outer wall of the lungs and the inner wall of the chest. The pericardium can also be visualized. Inflating gas is used for better visual resolution. Thorascopy is used to detect infections, cancer, and pneumothorax (a ruptured alveolus allows breathed air to enter the pleural cavity, which may collapse a lung).

In the early 1900s, endoscopes were lighted with incandescent lamps, and had straight tubes. Although crude by today's standards, straight-tube endoscopes permitted the introduction of hand-manipulated instruments to take biopsies and to remove foreign objects, polyps, etc. Magnifying lenses could be used to see tissue details. In the 1930s, semi-flexible gastroscopes were introduced that used multiple cylindrical rod lenses. The optical quality of their images was of low quality. The first FO endoscope was developed at the University of Michigan in 1957 by Basil Hirschowitz; its widespread use began in the 1960s (Imaginis, 2000). More recently, miniature digital charge-coupled device (CCD) cameras have been adapted to both straight-tube and FO endoscopes. In some models, the CCD camera is located at the tip of the endoscope, and is optically coupled to the object by a short length of coherent FO cable. Illumination light is coupled to the tip of the endoscope by an FO cable from a 150- to 300-W xenon light source. Some CCD cameras use an automatic exposure control to preserve image contrast over a wide range of illumination conditions. Figure 2.5 illustrates the operator's end of a Pentax® model FS-34V sigmoidoscope, as well as its tip. Note the extreme movement range of the tip. This endoscope is not shown equipped with a camera.

Ultrathin FO endoscopes called needlescopes have diameters of 0.2 to 0.5 mm that contain 2,000 to 6,000 pixels. Such needlescopes have been inserted into mammary glands to detect breast cancer at early stages, and also inserted into the eye to view the back side of the iris, and the posterior chamber. They also have been used to visualize heart valves in action, and plaque in coronary arteries (Nanoptics, 1999).

A coherent FO bundle is effectively a spatial sampling array that operates on the object. Because each optical fiber has an acceptance cone for input rays, a spatial low-pass filter is introduced in series with the 2-D spatial sampler. Generally, the smaller the diameter of individual optical fibers, the higher the spatial resolution, with some limits. According to Nanoptics, 1999:

"For a (coherent) fiber optics bundle, the resolution can be defined by about half a line pair per fiber core. For example, if the individual fiber diameter is 50 μm, cores could resolve 10 line pairs per millimeter (10 lp/mm). Generally, the smaller the fiber core diameter, the greater the image resolution in a unit area of image fiber bundle. However, there are some phenomena which lead to reduced resolution, such as cross-talk between individual (adjacent) fibers, and leaky rays from individual fiber (sic). These phenomena may deteriorate image quality and can be the main reason for reduction in spatial resolution. These phenomena become more important as the core diameter is increased [Northrop query: decreased?]. Therefore, the

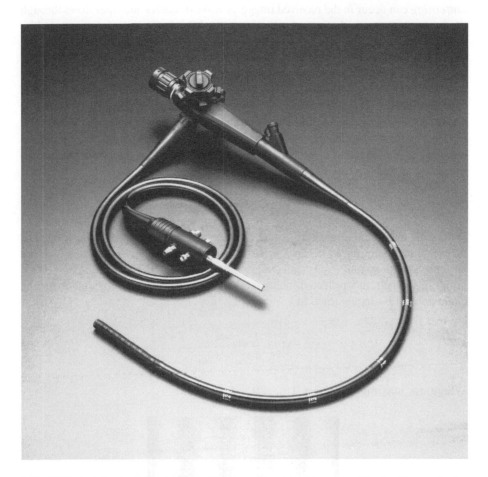

FIGURE 2.5 A Pentax® Model FS-34V fiber optic sigmoidoscope. (Used with permission of Pentax Precision Instrument Co.)

optimum core diameter for a given desired resolution depends on parameters such as cladding thickness, refractive index of the core and cladding and the wavelength of the incident ray."

The packing fraction of an FO bundle is defined as the total FO core surface area divided by the total area of optical fibers (core plus cladding). The packing fraction is proportional to the light-gathering efficiency of the FO bundle because all light entering the cladding is lost. In practice, the minimum cladding thickness is about 1 μm. Thus, if the core diameter is 4 μm, the fiber end area is $\pi(3 \ \mu m)^2 =$ 28.27 μm², and the core area is $\pi(2 \ \mu m)^2 = 12.57 \ \mu m^2$. Thus, the packing fraction is 12.57/28.27 = 0.445.

Another optical engineering tradeoff in the design of FO endoscopes with CCD cameras involves matching the discrete fiber outputs to the discrete pixel inputs of the CCD chip. Because of optical interference effects between adjacent optical fiber outputs viewed by individual CCD pixel sensors, a phenomenon known as *Moiré patterning* can occur in the received image. A wave of colors and lines flows through the image as the endoscope is moved. Often, the Moiré effect can be suppressed by defocusing the CCD camera and rotating it with respect to the FO bundle, or by the use of a special *anti-Moiré filter* between the camera and the end of the FO bundle.

An important figure of merit for any imaging system is its modulation transfer function (MTF), S(u), also called its contrast transfer function. The MTF concept can be applied to any component of, or an entire imaging system; X-ray systems, endoscopes, CCD cameras, film, etc., can all be characterized by a MTF. The MTF is a normalized spatial sinusoidal frequency response comparing the amplitude response of the image to a spatial sinusoidal (+ dc) object. In the x dimension, the object's sinusoidal intensity is given by:

$$I(x) = (I_o/2)[1 + \cos(2\pi u x)] \qquad 2.1$$

Where the maximum intensity is I_o and u is the spatial frequency in cycles/mm. The dc component is required because light intensity is non-negative. Figure 2.6 shows an approximate spatial (1-D) sinusoidal object pattern, and Figure 2.7(A) shows a graph of the pattern's reflected intensity as a function of x. The object can also be characterized by its contrast, M_o.

$$M_o = \frac{I_{o\,max} - I_{o\,min}}{I_{o\,max} + I_{o\,min}} \qquad 2.2$$

Where, for maximum contrast, $I_{omin} \equiv 0$.

FIGURE 2.6 An 8-bit 1-D spatial sinewave MTF test pattern object for endoscopes, cameras, etc.

Figure 2.8 shows a typical sinusoidal image as processed by an optical system. A plot of the x-axis intensity of Figure 2.8 is shown in Figure 2.7(B). Note that the average intensity is the same for both input and output graphs. Also note that the image contrast, M_i, is generally lower than the object contrast, M_o, especially at high spatial frequencies. M_i is given by:

$$M_i(u) = \frac{I_{i\,max} - I_{i\,min}}{I_{i\,max} - I_{i\,min}} \qquad 2.3$$

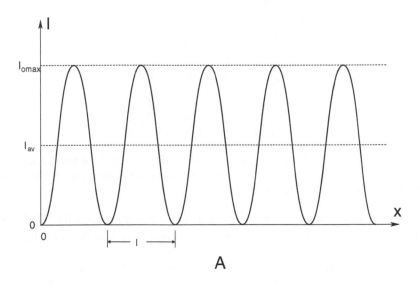

A

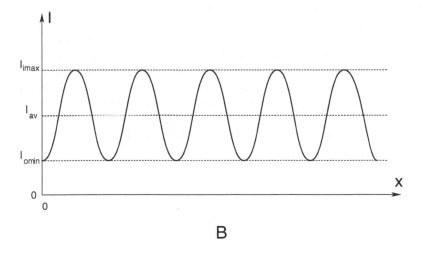

B

FIGURE 2.7 **(A)** A graph of the intensity in the x-direction of the test object of Figure 2.6. **(B)** A graph of the intensity of the image, given the test object as the input. Note that the average intensity is the same for both object and image.

The MTF of the optical system is defined by:

$$S(u) \equiv \frac{M_i(u)}{M_o}$$

2.4

FIGURE 2.8 A simulated optical system's output (image), given the sinusoidal test object of Figure 2.6 as the input. Note that the spatial sinewave input is attenuated by the system's MTF. Peak contrast is also reduced.

The MTF response of an optical system at dc (u = 0) is generally 1 (or 100%), even though there may be a neutral density attenuation of the average intensity of the object. At very low spatial frequencies, the image contrast is basically that of the object. As the spatial frequency, u, of the object is increased, the general spatial low-pass nature of diffraction-limited optics causes the image contrast to decrease, causing S(u) → 0 as u → ∞. Figure 2.9 illustrates the MTF of an ideal diffraction-limited lens system along with the MTF of a practical imaging system. Note that high spatial frequencies are lost in a practical imaging system from a variety of conditions, including the spectral distribution of the light, the system's numerical aperture, f-stop, the angle of the axis along which the test sine object is displayed, and nonlinear optical effects such as various aberrations, coma, astigmatism, distortion (barrel vs. pincushion) and spatial sampling by packed optical fibers.

In many imaging systems, it is inconvenient to generate a sinusoidal (+ dc) object; instead, a 1-D square wave object is used of the form:

$$I(x) = (I_o/2)[1 + SGN\{sin(2\pi x/\lambda)\}] = I(x + \lambda) \qquad 2.5$$

This periodic object can be represented by the Fourier series:

$$I(x) = B_o + \sum_{\substack{n=1 \\ n\ odd}}^{\infty} A_n \sin(n v_o x) \qquad 2.6$$

Where the fundamental spatial frequency in radians/mm is given by: $v_o = 2\pi/\lambda$. B_o is the average value of the object's intensity, equal to $I_o/2$. The sine term (odd) Fourier series coefficients, A_n, are given by:

$$A_n = (1/\pi) \int_{-\pi}^{\pi} I(x) \cos(n v_o x) \, d(v_o x) \qquad 2.7$$

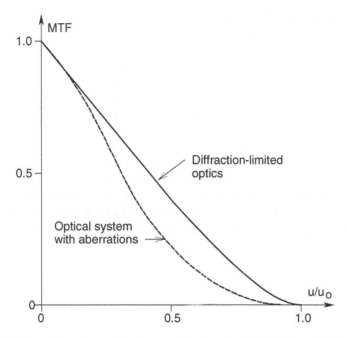

FIGURE 2.9 Examples of a modulation transfer function (MTF) of an ideal lens system (upper curve) and a non-ideal imaging system (lower curve).

For example, the third harmonic coefficient, A_3, can be calculated:

$$A_3 = (1/\pi)\int_0^\pi (I_o/2)\sin(3v_o x)\, d(v_o x) - (1/\pi)\int_\pi^{2\pi} (I_o/2)\sin(3v_o x)\, d(v_o x)$$

$$\qquad\qquad 2.8$$

$$= (I_o/2)/(3\pi)\left\{ \left[-\cos(3v_o x)\right]\Big|_0^\pi - \left[-\cos(3v_o x)\right]\Big|_\pi^{2\pi} \right\} = 4(I_o/2)/(3\pi)$$

Thus, the Fourier series for the square wave object can be written out in terms of its odd harmonics:

$$I(x) = (I_o/2) + [4(I_o/2)/\pi]\sin(v_o x) + [4(I_o/2)/(3\pi)]\sin(3v_o x)$$

$$+ [4(I_o/2)/(5\pi)]\sin(5v_o x) + \ldots \qquad\qquad 2.9$$

The relation for the MTF (Equation 2.4) can still be used to characterize the optical system when a square wave object is used, but obviously the MTF derived is the result of the superposition of the responses to all of the harmonics making up the "sine" square wave. As the period of the spatial square wave object is made smaller, the optical image responds to fewer and fewer of the high spatial harmonics; the image becomes a rounded square wave. At limiting spatial resolution, the optical system responds only to the dc + fundamental frequency term in the series, and the image is basically a low-contrast intensity sine wave.

An automated test system for FO endoscopes operating on a PC using Lab-VIEW® software and a National Instruments' IMAQ-PCI-1408 frame-grabber interface card was described by Rosow, Beatrice and Adam, 1998. Their EndoTester® system measures the following properties of an endoscope: 1) Relative light loss. 2) Geometric distortion. 3) Modulation transfer function (MTF). 4) Reflective symmetry. 5) Percent of lighted (good) fibers. The EndoTester is produced by Premise Development Corp., West Hartford, Connecticut.

We have seen that endoscopes can be guided to and focused on specific tissues. They also can be used to guide the taking of tissue samples for biopsy (to determine whether certain cells are cancerous). In some endoscopes, tissue is actually cut off and sucked into the endoscope for collection. Another method is to dislodge the targeted cells by abrasion with a brush operated through the endoscope. The loose cells are then drawn into the end of the endoscope for collection and examination.

2.4 CCD CAMERAS

In many medical imaging applications, the charge-coupled device (CCD) camera is replacing photographic film, including X-ray film. CCD cameras come in various styles and sizes.

Some CCD sensors are responsive to colored objects, others produce monochrome images. Color is of paramount interest in medical imaging applications because, in the case of endoscopy, the physician is looking for color changes indicating inflammation, infection, tumors, etc. When fluorescence techniques are used to detect cancers, bacterial infections, etc., the operator needs to see the colored fluorescent object against an otherwise normal background.

Figure 2.10 illustrates a typical CCD camera chip. A rectangular array of photodiode photosensors forms the basic transducer matrix. Depending on application, there can be as few as 180 h × 120 v photodiodes in the CCD array, to over 1280 h × 1024 v sensors. (The image aspect ratio is generally 4:3.) The Kodak KAF-0401(L) monochrome CCD chip has a sensor array of 768 × 512; each photosensitive pixel measures 9 × 9 μm, and the entire array is 6.9 × 4.6 mm (h × v). The Kodak KAF-4202 monochrome CCD sensor series has 2032 h × 2044 v pixels, each 9 μm square, arranged in an 18.29 × 18.40 mm (nearly square) array. The Kodak KAF-3000CE color CCD sensor chip has a 2016 × 1512 pixel array arranged in an 18.1 × 13.6 photosensitive array. The presence of anti-blooming conductors makes the fill factor 70% for this chip.

Light from the object is focused on the flat surface of the CCD array. Photons striking the pn junction of a photodiode cause photoelectrons to be generated. These photoelectrons are collected in "storage wells" in the proximity of each of the illuminated pn junctions. The number of electrons in a given well is proportional to the light intensity times the integration time or exposure (generally c. 1/60 second). At frame readout time, the charge in each photodiode's storage well is sequentially shifted out to a charge-to-voltage converter circuit by a system of vertical shift registers (one for each vertical column of sensors) that feed into a common horizontal

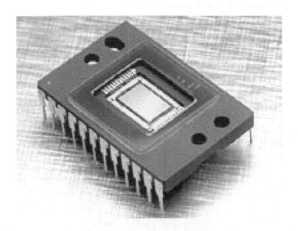

FIGURE 2.10 A Kodak CCD array IC. The photosensor matrix is on the inner rectangle. (Used with permission of Kodak.)

shift register. As each pixel's voltage is generated, it goes to a track-and-hold circuit that feeds an analog-to-digital converter (ADC). The ADC sequentially generates a 14 or 16-bit word for each pixel, for each frame. The CCD camera's digital output is fed to a computer for further image processing and image display generation. Figure 2.11 illustrates the organization of the CCD camera's shift registers and ADC. Not shown are the complex clock waveforms necessary to effect read-out and reset the wells to zero charge at the beginning of the next frame cycle.

If the exposure (time × intensity) of a given pn junction is too large, a phenomenon known as blooming occurs. The overexposure causes so many photoelectrons to be produced that they exceed the capacity of the well to hold them, and leak out into neighboring wells, corrupting the image. There are two ways to avoid blooming: One is to incorporate electron "gutters" that surround each well and carry off the electron overflow into the CCD chip design. This method uses up about 30% of the effective pixel area and reduces both well depth and sensitivity. Another method to reduce blooming is to limit exposure, take multiple frames and use signal averaging on the image to improve the signal-to-noise ratio.

In one strategy to make a CCD array responsive to color, each cluster of four pixels is given a color filter, as shown in Figure 2.12. In a CCD chip described by Cirrus Logic, 1998, a pattern of four bandpass filters is used: Magenta (purplish red), Yellow, Cyan (greenish blue) and Green. A special DSP chip, such as the Cirrus Logic® Crystal® CS7666, converts the four-color MYCG data to YCrCb-formatted component digital video. (YCrCb stands for Luma, Chroma Red, Chroma Blue.) Note the overlapping and repeating pattern of four color filters in the figure.

The Kodak KAF-3000CE color CCD uses three color filters in a repeating pattern over adjacent pixels. The filters pass red, green and blue light. The blue filter's transmission peaks at about 450 nm, and is about 100 nm wide. The green filter peaks at c. 530 nm, and is c. 100 nm wide. The red filter peaks at c. 625 nm and

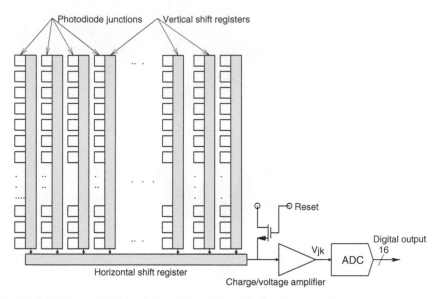

FIGURE 2.11 Functional organization of a CCD imaging IC. The photosensor elements are organized into N columns of M sensors. The sensors load the N analog, charge-coupled shift registers in parallel, then each shift register is sequentially downloaded in parallel, one pixel at a time, into the horizontal output shift register where each pixel is output, one at a time, until all N × M pixels have been digitized and downloaded to the image-processing computer. Typical maximum frame rate is 30–60 fps (to download and digitize all N × M pixels).

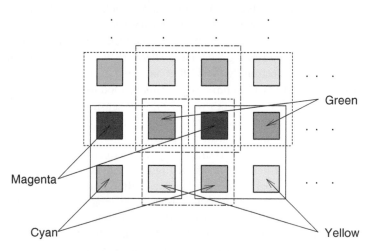

FIGURE 2.12 Cell layout of of a Cirrus Logic® color CCD imaging array.

is c. 100 nm wide. How the outputs from the various color pixels are combined to create a color image on a TFT or CRT display is beyond the scope of this section.

CCD cameras are available as integrated packages with lenses, board-level do-it-yourself systems, and as chips. Some integrated CCD cameras are configured as

30 frame/second, TV cameras using the IEEE1394-1995 standard interface. Some, like the Sony DFW-V300 camera give VGA (640×480) resolution with a 200 Mbps data transfer rate. A wide variety of CCD cameras and systems are made by Adimec, Cohu, Cooke Corp, Crystal® (Cirrus Logic®), EG&G Reticon, Hamamatsu, Images Co., Kodak, Optronics, Panasonic, Pulnix America Inc., Sony, etc. Some cameras are suitable for fluorescence microscopy, and all forms of endoscopy. The wide popularity and application of CCD imaging systems stems from their ability to produce high-resolution images almost instantaneously (e.g., in 1/30 second) in high-resolution digital format that can then be stored compactly in that form and manipulated by various picture-processing algorithms to improve picture quality and to extract image features.

One way of characterizing the resolution of CCD imaging systems is by the MTF, described in Section 2.3. Another way, analogous to transient testing of a temporal signal processing system, is to examine the camera's resolution of line pair objects and pairs of dots. This is analogous to seeing how narrow and how close together two input pulses must be before they cannot be resolved at an amplifier's output. The line-and-dot test objects are generally made black on white (or white on black), with 100% contrast.

2.5 NONINVASIVE DIAGNOSIS OF SKIN LESIONS

2.5.1 INTRODUCTION

Skin lesions and lesions on the surface of internal tissues viewed with endoscopes are indicative of disease conditions. In the case of skin lesions, the cause can be inflammation caused by a lodged foreign object, an infection, an insect bite, a benign growth, or a cancer. A lesion is detectable by eye because it generally involves some sort of swelling, a color that differs from the surrounding tissues, and a different texture. Noninvasive diagnosis of the type and cause of the lesion is the challenge. Diagnoses of lesions of this type are traditionally experience-based personal observations. In the case of skin melanomas, a physician with more than ten years of experience can diagnose correctly about 80% of the time. The diagnostic accuracy rate for physicians with three to five years of diagnostic experience and one to two years of experience is 62% and 56%, respectively. As you will see, some work has been done to devise machine-vision-based expert systems to diagnose malignant melanomas vs. benign nevi and other lesions (Grin et al., 1990).

The following section will focus attention on the detection of malignant melanomas.

2.5.2 MALIGNANT MELANOMA

Melanocytes are non-dermal cells derived embryologically from the tissue matrix for the brain and medullary spine; they migrate during fetal development into the skin, where they settle within the epidermal layer. Melanocytes are characterized by the ability to produce the pigment melanin in response to UV radiation to protect the skin from sunburn damage (tanning). They also respond to other biochemical signals (e.g., certain hormones).

There are three major categories of skin cancer:

1. Melanoma
2. Squamous cell carcinoma, derived from malignant keratinocytes
3. Basal cell carcinoma, derived from malignant basal keratinocytes (Tustison, 1999)

Skin cancer of various types affects about one million persons in the United States per year. 41,600 individuals were expected to develop melanoma in the United States in 1998; of those, some 7,300 are expected to eventually die from it.

Friedman, 1985, set forth an "ABCD Rule of Visual Melanoma Diagnosis." This can be stated:

A = Asymmetry in lesion in 0, 1, or 2 axes.
B = Border irregularity. Abrupt cut-off of pigment pattern at the border in up to 8 segments.
C = number of Colors present (white, red, blue-gray, light and dark brown, black).
D = number of Dermatoscopic structural elements: Areas without any structures, network, branched streaks, dots and globules.

The dermatoscopy score, S, is calculated from the single values for A, B, C, & D by the following formula: $S = 1.3A + 0.1B + 0.5C + 0.5D$. If $S > 5.45$, a melanoma can be highly suspected (Specificity c. 75%, Sensitivity c. 90%). Melanocytic lesions with $S < 4.75$ are probably benign nevi, while those with $4.74 < S < 5.45$ are suspicious and should be removed and be checked microscopically. Example: A = 2, B = 0, C = 3 (light brown, dark brown, black), D = 4 (network, branched streaks, structureless areas, globules); so S = 6.1.

The real challenge is accurate, differential diagnosis of melanomas from large moles (nevi), seborrheic keratosis lesions, etc. The gold standard is biopsy, where the lesion is surgically removed and it cells examined microscopically. Some workers have designed prototype, machine vision-based computer programs to extract the common features of melanomas. The input device is generally a high-resolution color CCD camera focused on the lesion, which is well illuminated with white light. One such system, described by Ercal et al., 1994, used a modified ABCD rule with a multi-layered feed-forward neural network trained using the generalized delta rule (back-propagation training algorithm) to obtain better than 80% differential success on digitized real melanoma images. The neural network was given the following 14 inputs:

• Irregularity index (1)
• Percent asymmetry (1)
• R, G and B color variances (3)
• Relative chromaticity (R, G & B) (3)
• Spherical color coordinates (L, α, β) (3)
• (L*, a*, b*) color coordinates (3)

An up-to-date review of algorithmic detection of melanomas from digital color images can be found in the 1999 MS thesis by H.V. Le, who presents his own concatenated image processing algorithms for differentiating tumor images. His approach is also based on the good old ABCD rule. First,a process called peer group filtering is executed, then color quantization, followed by region merging, and object localization. The processed image produced can next be sent to a feature extraction algorithm. Le designed an image processing "front end" for melanoma identification that evidently worked well; he suggested that the feature analysis could be done by a neural network.

Another approach to quantifying skin melanomas uses the optical reflectance characteristics at different wavelengths of the components of these lesions. Wallace et al., 2000, described a spectrophotometric approach to skin tumor classification. An area 1.5 mm in diameter was illuminated with broadband white light from a 75 W xenon arc lamp passed through 18 quartz fibers, each with a 200 μm core diameter and a NA = 0.2. Twelve quartz fibers in the same 30-fiber bundle traveled from the common object (skin) end to a monochromator with an output wavelength that could be scanned between 320 to 1,100 nm. Wallace et al. measured reflectance spectra for normal skin, skin near the lesions, and various types of lesions, including malignant melanoma. The reflectance fraction, $R(\lambda)$, was defined as:

$$R(\lambda) = \frac{S(\lambda) - D}{S_{ref}(\lambda) - D} \qquad\qquad 2.10$$

Where $S(\lambda)$ is the sensor current from the measured, reflected intensity at wavelength λ, D is the dark current, and $S_{ref}(\lambda)$ is the sensor output at λ when the probe is directed at a white calibration object. The following number of spectra were obtained for the following types of pigmented skin lesions:

- Malignant melanoma (15 cases, 55 spectra)
- Melanoma *in situ* (9, 33)
- Dysplastic nevus (11, 36)
- Compound nevus (32, 98)
- Seborrheic keratosis (14, 42)
- Basal cell carcinoma (5, 15)
- "Other" (37, 120)

In summary, following application of a statistical classification rule, the authors claimed results comparable with an expert dermatologist; the sensitivity was 100%, and the specificity was 84.4%. Note that lesion size, shape and fine structure did not enter into the analysis of Wallace et al.

2.5.3 DISCUSSION

In the future, we expect to see improvements in automated detection of malignant melanoma lesions. Combining spectral analysis with the ABCD method may hold promise. Also, it is known that the metabolisms of malignant melanocytes differ from normal cells, so it is possible that tagging malignant cells with fluorescent antibodies or radioactive metabolites may yield good results. Raman spectroscopy of the malignant cells is another approach that may be tried. (See Section 15.9 of this text for a description of some applications of Raman spectroscopy to medical diagnosis.)

2.6 SUMMARY

Diagnosis by direct visual inspection of tissue surfaces has been used by physicians since earliest times. The medical importance of a lesion lies in its color(s), swelling, size, texture, any exudate, etc. Such diagnosis is experience-based; an inexperienced person can easily differentiate between a wart, a boil, or an impetago lesion, but diagnosis of suspect skin cancers by eye is not easy. Fortunately, there are comprehensive data bases available for various skin lesions and retinal pathologies. Visual inspection is generally just the beginning of diagnosis of skin cancer; initial impressions are verified by biopsy or DNA analysis.

We have seen that there are a number of optical aids that have been developed in the past 150 years or so for visual inspection of various body parts. The least invasive are the ophthalmoscope, slit lamp and the otoscope. Recently, the development of fiber optic endoscopes have permitted the inspection of the surfaces of internal mucous membranes that are continguous with the body's surface. Such procedures are generally semi-invasive, because sterile technique is required, and the patient is generally given local or general anesthesia. It was discovered recently that there is differential fluorescence between normal and tumorous tissues, and near-UV light can be delivered, by the endoscope to the target lesion. Other spectrophotometric techniques can also be used with endoscopes. For example, Raman spectroscopy may prove useful in differentiating between normal and cancerous tissues (See Section 15.9).

Computers have made it easy for diagnosticians to download digital photographs of suspect lesions from CCD color cameras, and compare them with known figures in a database. CCD images have also expedited data storage to track the course of an infection or lesion being treated, giving an objective measure of progress.

3 Noninvasive Diagnosis Using Sounds from Within the Body

3.1 INTRODUCTION

3.1.1 BACKGROUND

Many endogenous sources of acoustic energy have diagnostic significance. These include:

- Heart sounds (valves, blood turbulence, pericardial friction rub)
- Lungs (rales, rhonchi, squeaks, crepitations, gurgling, pleural friction rub, silence)
- Arteries (*bruit* aka turbulence sounds caused by a *stenosis*)
- Stomach and intestines (sounds of digestion)
- Joints (arthritic friction rub, tendon snap, etc.)
- Inner ear (*otoacoustic emissions*)

Most of these sounds have acoustic spectral energy in the lowest range of human hearing, as well as at audible low frequencies. Some have origin in the elastic vibrations of dense tissues, or vibrations induced in arteries by blood turbulence, or vibrations induced by blood passing through small apertures. All such sound vibrations propagate through the body's tissues with losses, reflections and refractions to the skin, in which perpendicular vibrations are introduced. Stethoscopes and microphones respond to the sound waves that the vibrating skin radiates into the air. Surface vibrations can be measured directly by accelerometers on the skin surface, or laser Doppler sensors in which the Doppler shift in a laser beam reflected from the skin is detected. The Doppler frequency shift is proportional to skin velocity, so this signal must be integrated to obtain a signal proportional to vibration amplitude.

To make an effective NI diagnosis, medical professionals listening with a stethoscope must: 1) be able to hear the tones of the sound, and 2) have stored in their memories the acoustic patterns of many normal vs. abnormal sounds for the source of sound being heard. As an alternative, the sound can be picked up electronically by an accelerometer, low-frequency microphone, or laser Doppler microphone, amplified, digitized, and processed by computer into a *time-frequency spectrogram* that can be compared with normal spectrograms stored in the computer's memory.

3.1.2 STETHOSCOPES

Aside from the white lab coat, the symbol the public probably associates most with physicians and nurses is worn around the neck — the stethoscope. The modern acoustic stethoscope has evolved from its original format invented in 1816 by the French physician R.T.H. Laennec, who invented the stethoscope not only to improve the perception of endogenous sounds, but so physicians would not have to place their ears directly on the chests of the patients. To quote Laennec: "Direct auscultation was as uncomfortable for the doctor as it was for the patient, disgust in itself making it impracticable in hospitals. It was hardly suitable where most women were concerned and, with some, the very size of their breasts was an obstacle to the employment of this method." (Ornadel, 2000)

Laennec's original stethoscope was a hollow wooden cylinder with a funnel-like termination (a bell, or inverse horn) at the end that touched the patient. The distal end fitted into the doctor's ear canal. In its modern form, the stethoscope has two types of chest pieces, a shallow bell (for acoustic impedance matching), and a stiff, vibrating diaphragm (over a small bell chamber) that makes direct contact with the skin. The latter form is called a cardiology stethoscope. The chest piece (at the apexes of the bells) is attached to two flexible tubes, 25 to 30 cm in length, that, in turn, connect to two metal ear tubes that insert into the clinician's ears. The ear tubes are spring-loaded to hold them in place. The flexible tubes can be neoprene, plastic, or even latex. Their material will affect the frequency response of acoustic transmission from the body surface to the ears. The frequency responses of the acoustic transmission of modern acoustic stethoscopes have been measured by several workers (Jacobsen and Webster, 1977; Korhonen et al., 1996). Figure 3.1 illustrates the magnitude of the acoustic transmission in dB: $20 \log_{10}$ (rms sound pressure out/rms sound pressure in). The trace with one major peak is for the diaphragm-type cardiology chest piece alone (no tubes or ear pieces). The single peak at c. 800 Hz may be due to diaphragm mechanical resonance, or a series Helmholz resonance involving the bell chamber. The acoustic transmission of the same chest piece given tubes and ear pieces shows multiple peaks due to transmission-line-type resonances of the tubes. Note that the peaks do not appear to be related as simple harmonics. Figure 3.2 shows the difference in transmission between a conventional bell-type chest piece, and one with a diaphragm. The simple bell shows more than 15 dB attenuation relative to the diaphragm stethoscope in the frequency range from 15 to 60 Hz.

Thus, what clinicians hear through modern acoustic stethoscopes is "flavored" by the complex frequency transmission caused by its acoustic elements. Interns learn to recognize certain sounds associated with a healthy body, as well as pathologies using acoustic stethoscopes. Thus, when a broad-band electronic acoustic sensor is used, with its output amplified linearly and presented through high fidelity headphones, a person trained with an acoustic stethoscope may find the sounds unrecognizable. Surely Laennec's original tube had a flatter frequency response than a modern acoustic stethoscope because it had no 30-cm lengths of elastic tubing to resonate.

Electronic stethoscopes that avoid the worst of the tube resonance problem are now available. The chest piece contains a broad-band microphone, amplifier power

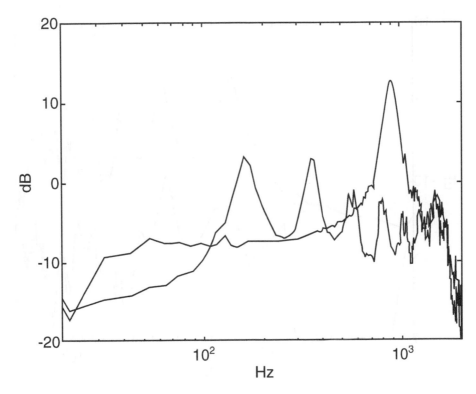

FIGURE 3.1 Measured acoustic transmission frequency response of a modern diaphragm-type stethoscope chestpiece (one large peak at c. 900 Hz). The transmission frequency response of a complete stethoscope is shown on the same axes; note the many peaks and nulls caused by the tubes. (Used with permission of Korhonen et al., 1996.)

supply, and frequency bandwidth and volume controls. The conditioned amplifier output is sent to a miniature loudspeaker, or headphones. The loudspeaker is coupled directly to the spring-loaded metal earpieces; the headphones are worn directly over the ears. For example, the Littmann electronic stethoscope, model 2000, offers amplification of 15 to 20 dB over an acoustic instrument, bandwidth settings of 20–200 Hz, 100–500 Hz and 100–1 kHz. The Cardionics® E-scope® has a selectable 20–1 kHz bandwidth for heart sounds, and a 70–2 kHz bandwidth for breath (lung) sounds. Its conditioned electrical output can power a speaker feeding the metal earpieces, headphones and a tape recorder. It has a variable volume control, and a selection of diaphragms and bells to couple sound from the skin to the microphone. Because of its good acoustic isolation, the manufacturer claims it is useful in noisy environments such as medivac helicopters and ambulances.

3.1.3 MICROPHONES

Several types of microphones are suitable for picking up air-coupled body sounds from the skin. These include:

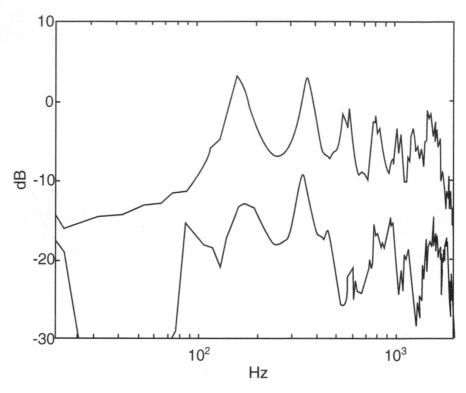

FIGURE 3.2 Measured acoustic transmission frequency response of two complete stethoscopes; one with a simple bell chestpiece, the other with a diaphragm chestpiece. The bell chestpiece stethoscope rejects low frequencies from c. 15 to 60 Hz. (Used with permission of Korhonen et al., 1996.)

- *Capacitor microphones*, where the induced vibration of a metalized mylar film forming one plate of a capacitor changes the capacitance between it and a fixed plate, inducing a change in the capacitor voltage under conditions of constant charge.
- *Crystal* or *piezoelectric microphones*, in which air-coupled sound pressure vibrates a piezo-crystal, directly generating a voltage proportional to dp/dt, where p is the sound pressure at the microphone.
- *Electret microphones* are variable capacitor sensors in which one plate has a permanent electrostatic charge on it; the moving plate varies the capacitance, inducing a voltage which is amplified. Electret microphones are small in size, and found in hearing aids, tape recorders, computers, etc.

Microphones generally have a high-frequency response that is quite adequate for endogenous body sounds. It is their low-frequency response that can be lacking. Indeed, some heart sounds are subsonic, ranging from 0.1 Hz to 20 Hz (Webster, 1992), while 0.1 to 10 Hz is generally inaudible, and sound with energy from 10 to

20 Hz can be sensed as subsonic pressure by some listeners. To record body sounds, the author modified a pair of B&K model 4117 piezoelectric microphones to cover down to < 1 Hz by inserting a fine, stainless steel wire into the pressure relief hole that vents the space in back of the piezo-bender element. The wire increased the acoustic resistance of the vent hole and thus increased the low-frequency time constant of the microphone from about 0.05 seconds (corresponding to a −3dB frequency of c. 3 Hz) to > 0.15 seconds, giving a −3 dB frequency < 1 Hz. The high −3 dB frequency of the 4117 microphones was c. 10 kHz. The voltage sensitivity of the 4117 microphone at mid-frequencies is about 3 mV/Pa, or 3 mV/10 μbar.

Another high-quality B&K microphone used by the author was the model 4135 quarter-inch condenser microphone. This research-grade device had a high-frequency −3 dB frequency in excess of 100 kHz, a total capacitance of 6.4 pF with a diaphragm-to-plate spacing of 18 μm. For body sounds, the low-frequency end of the 4135's frequency response is of interest. Three factors affect the 4135 microphone's frequency response:

1. The acoustic time constant formed by the acoustic capacitance (due to the volume between the moving (front) diaphragm and the insulator supporting the fixed plate), and the acoustic resistance of the small pressure equalization tube venting this volume. As in the case described above, the acoustic resistance can be increased by inserting a fine wire into the tube; this raises the acoustic time constant, and lowers the low −3 dB frequency.
2. The low −3 dB frequency is affected by the electrical time constant of the parallel RC circuit shunting the microphone capacitance (see Figure 3.3).
3. The mechanical resonance frequency of the vibrating membrane and its mass generally set the high-frequency end of the microphone's response. The smaller and thinner the diaphragm, the higher will be its upper −3 dB frequency.

In the circuit of Figure 3.3B, C_o is the 6.4 pF microphone capacitance, C_{in} is the signal-conditioning amplifier's input capacitance plus any wiring (stray) capacitance, R_{in} is the input resistance of the amplifier (greater than 10^{12} Ω), and R_s is the Thevenin source resistance of the source charging the capacitor to its fixed polarizing voltage. Olson (1940) analyzed the electrical circuit of a capacitor microphone, showing that, under certain assumptions, it could be reduced to one simple series loop containing the dc polarizing voltage source, V_s, in series with the average value of the microphone's capacitance, C_o, plus C_{in} (see Figure 3.3C). (Normally, $C_o \gg C_{in}$ so we will call the capacitance C_o.) The amplifier's R_{in} is normally $\gg R_s$, so the ac output voltage of the microphone is assumed to be developed across R_s. Let us write a loop equation for the simplified loop:

$$V_s - i R_s - C^{-1} \int i \, dt = 0 \qquad 3.1$$

Now the sound pressure vibrates the capacitor's diaphragm; we assume that it modulates the capacitance sinusoidaly. Thus:

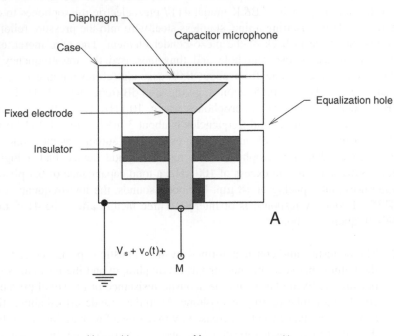

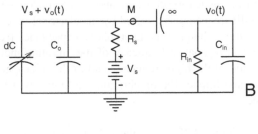

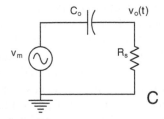

FIGURE 3.3 (A) Schematic cross-section of a capacitor microphone. (B) Equivalent circuit of the capacitor microphone. (C) Simplified linear circuit of the capacitor microphone.

$$C(t) = C_o + \delta C \, \sin(\omega t) \qquad\qquad 3.2$$

This expression for C(t) is substituted in Equation 3.1, and the resulting equation is differentiated with respect to time. This results in a first-order nonlinear ODE in the loop current, i(t), which is solved to yield a frequency response function, from which we can write:

$$i(t) = \frac{V_s \, \delta C/C_o}{\sqrt{\left[R_s^2 + 1/(\omega C_o)^2\right]}} \sin(\omega t + \varphi_1)$$

$$-\frac{V_s R_s \, \delta C/C_o^2}{\sqrt{\left[4R_s^2 + 1/(\omega C_o)^2\right]}\sqrt{\left[R_s^2 + 1/(\omega C_o)^2\right]}} \sin(2\omega t + \varphi_1 - \varphi_2) \qquad 3.3$$

+ Other higher - order harmonics.

Note that $\varphi_1 = \tan^{-1}[1/(\omega R_s C_o)]$ and $\varphi_2 = \tan^{-1}[1/(\omega 2 R_s C_o)]$. When $\delta C/C_o \ll 1$, the fundamental frequency term dominates, and the ac small-signal output of the microphone (superimposed on the dc voltage, V_s, can be written as a frequency response function:

$$\frac{V_o}{\delta C}(j\omega) = \frac{V_s R_s \omega}{\sqrt{\left[1 + (\omega C_o R_s)^2\right]}} \angle \varphi_1 \qquad 3.4$$

Olson points out that this is the same result obtained if we place an open-circuit (Thevenin) voltage of $v_{oc} = v_s\,(\delta C/C_o) \sin(\omega t + \varphi_1)$ in series with C_o and R_s in the loop, and observe $v_o(t)$ across R_s. From Equation 3.4, we see that the low corner frequency is $f_{Lo} = 1/(2\pi R_s C_o)$ Hz. For example, if $C_o = 7$ pF, and $R_s = 10^{10}$ ohms, then $f_{Lo} = 2.3$ Hz.

3.1.4 Acoustic Coupling

No matter which kind of sensor is used to detect endogenous sounds over the skin, there is a problem in efficiently coupling the sound vibrations from within the body to the microphone (or the eardrum). Since the days of Laennec and his first stethoscope, a bell-shaped or conical interface has been used to effectively couple a relatively large area of low-amplitude acoustic vibrations on the skin to a small area of larger amplitude vibrations in the ear tube(s). This bell-shaped interface is in fact an *inverse horn* (at that time, literally cow horns), which were used pre-20th century as hearing aids. Note that the pinna of the human ear is an effective inverse horn, matching the low acoustical impedance of open space to the higher impedance of the ear canal and eardrum. Like all horns, the pinna exhibits comb-filter properties, attenuating certain high frequencies in narrow bands around 8 and 13 kHz (Truax, 1998).

Regular horns were first used as speaking trumpets, later as output devices for early mechanical record-players; here the lateral displacement of the needle on the disk vibrated a mica diaphragm (c. 2 in. in diameter). A horn was used to couple those vibrations to a room and listeners. Most acoustics textbooks describe horns in the role of coupling sound from a small-diameter, vibrating piston to a large-diameter opening into free space (the room). In examining endogenous body sounds, the opposite events occur. A large area of small-amplitude acoustic vibrations on the skin is transformed by the inverse horn to a small area of large-amplitude vibrations (at the eardrum or microphone). It is beyond the scope of this section to mathematically analyze the acoustics of direct and inverse horns. However, we will examine them heuristically.

Basically, horns and inverse horns are acoustic impedance-matching systems. They attempt to couple the acoustic radiation impedance of the source to the acoustic impedance of the horn termination. The termination in the case of a stethoscope is the rather complex input impedance of the coupling tubes (or tube, in Laennec's instrument); in the case of a microphone, it is the moving diaphragm. If impedances are not matched, sound transmission will not be efficient, because there will be reflections at interfaces between any two media with different *characteristic acoustic impedances*; e.g., at the skin–air interface, and at the air–microphone interface. The characteristic acoustic impedance of a medium is a real number defined simply by (Truax, 1999):

$$Z_{ch} = \rho c \text{ cgs ohms } (ML^{-2}T^{-1}) \qquad 3.5$$

For air, the density, ρ, is a function of atmospheric pressure, temperature, and relative humidity. The velocity of sound, c, in air is not only a function of atmospheric pressure, temperature, and relative humidity, but also of frequency. Thus, the Z_{ch} of air can vary over a broad range, varying from c. 40 to 48 cgs ohms (43 is often taken as a compromise or "typical" value). An average Z_{ch} for body tissues (skin, muscle, fat, connective tissue, organs, blood) is c. 2×10^5 cgs ohms. Thus, we see that there is an enormous impedance mismatch in sound going from the body to air, and much intensity is reflected back internally. Clearly, there will be better sound transmission through the skin when the skin sees a much larger acoustical impedance looking into the throat of the inverse horn. As far as the author knows, there has been no scientific attempt to optimize the shape of the inverse horn used with the acoustic stethoscope, or, for that matter, any attempt to design a more efficient pressure microphone pick-up.

The acoustic impedance on one side of a vibrating piston set in an infinite baffle has been shown to be (Olson, 1940):

$$z_A = \left[\rho c / (\pi R^2)\right]\left[1 - \frac{J_1(2kR)}{kR}\right] + j\omega\left[\rho / (2\pi R^4 k^3)\right] K_1(2kR) \qquad 3.6$$

cgs acoustic ohms

Where: ρ is the air density ($\cong 1.205 \times 10^{-3}$ g/cm^3), c is the speed of sound in air ($\cong 2.877 \times 10^4$ cm/sec), R is the piston radius (cm), $k \equiv 2\pi/\lambda = \omega/c$, $J_1(2kR)$ is the first-order Bessel function of the first kind, $K_1(2kR)$ is a first-order modified Bessel function of the second kind. (Bessel function values can be found from tables or calculated from infinite series.) Note that πR^2 is the piston area. Figure 3.4 plots the normalized real and imaginary parts of $z_A(kR)$. Note that Re$\{z_A(kR)\}$ and Im$\{z_A(kR)\}$ increase with frequency until $\omega > c/R$. The Bessel functions contribute to the ripples at high ω.

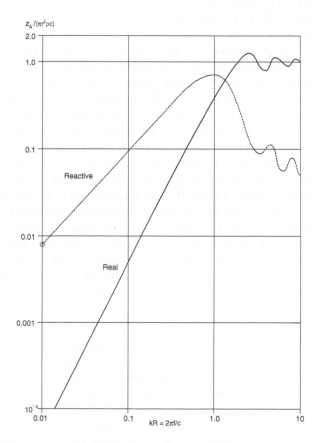

FIGURE 3.4 Plot of the scaled, real, and imaginary parts of the acoustic driving-point impedance of a vibrating cylindrical piston. (Adapted from Olson, 1940.)

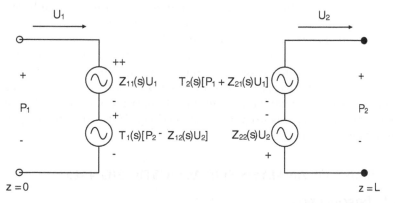

FIGURE 3.5 Two-port equivalent analog electrical circuit describing the transmission behavior of acoustic horns.

Horns can be classified as conical, parabolic, exponential, catenoidal, or hyperbolic, depending on how their cross-sectional area varies with z, the distance from the throat. For regular horns, A(z) *increases* monotonically with z; A(z) *decreases* monotonically with z for inverse horns. Leach (1996) developed a closed-form mathematical analysis for a class of horns known as *Salmon's family* (these include conical, catenoidal, exponential and hyperbolic forms). Leach's analysis employs the formalism of two-port circuit analysis; he used PSpice for his simulations. Leach gives expressions for: $Z_{11}(\omega)$, $Z_{12}(\omega)$, $Z_{21}(\omega)$ and $Z_{22}(\omega)$, in terms of the horn's propagation constant, $\gamma(\omega)$, the horn area at the throat (input, or z = 0) end, A_0, the horn area at its output end (z = L), A_L, and dA(z)/dz evaluated at z = 0 and z = L (A_0', and A_L', respectively). He also gives expressions for the transfer functions, $T_1(\omega)$ and $T_2(\omega)$. Figure 3.5 shows the equivalent controlled-source analog circuit for horn input and output pressures (P_1 and P_2), (analogous to sinusoidal voltages V_1 and V_2). The volume velocities U_1 and U_2 are analogous to the ac currents I_1 and I_2 in the two-port. Note that, normally, a load impedance, Z_L, must appear across the output terminals of the two-port circuit to represent the impedance the horn is driving. Without belaboring the details of Leach's analysis, the reader can appreciate its complexity. The utility of Leach's analysis is that one can analyze inverse horns, i.e., those in which the throat is larger than the output end.

3.1.5 DISCUSSION

We have stressed that, to sense endogenous sounds from the body, air-coupled sound pressure waves must be coupled to the sound sensor (microphone or eardrum) using some type of an inverse horn as an acoustic impedance-matching device. The price paid for using an inverse horn is that it inserts a comb filter-type of frequency response into the sound air transmission path. Typically, the pressure transfer function for a horn is poor at low frequencies (e.g., below 100 Hz), then rises abruptly with increasing signal frequency. The high-frequency part of the transfer function generally has a comb filter ripple on it, giving enhanced transmission at frequencies determined by the Bessel functions inherent in $z_A(2\pi f)$.

To overcome the low-frequency loss in transmission inherent in horns, some workers have placed vibration sensors directly on the skin in order to record subsonic (and sonic) vibrations efficiently. Such sensors can be piezoelectric accelerometers which respond to the second derivative of the skin displacement, $\ddot{x}(t)$. A double integration is required to recover x(t), which produces the sound. If the peak vibration, δx, is $< \lambda/4$ of the laser used, an *interferometer* such as a Fizeau or a Michelson can be used to directly measure x(t) of the skin. When a laser Doppler technique is used on the skin (Hong, 1994), then the output signal is proportional to $\dot{x}(t)$.

3.2 MEANS OF ANALYSIS FOR ACOUSTIC SIGNALS

3.2.1 INTRODUCTION

An audio-frequency signal from an endogenous body sound can be processed in several ways. On the qualitative side, we can observe a microphone output voltage on an oscilloscope vs. time. Very little useful information is gained by doing this. Another way is to listen to it, either with a stethoscope or using headphones. The amplitude, pitch, and rhythm of a complex physiological sound are features that the brain can store, identify, and compare. Clearly, some individuals are inherently better at this than others. People with "trained ears," such as musicians, are better at making diagnoses with acoustic stethoscopes than others. Recall that the stethoscope in its earliest 19th-century form was probably less distorting to body sounds than the modern instrument. As we have seen, all stethoscopes impose a transfer function on the input sound that has low transmission at low frequencies, and a comb filter-type response at higher frequencies.

To remove the problem of inverse horn- and tube-transfer functions, plus human psychoacoustics, body sounds may be better sensed directly from skin vibrations by laser interferometry. The signal so derived is proportional to the skin displacement, hence is at the endogenous sound frequency and can then be displayed in the frequency domain after digital processing as its average *root power density spectrum* (the spectrum must be averaged over several cardiac cycles, or breath cycles if the lungs are involved). Interferometric signals tend to be noisy, however, and the apparatus is expensive and delicate.

When the laser Doppler technique is used on skin, the resulting (mixed) output signal's frequency is given by $f_D = 2 |\dot{x}| / \lambda$ Hz. Note that the frequency of the Doppler signal is proportional to the *magnitude of the skin velocity,* and is not the sound originating in the patient's body. A simple laser Doppler system cannot differentiate between a positive and a negative frequency shift (due to $\dot{x} > 0$ and $\dot{x} < 0$, respectively).

Probably the two best ways to sense body sounds are:

1. Use a well-designed inverse horn to couple the skin vibrations through the air to a capacitor microphone's diaphragm. The signal so acquired, after amplification and filtering to improve the signal-to-noise ratio, can be listened to with headphones (a high-fidelity electronic stethoscope), or processed by a computer to form an average *root-power density spectrogram* or a *time-frequency spectrogram* (TFS).
2. Miniature IC accelerometers can be attached to the skin to measure vertical (sound) vibrations. Variations of the fast Fourier transform (FFT) are used to calculate the sound (average) spectrogram and the TFS. Diagnostic information about the heart can be obtained by examining anomalies in the cardiac power spectrogram or the TFS. The TFS shows how sound frequencies and intensity are distributed in time over the events that produce the sound.

3.2.2 THE DISCRETE FOURIER TRANSFORM AND THE POWER DENSITY SPECTRUM

The power density spectrum (aka autopower spectrum) is used to characterize the spectral (frequency) content of *stationary signals* in the frequency domain. A stationary signal is one in which the physical processes and environmental conditions giving rise to the signal do not change with time. Another way to view stationarity is to note that the statistics governing the production of the signal are constant. Signals derived from physiological systems are, in general, nonstationary. In a physiological system, an approximation to stationarity may exist for the short time over which data is recorded.

When we digitize and calculate an estimate to the power spectral density of heart sounds over many cardiac cycles, the spectrum will contain a peak at the mean heartbeat frequency, plus peaks at all the frequencies of all the sounds in the cardiac cycle. Information is lost on the spectral content of individual sounds (such as from mitral valve closing), and on when in the cardiac cycle these sounds occur. One way to examine the spectra of individual sounds as they occur is to synchronize the sampling of the cardiac sound signal with the ECG waveform to gate only those sounds of interest. The display of the phonocardiogram spectrum is usually presented as a root power density spectrogram (a spectrogram is computed from finite length data). Because many spectrograms are averaged to reduce noise, the display generally shows *mean* rms volts/√Hz.

To gain an understanding of the theory behind the calculation of a power density spectrum, we will first review the basics of the continuous Fourier transform (CFT) and the autocorrelation function. The CFT pair for a stationary signal is well-known:

$$X(j\omega) \equiv \int_{-\infty}^{\infty} x(t) \exp[-j\omega t]\, dt \qquad\qquad 3.7$$

$$x(t) \equiv (1/2\pi) \int_{-\infty}^{\infty} X(j\omega) \exp[+j\omega t]\, d\omega \qquad\qquad 3.8$$

The autocorrelation of a stationary signal, x(t), is defined as:

$$r_{xx}(\tau) \equiv (1/2T) \int_{\lim T \to \infty}^{T} \!\!\!\!\!\!\!\!\!{}_{-T} x(t)\, x(t+\tau)\, dt \qquad\qquad 3.9$$

The autocorrelation function has many interesting properties; the most important here is the fact that it is real and even in τ. The autopower spectrum is simply the CFT of the autocorrelation function:

$$S_{xx}(2\pi f) \equiv S_{xx}(f) = \int_{-\infty}^{\infty} r_{xxf}(\tau) \exp[-j2\pi f\tau]\, d\tau \qquad\qquad 3.10$$

$S_{xx}(f)$ is a *two-sided, even, positive-real function of frequency*. It has the units of mean squared volts/Hz. Depending on the form of x(t), there are many mathematical models for power density spectra, for example: white noise, 1/f noise, Gaussian, exponential, Markov, etc. (Lee, 1960).

In the real world, the power density spectrum is approximated by the use of finite data. It is also calculated using periodic samples of the time function. The calculation of a root power density spectrogram begins with acquiring a long analog record of the sound under study. This signal is often analog bandpass-filtered to improve its signal-to-noise ratio. The high-frequency filter cut-off is adjusted to prevent *aliasing*. That is, the conditioned analog signal is low-pass-filtered to remove any spectral energy at or above one-half the sampling frequency (the Nyquist frequency, f_N). The signal is then digitized (sampled) periodically; a total of N samples are taken spaced T_s seconds apart. Each sample is converted to a digital number by an analog-to-digital converter (ADC), and the samples are stored in computer memory. Thus, a *signal epoch* of duration $T_E = (N-1)T_s$ is required (sample 0 is taken at $t = 0$, sample $(N-1)$ is taken at $t = T_E$). For computational convenience, N is always made a power of 2, i.e., $N = 2^B$, in order to be able to use an FFT algorithm. Typically, B might be 12, so $N = 4,096$ samples. In the frequency domain, the spectrogram will have data values spaced at $\Delta f = 1/((N-1)T_s)$; the maximum useful frequency of the spectrogram will be $f_s/2 = f_N$, the Nyquist frequency.

The discrete Fourier transform (DFT) of a sampled finite-length signal is given by:

$$X(k\Delta f) = X(k) = (1/N) \sum_{n=0}^{N-1} x(n) \exp\left[-jk(2\pi/N)n\right] \qquad 3.11$$

$k = 0, 1, 2 \ldots (N-1)$. n is sample number.

or:

$$X(k) = (1/N) \sum_{n=0}^{N-1} x(n) \cos(kn\, 2\pi/N) - j(1/N) \sum_{n=0}^{N-1} x(n) \sin(kn\, 2\pi/N) \qquad 3.12$$

Note that X(k) is, in general, complex, with a real and imaginary part for every k. X(k) is generally calculated using one of the efficient fast-Fourier transform (FFT) algorithms. Calculation of the *power density spectrogram* can proceed by several methods. First, an array of N samples of x, (x_N), is made and stored (N even). The array elements (samples) are renumbered so they extend from $-(N/_2 - 1)$ to $+N/2$. Next, the *discrete autocorrelogram* of x, $r_{xx}(k)$ can be calculated in the time domain by the following function (Papoulis, 1977):

$$r_{xx}(k) = \frac{1}{N-k} \sum_{n=[-(N/2-1)+|k|/2]}^{(N/2-|k|/2)} x(n+k/2)\, x(n-k/2) \qquad 3.13$$

Note that, ideally, $r_{xx}(k)$ is even in k. Papoulis (1977) shows that $r_{xx}(k)$ is an unbiased estimator of the discrete autocorrelation, $R_{xx}(k)$. The Autopower spectrogram, $S_{xx}(q)$ is simply the DFT of $r_{xx}(k)$. That is:

$$S_{xx}(q) = (1/N) \sum_{k=-N/2}^{N/2-1} r_{xx}(k) \exp[-jq(2\pi/N)_k],$$

$$(q = 0, \pm 1, \dots \pm N/2) \quad msV/Hz$$

3.14

$S_{xx}(q)$ is positive-real and even in q.

$S_{xx}(q)$ is computed M times (e.g., M = 16) from M epochs of $\overline{N}$ samples of x(t) (sound) data, and corresponding points are averaged to form $\overline{S_{xx}(q)}$ with reduced noise. The root power spectrogram is simply:

$$s_{xx}(q) = \sqrt{|\overline{S_{xx}(q)}|} \quad rms \ volts/\sqrt{Hz}$$

3.15

The autopower spectrogram of x(t) can be computed using a number of algorithms. In the Blackman-Tukey method, the sample autocorrelogram is *windowed* before the autopower spectrogram is computed. A *windowing function*, w(n) weights the sampled data array to form the product:

$$z(n) = x(n) \ w(n), \quad -N/2 \leq n \leq (N/2 - 1)$$

3.16

Windowing functions are used on finite-length sampled data before DFTing to minimize some function of the spectral error, $E(q) = X(q) - X_w(q)$, where X(q) is the DFT of x(t) as N → ∞, and $X_w(q)$ is the DFT of x(n)w(n). There is a trade-off between spectral resolution and spectral smoothness for windows other than rectangular. One way to appreciate what a window does is to take the DFT of a pure sine wave given a rectangular window. We see a sharp peak at the fundamental frequency of the sine wave, and also smaller sidelobe peaks on either side of the main peak. The sidelobe peaks are artifactual; no such frequencies exist in the analog signal. The use of a windowing function reduces the sidelobe artifacts, but generally at the expense of broadening the fundamental frequency peak and thus decreasing spectral resolution.

The simplest windowing function is, of course, the *rectangular window*, which is inherent in all finite data arrays, (x_N). Here $w_r(n) = 1$ for $-N/2 \leq n \leq (N/2 - 1)$, and 0 for $|n| > N/2$. Other windows include the *Bartlett* or *triangular window*: $w_b(n) = (1 - |n|/(N/2 + 1))$ for $-N/2 \leq n \leq (N/2 - 1)$, and 0 for $|n| > N/2$. The *Hanning* window is also widely used: $w_h(n) = 1/2 (1 + \cos(2\pi n/N))$ for $-N/2 \leq n \leq (N/2 - 1)$, and 0 for $|n| > N/2$. Many other types of windows exist, including the *Parzen, Hamming, Tukey, Kaiser* and *Parabolic* (Papoulis, 1977; Williams, 1986).

The *Blackman-Tukey spectrogram function* can be written:

$$S_{xx}(q) = \sum_{k=-N/2}^{N/2} r_{xy}(k) \ w(k) \exp[-jq(2\pi/N)k] \quad q = 0, 1, \dots \pm N/2$$

3.17

Where w(k) can be one of the window functions described above.

In summary, there are many ways to compute the power density spectrogram of a recording of body sounds. For example, the Matlab® Signal Processing Toolbox has a utility, P = spectrum(x,m) that uses the *Welch method* (Proakis & Manolakis, 1995) to calculate the autopower spectrogram of a sampled (discrete) signal array, (x_N). The Hanning window is used on each epoch of m samples before the calculation; m is also the number of points in the FFT. Note that N = km, where k is the (integer) number of epochs in (x_N) FFTd, and m = 2^B. The routine automatically averages the k spectrograms. Other Matlab spectrum functions calculate the cross-power spectrogram of two time signals, (x_N) and (y_N). A root spectrum is calculated by:

$$\sqrt{S_{xy}(q)} = \sqrt{\left[\text{Re}\{S_{xy}(q)\}\right]^2 + \left[\text{Im}\{S_{xy}(q)\}\right]^2} \qquad 3.18$$

That is, it is the square-root of the mean-squared real part of $S_{xy}(q)$ plus the mean-squared imaginary part of $S_{xy}(q)$. $S_{xx}(q)$ is positive-real, i.e., it has no imaginary terms.

Many stand-alone digital sampling oscilloscopes (DSOs) not only allow data capture and visualization, but they also come with utilities that compute root power spectrograms of signals. The operator can choose the sampling rate, the window, the number of samples, and the number of spectrums to be averaged together to reduce noise. National Instruments' Lab View® data acquisition and signal processing software for PCs and laptop computers also will compute spectrograms.

Because heart sounds occur sequentially, each is associated with a physical event in the cardiac cycle, and information is lost if we pool these periodic events in a common spectrogram. In the following section, we examine the interesting DSP algorithms associated with time-frequency analysis, first used to analyze speech and animal sounds.

3.2.3 Time-Frequency Analysis for Transient Sounds

This section will examine the techniques used to make *time-frequency spectrograms* (TFSs). The first use of TFSs was to characterize the frequency content vs. time in human speech (the "voice print"). This application was soon extended to the analysis of animal sounds used for navigation, prey location, and communication (e.g., whales, dolphins, bats, birds). The original speech spectrograph was an all-analog system. In the earliest sound spectrographs, the sound signal was recorded on analog magnetic tape. The tape was passed over a rapidly spinning drum containing the playback head (one rotation defined the time window). The resulting analog signal from the rotating head was sent to a narrow-bandpass filter whose center frequency was proportional to the height of the recording stylus on the spectrogram chart. The higher the peak voltage at the BPF output , the darker the data point on the spectrogram. This procedure is time consuming, and there is the obvious trade-off on filter rise time, which is inversely related to filter bandwidth.

TFSs are the preferred form of spectral analysis when the sounds being studied are short-term, nonstationary, or transient in nature. Because time-frequency analysis displays a signal recorded in time in both time and frequency, it can be shown that there is an ultimate trade-off between the time- and frequency resolution of any TFS. This tradeoff is analogous to Heisenberg's uncertainty principle in quantum physics. It can be stated simply as $\Delta f\, \Delta t \geq 1$. Δf is the frequency resolution, and Δt is the length of signal used to calculate the TFS (Stanford Exploration, 1997).

A number of discrete algorithms calculate TFSs: The *short-term Fourier transform* (STFT), the *Wigner Transform,* the *Wigner-Ville transform* (WVT), the *Binomial Transform* (BT), the *Choi-Williams transform* (CWT), the *Gabor transform* (GT), and the *adaptive Gabor transform* (AGT). Each transform has its advantages and disadvantages, however, for sources that contain overlapping (additive) sound sources in time, it has been remarked by Wood et al. that the BT ... "provides higher joint resolution of time and frequency than the spectrograph and spectrogram (STFT) and better interpretability than other time-frequency transforms such as the Wigner-Ville" (Wood et al., 1992; Wood and Barry, 1995). The BT evidently is an efficient algorithm with very good cross-term suppression properties.

We will first examine properties of certain TFS algorithms. For pedagogical purposes we will first treat them in integral rather than discrete forms. The CFT of a time signal, x(t), is given by the well-known integral:

$$\mathbf{X}(f) = \int_{-\infty}^{\infty} x(t)\exp[-j2\pi ft]\,dt \quad (\mathbf{X}(f) \text{ is in general complex.}) \qquad 3.19$$

The first TFS algorithm to be considered here is the *short-term Fourier transform* (STFT) which has been used since the 1950s to calculate spectrograms to characterize human speech and was first applied to the TFS analysis of heart sounds by McCusik et al. (1959). The STFT spectrogram is calculated by:

$$\text{STFT}(t, f) = \left| \int_{0}^{\tau} x(t)\, g(t-\tau)\, \exp[-j2\pi ft]\,dt \right|^{2} \qquad 3.20$$

Where x(t) is the audio signal and w(t) is a *windowing* or *gating function.* g(t) is slid along x(t) by fixing τ. If the gating function is Gaussian, then the STFT is called a *Gabor* transform. (Some workers have used a Hanning gating function in their discrete data realization of the STFT TFS.) (The discrete form of the STFT can be written:

$$\text{STFT}(n, q) = \left| \sum_{m=-L/2}^{(L/2)-1} x(m)\, g(n-m)\exp[-j(2\pi/L)mq] \right|^{2} \qquad 3.21$$

Where L is the length of the sliding window, g(n), and g(n) is an even function around $n - m = 0$. The STFT is positive and has no problem with cross-term interference. However, its frequency resolution is inferior to the WV and CW TFSs. The *Wigner transform* (WT) is given by CFT of the time-shifted product:

$$W(t, f) = \int_{-L/2}^{L/2} \left[x(t + \mu/2) \, x * (t - \mu/2) \right] \exp\left[-j2\pi f\mu\right] d\mu \qquad 3.22$$

Where: $\mu/2$ is the shift, L is the duration of the integration, and x* is the complex conjugate of x (x is real, so this notation is meaningless in this case). The integral is computed many times for $t = k\Delta t$, $k = 1, 2, 3 \ldots M$. There is an equivalent definition of WV(t, f) in the frequency domain as an inverse CFT:

$$WV(t, f) = (1/2\pi) \int_{-\infty}^{\infty} X(f + v/2) \, X * (f - v/2) \exp\left[+jvt\right] dv \qquad 3.23$$

Note that the WVT is real, although it can go negative. Because the WVT depends quadratically upon the signal, a signal composed of sums of frequencies will produce a WVT containing cross-terms from the sums and differences of the component frequencies. This means that certain signals that are the sums of several frequencies occurring at the same time will produce "fuzzy" WVTs. If the signal is statistical, instead of sums of sinusoids, then the signal's autocorrelation function, $R_{xx}(\tau_1 - \tau_2)$ can replace the product, $[x(t + \mu/2) \, x*(t - \mu/2)]$, in the CFT integral, with the τs replaced by $R_{xx}[(t + \mu/2), (t - \mu/2)]$, or $R_{xx}(\mu)$ (Bastiaans, 1997).

When x(t) in the WT is replaced with the *analytical signal*, $Ax(t) \equiv x(t) + j[HX(t)]$, the WT is called the *Wigner-Ville* transform (WVT). HX(t) is the *Hilbert transform* of x(t), defined as (Papoulis, 1977):

$$HX(t) \equiv (1/\pi) \int_{-\infty}^{\infty} \frac{x(\tau)}{\pi(t - \tau)} d\tau = (1/\pi) \, x(t) \otimes (1/t) \qquad 3.24$$

It can be shown that the Hilbert transform filters out the negative frequencies in the analytical signal. The discrete form of the WVT is given by:

$$WVT(k, q) = 2 \sum_{m=-L/2}^{(L/2)-1} Ax(k + m) \, Ax * (k - m) \exp\left[-j(2\pi/L)mq\right] \qquad 3.25$$

Here, L is the block length over which the DFT is calculated, and Ax(k) is an analytical sequence computed from a discrete Hilbert transform. The WVT possesses the highest resolution of the TF algorithms, however it suffers the most serious interference problems, and can go negative.

Finally, let us examine the CFT version of the Binomial transform (BT) TFS. First, we find the running estimate of the signal's autocorrelation at various times, t: $r_{xx}(t, \tau)$. This autocorrelation function is then convolved in the time domain with a binomial smoothing function, given by:

$$R_{cxx}(t, \tau) = r_{xx}(t, \tau) \otimes h_{bin}(t, \tau) \qquad\qquad 3.26$$

Hence

$$BT(t, f) = \int\limits_{-\infty}^{\infty} R_{cxx}(t, \tau)\exp[-j2\pi ft]\, dt \qquad\qquad 3.27$$

$$\text{In discrete form, } h_{bin}(m, k) = \left(\left|\frac{|k|}{m + |k|/2}\right|\right)^{2-|k|} \qquad\qquad 3.28$$

According to Wood et al. (1992), "The Binomial transform uses a binomial approximation to the exponential (Gaussian), and is particularly efficient because the convolution in (6) (Equation 3.26) may be implemented using shift and add operations alone, avoiding floating point multiplication."

In summary, the choice of algorithm for time-frequency analysis of a non-stationary time signal will depend on the desired resolution in time and frequency, and the presence of superimposed frequencies or noise in the signal. There is no single good universal method.

3.2.4 DISCUSSION

Body sounds are non-stationary in nature and generally periodic. If we take the Fourier transform of the sound over several cycles, the resultant spectrogram contains all the spectral energy in the sound, but tells us nothing about when a given spectral component occurred. Time-frequency analysis (TFA) had its origin in the early analog spectrograms used for "voice-print" analysis. Today, TFA is done digitally with a wide choice of algorithms and display modalities. TFA is particularly useful in aiding the analysis of heart and breath sounds. It provides a visual quantitative record of what spectral components occurred when. TFA algorithms are included in Matlab's Signal Processing Toolbox™, and in the National Instruments signal processing software. Expect to see an increasing reliance on TFA as a signal descriptor in medical diagnosis.

3.3 HEART SOUNDS

3.3.1 INTRODUCTION

One of the earliest noninvasive measures of health in humans was the sounds made by the beating heart. After Laennec's invention of the stethoscope, it became apparent that heart sounds could be more complex than a simple "lub dub". By observing the action of a beating heart in surgically opened animal chests, early workers could correlate features in the heart sounds with specific events in the cardiac cycle. For example, the "lub" sound comes from the closing of the tricuspid and mitral (A-V) valves at the beginning of systole. The "dub" is associated with the sudden closure of the aortic and pulmonary (semilunar) valves at the end of systole. The sounds are now known to come not from the valves alone, but from kinetic energy stored in moving blood being transformed into elastic stretch of the valves' and the heart's walls, causing them to vibrate when the valves abruptly stop the moving blood. In the case of the first heart sound (lub), the initial contraction of the ventricles forces the tricuspid and mitral valves to close and then bulge toward the atria until their leaves are snubbed by the *chordae tendineae*. The elastic tautness of the valves then causes the moving mass of the blood, which is incompressible, to cause the ventricular walls and closed valves to vibrate. There is also vibrating turbulence in the blood. These vibrations have a low-frequency content; they are transmitted through the chest tissues to the chest wall, where they cause the skin to vibrate perpendicularly.

The second heart sound (dub) occurs at the end of systole when the aortic and pulmonary (semilunar) valves close. At this point, the pressure in the aortic arch exceeds that in the left ventricle, even though the blood is still moving in the aorta. Again, kinetic energy of the blood and potential energy of stretched blood vessels interact. The outward-moving blood in the aorta is forced back against the valves; their elastic stretch redirects the blood outwardly. The valves and the aorta walls are under tension, and so vibrate at subsonic and low sonic frequencies when excited by the moving mass of the aortic blood. The timing of these events, the aortic blood pressure, and the ECG waveform, are shown in Figure 3.6.

When heart sounds are recorded directly from the heart surface with miniature accelerometers, or with good acoustic coupling from the chest wall to a broad-band microphone with good low-frequency response, further details of normal heart sounds can be heard, seen on a CRT monitor (oscilloscope), or viewed as time-frequency spectrograms. Interestingly, the best points to listen to or record specific heart sounds are not directly over the involved valve's direct projections to the chest surface. For example, the auscultation point for sounds associated with the opening and closing of the aortic semilunar valve is at the second intercostal space at the right edge of the sternum. The sounds from the pulmonary semilunar valve are best heard at the left side of the sternum at the second intercostal junction. Listen at the lower left tip of the sternum for sounds from the tricuspid valve (between the right atrium and right ventricle). To best hear the sounds from the bicuspid valve (between the left atrium and left ventricle), listen at the fifth intercostal space on the left mid-clavicular line.

In Figure 3.6, the first (normal) heart sound, S_1, has several components: vibrations introduced by the closure of the tricuspid and mitral valves between the atria and ventricles when the ventricles begin their forceful contraction. There may also be turbulence sounds as blood is forced into the aorta. The sound originating with the closure of the mitral valve is generally louder than the tricuspid sound. This difference is because the pressure in the left ventricle is higher than that in the right, and the mitral valve and heart walls are under more tension. Under conditions of inspired air (expanded lungs) it is sometimes possible to hear a "split" between the two, A-V valve sounds. That is, the louder sound caused by the mitral valve precedes the softer sound caused by the tricuspid valve.

The second heart sound, S_2, is associated with the closure of the aortic valve between the left ventricle and the aorta, and the closure of the pulmonary valve

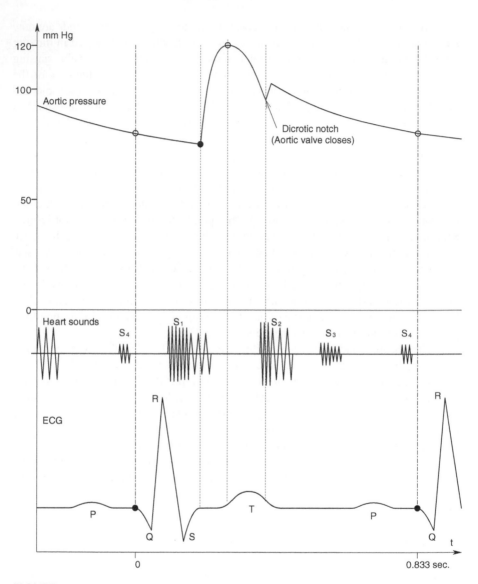

FIGURE 3.6 Timing diagram showing the times in the cardiac cycle when various heart sounds occur compared with a lead II ECG waveform, and a typical aortal blood pressure waveform.

between the right ventricle and the pulmonary artery. The frequency content of S_2 is higher because there is greater elastic tension on the associated valves, the ventricles, and the walls of the aorta and pulmonary artery. S_2 can also exhibit a split between the sounds associated with the two valves. The louder aortic valve closes slightly before the pulmonary valve when the chest is inflated. The sounds are virtually coincident with an expired chest.

The third heart sound, S_3, is a weak, very low-frequency sound caused by atrial blood's being forced into the ventricles. It is considered normal in children and young adults, but can indicate left ventricular hypertrophy or ventricular dysfunction in adults over 40. S_3 occurs in the last third of diastole (Tilson-Chrysler, 2000).

The S_4 sound or "atrial gallop" precedes S_1, and is due to blood's being forced into the ventricles by vigorous atrial contraction. It contains frequencies no higher than about 20 Hz and is therefore almost inaudible. It can be seen on oscilloscope displays and by time-frequency spectrograms. S_4 is found in patients with hypertension, aortic stenosis, acute myocardial infarction or left ventricular hypertrophy (Guyton, 1991).

3.3.2 ABNORMAL HEART SOUNDS

There are many cardiac defects that can lead to the production of additional or modified heart sounds. Some of these will be discussed below. There are many web sites where one can download and listen to electronically recorded heart sounds as *.wav files. Also, in Canada, McGill University's Physiology and Music Departments have an unique Medical Informatics web site at which the viewer can listen to various cardiac sounds (normal and abnormal) at different chest recording sites. In addition, the viewer can download 3-D, colored-mesh, time-frequency spectrograms covering several cardiac cycles of a particular sound, as well as read text about the source and significance of the sound (Glass, 1997).

A major source of anomalous heart sounds is damaged heart valves. Heart valves, in particular, the left heart valves, can either fail to open properly (they are *stenosed*) or they cannot close properly, causing a backflow of blood, or *regurgitation*. A major source of heart valve damage can be infection by a group A hemolytic streptococcus, such as scarlet fever, sore throat, or middle ear infection. A serious complication of group A strep infections is rheumatic fever, one of the characteristics of which is *carditis* and valvular damage. The streptococcus bacteria manufacture a protein called the "M antigen," to which the immune system forms antibodies. Unfortunately, these antibodies also attack certain body tissues, notably the joints and the heart. Guyton (1991) states: "In rheumatic fever, large hemorrhagic, fibrinous, bulbous lesions grow along the inflamed edges of the heart valves." The scarring from this autoimmune inflammation leaves permanent valve damage. The valves of the left heart (aortic and mitral) are the most prone to damage by antibodies.

In *aortic valve stenosis*, the valve cannot open properly; there is an abnormally high hydraulic resistance against which the left ventricle must pump. Thus, the peak left ventricular pressure can rise as high as 300 mmHg, while the aortic pressure remains in the normal range. The exiting blood is forced through the small aperture at very high velocity, causing turbulence and enhanced vibration of the root of the aorta. This vibration causes a loud murmur during systole that is characteristic of aortic stenosis.

Aortic regurgitation, on the other hand, occurs because the damaged aortic valve does not close completely. Again, there is a high-velocity jet of blood forced back into the left ventricle by aortic back-pressure during diastole (when the left ventricle is relaxed). This back-pressure makes it difficult for the left atrium to fill the left ventricle, and, of course, the heart must work harder to pump a given volume of blood into the aorta. The aortic regurgitation murmur is also of relatively high pitch, and has a swishing quality (Guyton, 1991).

In *mitral valve stenosis,* the murmur occurs in the last two thirds of diastole, caused by blood's jetting through the valve from the left atrium to the left ventricle. Because of the low peak pressure in the left atrium, a weak, very low-frequency sound is produced. The mitral stenotic murmur often cannot be heard; its vibration must be felt, or seen on an oscilloscope from a microphone output. Another audible clue to mitral stenosis is an "opening snap" of the mitral valve, closely following the normal S_2.

Mitral valve regurgitation takes place during systole. As the left ventricle contacts, it forces a high-velocity jet of blood back through the mitral valve, making the walls of the left atrium vibrate. The frequencies and amplitude of mitral valve regurgitation murmur are lower than aortic valve stenosis murmur because the left atrium is not as resonant as the root of the aorta is. Also, the sound has farther to travel from the left atrium to the front of the chest.

Another cardiac defect that can be diagnosed by hearing the S_2 sound "split" is a left or right *bundle branch block.* The synchronization of the contraction of the muscle of the left and right ventricles is accomplished by the wave of electrical depolarization that propagates from the AV node, down the *bundle of His,* which bifurcates into the left and right bundle branches that run down on each side of the *ventricular septum.* Near the apex of the heart, the bundle branches branch extensively into the *Purkinje fibers,* which invade the inner ventricular cardiac muscle syncytium, carrying the electrical activity that triggers ventricular contraction. See Figure 3.7 for a schematic cut-away view of the heart, and Figure 3.8 for a time-domain schematic of where certain heart sounds occur in the cardiac cycle.

If the bundle branch fibers on the right side of the septum are damaged by infection, the contraction of the right ventricle will lag that of the right, and the sound associated with the aortic valve's closing will lead that caused by the pulmonary valve. This split in sound S_2 is heard regardless of the state of inhale or exhale. A left bundle branch block will delay the contraction of the left ventricle, hence delay the aortic valve sound with respect to that of the pulmonary valve. This condition causes reverse splitting of S_2 during expiration, but is absent on inspiration. Other causes of the reverse split include premature right ventricular contraction (as opposed to a delayed left ventricular systole), or systemic hypertension (high venous return pressure).

3.3.3 DISCUSSION

Because of the subtlety of the patterns and timing of cardiac sounds, and the fact that some of their frequencies are too low to be heard by a typical human ear, there is an increased reliance on either observing the sound waveforms on an oscilloscope, or using a time-frequency spectrogram to observe the fine frequency structure of the component sounds as they occur. There is certainly more information in the latter class of display.

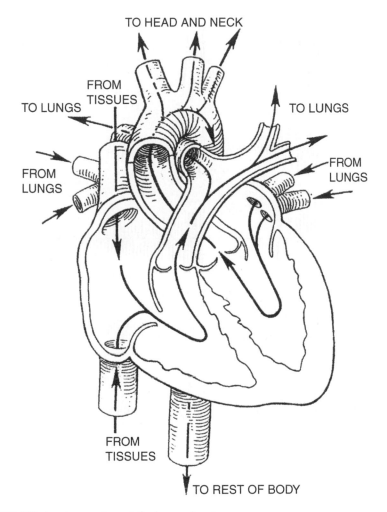

TO HEAD AND NECK

FROM TISSUES

TO LUNGS

TO LUNGS

FROM LUNGS

FROM LUNGS

FROM TISSUES

TO REST OF BODY

FIGURE 3.7 A cutaway view of the human heart.

3.4 BREATH SOUNDS

3.4.1 INTRODUCTION

As air passes in and out of the normal respiratory system during normal breathing, certain sounds can be heard by auscultating the back and chest over the lungs, trachea, and bronchial tubes with an acoustic or electronic stethoscope. As in the case of heart sounds, it requires a good ear and much experience to use breath sounds effectively for noninvasive diagnosis. The normal sounds perceived are due in part to air turbulence, air turbulence exciting damped mechanical resonances in connective tissues, and alveoli stretching open on inspiration, and shrinking on expiration. Normal breath sounds are classified as *tracheal, bronchial, broncovesicular* and *vesicular*. Tracheal sounds are heard over the trachea; they have a harsh quality and

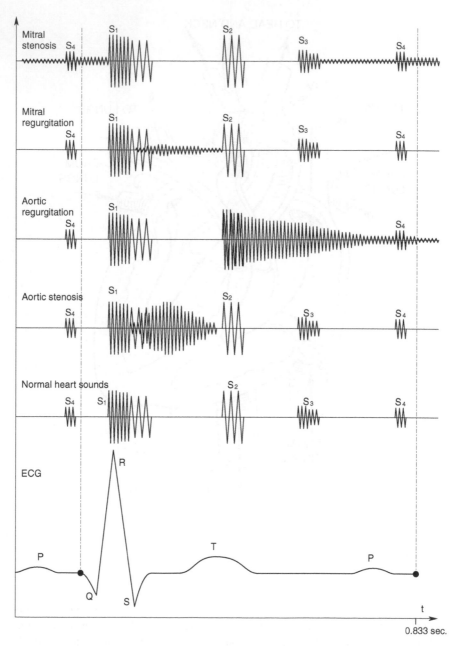

FIGURE 3.8 A schematic timing diagram of heart sounds for normal and various heart pathologies referenced to the lead II ECG waveform.

sound like air moving through a pipe. Heard over the anterior chest over the sternum and at the second and third intercostal spaces, the bronchial sounds originate in the bronchial tubes (see Figure 3.9) and have a more hollow quality, not as harsh as tracheal sound. They are generally louder and higher in pitch; expiratory bronchial sounds last longer than inspiratory sounds, and there is a pause at peak inspiration. Bronchovesicular sounds are heard in the posterior chest between the scapulae, and also in the center of the anterior chest. They are softer than bronchial sounds and also have a tubular quality. Vesicular sounds are soft, breezy or rustling in nature, and can be heard throughout most of the lung fields. Heard throughout inspiration, they continue with no pause through the beginning of expiration, and fade away about one third of the way through expiration.

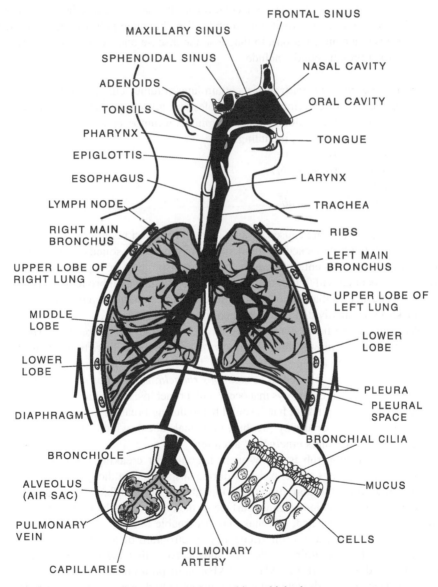

FIGURE 3.9 Anatomy of the lungs, trachea, and bronchial tubes.

Several web sites for medical and nursing students have on-line audio samples of normal and abnormal breath (and heart) sounds that can be played on your computer's audio system. The McGill web site (Glass, 1997) is particularly good because it gives time-frequency spectrograms as well as the real-time audio for each type of sound.

3.4.2 ABNORMAL BREATH SOUNDS

Almost all diseases of the lungs are characterized by certain classes of abnormal breath sounds. Also, certain systemic conditions, such as congestive heart failure or high altitude disease, can affect lung sounds. The challenge is to use the abnormal sounds (plus other information), to diagnose the disease and evaluate its severity.

Abnormal breath sounds include:

1. The *absence of sounds* over a certain lung volume. This generally means that air is not entering the bronchioles and alveoli in that lung volume; this can be due to fluid filling the volume, a tumor, etc.
2. *Adventitious sounds*, including:
   - *Crackles* (or *rales*)
   - *Wheezes* (or *rhonchi*)
   - *Stridor*
   - *Pleural friction rub*

Crackles, or rales, are caused by air's being forced past respiratory passages that are narrowed (but not blocked) by fluid, mucus or pus. These sounds are intermittent, non-musical and transient; they can be heard on inspiration or expiration. Crackles are often associated with inflammation or infection of the small bronchi, bronchioles and alveoli. Crackles that do not clear with coughing can indicate pulmonary edema. Crackles can be subdivided into fine, medium and coarse.

Wheezes can be heard continuously through inspiration or expiration. They are produced when air moves through airways narrowed by constriction or swelling. Squeaky wheezes are called *sibilant rhonchi*, lower-pitched wheezes with a moaning or snoring quality are referred to as *sonorous rhonchi*. A cause of sonorous rhonchi is secretions in the larger airways that occur with bronchitis, bronchial pneumonia, etc.

Stridor is a high-pitched, harsh sound heard during breathing. It is caused by an obstruction in an upper airway (trachea, bronchial tubes), which can be an inhaled foreign object. It requires emergency attention.

A pleural friction rub is a low-pitched, grating or creaking noise that occurs mostly when the lungs are expanding during inspiration, although some rubbing sound is heard on expiration. Its cause is the rubbing of the inflamed outside surface of the lung with the inflamed inner surface of the chest wall. (Normally the pleural surfaces are well lubricated, and make no discernable noise.)

Figure 3.10 illustrates a time-frequency spectrogram of lungs producing sonorous rhonchi. Two breathing cycles are shown. Note that the band of significant sound power density is from 2 kHz to 3 kHz on inspiration, while, when exhaling, the frequencies of the rhonchi having significant sound power are from 400 Hz to 1.3 kHz. We can also see that the dominant frequencies on exhale tend to die out.

(A graph of tracheal air velocity (or volume) vs. time would be useful in interpreting this diagram.) Sonorous rhonchi are a symptom of bronchitis or asthma.

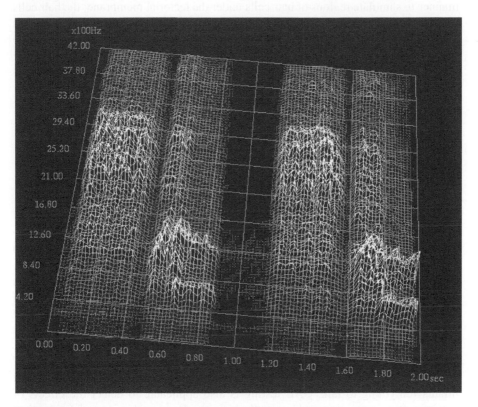

FIGURE 3.10 Time frequency spectrogram of lungs producing sonorous rhonchi; two breaths are shown. (Used with permission of the McGill sound web site.)

3.4.3 DISCUSSION

Diagnosis of respiratory diseases and conditions by their sounds is an art. Clearly, the listener must be able to discriminate different frequencies, i.e., have a musician's ear, for best effect. It goes without saying that diagnosticians or listeners must have extensive clinical experience on which to base their judgment. Viewing a T-F spectrogram of the sound can aid in the diagnostic decision, but interpretation of the T-F spectrogram by itself also requires an extensive experience database with this modality. The comb filter properties of the traditional stethoscope would only appear to complicate this diagnostic process.

3.5 OTOACOUSTIC EMISSIONS

3.5.1 INTRODUCTION

Traditionally, the human hearing mechanism has been viewed as a purely passive process with no efferent feedback from the CNS. Sound waves impinging on the eardrum vibrate it, causing the three ossicles in the middle ear to vibrate, in turn, the oval window of the cochlea. The vibrations in the cochlea act in a complex manner to stimulate regions of hair cells under the tectorial membrane; the hair cells in turn send neural signals along the eighth cranial nerve to the CNS. As it has developed, the hearing process may also involve efferent neural signals from the CNS.

Otoacoustic emissions (OAEs), first reported by Kemp 1978, are narrow-band acoustic signals generated in the inner ear by certain outer hair cells. Presumably these hair cells vibrate in response to some sort of local active nonlinear feedback mechanism. There are three classes of OAEs:

1. Spontaneous continuous-wave (CW) emissions
2. Click or tone-burst-evoked transient emissions (TOAEs)
3. Distortion product emissions ($(2f_1 - f_2)$ DPOAEs) in response to CW stimulation by two sinusoidal frequencies

Spontaneous CW emissions are pure tone, and occur in about 68% of infants under 18 months, decreasing to 35% in adults under 50 and to 20% in persons over 50 who have normal hearing (Redhead, 1998). All normal human ears emit reflex TOAEs to clicks and tone bursts, and DPOAEs to CW, two-frequency stimuli. OAEs have also been found in such diverse animals as frogs (*Rana sp.*), bats, gerbils, barn owls, opossums, mice, kangaroo rats, lizards, and chinchillas (see www.aro.org/ abstracts.html, 1996).

Most hearing impairment is associated with a decrease or loss of OAEs. Thus. several companies have developed noninvasive instruments to test the OAE reflex. Such tests are particularly useful in diagnosing hearing impairment in neonates and infants too young to talk. OAE testing is also applicable to detect the effects of ototoxic drugs (e.g., tetracycline) on hearing, to detect early signs of loud-noise-induced deafness in teenagers and industrial workers, to check hearing following episodes of Meniere's disease, and to detect lesions affecting the eighth nerve or cochlea.

To perform a DPOAE test, a probe, much like a hearing aid earpiece, is inserted into the end of the ear canal. The probe contains a miniature microphone and two miniature earphones. In a typical DPOAE test, the CW sound stimuli from the headphones are $f_1 = 2.0$ kHz and $f_2 = 2.5$ kHz, at 70 dB SPL. Thus the DPOAE is at $(2f_1 - f_2) = 1.5$ kHz, typically at c. 8 dB SPL, or 62 dB weaker than the stimuli's sound pressure (less than 1/1000 the sound pressure of the stimuli) (Leonard et al., 1990).

Leonard et al. showed that the $(2f_1 - f_2)$ CW, DPOAE follows the input dB SPL with a sigmoid curve. There is a threshold input dB SPL below which no DPOAE is produced. This threshold is frequency- and individual-dependent; covering a wide range from 35 to 58 dB. The threshold is higher in ears with hearing loss, and the dB level of the DPOAEs is lower. The loudest stimuli used were 80 dB SPL; these typically produced an OAE as loud as c.15 dB SPL in normal ears.

3.5.2 OTOACOUSTIC TESTING

There are many different scientific parameters that can be used to characterize OAEs. In the case of click-evoked transient emissions, an obvious analysis modality is the time-frequency spectrogram; the response latency as a function of stimulus amplitude is also of interest. The click is basically the impulse response of the miniature loudspeaker used to stimulate the ear. Its pressure waveform can be approximated as the impulse response of an underdamped, second-order, low-pass system. That is: $p(t) = P_o \exp(-\xi \omega_n t) \sin[\omega_n \sqrt{(1 - \xi^2)} t]$. ξ is the loudspeaker's damping factor, and $\omega_n = 2\pi f_n$ is the natural resonant frequency of the loudspeaker in r/s. f_n is made as high as possible, and $\xi \to 0.5$, so the frequency content in $p(t)$ is high, as seen from its Fourier transform, $P(j\omega)$. The click is thus a broad-band transient stimulus.

DPOAEs are the result of steady-state, f_1 and f_2 stimulation. Thus, the power density spectrogram of the DPOAE is of interest; it will show not only the established $2f_1 - f_2$ product, but any other residual terms such as $2f_1 + f_2$, $2f_2 \pm f_1$, $3f_1$, $3f_2$, $f_2 \pm f_1$, $2f_1$ and $2f_2$. (The last three terms are the result of a square-law nonlinearity, the others from a cubic nonlinearity operating on the $p_{in} = A \sin(2\pi f_1 t) + B \sin(2\pi f_2 t)$ input.)

An example of a commercially available TOAE testing system is the ILO88 transient emission tester made by Otodynamics, Ltd., Hertfordshire, England. 260 repetitions of 80 dB clicks, each lasting 1 ms and spaced about 0.25 seconds apart are given, and the evoked, TOAEs are recorded. The first 20 ms of each alternate TOAE is averaged to form two alternate arrays, each made from the average of 130 responses. The machine then computes a correlation coefficient between the two arrays. If the TOAE response is 100% consistent, the correlation will be 1.0, or 100%. Variability between successive TOAEs will cause a lower correlation, called the "Waverepro%." The Waverepro% needs to be below c. 35% before hearing loss is detectable by conventional audiometry. On-line excerpts from the *Australian Medical Journal*, (Redhead, 1998) show how the Waverepro% declines with age, and also how it decreases with cumulative exposure to industrial noise and loud personal stereo use.

Intelligent Hearing Systems of Miami, Florida, markets the SmartOAE™, a computer-based, CW OAE testing system. This is a research-grade instrument that displays the root power density spectrogram of the DPOAE. It also displays the DPOAE signal-to-noise ratio, noise statistics, testing parameters, etc. The input dB SPL can be set from 0 to 75 dB SPL, and input frequencies can be varied from 500 Hz to 8 kHz.

3.5.3 DISCUSSION

The measurement of the $(2f_2 - f_1)$ OAE has found use in the noninvasive diagnosis and quantification of hearing loss from various causes, including Meniere's disease, tetracycline toxicity, lesions affecting the eighth nerve or cochlea, etc., or idiopathic causes. Otoacoustic testing is particularly valuable in evaluating the hearing of infants too young to speak. The $(2f_2 - f_1)$ product is "hard-wired" in the auditory system; it does not habituate or fatigue, and thus provides a valuable objective test of the closed-loop auditory system.

3.6 SUMMARY

One of the basic low-cost modalities of noninvasive diagnosis is the analysis of sounds originating from within the body. It is well known that the sound transmission properties of the body act as a low pass filter to internal sound sources as they propagate to the body surface. In addition, the traditional physician's stethoscope imposes a comb filter type transmission on sounds it couples from the skin to the listener's ears. Even with these handicaps, an experienced cardiologist or respiratory specialist can recognize abnormal sounds and correlate them with suspect pathologies.

The modern approach to analyzing heart and breath sounds is to use an electronic stethoscope that eliminates the spectral distortions caused by the conventional stethoscopes's coupling tubes. We have seen that a great visual aid in analyzing non-stationary body sounds is the time-frequency spectrogram (TFS). We reviewed several ways of computing TFSs and their relative merits. The TFS plots the spectral components of sounds vs. time, providing a quantitative graphical description of sounds to complement the subjective impression of the listener.

This chapter has considered heart and breath sounds and the pathologies that can be diagnosed from them. Otoacoustic emissions were also covered, and their potential importance in diagnosing hearing problems was described. Several medical school web sites provide audio clips of body sounds and their corresponding TFSs.

4 Measurement of Electrical Potentials and Magnetic Fields from the Body Surface

4.1 INTRODUCTION

It has long been known that electric fields generated by action potentials accompanying the conduction of nerve impulses, and the depolarization of muscle membranes can propagate through the various volume conductor layers of the body and be sensed on the skin surface. Such potentials are given names according to their sources: from muscles, we have the *electromyogram* (EMG); from the brain, the *electroencephalogram* (EEG) and evoked cortical potentials (ECPs); from the eyes, the *electrooculogram* (EOG) and the *electroretinogram* (ERG); from the ear, the *electrocochleogram* (ECocG); and from the heart, the *electrocardiogram* (ECG or EKG).

All of these potentials have frequency spectra that basically span the audio range of frequencies, and, in some cases, very low, subsonic frequencies as well. Their amplitudes are basically in the range of 10s of microvolts to 10s of millivolts. All bioelectric signals are noisy, i.e., they are recorded with bioelectric background noise, as well as measurement noise from electrodes, amplifiers and the surrounding electrical environment. Signal averaging is often used to improve the signal-to-noise ratio of evoked transient signals such as ECPs and ERGs.

Probably the most widely exploited bioelectric signal for diagnostic purposes is the ECG. It is easy to record and can be displayed in 3-D vector form to aid diagnosis. Changes in the ECG vector display occur when an area of heart muscle is starved for oxygen or necrotic because of a previous infarct. The reason ECG analysis is so effective is that the cardiac pumping cycle involves the synchronized, spatiotemporal spread of electrical activity through the volume of the heart muscle. Thus, a region of damaged muscle shows up as a reduced potential when the wave of activity reaches that region. Another sign of damage is the inability of damaged heart muscle to electrically repolarize in a normal manner after contraction has occurred.

The following sections describe the electrodes and amplifiers used to record bioelectric potentials, the sources of the potentials, and what they tell us. Along with the section on signal conditioning, sources of noise and low-noise amplifier design are treated. Special medical isolation amplifiers are described.

Also covered is the recording of the very small transient magnetic fields resulting from the transient flow of ionic currents accompanying nerve and muscle action potentials. The *super-conducting quantum interference device* (SQUID) is introduced, and we show how it is used to monitor brain activity, etc. SQUIDS are generally used experimentally, and, as in the case of MRI, the cost of running a SQUID array is considerable (it requires a magnetically shielded room, a source of liquid helium, and extensive electronics). On the plus side for magnetoencephalography (MEG) is that it truly is a no-touch recording method. From multiple SQUID recordings, volumes of magnetic activity in the brain can be generated by computer and colored according to their intensity. Magnetic voxel resolution is highest in the cortex, and decreases with increasing depth into the brain.

4.2 ELECTRODES

4.2.1 INTRODUCTION

The noninvasive measurement of bioelectric potentials from the body surface (skin) generally makes use of electrochemical electrodes to couple the electrical potentials at points on the skin to the copper wires that connect to the signal-conditioning amplifier. A good electrochemical electrode must have as low an impedance as possible in the range of frequencies occupied by the signal. The reason for needing low electrode impedance is that thermal noise is produced by the real part of the electrode's impedance. A high-impedance electrode is, in general, noisier than a low-impedance electrode, and can limit signal resolution. The input impedance of a modern medical isolation amplifier used to condition the biomedical signal is generally so high ($> 10^9 \, \Omega$) that a few tens of kilohms of electrode impedance has little effect on attenuating the bioelectric signal. In the late 19th and early 20th centuries, before the invention of high-gain, high-input impedance amplifiers, ECG measurement was done with sensitive galvanometers that were driven by ECG currents from the body. Thus. early ECG electrodes needed really low impedances. The patient placed a foot into a large jar of salt water that was connected to the galvanometer by a wire attached to a large carbon rod electrode that was also in the jar. The other contact with the body was a hand placed in a jar of salt water and similarly connected to the galvanometer. A roving electrode was made from a saline-soaked sponge.

With modern electrode systems, a water-based electrolyte paste, cream or gel containing sodium, potassium and chloride ions is used to galvanically couple the skin to the electrode's metal-salt surface. The electrolyte may also contain an organic gelling agent to prevent it from running, and a preservative to inhibit mold and bacteria growth. Synapse® conductive electrode cream made by Med-Tek Corp, Northbrook, Illinois, lists the following ingredients: water, sodium chloride, propylene glycol, mineral oil, glyceryl monostearate, polyoxyethelene stearate, stearyl alcohol, calcium chloride, potassium chloride, methylparaben, butylparaben, propyl paraben, perfume, and D and C Red #19. The electrolyte gel is largely responsible for maintaining low electrode impedance, hence low thermal noise, and also for reducing electrical motion artifacts from relative motion of the electrode with the skin. Early body-surface electrodes were held in place by rubber straps. A modern recording electrode has a self-adhesive "skirt" surrounding the electrolyte-gel-filled center cup, which contains the silver chloride contact electrode. Some of the newer temporary electrodes, such as the Burdick CardioSens/Ultra® II, and the Medtronic Fastrace® 4, use a conductive latex adhesive over the entire 1-in.-square active area of the electrode to attach it to the skin.

Nearly all modern stick-on skin electrodes interface the electrons in the copper wire to a thin layer of silver chloride deposited on a thin layer of silver metal bonded to the electrode. The principal ions carrying charge through the skin are sodium, potassium and chloride. These ions are in serum (extracellular fluid) and sweat. They have different mobilities; i.e., they travel at different speeds in a given medium in the same electric field. The electrolyte paste or adhesive couples these ions to the Ag | AgCl layer where the half-cell reaction that involves electrons occurs. Note that there are no free electrons in the electrolyte, and no anions and cations in the solid phase (metal, metal salt) of the electrode. Charge transfers at electrode surfaces make 1/f noise, so it is important that very little current flows in the wire and the electrode interface.

4.2.2 THE ELECTRODE HALF-CELL POTENTIAL

Two different electrodes coupled by a common electrolyte form an *electrochemical cell*. This cell has a measurable electrochemical *open-circuit dc EMF* associated with it, which is a function of the ion activities in the electrolyte and on the electrode surfaces. The cell EMF is also a function of the Kelvin temperature, and is the algebraic sum of the *half-cell potentials* of the two electrodes. Half-cell potentials are found by measuring the EMF of a cell consisting of a so-called *hydrogen electrode* half-cell, defined to have 0 V fixed *standard half-cell potential* ($E_H^0 = 0$). The other half-cell is the one under measurement. By convention, a hydrogen half-cell electrode is made by bubbling H_2 gas at p = 1 atmosphere over a platinum screen electrode covered with platinum black. The Pt screen is immersed in an aqueous electrolyte having temperature T °K, and some pH. Note that pH is defined as: pH $\equiv -\log_{10}(a_{H+})$, where a_{H+} is the hydrogen ion *activity* in the electrolyte of the hydrogen half-cell. It can be shown (Maron and Prutton, 1958) that if the gas pressure is 1 atmosphere, the Hydrogen electrode's half-cell potential varies with temperature and pH according to:

$$E_H = -\frac{RT}{F}\ln(a_{H+}) = -\frac{2.303\,RT}{F}\log_{10}(a_{H+}) = \frac{2.303\,RT}{F}\,pH \quad \text{Volts} \quad 4.1$$

Where F is the Faraday number (96,500 Cb/equivalent), T is the Kelvin temperature, and R is the MKS gas constant (8.31 joule/mole °K). Standard half-cell potentials have been tabulated for many metal | metal salt half-cells, including the ubiquitous silver | silver chloride electrode; several are shown in Table 4.2.2.1.

The half-cell potential of a silver | silver chloride electrode can be shown to be given by:

TABLE 4.2.2.1
Oxidation Half-Cell Potentials vs. a Standard Hydrogen Electrode

Electrode	Oxidation Electrode Reaction	Std. Half-Cell Potential, E^0, @ 25°C
$H_2 \mid H^+$	H_2 (g, 1 atm.) $= 2H^+ + 2e^-$	0.000 V
$Ag \mid AgCl$	$Ag(s) + Cl^- = AgCl(s) + e^-$	-0.22233
$Ag \mid Ag^+$	$Ag(s) = Ag^+ + e^-$	-0.7991
$Hg \mid HgCl_2(s), Cl^-$	$2\,Hg(l) + 2Cl^- = Hg_2Cl_2 + 2e^-$	-0.2680
$Pb \mid PbSO_4(s), SO_4^=$	$Pb(s) + SO_4^= = PbSO_4(s) + 2e^-$	$+0.3546$

Note: When the reactions are written as reductions, the standard potentials have reversed signs.

$$E_{Ag/AgCl} = E^0_{Ag|AgCl} + \frac{RT}{F}\ln\left(a_{Cl-}\right) \qquad\qquad 4.2$$

That is, it depends on the activity (concentration) of the chloride ions surrounding the electrode. The concentration of chloride ions is held relatively constant by the electrode gel over the silver chloride surface. Because two identical silver chloride electrodes are used to measure biopotentials, their nearly identical half-cell potentials oppose each other, giving a dc "skin cell" potential of a few microvolts. Most biopotentials recorded from the skin (e.g., ECG, EEG, EMG) do not require dc coupling however, hence the small dc potential unbalance between a pair of silver chloride electrodes is not important. What is important is that the electrodes should have low impedance and not generate excessive motion artifact noise. A major component of motion artifact noise is low-frequency in nature, and arises when the electrode suddenly "sees" a change in chloride ion concentration, modulating $E_{Ag/AgCl}$.

4.2.3 EQUIVALENT CIRCUITS FOR AGCL SKIN ELECTRODES

One should never try to measure an electrochemical electrode's dc resistance with an ohmmeter. An ohmmeter passes a dc current through the electrode that causes ions to migrate toward or away from the AgCl/electrolyte interface, which alters the local concentration of chloride, which affects the electrode's half-cell potential. In addition, if the potential imposed across the electrode's interface by the ohmmeter is large enough, oxidation or reduction reactions can occur at the electrode's surface, further altering the passage of current and the electrode's half-cell potential. Thus, we see that, if any dc current is forced through the electrode by an ohmmeter or by an amplifier's dc bias current, irreversible chemical changes can occur at the electrode's interface, altering its half-cell potential and generally increasing its resistance. An electrode's dc resistance is, in general, nonlinear; it does not obey Ohm's law. Thus, the electrical characterization of electrodes is best done by using small ac voltages with varying frequency and measuring the magnitude and phase of the small currents that flow. The use of ac voltage avoids the problems of net ion migrations in the electrolyte, and irreversible oxidation or reduction reactions at the interface.

The electrical impedance of a silver│silver chloride skin electrode used to record bioelectric potentials consists of frequency-dependent real and imaginary parts. Take two identical AgCl electrodes with electrolyte gel and place them face to face, as shown in Figure 4.1(A). Thus, the impedance measured with a low ac current will be $2\,Z_e(f)$. A plot of the electrode's impedance magnitude vs. frequency, $|Z_e(f)|$ follows the shape shown in Figure 4.1(B). The shape suggests a simple parallel R-C circuit in series with a second resistor, as shown in Figure 4.1(C). Parameter constancy in this model is a gross approximation because C_i, R_i and R_G are all functions of frequency and ac current density. Nevertheless, at frequencies above 10 kHz, Z_e is relatively constant, and, in this example, is approximated by $R_G \cong 65$ ohms. At very low frequencies, C_i is basically an open-circuit, and $Z_e = R_i + R_G \cong$ 2,000 ohms. Thus $R_i \cong 1,935$ ohms. The first break frequency occurs at $f_b \cong 300 = 1/(2\pi R_i C_i)$ Hz, so $C_1 \cong 0.274\ \mu F$.

When two AgCl electrodes are attached to the skin, the equivalent circuit becomes more complex. Each input of the recording amplifier sees the series-parallel RC circuit describing the AgCl/electrolyte interface, in series with another parallel RC circuit modeling the interface between the conductive gel and the *stratum corneum* of the epidermis. The dermis and subcutaneous layer of the skin, plus the complex subcutaneous tissues, are modeled electrically by a simple resistance, R_T. Figure 4.2 illustrates the simplified Thevenin impedances seen by a differential biomedical amplifier used to record a biopotential such as an ECG, EMG or EEG. A major source of the resistive component of this Thevenin impedance is the natural oil and dead skin cells in the *stratum corneum*. If the oil is removed by rubbing with a solvent such as ethanol or acetone, and the surface cells are debrided with an abrasive such as fine sandpaper, a considerable reduction in R_s occurs.

4.2.4 Dry Electrodes

Instead of galvanically coupling the internal biopotential to the amplifier through the skin with a pair of reversible, electrochemical electrodes, it is possible to coat a metal electrode with a micron-thin insulating layer of oxide (e.g., SiO_2), or use a high-dielectric constant film over the electrode to conductively isolate it from the skin and body. The equivalent input circuit of a dry electrode amplifying system is shown in Figure 4.3. The insulated dry electrode appears as a capacitor, C_d, on the order of 1 nF. Because of the very high input impedance of the amplifier's headstage ($R_{in} > 10^{10}\ \Omega$, $C_{in} < 1$ pF) and dry electrodes, this system is very subject to electrode motion artifacts, triboelectric artifacts from lead motion, and to static electricity in the space around the electrodes. To minimize these effects, the amplifier's headstages are mounted directly over each electrode. In spite of their simplicity, dry electrodes are not used in clinical practice because the system is very noisy, and their expense precludes throwing away electrodes or amplifiers after use. It is much easier to use disposable film-type AgCl/electrolyte electrodes.

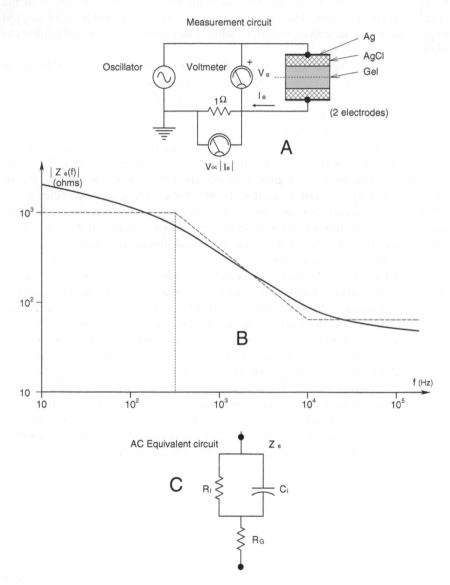

FIGURE 4.1(A) Test circuit for measuring the impedance magnitude of silver | silver chloride skin electrodes; the voltmeter-ammeter method is used with a sinusoidal VFO. (B) Plot of the typical impedance magnitude of a silver | silver chloride skin electrode. Bode asymptotes are shown. (C) Equivalent lumped-parameter circuit model for the electrode.

4.2.5 INVASIVE ELECTRODES

Because this text is about noninvasive measurements, we will mention only some of the electrode types that penetrate the skin when used in medical diagnosis. Needle electrodes and wire hook electrodes are inserted through the skin into muscle fibers

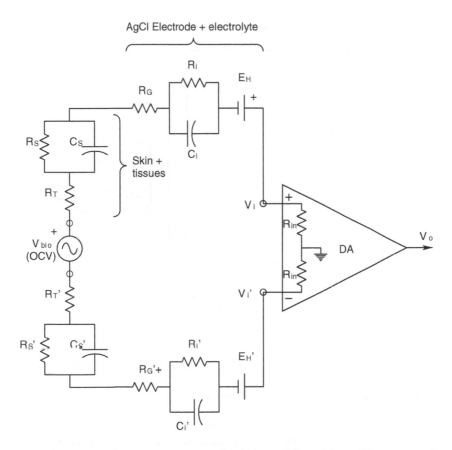

FIGURE 4.2 A complete equivalent input circuit for a differential amplifier connected to two silver | silver chloride skin electrodes, showing the CGR equivalent circuits for the skin and the Thevenin open-circuit voltage of a biopotential.

to record from single motor units and small groups of motor units. Their purpose is to record muscle action potentials and verify motor innervation. These electrodes are made from a mechanically tough, chemically inert — or relatively inert — material such as platinum —10% iridium alloy, tungsten, or stainless steel. A small hook in the end of the wire holds it in place, but it is thin and flexible enough to allow the electrode to be pulled out with minimum tissue damage.

Many other types of invasive electrodes are used in biomedical research, including suction electrodes used to pick up nerve fibers without damaging them. Pairs of hook electrodes are used for the same purpose. For extracellular recording of neuron action potentials in the brain or spinal cord, insulated metal microelectrodes are used. Their tips are bare and generally coated with platinum black to reduce their impedance. Saline-filled glass micropipette electrodes are used to record the transmembrane potential from single neurons and other cells. They penetrate the cell wall, which seals around them. Glass micropipette electrodes can have equivalent

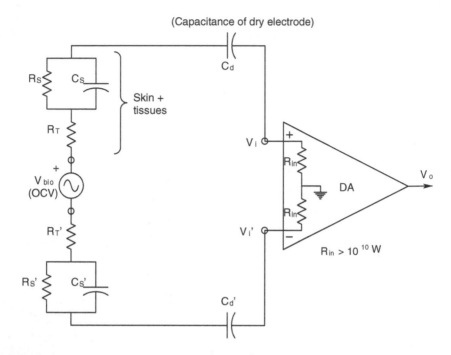

FIGURE 4.3 An equivalent circuit for a DA connected to two "dry" electrodes on the skin. Note that the dry electrodes are modeled by simple capacitors, while the skin and biopotential OCV have the same models as shown in Figure 4.2.

Thevenin resistances ranging from 10^7 to more than 10^8 ohms, depending on tip diameter and the filling electrolyte composition. Tip diameters can be made a fraction of a micron to penetrate axons and small cells. Ag$\,|\,$AgCl wire is used to interface with the electrolyte in glass micropipette electrodes.

4.3 BIOPOTENTIAL AMPLIFIERS

4.3.1 INTRODUCTION

In this section, we will examine the systems properties of biopotential amplifiers, while giving minimal attention to the electronic circuit details of their innards. Specifically, we will describe them by the equivalent circuits of their inputs, including input resistance, input capacitance, dc input bias current, dc input offset voltage, equivalent short-circuit input voltage noise source, and the equivalent input current noise source. At the output, we will either use the Thevenin model (open-circuit voltage and Thevenin series resistance) or the Norton model (short-circuit current source in parallel with the Norton conductance). The Thevenin or Norton sources are related to the input voltage by a transfer function (generally a Laplace rational polynomial) or a frequency response function used for steady-state sinusoidal input voltages.

Amplifiers used for biopotential recording fall into two categories, those with single-ended inputs, and those with differential (or differencing) inputs. Both types will be considered, including special-purpose instrumentation and biopotential amplifiers, as well as amplifiers made with op amps as building blocks. Single-ended and differential amplifiers can be further subdivided into those that are reactively coupled (RC) and do not pass dc, and direct-coupled (DC) amplifiers that amplify dc signals. For example, op amps are DC differential amplifiers, while ECG amplifiers are generally RC differential amplifiers.

Because the noise performance of an amplifier system is generally set by the noise injected by the first stage of amplification, i.e., the headstage, we will also discuss the factors contributing to low noise amplifier design at an electronic systems level.

4.3.2 SINGLE-ENDED AMPLIFIERS

A single-ended input amplifier can be characterized by the equivalent circuit shown in Figure 4.4. It can easily be made up from an op amp, as shown in Figure 4.5. When the op amp is operated in the non-inverting mode, the equivalent input circuit is that of the op amp, and the transfer function is given approximately by:

$$\frac{V_o}{V_{in}}(s) \cong \frac{\left(1 + R_F/R_1\right)}{\left(1 + s\,\tau_a\right)} \qquad\qquad 4.3$$

Where $\tau_a = (1 + R_F/R_1)/(2\pi f_T)$ seconds; f_T is the op amp's Hz *gain-bandwidth product*, aka *unity gain frequency* (Northrop, 1990,1997). Most bioelectric signals (with the exception of EMGs) have little spectral energy above 1 kHz, so amplifier f_T is generally not critical, as long as it is above 1 MHz. Single-ended amplifiers are used as interstages in multistage amplifiers, and as headstages for applications where the biosignal's SNR is good. That is, there is little interference picked up by the recording electrodes and wiring connecting them to the amplifier. This is usually not the case, however, and differential amplifiers are generally used for headstages in recording low-level signals from the skin, such as EEG, ECG, EMG, EOG, etc.

If one is measuring dc or very low frequency biopotentials such as EEG, body surface or bone potentials, the DC headstage amplifier used must be free of temperature-caused dc drift. *Chopper stabilization* is one technology used to achieve high dc drift stability. Reactive coupling avoids the dc drift problem when dc and very low frequency potentials are not being measured. Reactive coupling is generally used with EEG and EMG signals because of their higher bandwidths and lack of dc signal information. In RC amplifiers, successive gain stages are coupled with capacitor-resistor high-pass filters.

4.3.3 DIFFERENTIAL AMPLIFIERS

Differential amplifiers (DAs) are widely used for biopotential recording because of their ability to reduce or cancel common-mode interference and noise. A DC DA has a frequency response function that can be approximated by:

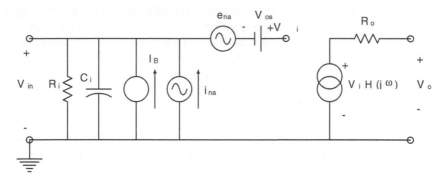

FIGURE 4.4 Equivalent circuit of a single-ended amplifier, showing dc offset voltage and bias current, as well as the equivalent short-circuit input, noise voltage root power spectrum and noise current root power spectrum. A Thevenin output model is shown.

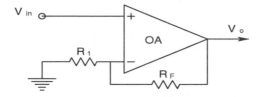

FIGURE 4.5 A non-inverting op amp. Ideally, $V_o/V_{in} = 1 + R_F/R_1$.

$$V_o = \frac{K_1}{(1 + j\omega\tau_1)} V_1 - \frac{K_2}{(1 + j\omega\tau_2)} V_i{}' \qquad 4.4$$

Ideally, K_1 is made equal to K_2, and $\tau_1 = \tau_2$, thus any interference signal that appears simultaneously at input V_i and $V_i{}'$ is cancelled by vector subtraction. Such interference and noise can include capacitively coupled 60 Hz hum, magnetically induced 60 Hz hum, ignition noise from gasoline engines, noise from fluorescent lights, etc. Noise that is common to both DA inputs is called a *common-mode signal*, which is defined formally as:

$$V_{ic} \equiv (V_i + V_i{}')/2 \qquad 4.5$$

The *difference mode input signal* is similarly defined:

$$V_{id} \equiv (V_i - V_i{}')/2 \qquad 4.6$$

The amplifier output can be written in terms of V_{ic} and V_{id}:

$$V_o = V_{id} A_D + V_{ic} A_C \qquad 4.7$$

In general, the complex common-mode gain, A_C, is very small, and increases at high frequencies. The difference-mode gain, A_D, can be approximately $2K_1/(1 + j\omega\tau_1)$. A figure of merit for all DAs is the common-mode rejection ratio (CMRR), usually given in dB, defined by:

$$CMRR \equiv 20 \log_{10} |A_D/A_C| \; dB \qquad\qquad 4.8$$

Note that the CMRR is a function of frequency. It is very large at low frequencies, e.g., >100 dB, and generally decreases steadily for $f > f_T/K_1$. An *Ideal DA* has $A_C \to 0$. Manufacturers usually specify the CMRR at a low frequency where it is maximum, such as 60 Hz. Another, more general, way to define CMRR is:

$$CMRR \equiv 20 \log_{10} \left\{ \frac{V_{ic} \text{ to produce a certain } V_o}{V_{id} \text{ to produce the same } V_o} \right\} \qquad\qquad 4.9$$

We will use the definition of Equation 4.9 to show how unbalances in Thevenin source resistance can affect the CMRR of the amplifier connected through electrodes to a biopotential source. The numerical argument of CMRR is always taken as a positive number.

As you can see from Figure 4.6, the input impedance for DAs is lower for DM input signals than it is for CM input signals because R_{id} carries current for DM inputs. This is ordinarily not a problem because the Thevenin source resistances are generally several orders of magnitude less than either the DM or CM input resistances. In situations where the bioelectrode impedances approach the input impedances of the amplifier, it is shown below that the effective CMRR of the amplifier *as connected* can be significantly lower (or higher) than the CMRR specified by the manufacturer for the basic DA alone. Figure 4.7 illustrates the simplified input circuit of a DA connected to a generalized two-source biosignal. When the two sources are equal and add, there is a DM open-circuit input voltage, v_{sd}. When the two sources are equal and oppose each other, there is a CM open-circuit input voltage, v_{sc}. If the input circuit is perfectly balanced, i.e., $R_{ic} = R_{ic}'$, and $R_s = R_s'$, then the CMRR of the system is the same as that of the amplifier, i.e., $CMRR_{sys} = CMRR_A$. If one of the Thevenin source resistances is larger or smaller than the other, i.e., $R_s' = R_s + \Delta R$, then a purely CM v_{sc} will produce a DM component, V_{id}, at the DA's input nodes, as well as a CM component, V_{ic}, and a purely DM v_{sd} will produce a CM component at the DA's input nodes, as well as a DM component. These unwanted components affect the CMRR of the overall system, as shown below. The overall or system CMRR is then defined as:

$$CMRR_{sys} \equiv 20 \log_{10} \left\{ \frac{V_{sc} \text{ to produce a certain } V_o}{V_{sd} \text{ to produce the same } V_o} \right\} \quad \textbf{CMRRsys} \qquad 4.10$$

To calculate the CMRRsys, we first let $V_s = V_s'$, so the input is pure CM, i.e., $V_{sc} = V_s$. Now from Figure 4.7, we see that:

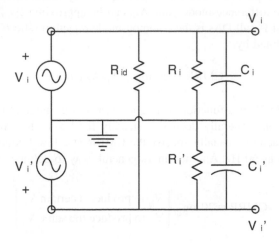

FIGURE 4.6 Equivalent input impedance model for a difference amplifier. R_{id} carries no current for a pure common-mode input.

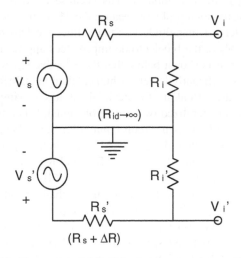

FIGURE 4.7 Simplified input circuit of a DA, showing two unequal Thevenin sources.

$$V_i = V_{sc}\, R_i/(R_i + R_s) \qquad\qquad 4.11A$$

$$V_i' = V_{sc}\, R_i/(R_i + R_s + \Delta R) \qquad\qquad 4.11B$$

V_{ic} and V_{id} can be found for the V_{sc} input:

$$V_{ic} \equiv \left(V_i + V_i'\right) / 2 = \left(V_{sc} R_i / 2\right) \left[\frac{1}{R_i + R_s} + \frac{1}{\left(R_s + R_i\right)\left(1 + \Delta R / \left(R_i + R_s\right)\right)} \right] \quad 4.12$$

Because $R_i \gg R_s$, the $\Delta R / (R_i + R_s)$ term is $\ll 1$ and we can finally write:

$$V_{ic} \cong \frac{V_{sc} R_i}{R_i + R_s} \quad\quad 4.13$$

Similarly, we can find V_{id} given V_{sc}:

$$V_{id} \equiv \left(V_i - V_i'\right) / 2 = \frac{V_{sc} R_i R_s}{\left(R_i + R_s\right)^2} \frac{\Delta R}{R_s} \quad\quad 4.14$$

Now the amplifier output is:

$$V_o \cong A_D \frac{V_{sc} R_i R_s}{\left(R_i + R_s\right)^2} \frac{\Delta R}{R_s} + A_c \frac{V_{sc} R_i}{\left(R_i + R_s\right)} \quad\quad 4.15$$

Now we let $V_s' = -V_s$ to create pure V_{sd}. In the manner used above, we find:

$$V_i = V_{sd} R_i / (R_i + R_s) \quad\quad 4.16A$$

$$V_i' = - V_{sd} R_i / (R_i + R_s + \Delta R) \quad\quad 4.16B$$

The DA's DM input is approximately:

$$V_{id} \cong V_{sd} R_i / (R_i + R_s) \quad\quad 4.17$$

And the CM input is:

$$V_{ic} \cong \frac{V_{sd} R_i R_s}{\left(R_i + R_s\right)^2} \frac{\Delta R}{R_s} \quad\quad 4.18$$

Using Equation 4.7, we can write the expression for V_o in terms of V_{sd}:

$$V_o \cong A_D \frac{V_{sd} R_i}{\left(R_i + R_s\right)} + A_c \frac{V_{sd} R_i R_s}{\left(R_i + R_s\right)^2} \frac{\Delta R}{R_s} \quad\quad 4.19$$

Now in Equations 4.19 and 4.15, we let $V_o = 1$, and solve for V_{sd} and V_{sc}, respectively, and substitute these expressions into Equation 4.10 for the log argument. After some algebra, the log argument (numerical value of the $CMRR_{sys}$) is found to be:

$$\arg CMRR_{sys} \cong \left| \frac{\arg CMRR_A}{\left(\arg CMRR_A \right) \Delta R / \left(R_i + R_s \right) + 1} \right| \qquad 4.20$$

Where $\arg CMRR_A \equiv |A_D / A_C|$. Note that $\arg CMRR_{sys}$ can go to ∞ (i.e., make an ideal DA) if

$$\frac{\Delta R}{R_s} = \frac{-\left(1 + R_i / R_s \right)}{\arg CMRR_A} \qquad 4.21$$

Figure 4.8 is a plot of $|\arg CMRR_{sys}|$ vs. $\Delta R/R_s$. As a numerical example, assume that $CMRR_A = 100$ dB, so $\arg CMRR_A = 10^5$. Let $R_i = 10^8 \ \Omega$, and $R_s = 10^4 \ \Omega$. To get $\arg CMRR_{sys} \to \infty$, ΔR must be $= -10^3 \ \Omega$. Note that it is more practical to add 1 k externally in series with R_s, instead of subtracting 1 k from R_s'. Also note from Figure 4.8 that when $\Delta R \to 0$, $CMRR_{sys} = CMRR_A$.

The lesson the development above teaches us is that even if we spend extra money to buy a DA with a very high $CMRR_A$, hidden source impedance unbalance can significantly reduce its actual effective value. On the other hand it is possible to make a silk purse out of a sow's ear; an inexpensive DA with a modest $CMRR_A$ can be made to have a very high $CMRR_{sys}$ by manipulating the apparent source resistances by adding a fixed external resistor in series with one electrode and the corresponding amplifier input. In practice, the shunt capacitances associated with the input leads, and the DA's input capacitances can further unbalance the input circuit and can reduce the CMRR at high frequencies.

4.3.4 Op Amps Used for Signal Conditioning

The well-known non-inverting op amp configuration shown in Figure 4.5 above generally has a very high input impedance (set by the op amp), and its -3 dB frequency f_b is given by

$$f_b = f_T / (1 + R_F/R_1) \qquad 4.22$$

That is, the higher the dc gain, the smaller the amplifier's bandwidth. This trade-off of bandwidth for gain is a general property of conventional op amps.

Another op amp property that can figure in the choice of a given type of op amp for a given application is the op amp's *slew rate,* η. The units of η are volts/microsecond or volts/sec. It is a large-signal parameter that gives the maximum magnitude of the rate of change of the output voltage, and is determined by the internal electronic circuitry of the op amp, typically ranging from ca. 10 V/μs to more than 1,000 V/μs in really fast op amps. Op amps that have high ηs generally also have high f_Ts.

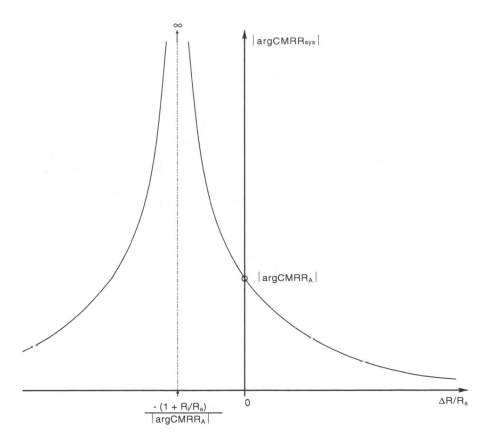

FIGURE 4.8 Plot of the magnitude of the numerical common-mode rejection ratio vs. the fractional unbalance in the sources' Thevenin resistors. Note that, in theory, it is possible to manipulate $\Delta R/R_s$ to make the CMRR $\to \infty$.

Op amps can be used to make differential amplifiers suitable for recording biopotential signals. Such circuits are called *instrumentation amplifiers* (IAs). A common IA circuit design is shown in Figure 4.9. In this circuit, high CMRR is obtained by matching the primed and non-primed resistor pairs precisely. If they are made equal, and the op amps are assumed ideal, then pure CM excitation ($V_i = V_i'$ $= V_{ic}$) will make $V_2 = V_2' = V_{ic}$, and zero current will flow in R_1 and R_1'. Thus R_1 and R_1' can be removed, and it is clear that $V_3 = V_3' = V_{ic}$, hence the ideal op amp, OA-3, connected as an ideal DA, gives $V_o = 0$. Thus $A_C = 0$. When $V_i' = - V_i$, there is ideal DM excitation with $V_{id} = V_i$. Hence $V_2 = V_i$ and $V_2' = - V_i$; thus there is $2V_{id}$ across $R_1 + R_1'$. Because $R_1 = R_1'$, using superposition it is easy to see that $V_c = 0$, effectively at ground potential. Now $V_3 = V_{id}(1 + R_2/R_1)$, and $V_3' = - V_{id}(1 + R_2/R_1)$. V_o is found from superposition:

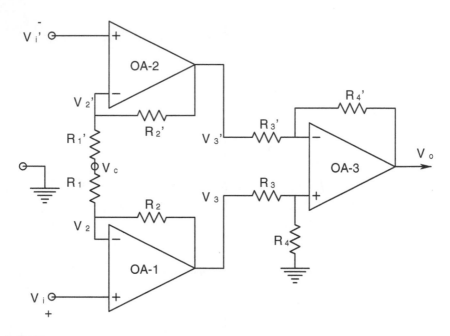

FIGURE 4.9 The well-known three-op amp instrumentation amplifier circuit. The resistors must be accurately matched to maximize the IA's CMRR.

$$V_o = V_3 \frac{R_4}{(R_4 + R_3)}(1 + R_4/R_3) + V_3'\left(-\frac{R_4}{R_3}\right)$$

↓   4.23

$$V_o = V_{id} \frac{2 R_4 (R_1 + R_2)}{R_3 R_1}$$

Thus, $A_D = 2R_4(R_1 + R_2)/(R_3 R_1)$ for this op amp IA circuit. In practice, the op amps are not ideal, they have finite $CMRR_A$s, and the resistors will not be perfectly matched, so the IA will have a finite $CMRR_{sys}$. To maximize the $CMRR_{sys}$, it is possible to deliberately introduce a small amount of asymmetry into the circuit, e.g., by making R_1' variable around the fixed R_1 value.

Another IA architecture uses only two op amps and matched resistors. The circuit is shown in Figure 4.10. To analyze this circuit, we will use superposition. First, we let $V_i' > 0$ and $V_i = 0$. By the ideal op amp assumption, $V_2 = V_i'$ and $V_3 = 0$. Node equations are written for the V_2 and V_3 nodes:

$$V_2(2G + G_F) - V_4G - V_3G_F = 0 \qquad\qquad 4.24A$$

$$V_3(2G + G_F) - V_4G - V_2G_F - V_oG = 0 \qquad\qquad 4.24B$$

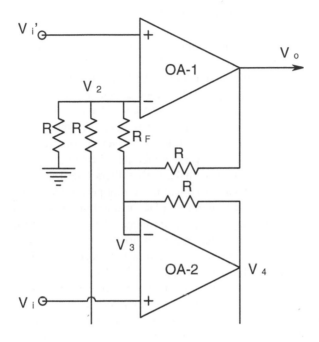

FIGURE 4.10 A two-op amp IA circuit. Resistors, R, must be accurately matched.

From the ideal op amp assumptions,

$$V_i'(2G + G_F) - V_4G = 0 \qquad 4.25$$

$$- V_4G - V_i'G_F - V_oG = 0$$

$$\downarrow$$

$$-V_i'(2G + G_F) - V_i'G_F = V_oG$$

$$\downarrow$$

$$V_o = - V_i'2(1 + R/R_F) \qquad 4.26$$

Next, we let $V_i > 0$ and set $V_i' = 0$. Thus by the ideal op amp assumption, $V_3 = V_i$ and $V_2 = 0$. Again, we write the node equations for the V_2 and V_3 nodes and solve for V_o:

$$V_o = + V_i\,2(1 + R/R_F) \qquad 4.27$$

By superposition we can finally write:

$$V_o = (V_i - V_i') \, 2(1 + R/R_F) = V_{id} \, 4(1 + R/R_F) \qquad\qquad 4.28$$

Thus $A_D = 4(1 + R/R_F)$, with a minimum of 4, and due to resistor matching and ideal op amps, $A_C = 0$.

One advantage of using op amps to make IAs is that the final cost is generally lower than a commercial single-chip IA. Another benefit is that some very low-noise op amps are available, so that the op amp IA can often be designed to have a better output signal-to-noise ratio (SNR) than a commercial counterpart. A disadvantage is that, in addition to two or three op amps, five to seven discrete resistors are needed (usually one or two are needed for a commercial IC IA to set the gain).

Op amps can also be used to make active filters (AFs) to improve the output SNR of recorded biopotentials. A typical noise root power density spectrum (PDS), such as might be found at the output of a DC bioamplifier, is shown in Figure 4.11; note that at low frequencies, the spectrum has an 1/f component that is present in all amplifiers at low frequencies, and often arises with the signal because of ion reactions at electrode wet interfaces. The root PDS also has spikes from coherent interference from power lines at 60 and 120 Hz. The center part of the root PDS remains flat to frequencies well-above the normal biomedical range. Thus because a biopotential signal has a root PDS that lies within the noise root PDS, the output SNR can be improved by passing only the signal spectral bandwidth, excluding high- and low-frequency noise, where applicable. Thus the amplified biopotential signal plus noise can be band-pass or low-pass filtered by op amp active filters, and notch AFs can be used to remove coherent interference. The spikes shown in Figure 4.11 are from coherent interference (e.g., 60- and 120-Hz power line fields).

4.3.5 Noise and Low Noise Amplifiers

An unfortunate property of all electronic amplifiers is that they introduce noise into the amplified signal. This noise provides a fundamental limitation to the resolution of very small signals, as determined by the SNR at the amplifier's output. In this section, we will examine how amplifier noise can be described, and how SNR at the amplifier's output can be maximized. First, let us make a distinction between *noise* and *interference,* both of which degrade output SNR. Interference is generally *coherent,* i.e., periodic in nature, and usually comes from some man-made source such as power lines, fluorescent lights, or automobile ignitions. Noise, as we define it, is completely random; it is the result of the random motion of many, many electrons in resistors and semiconductor devices (diodes, BJTs, and FETs). The descriptor of noise that we will use in this section is the *one-sided power density spectrum* (PDS). The significance of a PDS can be interpreted heuristically by referring to Figure 4.12. A random noise voltage source, $e_N(t)$, is connected to an *ideal low-pass filter* whose cut-off frequency, f_c, is variable between 0 and ∞. A broad-band, true rms voltmeter is connected to the filter output. We slowly increase the filter's cutoff frequency from zero and plot the squared meter reading vs. the cut-off frequency. Figure 4.13 shows the plot of the cumulative mean-squared volts vs. f_c. Note that this

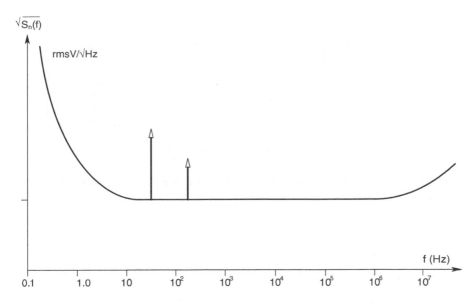

FIGURE 4.11 A typical noise voltage root power density spectrum seen at the output of a high-gain amplifier. The root spectrum's units are rms Volts /√Hz.

plot is not the PDS. To find the PDS, we must find the slope of the cumulative msV plot. That is,

$$S_n(f) = \frac{d\ v_{on}^2(f)}{df} \quad \begin{array}{l} \text{mean squared volts / Hz} \\ f_c \to f \end{array} \qquad 4.29$$

$S_n(f)$ is the one-sided PDS of the noise source; it is nonnegative. The *root PDS* is simply $\sqrt{S_n(f)}$.

Electrical engineers like to work with idealized components, amplifiers, voltage sources, etc. Noise is no exception. One idealized noise source makes *white noise*. A white noise PDS is constant over $0 \le f \le \infty$. That is, its PDS is $S_{Wn}(f) = \eta$ msV/Hz. An 1/f noise PDS is of the form: $S_{n/f}(f) = b/f$ msV/Hz. When a real noise PDS has a long, flat region, we say it is "white" in that range. White and 1/f PDSs can be added together to form a composite PDS. Note that superposition of noise PDSs can only be done using mean-squared quantities. It is not technically correct to add root spectra; the PDSs must be added, then the square root taken to get the combined root PDS. A large source of noise in circuits is from resistors (capacitors and ideal inductors do not make noise, although they can contribute to the shaping of a PDS). Resistors make white, *thermal* (or Johnson) noise; statistical thermodynamics tells us that the PDS for a resistor's thermal noise is given by:

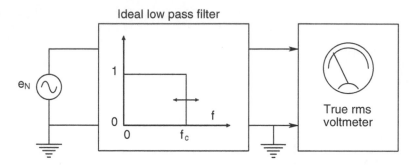

FIGURE 4.12 Basic set-up for measuring the one-sided mean-squared power density spectrum of a noise source.

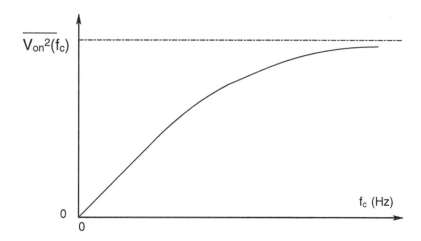

FIGURE 4.13 A representative plot of the cumulative mean squared noise voltage obtained with the circuit of Figure 4.12 as f_c is increased from zero.

$$S_{Rn}(f) = 4kTR \; msV/Hz \qquad\qquad 4.30$$

Where k is Boltzmann's constant (1.38×10^{-23} joule/°K), T is the Kelvin temperature, and R is the resistor value in ohms. (At VHF, resistor lead inductance and shunt capacitance cause the real thermal noise spectrum from a resistor to drop off to zero.) If two resistors are in series at different temperatures, the total PDS across them is: $S_{Rn}(f) = 4k(T_1R_1 + T_2R_2) \; msV/Hz$. If the two resistors are in parallel, the PDS is:

$$S_{Rn}(f) = 4kT_1R_1[R_2/(R_1 + R_2)]^2 + 4kT_2R_2[R_1/(R_1 + R_2)]^2 \; msV/Hz \qquad 4.31$$

See Figure 4.14 for a summary of how thermal noises from resistors combine. Note that when an average or dc current, I, passes through a resistor, it also emits 1/f noise in addition to its thermal noise. That is:

$$S_{Rn}(f) = 4kTR + A\ I^2/f \text{ msv/Hz} \qquad 4.32$$

Certain resistor materials have lower As than others. Wire-wound resistors have a lower A coefficient than do carbon composition resistors.

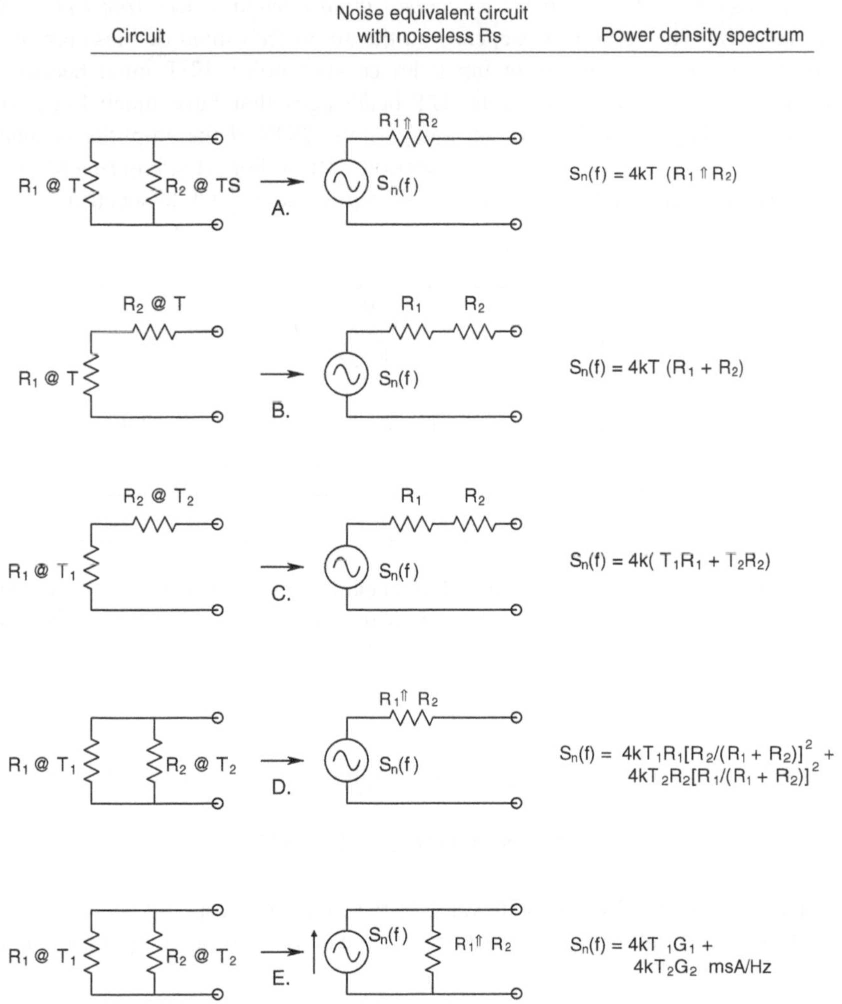

FIGURE 4.14 Five examples of how the thermal noise power spectrums from pairs of resistors combine. In the Thevenin equivalent circuits, the resistors are noiseless.

   The bad news is that every resistor, transistor and diode in IC op amps, DAs, and IAs makes noise. As you will see, the good news is that components in the first stage (input, or headstage) of an amplifier are mostly responsible for the overall amplifier's output noise. The total output noise of an amplifier is always referred to its input terminals with the *two-noise-source model* (Figure 4.15), e_{na} is really $e_{na}(f)$, e_{na} is the *equivalent short-circuited input noise root power density spectrum* and $e_{na}(f)$ has the units of $rmsV/\sqrt{Hz}$. A typical $e_{na}(f)$ plot is shown in Figure 4.16. Note that it has an 1/f region and a white region, and increases again at high-frequencies. e_{na} accounts for the amplifier's output noise when its input is short-circuited; when open circuited, two other sources must be considered — the thermal noise from the input resistance, R_1 @ T, and the *equivalent input current source root PDS*, $i_{na}(f)$, in $rmsA/\sqrt{Hz}$. The value of i_{na} depends on the amplifier's input dc bias current, I_B, because most of i_{na} comes from input device shot noise. FET input headstages generally have very low i_{na}s, while BJT headstages that have much larger bias currents have larger i_{na}s. The output voltage noise PDS of the amplifier is shaped by the amplifier's frequency response function, $H(j\omega)$. For an *open-circuited input* amplifier, the PDS at the V_i node can be written (assuming white spectra):

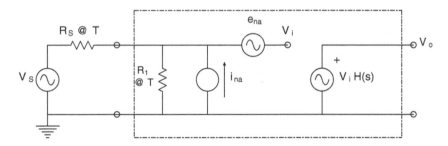

FIGURE 4.15 The two-source noise model for amplifiers and transistors. $e_{na}(f)$ is the equivalent input short-circuit voltage noise, root power spectrum in $rmsV/\sqrt{Hz}$. $i_{na}(f)$ is the equivalent input noise current root power spectrum in $rmsA/\sqrt{Hz}$.

$$S_{Vin}(f) = e_{na}^2 + 4kTR_1 + i_{na}^2\, R_1^2 \quad msV/Hz \qquad\qquad 4.33$$

It can be shown that the noise PDS at the amplifiers output is (Papoulis, 1965):

$$S_{Von}(f) = S_{Vin}(f)\,|\,H(j2\pi f)\,|^2 \quad msV/Hz \qquad\qquad 4.34$$

Note that the square of the absolute value of the frequency response vector, $H(j2\pi f)$, is used. Now the total mean-squared noise voltage at the amplifier output is found by:

$$\overline{v_{on}^2} = \int_0^\infty \left[e_{na}^2 + 4kTR_1 + i_{na}^2 R_1^2 \right] \left| H(j2\pi f) \right|^2 df \quad msV \qquad\qquad 4.35$$

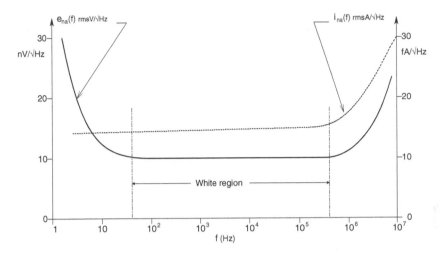

FIGURE 4.16 Plots of $e_{na}(f)$ and $i_{na}(f)$ for a typical FET input amplifier. Note that in the mid-band range of frequencies, e_{na} and i_{na} can be considered to be "white." Amplifiers having BJT headstages typically have a lower e_{na} and a larger i_{na}; also, i_{na} has a $1/\sqrt{f}$ component at low frequencies not seen in FET input amplifiers.

That is, the output noise PDS is integrated with respect to Hz frequency from 0 to ∞. If we include the amplifier's input capacitance in parallel with R_1, a low-pass filter is formed for the thermal noise current from R_1, and from i_{na}. The output PDS is then:

$$S_{Von}(f) = e_{na}^2 \left|H(j2\pi f)\right|^2 + \left[i_{na}^2 + 4kTG_1\right]\frac{R_1^2}{\left|1 + j2\pi fC_1 R_1\right|^2}\left|H(j2\pi f)\right|^2 \qquad 4.36$$

Note that the low-pass filter's frequency response magnitude squared must be included as a factor for the noise currents with the amplifier's frequency response magnitude squared. The integral of $S_{Von}(f)$ over $0 \le f \le \infty$ gives the total output ms noise voltage for this open-circuited model. When the amplifier is connected to a Thevenin signal source, as shown in Figure 4.15, R_s is in parallel with R_1. We can generally assume that $R_1 \gg R_s$, so R_1 can be set equal to ∞ (an open circuit), and we can neglect C_1. We also assume that e_{na} and i_{na} are white to simplify calculations. The ms output noise is then given by:

$$\overline{v_{on}^2} = \left[e_{na}^2 + 4kTR_s + i_{na}^2 R_s^2\right]\int_0^\infty \left|H(j2\pi f)\right|^2 df \quad \text{msv} \qquad 4.37$$

The integral in Equation 4.37 is called the *gain² noise bandwidth* (G²BW) function of the frequency response function. It can be expressed, in general, as $K_v^2 B$, where

K_v is the amplifier's low frequency gain if it is a DC amplifier, or the amplifier's midband gain if it is an RC (ac) amplifier. B is the *equivalent noise bandwidth* in Hz. A table of K_v^2 B functions for common amplifier transfer functions can be found in Northrop, 1997. A simple band-pass amplifier, such as used for ECG recording, has a frequency response that can be modeled by:

$$H(j2\pi f) = \frac{K_v\, 2\pi f \tau_L}{(1 + j2\pi f \tau_L)(1 + j2\pi f \tau_H)} \qquad 4.38$$

The G^2BW function for this amplifier can be shown to be:

$$G^2BW = K_v^2 \left[\frac{1}{4\tau_H(1 + \tau_H/\tau_L)} \right] \qquad 4.39$$

The term in brackets is the *noise bandwidth*, B, in Hz. K_v^2 is the midband gain squared, τ_L is the time constant of the low-frequency pole, and τ_H is the time constant of the high-frequency pole, in seconds.

Now let a *sinusoidal signal* of V_s peak volts be applied to the amplifier [$v_s(t) = V_s \sin(2\pi f_s t)$]. Assume its frequency, f_s, is in the mid-frequency or passband range of $H(j2\pi f)$, so it gets multiplied by the midband gain, K_v. Thus the *mean-squared output signal* is simply:

$$\overline{V_{os}^2} = (V_s^2/2)K_v^2 \quad msV \qquad 4.40$$

The *mean-squared output SNR* is then:

$$SNR_o = \frac{(V_s^2/2)K_v^2}{\left[e_{na}^2 + 4kTR_s + i_{na}^2 R_s^2\right]K_v^2 B} \qquad 4.41$$

Examining Equation 4.41, we see that decreasing the noise bandwidth, B, around the frequency of the signal, f_s, raises the SNR_o. A noise figure of merit for an amplifier is its *noise factor*, defined as:

$$F \equiv \frac{SNR_{in}}{SNR_o} \qquad 4.42$$

Its *noise figure* is given in dB:

$$NF \equiv 10\, \log_{10}(F) \qquad 4.43$$

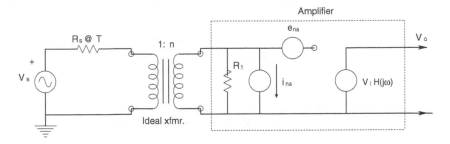

FIGURE 4.17 Equivalent circuit for an amplifier using an (ideal) transformer to maximize its output SNR ratio at the same time it minimizes its noise figure. The transformer's turns ratio, n, is varied to maximize the SNR_{out}.

For the case of the sinusoidal input at f_s, the output SNR is given by Equation 4.41. The input mean-squared SNR is defined as:

$$SNR_{in} \equiv \frac{\left(V_s^2/2\right)}{4kTR_s B} \qquad\qquad 4.44$$

In this case, the only noise assumed to accompany the signal is the thermal white noise from its Thevenin resistor, R_s. This noise must be given the noise bandwidth of the amplifier, B. Using the definition for noise factor, we find the well-known result (Northrop, 1997):

$$F = 1 + \frac{e_{na}^2 + i_{na}^2 R_s^2}{4kTR_s} \qquad\qquad 4.45$$

Manufacturers of low noise amplifiers typically specify an NF in dB. Along with this number, the R_s, B, and T must also be given. An ideal noiseless amplifier has $F = 1$. The larger F is, the poorer the noise performance of the amplifier. The bottom line in designing signal conditioning systems, however, is not the minimization of amplifier F, but the maximization of amplifier SNR_o. One way SNR_o can be maximized for ac (bandpass) signals is through the use of a precision impedance-matching transformer to couple the Thevenin circuit of the source to the amplifier. The transformer circuit is shown schematically in Figure 4.17. The mean squared signal at the output is:

$$S_o = \overline{v_s^2}\, n^2\, K_v^2 \quad msV \qquad\qquad 4.46$$

Note that the open-circuit source voltage is multiplied by the turns ratio, n, of the transformer on the amplifier side. The mean squared noise at the output is given by (Northrop, 1997):

$$N_o = \left[e_{na}^2 + i_{na}^2 \left(n^2 R_s \right)^2 + n^2 4kTR_s \right] K_v^2 B \quad msV \qquad 4.47$$

Note that the resistance i_{na} "sees" looking back into the transformer can be shown to be $n^2 R_s$. Thus the msSNR$_o$ of the circuit is:

$$SNR_o = \frac{\overline{v_s^2} n^2 K_v^2}{\left[e_{na}^2 + i_{na}^2 \left(n^2 R_s \right)^2 + n^2 4kTR_s \right] K_v^2 B} \qquad 4.48$$

$\downarrow$

$$SNR_o = \frac{\overline{v_s^2}}{\left[e_{na}^2 / n^2 + i_{na}^2 n^2 R_s^2 + 4kTR_s \right] B} \qquad 4.49$$

SNR$_o$ clearly has a *maximum* when its denominator has a *minimum*. When the denominator is differentiated with respect to n^2 and set equal to zero, we find that maximum SNR$_o$ occurs when the transformer turns ratio is:

$$n = n_o = \sqrt{e_{na} / \left(i_{na} R_s \right)} \qquad 4.50$$

The maximum SNR$_o$ is:

$$SNR_{o\,max} = \frac{\overline{v_s^2} / B}{4kTR_s + 2e_{na} i_{na} R_s} \qquad 4.51$$

Because real transformers are noisy (their windings have resistance that makes thermal noise, and their magnetic cores make Barkhausen noise), the actual SNR$_o$ never reaches the value given by Equation 4.51. In practice, transformer maximization of SNR$_o$ is justifiable only if (Northrop, 1997):

$$[e_{na}/(i_{na} R_s) + i_{na} R_s/e_{na}] > 20 \qquad 4.52$$

In all the developments above, we have assumed that both e_{na} and i_{na} are white, i.e., they have the values seen in the flat range of their plots vs. frequency. For example, if an Analog Devices' AD6251 IA is used, $e_{na} = 4 \text{ nV}/\sqrt{Hz}$ in the white region, and $i_{na} = 0.3 \text{ pArms}/\sqrt{Hz}$. Let the $R_s = 5,000$ ohms. Thus $[4 \times 10^{-9}/(3 \times 10^{-13} \times 5 \times 10^3) + (3 \times 10^{-13} \times 5 \times 10^3)/4 \times 10^{-9}] = 3.042 < 20$, and the use of a transformer would not be practical. Note that $e_{na}/i_{na} = 13.3 \text{ k}\Omega$ for this amplifier. Now let us use an FET input IA, the Burr-Brown INA1102, which has $e_{na} = 10 \text{ nVrms}/\sqrt{Hz}$ and $i_{na} = 1.8 \text{ fArms}/\sqrt{Hz}$. Again, let $R_s = 5 \text{ k}\Omega$. Thus $[1 \times 10^{-8}/(1.8 \times 10^{-15} \times 5 \times 10^3) + (1.8 \times 10^{-15} \times 5 \times 10^3)/1 \times 10^{-8}] = 1.11 \times 10^3 >> 20$, and the use of a transformer is justified. Its turns ratio should be: $n_o = \sqrt{1 \times 10^{-8}/(1.8 \times 10^{-15} \times 5 \times 10^3)} = 33.3$. $e_{na}/i_{na} = 5.56 \times 10^6\ \Omega$. It should be stressed that low-noise impedance-matching transformers are expensive, and their low-frequency −3 dB frequencies are ca. 3 Hz, limiting their usefulness for certain low-frequency bioelectric signal conditioning. When a high-gain amplifier is designed with two or more separate cascaded noisy amplifier stages, (Figure 4.18), the output ms SNR can be found. Assuming scalar gains, we have:

$$SNR_o = \frac{\overline{v_s^2}K_{v1}^2 K_{v2}^2 K_{v3}^2}{\left[\left(4kTR_s + e_{na1}^2 + i_{na1}^2 R_s^2\right)K_{v1}^2 K_{v2}^2 K_{v3}^2 + e_{na2}^2 K_{v2}^2 K_{v3}^2 + e_{na3}^2 K_{v3}^2\right]B} \qquad 4.53$$

Dividing by the overall gain gives us an instructive expression for the SNR_o:

$$SNR_o = \frac{\overline{v_s^2}/B}{\left(4kTR_s + e_{na1}^2 + i_{na1}^2 R_s^2\right) + e_{na2}^2/K_{v1}^2 + e_{na3}^2/\left(K_{v1}^2 K_{v2}^2\right)} \qquad 4.54$$

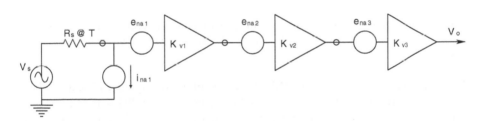

FIGURE 4.18 Three cascaded noisy stages are used to make a high-gain amplifier. The stage with the lowest e_{na} should be the headstage.

Thus, as long as $K_{V1} > 5$, the SNR_o of the amplifier cascade is approximately that of the headstage alone. That is, the headstage sets the noise performance of the cascaded amplifier. If, for some reason, a unity gain buffer stage is used as the headstage, the e_{na} of the second stage also becomes significant, and both it and the headstage must be chosen for low e_{na}s. As an example of calculating the output SNR of an amplifier, consider the non-inverting op amp shown in Figure 4.19. The mean squared output signal is:

$$S_o = \overline{v_s^2}\left(1 + R_2/R_1\right)^2 \quad msV \qquad 4.55$$

The ms output noise is:

$$N_o = B\left[\left(4kTR_s + e_{na}^2 + i_{na}^2 R_s^2\right)\left(1 + R_2/R_1\right)^2 + 4kTR_1\left(R_2/R_1\right)^2 + 4kTG_2 R_2^2\right] \qquad 4.56$$

Putting these expressions together and doing some algebra, we find:

$$SNR_o = \frac{\overline{v_s^2}/B}{4kTR_s + e_{na}^2 + i_{na}^2 R_a^2 + 4kT\,R_1 R_2/(R_1 + R_2)}$$ 4.57

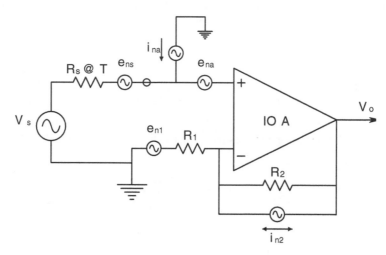

FIGURE 4.19 Non-inverting op amp amplifier showing the five noise sources contributing to the output noise. The resistors R_s, R_1 and R_2 all contribute white Johnson noise to the net ms input noise.

The expression is similar to the SNR_o for the amplifier of Figure 4.15, except there is an extra term derived from the thermal noise in R_1 in parallel with R_2. For high gain, we make $R_2 \gg R_1$, however, low absolute values should be used so $R_1 R_2/(R_1 + R_2)$ will be small. As we have seen, differential amplifiers have two active inputs, and thus can be assigned an independent i_{na} and e_{na} for both inputs. While two sources at each input are technically correct, it is more expedient to use only one equivalent e_{na} and i_{na} *at one input*. These are the parameters that manufacturers, in fact, give us in IA specs. Because, in general, the amplifier's $|A_D| \gg |A_C|$ in the operating range of interest, we can neglect the CM noise components resulting from using single sources at either the + or − inputs. Inspection of Figure 4.20 allows us to write an expression for the ms signal output,

$$S_o = \overline{v_{sd}^2} A_D^2$$ 4.58

given pure DM signal in. That is, $v_s' = -v_s$. The ms noise output is found from finding the mean squared value of $v_{id} = (v_i - v_i')/2$ for the noise voltages.

$$\overline{v_{id}^2} = \tfrac{1}{4}\left[\overline{v_i^2} - \overline{2v_i v_i'} + \overline{v_i'^2}\right] \rightarrow \tfrac{1}{4}\left[\overline{v_i^2} + \overline{v_i'^2}\right]$$ 4.59

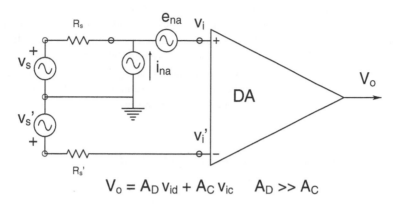

$$V_o = A_D V_{id} + A_C V_{ic} \qquad A_D \gg A_C$$

FIGURE 4.20 A differential amplifier's noise can be approximated as coming from only one input.

The mean cross-term $\rightarrow 0$ because the thermal noise sources from R_s and $R_s{}'$ are uncorrelated. $\overline{v_i{}'^2} = 4kTR_s{}'B$, and $\overline{v_i^2} = (e_{na}^2 + 4kTR_s + i_{na}^2 R_s^2) B$. Assuming that $R_s = R_s{}'$, the total mean-squared noise voltage at the output is:

$$N_o = A_D^2 B \left[e_{na}^2 + 8kTR_s + i_{na}^2 R_s^2 \right] / 4 \qquad 4.60$$

And the DA's ms output SNR is:

$$SNR_o = \frac{\overline{v_{sd}^2}(4/B)}{\left[e_{na}^2 + 8kTR_s + i_{na}^2 R_s^2 \right]} \qquad 4.61$$

The 4 factor in the numerator comes from the definition of v_{id}. As a numerical example, let us calculate the rms v_{sd} required to give an ms $SNR_o = 9$ (the same as an rms $SNR_o = 3$). Assume the noise sources are white and the noise bandwidth is 400 Hz, also, $e_{na} = 4$ nVrms/$\sqrt{Hz}$, $i_{na} = 0.3$ pArms/$\sqrt{Hz}$, $R_s = R_s{}' = 4{,}000 \ \Omega$, and $T = 300$ K.

$$9 = \frac{\overline{v_{sd}^2}(4/400)}{\left[1.6 \times 10^{-17} + 8 \times 1.38 \times 10^{-23} \times 300 \times 4 \times 10^3 + 9 \times 10^{-26} \times 1.6 \times 10^7 \right]} \qquad 4.62$$

$$\downarrow \qquad\qquad\qquad\qquad\qquad \downarrow$$

$$1.3248 \times 10^{-16} \qquad\qquad\qquad 1.44 \times 10^{-18}$$

$$\left[1.499 \times 10^{-16} \right]$$

Solving for $\sqrt{\overline{v_{sd}^2}}$, we find that an rms, DM input of 0.3673 µV will give an rms $SNR_o = 3$. In practice, this voltage may be significantly higher because $e_{na}(f)$ and $i_{na}(f)$ will have 1/f spectral components in the low end of the signal's bandpass region. We ignored the 1/f problem in this example for mathematical simplicity. To examine how the 1/f spectrum of e_{na} should be treated, let us return to the example illustrated above in Figure 4.19. We will assume that $e_{na}^2(f) = b/f + e_{naw}^2$; i_{na} and all resistor noises will be assumed to be white. The noise bandwidth, B, will be defined over the interval, $\{f_L, f_H\}$, i.e., $B = f_H - f_L$. Thus the output ms noise is:

$$N_o = \int_{f_L}^{f_H} \left[\left(b/f + e_{naw}^2 + 4kTR_s + i_{na}^2 R_s^2 \right)\left(1 + R_2/R_1\right)^2 \right.$$

$$\left. + 4kTR_1\left(R_2/R_1\right)^2 + 4kTG_2R_2^2 \right] df$$

$$\downarrow \hspace{9cm} 4.63$$

$$N_o = \left(1 + R_2/R_1\right)^2 \left\{ b\ln\left(f_H/f_L\right) + \left[e_{naw}^2 + 4kTR_s + i_{na}^2 R_s^2\right]\left(f_H - f_L\right) \right\}$$

$$+ \left[4kTR_1\left(R_2/R_1\right)^2 + 4kTR_2\right]\left(f_H - f_L\right)$$

The ms output SNR is then:

$$SNR_o = \frac{\overline{v_s^2}/B}{(b/B)\ln\left(f_H/f_L\right) + e_{naw}^2 + 4kTR_s + i_{na}^2 R_s^2 + 4kT\,R_1R_2/\left(R_1 + R_2\right)} \hspace{1cm} 4.64$$

The first term in the denominator above is the extra ms noise from the 1/f part of the e_{na}^2 spectrum. Good resolution of threshold low-frequency bioelectric signals requires the use of amplifiers with low e_{na}^2 1/f noise; not only should the parameter b be small (b has the units of ms volts), but the white component of e_{na}^2 should be small as well.

A low-noise amplifier is one that has $e_{na} < 10$ nV/$\sqrt{Hz}$ in its white region. The best low- noise amplifiers use BJT headstages in which the transistor biasing can be optimized to give the least e_{na}. In some low-noise BJT-input amplifiers, such as the LT1028 op amp, $e_{na} = 1$ nVrms/$\sqrt{Hz}$ @ 10 Hz, and 0.85 nVrms/$\sqrt{Hz}$ @ 10 Hz, and $i_{na} = 4.7$ pArms/$\sqrt{Hz}$ @ 1 Hz, and 1.0 pArms/$\sqrt{Hz}$ @ 10 Hz. The input impedance of the LT1028 is 20 MΩ (DM) and 300 MΩ (CM) and its input bias current is $I_B = 25$ nA. (Most JFET-input amplifiers have I_Bs on the order of pico amps, and corresponding i_{na}s on the order of fArms/$\sqrt{Hz}$. JFET op amps also have R_{in}s on the order of 10^{13} to 10^{14} ohms. A short table of properties of low-noise amplifiers (op amps, IAs and isolation amps) can be found in Northrop (1997).

4.3.6 MEDICAL ISOLATION AMPLIFIERS

All amplifiers used to record biopotential signals from humans must meet certain standards for worst-case voltage breakdown and maximum leakage currents through their input leads, which are attached to electrodes on the body, and maximum current through any driven output lead attached to the body. A variety of testing conditions or scenarios to ensure patient safety have been formulated by various regulatory agencies. The conservative leakage current and voltage breakdown criteria set by the National Fire Protection Association (NFPA) (Quincy, Massachusetts), and the Association for the Advancement of Medical Instrumentation (AAMI) have generally been adopted by medical equipment manufacturers and by hospitals and other health care facilities in the United States. A number of other regulatory agencies are also involved in formulating and adopting electrical medical safety standards: The International Electrotechnical Commission (ITC), the Underwriters Laboratories (UL), the Health Industries Manufacturers'Association (HEMA), the National Electrical Manufacturers'Association (NEMA) and the U.S. Food and Drug Administration (FDA). Most of the standards have been adopted to prevent possible patient electrocution — burns, the induction of fibrillation in the heart, muscle spasms, etc.

Space does not permit us to go into the effects of electroshock, and the many scenarios through which it can occur. Nor can we explore the technology of safe grounding practices and ground fault interruption. The interested reader should consult Chaper14 in Webster (1992) for these details.

If the threshold ac surface current required to induce cardiac fibrillation in 50% of dogs tested is plotted vs. frequency, it is seen that the least current is required between 40 to 100 Hz. From 80 to 600 µA rms of 60 Hz current will induce cardiac fibrillation when applied directly to the heart, as through a catheter (Webster, 1992). Thus the NFPA-ANSI/AAMI standard for ECG amplifier lead leakage is that *isolated* input lead current (at 60 Hz) must be < 10 µA between any two leads shorted together, < 10 µA for any input lead connected to the power plug ground (green wire) with and without the amplifier's case grounded. A more severe test is that isolation amplifier input lead leakage current must be < 20 µA when any input lead is connected to the high side of the 120 Vac mains. To meet these severe tests for leakage, the *medical isolation amplifier* has evolved.

Isolation is accomplished by electrically separating the input stage of the isolation amplifier (IA) from the output stage. That is, the input stage has a separate floating power supply and a "ground" that are connected to the output side of the IA by a resistance of more than 1000 megohms, and a parallel capacitance in the low picofarad range. The signal output of the input stage is also isolated from the IA's output by a similar very high impedance, although the Thevenin output resistance of the IA can range from milliohms to several hundred ohms.

Three major means effect the Galvanic isolation of the input and output stages of IAs:

1. Use a high-quality, toroidal transformer to magnetically couple regulated ac power from the output side to the isolated input stage where it is

rectified and filtered, and also is coupled to rectifiers and filters serving the output amplifiers. Frequencies in the range of 100 kHz to 750 kHz are typically used with transformer isolation IAs. The output signal from the isolated headstage modulates an ac carrier that is magnetically coupled to a demodulator on the output side.

2. Use photooptic coupling of the amplified signal; usually pulse-width or delta-sigma modulation of the optical signal is used, although direct linear analog photooptic coupling can be used. In optical type of IA, a separate isolated dc/dc converter must be used to power the input stage.

3. Use a pair of small (e.g., 1 pF) capacitors to couple a pulse-modulated signal from the isolated input to the output stage. A separate, isolated power supply must be used with the differential capacitor-coupled IA, too.

Table 4.3.6.1 lists some of the critical specifications of three types of medical-grade IAs.

TABLE 4.3.6.1
Comparison of Properties of Some Popular Isolation Amplifiers

Amplifier Iso. type Manufacturer	290A Transformer Intronics	BB3656 Transformer Burr-Brown	BB3652 Optical Burr-Brown	BB ISO121 Capacitor Burr-Brown	ISO-Z Transformer? Dataq
CMV isolation	±1500V continuous	±3500 continuous ±8000, 10 sec.	±2000 continuous ±5000, 10 sec	3500 rms	1500 V continuous 5000 V, 10 sec
CMRR @ 60 Hz	> 100 dB @ 60 Hz	108 dB	80 dB @ 60 Hz	115 dB IMR @ 60 Hz	> 100 dB @ 60 Hz
Gain range	1 – 100	1 – 100	1 to >100, by formula	1 V/V (fixed)	10 (fixed)
Leakage to 120 Vac mains	?	0.5 μA	0.5 μA 1.8 pF leakage capacitance	$I_{ac} = V2\pi fC$ $C \cong 2.21$ pF	< 5 μA, any input to ground
Noise	1 μV pkpk @ $K_v = 100$, 10 Hz BW	5 μV pkpk 0.05 – 100 Hz BW	8 μV pkpk 0.05 – 100 Hz BW	4 μVrms/ √Hz	< 4 μVrms, referred to input, "wideband"
Bandwidth	0 – 2 kHz	0 – 30 kHz, ± 3 dB	0 – 15 kHz, ± 3 dB	0 – 60 kHz (c. 200 kHz clock)	0 – 8 kHz
Slewrate	?	+0.1, –0.04 V/μs	1.2 V/μs	2 V/μs	?

The Burr-Brown, ISO121, differential capacitor-coupled IA is used with a separate, isolated clock to run its duty cycle-modulator. The clock frequency can be from 5 kHz to 700 kHz, giving commensurate bandwidths governed by the Nyquist criterion.

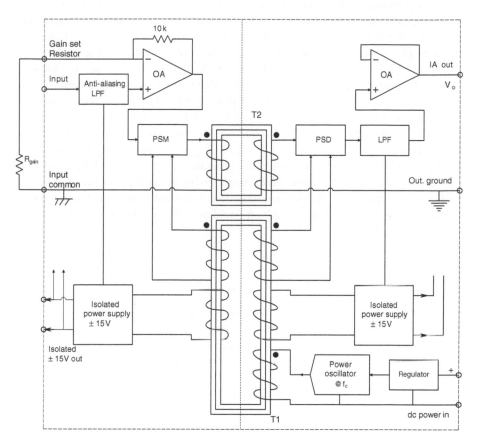

FIGURE 4.21 Simplified schematic circuit of an Analog Devices' magnetically coupled isolation amplifier (AD289). A transformer is used to couple power to the isolated headstage, and also to couple the isolated acquired signal back to the output.

A simplified schematic of an Analog Devices AD289 magnetically coupled IA is shown in Figure 4.21. Note that this IA has a single-ended input. The clock power oscillator drives a toroidal core, T1, on which are wound coils for the input and output isolated power supplies, and for the synchronizing signals for the double-sideband suppressed carrier (DSBSC) modulator and demodulator. A separate tor-oidal transformer, T2, couples the modulated output signal to the output side of the IA. This is basically the architecture used in the Intronics 290 and the Burr-Brown BB3656 IAs.

An unmodulated feedback-type analog optical isolation system is used in the Burr-Brown BB3652 differential optically coupled linear IA. This IA still requires a transformer-isolated power supply for the input headstage, and for the driver for the linear optocoupler. A feedback-type linear optocoupler, similar to that used in the BB3652, is shown in Figure 4.22. (In the B3652, OA1 is replaced with a high-input impedance DA headstage.) The circuit works in the following manner: The summing junction of OA2 is at 0 volts. DC bias current through R_{B1}, I_{B1}, drives the OA2 output negative, biasing the LED, D2, on at some I_{D20}. D2's light illuminates photodiodes D1 and D3 equally; the reverse photocurrent through D1 drives OA2's output positive, reducing I_{D2}. It thus provides a linearizing negative feedback around OA2, acting against the current produced by the input voltage, V_{in}/R_1. Because D1 and D3 are matched photodiodes, the reverse photocurrent in D3 equals that in D1, i.e., $I_{D10} = I_{D30}$, and $V_o = R_3 (I_{D30} - I_{B3})$. The bias current I_{B3} makes $V_o \to 0$ when $V_{in} = 0$. Now when $V_{in} > 0$, the input current, V_{in}/R_1, makes the LED D2 brighter, increasing $I_{D1} = I_{D3} > I_{D10} = I_{D30}$, increasing V_o. Thus $V_o = K_V V_{in}$. Note that analog opto-isolation eliminates the need for a high-frequency carrier, modulation, and demodulation, while giving a very high degree of Galvanic isolation. Unfortunately, the isolated headstage still must receive its power through a magnetically isolated power supply. It could use batteries, however, which would improve its isolation.

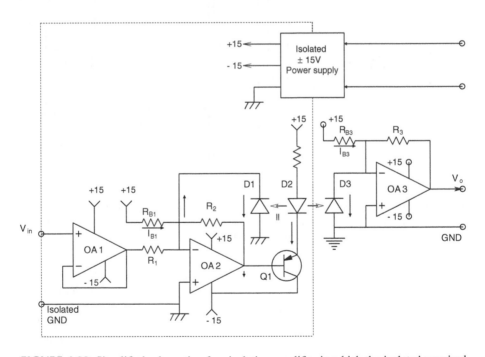

FIGURE 4.22 Simplified schematic of an isolation amplifier in which the isolated acquired signal is coupled to the output with a linearized, analog photocoupler. Power must be coupled to the headstage through an isolation transformer (not shown).

The third type of isolation uses high-frequency *duty-cycle modulation* to transmit the signal across the isolation barrier using a differential 1 pF capacitor coupling circuit. This type of IA also needs an isolated power supply for the input stages, the clock oscillator and the modulator. Figure 4.23 illustrates schematically a simplified version of how the Burr-Brown ISO121, capacitively isolated IA works. The signal

V_{in} is added to a high-frequency symmetrical triangle wave, V_T, with peak height, V_{pkT}. The sum of V_T and V_{in} is passed through a comparator that generates a variable-duty-cycle square wave, V_2. Note that the highest frequency in V_{in} is $\ll f_c$, the clock frequency, and $|V_{inmax}| < V_{pk}$. The state transitions in V_2 are coupled through the two 1 pF capacitors as spikes to a flip-flop on the output side of the IA. The flip-flop's transitions are triggered by the spikes. At the flip flop's output, $a \pm V_{3m}$ variable duty-cycle square wave, V_3, is then averaged by low-pass filtering to yield V_o.

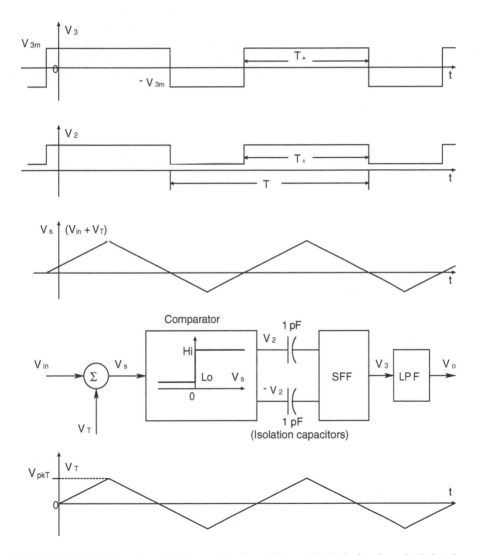

FIGURE 4.23 A duty cycle modulation system is used to couple the isolated acquired signal back to the output of the capacitively coupled IA. Power for the isolated headstage's subsytems (triangle wave generator, comparator, input preamplifier) must again be coupled to it by an isolation transformer.

The duty cycle of V_2 and V_3 can be shown to be:

$$\eta(V_{in}) \equiv T_+/T = (^1/_2 + V_{in}/2V_{pkT}), \; |V_{in}| < V_{pkT} \qquad 4.65$$

The average of the symmetrical flip-flop output is:

$$V_o = \overline{V_3} = V_{in}\left(V_{3m}/V_{pkT}\right) \qquad 4.66$$

Thus the output signal is proportional to V_{in}. The actual circuitry of the Burr-Brown ISO121 is more complex than described above, but the basic operating principle remains the same. Certified isolation amplifiers must be used in surgery and intensive-care hospital environments where cardiac catheters are used. While the scenarios for direct cardiac electroshock do not generally exist for outpatients, IAs are still used for ECG, EEG and EMG applications to limit liability in the unlikely event of an electroshock incident.

4.3.7 Driven-Leg ECG Amplifiers

In this section, we will examine the driven-leg ECG amplifier architecture and demonstrate that it acts to raise the overall ECG amplifier's common-mode rejection ratio (CMRR), making the ECG DA less sensitive to common-mode hum and interference. Figure 4.24 illustrates the schematic of a three-op amp DA connected as a Lead I ECG amplifier to the right and left arms. As we defined in Section 4.3.3, the ECG amplifier's output voltage can be written in terms of its difference-mode (DM) and common-mode (CM) gains and input signals.

$$V_o = v_{id} A_D + v_{ic} A_C \qquad 4.67$$

(We will use scalar gains and voltages to simplify the analysis.) The DM and CM input voltages are given as before:

$$v_{id} \equiv (v_i - v_i')/2, \; v_{ic} \equiv (v_i + v_i')/2 \qquad 4.68A \text{ and } B$$

When the input to the 3 op amp DA is *pure DM*, the current into the summing junction of OA-4 is zero, hence $v_5 = 0$. In the DA, we assume that $R_{in} \ggg R_S$, R_S' R_N and R_C. Also, the corresponding circuit resistors are matched ($R_S = R_S'$, etc.). Thus, any CM gain is the result of OA-3's finite CMRR. Consider first the two ECG input voltages, v_{LA} and v_{RA}, with v_{CN} and $v_5 = 0$. By definition, Lead I voltage, $v_I \equiv (v_{LA} - v_{RA})$, and

$$V_o = ((v_{LA} - v_{RA})/2)\, 2A_D + ((v_{LA} + v_{RA})/2)\, 2A_C$$

$$\downarrow$$

$$V_o = v_I A_D + ((v_{LA} + v_{RA})/2)\, 2A_C \qquad 4.69$$

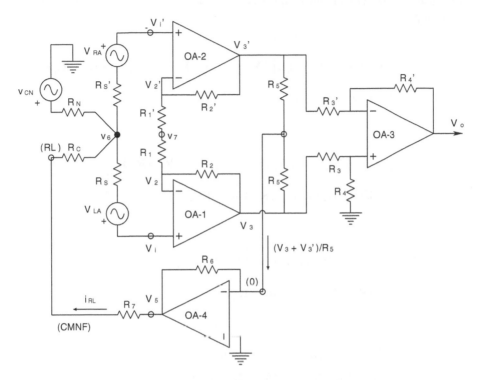

FIGURE 4.24 Simplified schematic of a driven-leg ECG amplifier similar to the system invented by Hewlett-Packard. Note that a three-op amp DA is used, from which it is easy to derive and amplify a common-mode signal between the two R_Ss. The amplified CM signal, V_5, injects a current into the v_6 common node. The net effect of the driven leg is to reduce output sensitivity to the CM noise, V_{CN}.

There is a small unwanted component of output voltage due to the input signal's CM component. If $v_{CN} \neq 0$, then there is a CM input component equal to v_{CN}. Thus V_o is now:

$$V_o = v_I A_D + [(v_{LA} + v_{RA})/2] 2A_C + v_{CN} A_C \qquad 4.70$$

With V_5 connected to the patient's right leg through resistor R_7, the ECG DA is given *common-mode negative feedback* (CMNF), which has the effect of raising the amplifier's CMRR (Northrop, 1990). The numerical CMRR of the DA without CMNF is simply $CMRR_{DA} = A_D/A_C$. The CMNF only affects the overall A_C, making it smaller; A_D is unchanged.

The current into OA-4's summing junction, which is effectively at ground potential, is simply $i_{4sj} = (V_3 + V_3')/R_5$. This same current flows through R_6, so by Ohm's law,

$$V_5 = -(V_3 + V_3')(R_6/R_5) \qquad 4.71$$

Because the DM DA output with CMNF is unchanged, we will examine only the CM output:

$$V_o = v_{ic}A_C = \left[(v_{LA} + v_{RA})/2\right]2A_C + v_{CN}A_C\left(R_C + R_7\right)/\left(R_C + R_7 + R_N\right)$$
$$+ V_5\, A_C R_N/\left(R_C + R_7 + R_N\right)$$

$\downarrow$

$$v_{ic}A_C = \left[v_{Ic}\right]2A_C + v_{CN}A_C\left(R_C + R_7\right)/\left(R_C + R_7 + R_N\right)$$
$$-\left(v_{ic}\right)2\left(R_6/R_5\right)A_C\, R_N/\left(R_C + R_7 + R_N\right)$$

$\downarrow$ 4.72

$$v_{ic}\left[1 + 2\left(R_6/R_5\right)R_N/\left(R_C + R_7 + R_N\right)\right] = \left[v_{Ic}\right]2$$
$$+ v_{CN}\left(R_C + R_7\right)/\left(R_C + R_7 + R_N\right)$$

$\downarrow$

$$v_{ic} = \frac{2\left[v_{Ic}\right] + v_{CN}\left(R_C + R_7\right)/\left(R_C + R_7 + R_N\right)}{\left[1 + 2\left(R_6/R_5\right)R_N/\left(R_C + R_7 + R_N\right)\right]}$$

The CMNF reduces not only the CM interference, but also the CM component of V_I. Clearly, we want to make $2(R_6/R_5)R_N/(R_C + R_7 + R_N) \gg 1$ to reduce the effective v_{ic}. To do this, (R_6/R_5) can be made $\gg 1$. We have little control of R_C, and no control of R_N.

For safety reasons, the current from OA-4 into or out of the right leg must not exceed 1 μA. In other words,

$$10^{-6}\,A \geq i_{cmf} = \frac{|V_5|}{\left(R_C + R_7\right)}$$ 4.73

Let us make $R_7 = 10^6\ \Omega$; then if we limit $|V_5| < (10^{-6}R_C + 1)$ volts, the $\pm$ 1 μA limit is met.

While the driven-leg ECG amplifier was an innovative solution to the problem of unwanted CM signals, its extra complexity is not generally warranted today. Modern ECG isolation amplifiers have CMRRs that are 140 to 160 dB. Such high inherent CMRRs are the result of laser trimming internal components during manufacturing to give component symmetry, which causes $A_C \to 0$. In some medical DA designs, CMNF is used internally in the circuit to reduce A_C.

4.3.8 Discussion

Biopotentials recorded noninvasively from the body surface have a range from single microvolts to more than 10 mV, depending on the source. Skeletal muscles and the heart are the stronger potential sources; the brain, the ECoG, ERG, and EOG have the weaker signals. For safety reasons, the amplifiers used clinically to record biopotentials are generally the isolation type. Many biopotential amplifiers are also RC-coupled differential amplifiers. They have low-noise, high-input impedance front ends and adjustable bandwidths to suit the signal being recorded and minimize output noise. Signals from the brain and heart generally require a high-frequency −3dB frequency of little more than 100 Hz; amplifiers used to condition EMG signals require more high-frequency bandwidth, generally ca. 5kHz at the most.

In this section, we have stressed the sources of amplifier noise and ways to calculate the output SNR for an amplifier system. Many EEG measurements have poor output SNR, and signal averaging must be used to recover an event-evoked brain potential. In the future, we can expect to see a continued slow improvement in low noise amplifier headstage noise. Twenty years ago, a "low-noise" amplifier's short-circuit input noise, $e_{na} = 12$ nV√Hz. Today, amplifiers are available with about one tenth that e_{na}, and better. It is often possible to design an IA from low-noise op amps that exceeds the noise specs of commercial units, and costs less as well.

4.4 THE ECG

4.4.1 Introduction

More than 150 years ago, the Italian physicist Carlo Matteucci showed that an electric current accompanies each heartbeat. The next year, in 1843, the German physiologist Emil Dubois-Reymond confirmed Matteucci's findings in frogs (Jenkins, 1997). A preparation was used called the "rheoscopic frog." Before the invention of the galvanometer to measure minute currents, the "action potentials" (a term invented by Dubois-Reymond) of muscles, including the heart, could be detected by placing a frog muscle on the contracting muscle and seeing it also contract with the stimulated muscle, or by placing a motor nerve innervating a frog muscle on an exposed heart ventricle, for example, and observing the muscle contract slightly in advance of the heart (Fye, 1998).

The first effective device that was used to measure the action potentials of the beating heart was the *mercury capillary electrometer*, invented by French physicist Gabriel Lippmann in 1872. A thin capillary tube was partially filled with mercury, with a layer of sulfuric acid above it. When the cardiac action potential was applied across the capillary column, the mercury column moved up and down with the potential. This displacement was so small that it had to be observed with a microscope. For the next 25 years or so, the capillary electrometer was the only means of measuring the ECG. In 1895, Dutch physiologist Willem Einthoven had refined the capillary electrometer and developed a correction formula to compensate for its poor frequency response so he could visualize the P, Q, R, S and T inflections seen in ECG waveforms recorded with modern instrumentation.

Einthoven went on to modify the *string galvanometer,* previously invented to receive telegraph signals in 1897 by French engineer Clement Ader. In 1901, Einthoven used his string galvanometer to measure the ECG. His first model had a huge heavy magnet, in the airgap of which ran a thin silk string under tension, made conductive by rubbing with powdered silver. The ends of the string were connected to two wires that led to two saline-filled jars in which the patient immersed either both hands, or a hand and a foot. Each wire was attached to a thick carbon electrode immersed in the jar to couple the ECG current to the galvanometer. The low impedance of the saline jar electrodes allowed a relatively large action current to flow through the galvanometer string. The solenoidal magnetic field surrounding the current-carrying string interacted with the linear magnetic field in the magnet's air gap, and the string experienced a differential force along its length given by the vector cross-product:

$$\mathbf{dF} = \mathbf{I}\ \mathbf{dl} \times \mathbf{B} \qquad\qquad 4.74$$

dF tries to force the string out of the airgap, as shown in Figure 4.25. A light beam is projected onto the string, which casts a shadow, the displacement of which is proportional to the galvanometer current. Note that a string under tension will tend to vibrate at a resonant frequency given by:

$$f_r = \frac{1}{2\,L}\sqrt{(s/\rho)} \quad \text{Hz} \qquad\qquad 4.75$$

Where L is the string length in meters, s is the stress on the string in Newton's/m², and ρ is the density of the string material in kg/m³. Evidently, Einthoven's string galvanometer's resonant frequency was high enough to not cause excessive artifacts on his recordings. Einthoven went on with his pioneering work to characterize heart pathologies from the *ECG Leads I, II,* and *III.* He was a pioneer in this area of noninvasive diagnosis, for which he earned the 1923 Nobel Prize in medicine. A picture and description of an Einthoven string galvanometer made by The Cambridge and Paul Instrument Co., Ltd., in the collection of the University of Toronto Museum of Science (UTMuSci) can be found at its URL (www.chass.utoronto.ca/cgi-bin/ utmusi/displayrec?/num=psy221). This particular galvanometer used a huge electromagnet. Its deflection sensitivity was 1 mm/10^{-7} A, and its period was ca. 0.005 seconds (f_r = 200 Hz).

Vacuum tube amplifiers were first applied to the measurement of the ECG in 1928 by Ernstine and Levine, and all subsequent ECG recordings have involved amplification of ECG voltage, rather than ECG current, direct use of which activated the string galvanometer (Jenkins, 1997).

Modern ECG amplifiers are reactively coupled and have standard corner (−3 dB) frequencies of 0.05 and 100 Hz (Rawlings, 1991). The recording medium is generally moving paper, and robust galvanometer movements with bandwidths from dc to more than 100 Hz move the writing element, making a graph of the ECG voltage vs. time. The ECG can be written with a pressurized ink pen, a moving hot

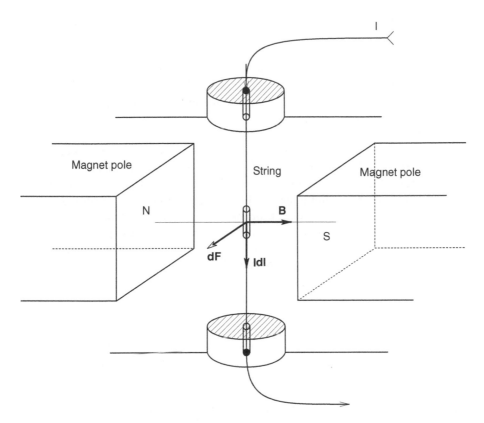

FIGURE 4.25 Schematic of a string galvanometer. The downward-flowing current causes the steady B field to force the string out of the airgap. String deflection is approximately proportional to I.

stylus (on special paper), a fixed hot stylus matrix (special paper moves past it), or a UV light beam (on special paper). The ECG record can also be digitized and stored in computer memory, and then displayed on a monitor in a moving display (seen in hospital ORs and ICUs), or as a static display. Such computer-processed displays can then be printed out by an inkjet or laser printer.

4.4.2 ELECTRODE PLACEMENTS

The original Lead I, II and III ECG electrode placements were defined by Einthoven in 1912. The electrode placement, called *Einthoven's triangle*; is still used today for routine ECG measurement. Electrodes are placed on the left leg (on the shin above the foot), on the right arm (about one quarter of the way from the wrist on the medial surface), and on the left arm in the same location. The potentials at these body locations will be denoted: v_{LL}, v_{RA} and v_{LA}, respectively. To avoid muscle electromyogram (EMG) artifacts, electrodes are purposely located away from large muscle groups on the calf or upper arm. ECG Lead I is the potential between the left arm

(+) and the right arm (−), i.e., $v_1 = v_{LA} - v_{RA}$. Lead II is taken between the left leg (+) and the right arm (−), i.e., $v_2 = v_{LL} - v_{RA}$, and Lead III is between the left leg (+) and the left arm (−), i.e., $v_3 = v_{LL} - v_{LA}$. These sites are remote from the heart, but they were determined originally in the 19th century as the only practical locations for the saline-filled jar electrodes in which the limbs were immersed. *Einthoven's law* is basically a statement based on the (now) well-known Kirchoff's voltage law of electrical circuits. Basically, it says that if any two of the three bipolar limb lead ECG voltages are known at any instant, the third voltage can be found by summing the known two with appropriate attention to algebraic sign.

The three *Augmented Unipolar Leads* are called aVR, aVL and aVF. Circuit connections needed to record these ECG voltages are shown in Figure 4.26. These voltages resemble Einthoven Lead I, Lead II and Lead III voltages respectively, except that the aVR waveform appears like an inverted Lead I waveform.

To focus on possible local defects in ventricular muscle or conduction problems, recordings are also made from *six precordial leads*. The recording set-up is shown in Figure 4.27. The resistances, R, are typically 5 kilohms. By writing a node equation on the v_T node, it is easy to show that the reference voltage, v_T, is:

$$v_T = (1/3)[v_{RA} + v_{LA} + V_{LL}] \qquad\qquad 4.76$$

Thus, the DA output is actually "v_k" = $[v_k - v_T] K_A$, k = 1... 6.

By using pairs of electrodes at various nonstandard locations on the chest, abdomen and back, it is possible at any point in time in the cardiac cycle to make a map of isopotential contours on the body. These contours describe how the skin surface potential varies in time during the cardiac cycle, and underscores the fact that, electrically, the heart is not a simple fixed dipole voltage source embedded in a homogeneous volume conductor, but rather a superposition of time- and space-varying dipoles embedded in an inhomogeneous volume conductor. As the lungs fill with air, the ECG decreases in amplitude and can change shape. Although ECG signals are voltages in time, they are recorded at different sites on the body surface (defining an internal volume), and so offer an opportunity to investigate the *volume variation* of cardiac potential in time.

The normal temporal features of a Lead II ECG waveform are shown in Figure 4.28. Because of the tremendous variability in individual anatomy, cardiac conditioning, and conditions under which an ECG is measured, there is considerable variability in "normal" Lead II ECGs. The P wave occurs as the atrial muscle is depolarizing; its mean peak amplitude is ca. 0.107 mV. There is a large variability in P waves seen; some individuals have no visible P wave, in others, it is as high as 0.3 mV. The duration of the P wave can range from 0 to 100 ms. This variability in amplitude and duration can be seen in normal individuals.

The *P-R interval*, I_{PR}, in Figure 4.28 relates to the depolarization of the atria, the AV node, the AV bundle and its branches and the Purkinje system. Its normal range is 120 to 200 ms. Sinus tachycardia can reduce I_{PR} to ca. 110 ms (Rawlings, 1991). The duration of the *Q wave* is normally < 30 ms. The amplitude of the Q wave can range from 0 to −25% of the R wave peak. The *R wave* amplitude can

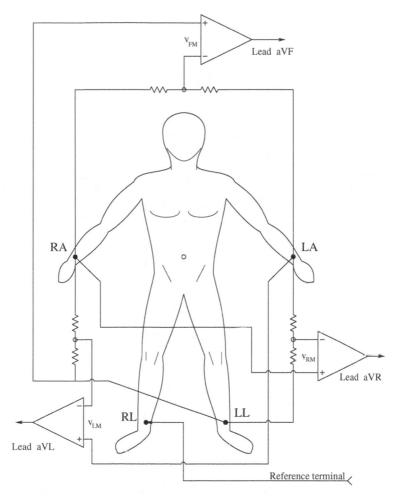

FIGURE 4.26 How the three ECG AV leads are measured. The resistors are equal, ca. 5 k ohms. The amplifiers are differential isolation amps (DIAs).

range from 0.05 mV to 2.8 mV and still be considered normal. The duration of the R wave (rise time) is usually < 70 ms. The fall time of the *S wave* is from 0 to 50 ms. The duration of the entire QRS complex in Lead II is 50 to 100 ms.

The duration of the *S-T segment,* S_{ST}, is from the end of the QRS complex to the onset of the T wave. The *Q-T interval,* I_{QT}, is the time it takes for the ventricles to depolarize, contract, relax and repolarize. Several formulas can predict its normal range from other intervals in the ECG cycle, but, in general, it should be shorter than 425 ms. The *T wave* occurs during ventricular muscle repolarization and is normally positive, having a duration of from 100 to 250 ms. Its normal mean peak amplitude is 0.267 mV, with a minimum of 0 and a maximum of 0.8 mV. In some individuals, a small *U wave* is seen following the T wave. Its origin is uncertain (Rawlings, 1991). Figure 4.29 illustrates one normal typical ECG cycle of Leads I,

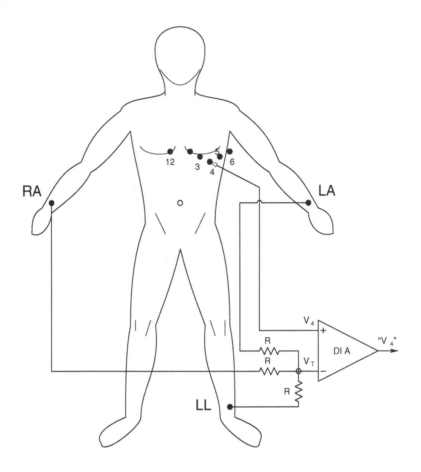

FIGURE 4.27 How the six precordial ECGs are obtained from the chest.

II and III, V_1, V_3 and aV_R. Note the inverted QRS spike in leads V_1 and aVR (also seen in V_2; not shown).

4.4.3 VECTOR CARDIOGRAPHY

Picture the human body described by three orthogonal axes: the y-axis is the vertical axis running from head to feet. The z-axis is the dorsal axis; it runs from the chest to the back. The x-axis is the horizontal axis running from the right hand to the left hand through the chest. Also consider three orthogonal planes that meet in the center of the chest: The *sagittal-* or *median plane* is defined by the y- and z-axes; it passes vertically through the center of the body. The coronal or horizontal plane contains the x- and z-axes; it is parallel to the ground. The frontal plane contains the x- and y-axes; it also runs from the head to the ground.

    Vector cardiography can be used to describe the electrical activity of the heart as ECG vector tip projections vs. time in the three planes described above. ECG vector projections in the frontal plane are probably more common, however. Natu-

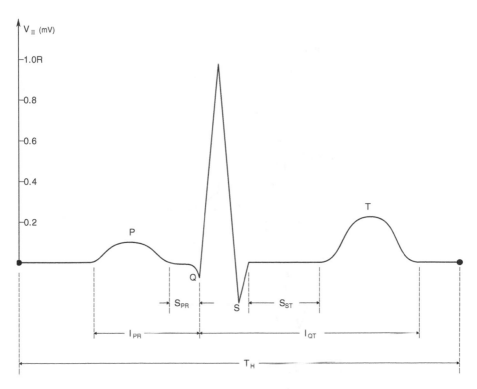

FIGURE 4.28 A normal Lead II ECG cycle, showing intervals and amplitudes used in diagnosis.

rally, the frontal ECG vector tip locus depends on the state of the cardiac cycle. The ECG Leads I, II and III, or aVR, aVL and aVF define a set of three vector axes spaced 60° apart, lying in the frontal plane. The three ECG voltages are treated as three vectors that, at any time, are resolved by vector addition to a vector or point at the vector + tip in the frontal plane. An example of a vector sum of V_I, V_{II} and V_{III} in the frontal plane at some time t_1 is shown in Figure 4.30. This is $\mathbf{V(t_1)} = \mathbf{V_I}(t_1) + \mathbf{V_{II}}(t_1) + \mathbf{V_{III}}(t_1)$. The vector axes are at 0°, −60°, and −120°. The (positive) tip of the vector $\mathbf{V(t_1)}$ defines a point. If the voltage vectors $\mathbf{V_I}$, $\mathbf{V_{II}}$ and $\mathbf{V_{III}}$ are sampled throughout the cardiac cycle, we can generate a closed curve connecting the points at the end of $\mathbf{V(t_k)}$. This curve is the *frontal plane vector cardiogram* (VCG). This type of vector cardiogram is easily calculated by computer. The voltages V_I, V_{II} and V_{III}, are sampled and converted into X and Y components:

$$\mathbf{V_x}(t_k) = V_I(t_k) + V_{II}(t_k)\cos(60°) + V_{III}(t_k)\cos(120°) \qquad 4.77A$$

$$\mathbf{V_y}(t_k) = V_{II}(t_k)\sin(60°) + V_{III}(t_k)\sin(120°)$$

(Note that positive Y is downward)   4.77B

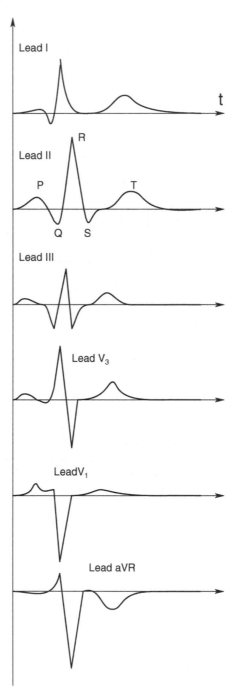

FIGURE 4.29 A summary of typical normal ECG wave-shapes recorded from various defined leads.

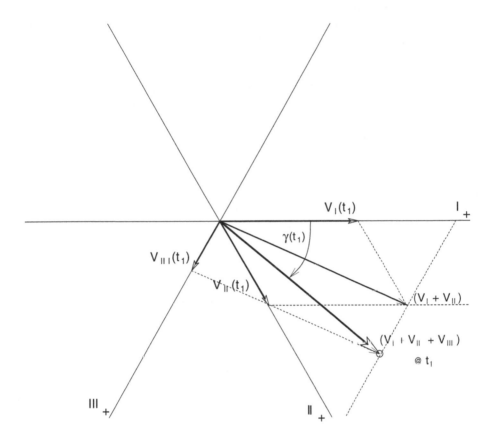

FIGURE 4.30 The vector addition of ECG waveforms from leads I, II and III in the frontal plane. Notice the three, fixed vector axes are spaced 60° apart.

Next, we put the net vector into polar form. Its magnitude is:

$$V(t_k) = \sqrt{V_x^2(t_k) + V_y^2(t_k)} \qquad 4.78$$

The angle of $\mathbf{V}(t_k)$ is:

$$\gamma(t_k) = \tan^{-1}\{V_y(t_k)/V_x(t_k)\} \qquad 4.79$$

So the VCG voltage at $t = t_k$ is:

$$\mathbf{V}(t_k) = V(t_k) \angle \gamma(t_k) \qquad 4.80$$

Note that, in this vector convention, positive $\gamma(t_k)$ is measured clockwise from the + x-axis.

Actually, there are three loops in the VCG, a very small one for the P-wave, another large one for the QRS complex, and a third small one for the T wave. Representative vector loops for the QRS and T waves in the frontal plane are shown in Figure 4.31. The large VCG loop from the QRS complex has great utility in diagnosing a multitude of cardiac problems, ranging from conduction blocks (bundle branch blocks) to ventricular hypertrophy, various ventricular myopathies, coronary artery ischemia, localization of infarctions, etc. (Guyton, 1991). VCG loops vary from beat to beat, and the cardiologist must take this small normal variability into consideration in making a diagnosis.

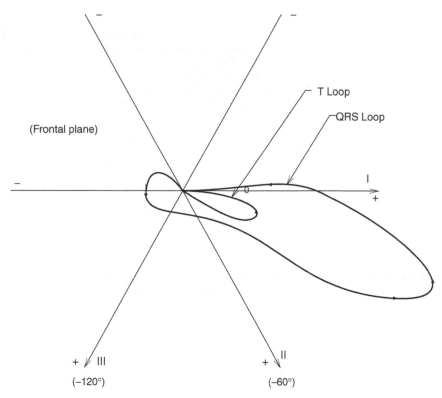

FIGURE 4.31 A typical frontal vectorcardiogram derived from lead I, II and III ECG voltages. Note that there are two loops, both traversed counterclockwise, one from the QRS complex, and the smaller one from the T-wave.

By recording from suitable electrodes lying in the median and horizontal planes, VCG plots can be created as closed curves lying in those planes, as well as in the frontal plane. From these three vector projections, a 3-D view of how the ECG vector varies in time can be constructed. The length of the resultant vector tip at $t = t_k$ in XYZ space is given by the pythagorean theorem, and its angles can be resolved by trigonometry. Figure 4.32 illustrates a representative, 3-D, VCG for one cardiac cycle.

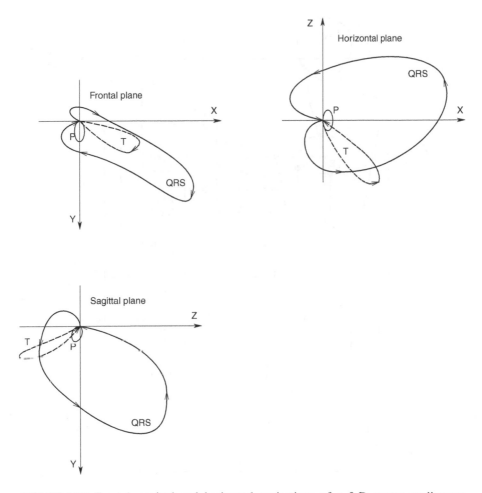

FIGURE 4.32 Frontal, sagittal and horizontal projections of a 3-D vector cardiogram recorded using a multiple 3-D electrode array such as the Frank system.

The *Frank VCG System* using seven electrodes is shown in Figure 4.33. Note the Frank axis convention where the positive x-axis points left, positive y is down, and positive z is points dorsal. The Frank system uses a resistive summing circuit to resolve the three orthogonal components of the VCG with 13% error, compared with a "gold standard" system that summed the outputs of 150 electrodes. The nine-electrode precordial system had 10% error compared with the 150-electrode system, and an experimental 30-electrode system gave only 1% error (Rawlings, 1991).

4.4.4 ECG ANALYSIS, FEATURE EXTRACTION AND DIAGNOSIS

An experienced cardiologist can read a standard set of ECG traces or a VCG and make a diagnosis based on education and experience. When one considers the many things that can go wrong with the heart, this diagnostic ability is remarkable.

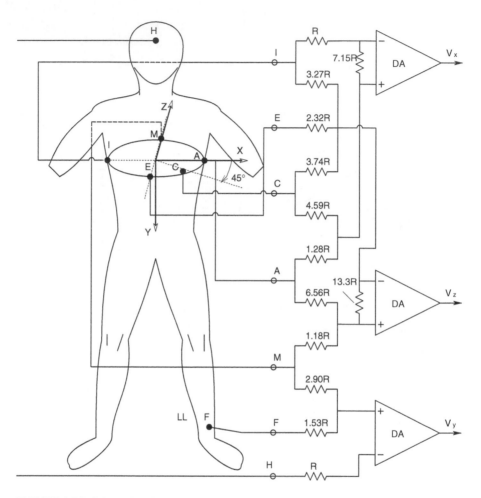

FIGURE 4.33 Schematic of the Frank VCG electrode system. The DAs are medical isolation amplifiers. The three analog voltages V_x, V_y and V_z are used to generate the 3-D VCG display.

Biomedical engineers, computer scientists, and cardiologists have tried since the days of the DEC PDP-series computers in the '70s to design pattern recognition software that could diagnose common cardiac pathologies, given various ECG lead voltages as inputs. Early ECG diagnostic programs would measure waveform features such as the various intervals and segment lengths associated with the PQRST elements of the lead II ECG waveform, and also examine peak heights and slopes, and then compare them with a standard database for statistical analysis. Certain sets of out-of-range ECG features could then be assigned probabilities for various cardiac diseases. Such programs were good for gross screening, but were nothing you would want to bet your life on.

More sophisticated techniques have now emerged for ECG analysis, including the use of Fourier-transformed ECGs, time-frequency analysis of ECGs (Clayton et al., 1998), and 2-D frequency-domain analysis of VCG loops (Lei et al., 1997). Work has also been done with trainable artificial neural networks (ANNs) for the diagnosis of cardiac pathologies, applying the trainable ANN to recognizing anomalies in the time-domain QRS complex (Barro et al., 1998).

4.4.5 DISCUSSION

As noninvasive diagnostic modalities, the ECG and VCG are probably among the more cost-effective presently available. The electrodes are simple and inexpensive, the ECG signals are conditioned by inexpensive differential isolation amplifiers, and their digitized outputs are easily processed by computer to form moving chart recorder displays or vector displays. Much can be learned from the various waveforms of the different ECG leads, and from the VCG about the state of the heart muscle over its surface, and the state of the internal excitation conduction system of the heart.

4.5 THE EMG

4.5.1 INTRODUCTION

An important bioelectric signal that has diagnostic significance for many neuromuscular diseases is the *electromyogram* (EMG), which can be recorded from the skin surface with electrodes identical to those used for electrocardiography, although, in some cases, the electrodes have smaller areas than those used for ECG (< 1 mm^2). To record from single motor units (SMUs), or even individual muscle fibers (several of which compose an SMU), needle electrodes that pierce the skin into the body of a superficial muscle can also be used. (This semi-invasive method obviously requires sterile technique.) EMG recording is used to diagnose some causes of muscle weakness or paralysis, muscle or motor problems such as tremor or twitching, motor nerve damage from injury or osteoarthritis, and pathologies affecting motor end plates.

Many of the problems associated with the motor system that can be diagnosed using EMGs arise from autoimmune causes (e.g., myasthenia gravis, Eaton-Lambert syndrome), others come from genetic disorders (e.g., the dystrophies: Duchenne, Becker, limb-girdle, Landouzy-Dejerine), and still others come from motoneuron problems that can be genetic in origin, from virus infection (Polio, coxsackievirus, and other enteroviruses). For a more detailed classification of motoneuron disorders, see Chapter 14 of the on-line *Merck Manual* (www.merck.com/pubs/mmanual/tables/section14/sec14.htm).

4.5.2 THE ORIGIN OF EMGS

There are several types of muscle in the body, e.g., cardiac, smooth, and striated. Striated muscle in mammals can be further subdivided into *fast* and *slow muscles* (Guyton, 1991). Fast muscles are used for fast movements; they include the two gastrocnemii laryngeal muscles, extraocular muscles, etc. Slow muscles are used for postural control against gravity; they include the soleus, abdominal muscles, back muscles, neck muscles, etc. EMG recording is generally carried out on both slow and fast skeletal muscles. It can also be done on less superficial muscles such as the extraocular muscles that move the eyeballs, the eyelid muscles, and the muscles that work the larynx.

Most striated muscles are innervated by motor neurons that have origin at various levels in the spinal cord. That is, motor neurons receive excitatory and inhibitory inputs from motor control neurons from the CNS, as well as excitatory and inhibitory inputs from local feedback neurons, from muscle spindles (responding to muscle length x and dx/dt), Golgi tendon organs (responding to muscle tension), and Renshaw cells (Northrop, 1999; Guyton, 1991). Individual motor neuron axons controlling the contraction of a particular striated muscle innervate small groups of muscle fibers called *single motor units* (SMUs). Many SMUs compose the entire muscle. The synaptic connections between the terminal branches of a single motor neuron axon and its SMU are called *motor end plates* (MEPs). MEPs are chemical synapses in which the neurotransmitter acetylcholine (ACh) is released presynaptically and then diffuses across the synaptic cleft or gap to ACh receptors on the sub-synaptic membrane. A schematic drawing of a motor end plate at different magnifications is shown in Figure 4.34. When a motor neuron action potential arrives at the MEP, it triggers the exocytocis or emptying of about 300 presynaptic vesicles containing ACh. (There are ca. 3×10^5 vesicles in the terminals of a single MEP; each vesicle is about 40 nm diameter.) Some 10^7 to 5×10^8 molecules of ACh are needed to trigger a muscle action potential (Katz, 1966). The ACh diffuses across the 20- to 30-nm synaptic cleft in ca. 0.5 ms, where some ACh molecules combine with receptor sites on the protein subunits forming the subsynaptic, ion-gating channels. Five high-molecular weight protein subunits form each ion channel. ACh binding triggers a dilation of the channel to ca. 0.65 nm. The dilated channels allow Na^+ ions to pass inward; however, Cl^- is repelled by the fixed negative charges on the mouth of the channel. Thus the sub-synaptic membrane is depolarized by the inward J_{Na} (i.e., its transmembrane potential goes positive from the ca. $- 85$ mV resting potential), triggering a *muscle action potential.* The local sub-synaptic transmembrane potential can go to as much as +50 mV, forming an *end plate potential* (EPP) spike fused to the muscle action potential it triggers, having a duration of ca. 8 ms, much longer than a nerve action potential.

The ACh in the cleft and bound to the receptors is rapidly broken down (hydrolized) by the enzyme *cholinesterase* resident in the cleft, and its molecular components are recycled. A small amount of ACh also escapes the cleft by diffusion, and is also hydrolyzed.

Once the post-synaptic membrane under the MEP depolarizes in a superthreshold end plate potential spike, a *muscle action potential* is generated that propagates along the surface membrane of the muscle fiber, the *sarcolemma.* It is the muscle action potential that triggers muscle fiber contraction and force generation. Typical muscle action potentials, recorded intracellulary at the MEP and at a point 2 mm from the initiating MEP, are shown in Figure 4.35. The muscle action potential propagates at 3 to 5 m/sec, its duration is 2 to 15 ms, depending on the muscle, and it swings from a resting value of ca. −85 mV to a peak of ca. +30 mV. At the skin surface, it appears as a triphasic spike of 20 to 2000 μV peak amplitude (Guyton, 1991).

To ensure that all of the deep contractile apparatus in the center of the muscle fiber is stimulated to contract at the same time and with equal strength, many transverse radially directed tubules penetrate into the center of the fiber along its

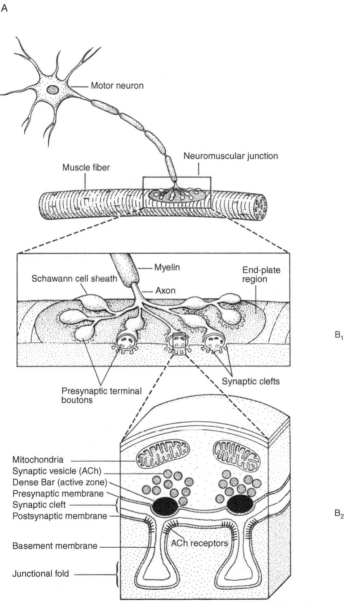

A

Motor neuron

Muscle fiber

Neuromuscular junction

Schawann cell sheath

Myelin

Axon

End-plate region

B₁

Presynaptic terminal boutons

Synaptic clefts

Mitochondria
Synaptic vesicle (ACh)
Dense Bar (active zone)
Presynaptic membrane
Synaptic cleft
Postsynaptic membrane

Basement membrane

Junctional fold

ACh receptors

B₂

FIGURE 4.34 A mammalian motor end plate (MEP) shown at different magnifications. At low magnification we see a myelinated motor neuron leaving the spinal cord and synapsing on a muscle fiber. In the middle panel, at medium magnification, we see how the presynaptic boutons from the motoneuron ending make contact with the post-synaptic membrane region of the muscle fiber. At highest (EM) magnification at the bottom of the figure, the ultrastructural details of the MEP and the basement membrane are shown. (From Kandel et al., 1991, *Principles of Neural Science*, 3rd ed. Appleton and Lange, Norwalk, CT. With permission from the McGraw-Hill Companies.)

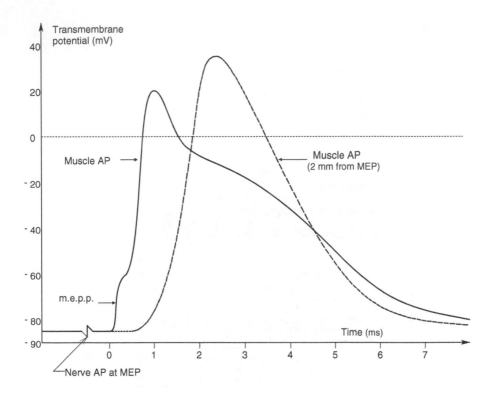

FIGURE 4.35 Representative intracellularly recorded muscle action potentials.

length. These *T-tubules* are open to the extracellular fluid space, as is the surface of the fiber, and they are connected to the surface membrane at both ends. The T-tubules conduct the muscle action potential into the interior of the fiber in many locations along its length.

Running longitudinally around the outsides of the contractile myofibrils that make up the fiber are networks of tubules called the *sarcoplasmic reticulum* (SR). The T-tubules and SR are shown schematically in Figure 4.36. Note that the terminal *cisternae* of the SR butt against the membrane of the T-tubes. When the muscle action potential penetrates along the T-tubes, the depolarization triggers the *cisternae* to release calcium ions into the space surrounding the myofibrils' contractile proteins. The Ca^{++} binds to the protein troponin C, which triggers contra-tion by the actin and myosin proteins. (We will not go into the molecular biophysics of the actual contraction process here.)

A synchronous stimulation of all of the motor neurons innervating a muscle produces what is called a *muscle twitch*; i.e., the tension initially falls a slight amount, then rises abruptly, then falls more slowly to zero again. Sustained muscle contraction is caused by a steady (average) rate of (asynchronous) motoneuron firing. When the firing ceases, the muscle relaxes. Muscle relaxation is actually an active process. Calcium ion pumps located in the membranes of the SR longitudinal tubules actively

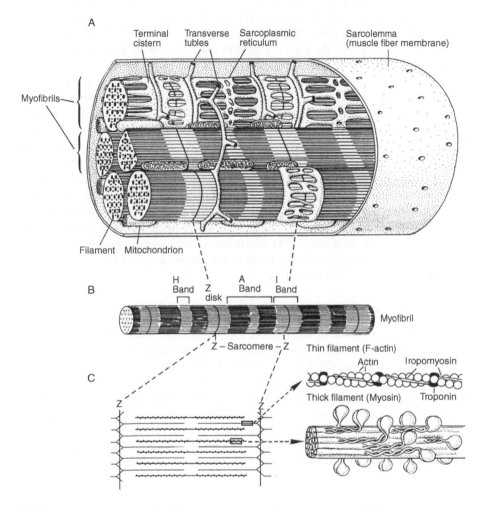

FIGURE 4.36(A) Schematic 3-D structure of a striated muscle fiber. (B) Structure of an individual myofibril showing bands. (C) Schematic cross-section of an individual sarcomere. The thick filaments are made up of arrays of myosin molecules. The myosin molecule has a stem region and a globular double head that protrudes from the stem. Thin filaments are composed of polymerized actin molecules. Note the complexity of this system. (From Kandel et al. 1991, *Principles of Neural Science*, 3rd ed. Appleton and Lange, Norwalk, CT. With permission from the McGraw-Hill Companies.)

transfer Ca^{++} from outside the tubules to back inside the SR system. It is the lack of Ca^{++} in proximity to troponin C that allows relaxation to occur. In resting muscle, the concentration, $[Ca^{++}]$, is about 10^{-7} M in the myofibrillar fluid (Guyton, 1991). In a twitch, $[Ca^{++}]$ rises to ca. 2×10^{-5} M, and in a tetanic stimulation, $[Ca^{++}]$ is about 2×10^{-4} M. It takes about 50 ms for the Ca^{++} released by a single motor nerve impulse to be taken up by the SR pumps to restore the resting $[Ca^{++}]$ level.

The Ca^{++} pumps require metabolic energy to operate; adenosine triphoshate (ATP) is cleaved to the diphosphate to release the energy needed to drive the Ca^{++} pumps. The pumps can concentrate the Ca^{++} to ca. 10^{-3} M inside the SR. Inside the SR tubules and cisternae the Ca^{++} is stored in readily available ionic form, and as a protein chelate bound to a protein, *calsequestrin.*

So far, we have described the events associated with a single muscle fiber. As noted above, small groups of fibers innervated by a single motoneuron fiber are called a single motor unit. In muscles used for fine actions, such as those operating the fingers or tongue, there are fewer muscle fibers in a motor unit, or, equivalently, more motoneuron fibers per total number of muscle fibers. For example, the laryngeal muscles used for speech have only two or three fibers per SMU, while large muscles used for gross motions, such as the gastrocnemius, can have several hundred fibers per SMU (Guyton, 1991). To make fine movements, only a few motoneurons fire out of the total number innervating the muscle, and these do not fire synchronously. Their firing phase is made random to produce smooth contraction. At maximum tetanic stimulation, the mean frequency on the motoneurons is higher, but the phases are still random to reduce the duty cycle of individual SMUs.

4.5.3 EMG Amplifiers

The amplifiers used for clinical EMG recording must meet the same stringent specifications for low leakage currents as do ECG amplifiers (see Section 4.3). EMG amplifier gains are typically X1000, and their bandwidths reflect the transient nature of the SMU action potentials. Typically, an EMG amplifier is reactively coupled, with low- and high-frequency −3 dB frequencies of 300 Hz and 3 kHz, respectively. With an amplifier having variable low- and high- −3 dB frequencies, one generally starts with a wide pass bandwidth, say 100 Hz to 10 kHz, and gradually restricts it until individual EMG spikes just begin to round up and change shape. Such an *ad hoc* adjusted bandwidth will give a better output SNR ratio than one that is too wide or too narrow.

4.5.4 What EMGs Can Tell Us

There are many diseases and conditions that can alter the normal operation of striated muscle. The problem can be in the CNS, or the spine where motoneuron activation occurs. Abnormal muscle action can also be due to a problem with the motor end plate, the ACh receptors, or the biochemical mechanisms coupling the MEP spike to muscle contraction. The major objective of EMG analysis is to sort out whether the problem lies with the motor nerve activation, the synaptic coupling from MEP to SR, or the contractile process itself. Often a superficial motor nerve (e.g., the ulnar nerve in the forearm) is stimulated electrically using skin surface electrodes, and needle electrodes are used to record SMU activity in a superficial muscle in the hand (e.g., the hypothenar muscle). This type of recording allows the neurologist to see if the synaptic coupling mechanism is normal from the latencies and amplitudes of the SMU action potentials.

When investigating the EMGs of large skeletal muscles such as the biceps or gastrocnemius, the motor nerves are not available for superficial external stimulation. EMG skin surface electrodes are commonly used, so the firing of many SMUs is picked up simultaneously. During a strong muscle contraction, their amplitudes and firing phases are superimposed to give an EMG that looks like a burst of noise. In addition, if the muscle is allowed to shorten under load, the active SMUs at muscle length L_0 can move away from the recording electrodes (fixed on the skin) and other SMUs will contribute to the net EMG at $L = L_0 - \Delta L$. If the behavior of certain SMUs is required, then the patient must do an *isometric muscle contraction* to minimize SMU motion relative to the recording electrodes.

Single motor fiber recording done on potentials from superficial hand muscles such as the *extensor digitorum communis*, can be used to diagnose diseases of the neuromuscular junction, including myasthenia gravis, Eaton-Lambert syndrome, botulism, etc. 25 μm diameter wires are inserted into the muscle mass through the skin using hypodermic needles. The fine wire electrodes contact one or two single muscle fibers from a common SMU. By measuring the "phase jitter" between two fibers and comparing it with the jitter of a normal reference muscle with the same load (level of contraction), diagnosis can be made (Healthgate, 1999).

The frequency, amplitude and duration of SMU triphasic spikes recorded with larger percutaneous wire electrodes can also be used to diagnose such conditions as anterior horn cell (motoneuron soma and dendrite) disease, demyelinating neuropathy, axonal neuropathy, neuromuscular transmission disorder, and myopathies (Cornwall, 1999). Figure 4.37 illustrates EMGs from an SMU in a partially denervated muscle.

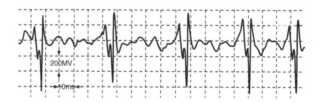

FIGURE 4.37 Top: Surface EMG recorded from a rapidly firing partially denervated SMU. Bottom: Another rapidly firing partially denervated, SMU. Note the curious multiple peaks on both EMGs. Can you explain why they are present?

A problem in recording from SMUs or single muscle fibers with wire electrodes is interference from action potentials on neighboring SMUs and fibers. These artifactual EMG spikes are generally smaller in amplitude than the desired spikes. It is possible to improve the SNR of the desired spikes by passing the recorded EMG signal, x(t), through an odd nonlinearity of the form:

$$y(t) = K \, \text{sgn}[x(t)] \, \{\exp[a \,|\, x(t)\,|\,] - 1\} \qquad 4.81$$

The slope of this nonlinearity for x > 0 is:

$$\frac{dy}{dx} = K\, a\, \exp[a\, x]\qquad\qquad 4.82$$

Thus, the larger values of x(t) get proportionally more amplification, suppressing noise and small EMG spikes recorded with the desired spikes. This type of nonlinearity distorts the desired spikes, but does not affect the timing or phase jitter which is of interest.

EMGs can be viewed in the *time domain* (most useful when single fibers or SMUs are being recorded), in the *frequency domain* (the FFT is taken from an entire surface-recorded EMG burst under standard conditions), or in the time-frequency (TF) domain (see Section 3.2.3). In the latter case, the TF display shows the frequencies in the EMG burst as a function of time. In general, a higher frequency content in the TF display indicates that more SMUs are being activated at a higher rate (Hannaford and Lehman, 1986). TF analysis can show how agonist–antagonist muscle pairs are controlled to do a specific motor task.

Still another way to characterize EMG activity in the time domain is to pass the EMG through a true rms (TRMS) conversion circuit, such as an AD637 IC. The output of the TRMS circuit is a smoothed positive voltage proportional to the square-root of the time average of $x^2(t)$. The time averaging is done by a single time-constant low-pass filter. For another time domain display modality, the EMG signal can be full-wave rectified and low-pass filtered to smooth it.

4.5.5 DISCUSSION

In this section, we have seen that the EMG, when recorded along with motor neuron activity or by itself, can be processed in the time, frequency, or TF domains to reveal evidence pointing to various neuromuscular diseases. Electrodes used for EMG recording from the skin surface are generally small Ag|AgCl types, similar to those used for ECG and EEG recording. Percutaneous wire electrodes, inserted into a superficial muscle mass by hypodermic needles, are used to record action potentials from single motor units and single muscle fibers. These electrodes are removable, and constitute a mildly invasive procedure that carries a small risk of infection.

For a comprehensive list of neuromuscular diseases, see the Washington University Medical School Neuromuscular Disease Web Site 2000 (www.neuro.wustl.edu/neuromuscular/index.html). This is a huge body of information on the topic. The overall perspective given from visiting this site and (www.neuro.wustl.edu/neuromuscular/lab/patterns.htm), is that motor nerve stimulation and EMGs provide a supporting role in diagnosis that is also heavily based on invasive procedures such as muscle biopsy, biochemical, histochemical and immuno-histochemical tests for autoantibodies.

4.6 THE ELECTROENCEPHALOGRAM (EEG)

4.6.1 Introduction

The EEG is a relatively low-frequency spontaneous electrical potential recorded from an electrode on the scalp (the second electrode can be on an earlobe or also on the scalp). The peak amplitude of the EEG can be as large as 150 μV peak-to-peak (delta waves), but, more typically, it is less than 50 μV ppk (alpha rhythm). The EEG was discovered by the German psychiatrist and electrophysiologist Hans Berger, whose initial discovery of EEG activity was made using a string galvanometer and surface electrodes on his son's scalp. At Jena, Berger went on to study EEGs in relation to brain diseases in the 1920s. In 1929, he published a paper entitled *Über das Electrenkephalogramm des Menschen* (visit the Biomagnetic Center Jena, Friedrich-Schiller University: http://jenameg10.uni-jena.de/nostalg.htm).

EEGs can be used to diagnose organic brain abnormalities such as abscesses, various forms of epilepsy, focal seizures, arteriovenous malformations (e.g., aneurisms, infarcts), tumors, hemorrhages, physical injury to brain tissue from head trauma, etc. Often, abnormal EEG results point to the need for detailed imaging studies such as dye-injection/X-ray fluoroscopy, CAT or MRI. EEGs are also used in brain research to localize brain volumes responsible for certain mental activities.

4.6.2 Sources and Classification of the EEG

Because of the EEG's low-frequency nature, it is evident that fast action potentials on the axons of brain neurons contribute little to its potential. The spiking axons run in various directions, and their very small external potentials tend to average out in the volume conductors of the brain, the meninges, and the skull and scalp. The generation of EEG potentials requires a neural source close to the inside surface of the skull that is coherent, i.e., all the neurons must be aligned similarly and act together electrically. It turns out that the pyramidal cells in the center layers of the cerebral cortex are, in fact, the major source of the EEG potentials. Figure 4.38 illustrates schematically the various cells found in a radial slice through the cerebral cortex, including the pyramidal cells. Note that the apical dendritic branches of the pyramidal cells lie in the outermost layer of the cortex, next to the skull. These dendrites receive excitatory or inhibitory inputs from surrounding neurons and ascending axons. If the apical dendrites are receiving excitatory inputs, some positive ion current carried by an ion such as Na^+ enters them, depolarizing the pyramidal cell toward firing. The inward apical J_{Na} is supplied by an extracellular current flowing outward from deeper layers in the cortex. This current flow is in response to the apical portions of the stimulated pyramidal cell's going negative, while the deep portions are positive, creating an effective dipole on the cortex around the stimulated cell. If the apical dendrites of a pyramidal cell receive inhibitory inputs, there is a net outward flow of positive ions (or a net inward flow of negative ions such as J_{Cl}). Thus, inhibition of a pyramidal cell causes its apex to go positive, reversing the external current flow and making the outer surface of the cortex positive

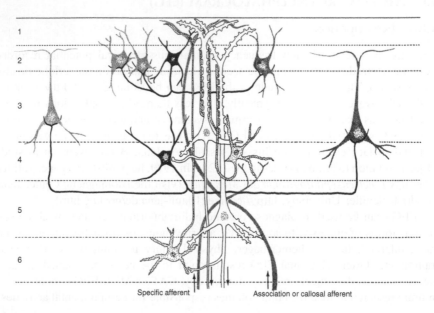

1

2

3

4

5

6

Specific afferent   Association or callosal afferent

FIGURE 4.38 A schematic radial slice down through the cerebral cortex showing the principal types of neurons, the layers in which they occur, and representative interconnections. The two large pyramidal cells whose somas lie in layers 3 and 5 receive multiple synaptic contacts from the star-shaped (stellate) cells (stippled) in layers 4 and 6. The basket interneurons (black) in layers 2 and 4 act inhibitorily on the neurons with which they synapse. Major cortical output is from pryamidal cells. (From Kandel et al., 1991, *Principles of Neural Science*, 3rd ed. Appleton and Lange, Norwalk, CT. With permission from the McGraw-Hill Companies.)

around the inhibited cell. Many pyramidal cells in a region of cortex surface must be excited or inhibited together to create a local dipole large enough to be sensed through the skull by an electrode on the scalp.

EEG potentials on the scalp are usually no more than 150 μV peak-to-peak. They are generally classified in the frequency domain by their power spectral content. The *spectrum* of *alpha waves* lies between 7.5 and 13 Hz; it is produced in adults when a person is in a conscious, relaxed state with the eyes closed. It disappears when attention is focused on a task and the eyes are opened. Alpha waves are best recorded from the posterior lateral parts of the scalp.

Beta waves have spectral energy of 14 Hz and greater. They are best recorded frontally. Beta activity is present when people are alert or anxious, with their eyes open.

Theta potentials are large-amplitude, low-frequency (3.5 to 7.5 Hz) waves. Theta is abnormal in alert adults but is seen during sleep, and in prepubescent children.

Delta waves have the largest amplitudes and the lowest frequency (≤ 3.5 Hz). It is a normal rhythm found in infants ≤ 1 year and in adults in deep sleep (stages 3 and 4). Delta activity may also occur when the patient has a subcortical brain lesion. In adults, normal delta waves occur in bursts called *frontal intermittent rhythmic delta activity* (FIRDA). All EEG waveforms are non-stationary and can be characterized in the frequency domain by short-term Fourier analysis.

4.6.3 EEG RECORDING SYSTEMS

As we have mentioned above, electrodes for EEG recording are generally small AgCl types that use a conductive coupling gel. In some cases, small saline-saturated sponges are used to couple the AgCl electrodes to the scalp. The hair is parted and pushed aside for good low-resistance electrode contact. EEG potentials can be recorded between pairs of electrodes on the scalp, or between a scalp electrode and a "remote" electrode attached to an earlobe. The voltage difference between any single electrode and the electronic average of the potentials from the rest of the electrodes can also be viewed.

A standard placement of EEG electrodes was adopted in 1958 called the *International 10-20 Electrode System* (Webster, 1998). This arrangement is shown schematically in Figure 4.39. Note that the odd electrode numbers are on the left side of the head. Electrodes C_3 and C_4 are placed to overlie the region of the central sulcus of the brain. The oval electrodes in the figure are on the vertical sides of the head (forehead, temples, etc.).

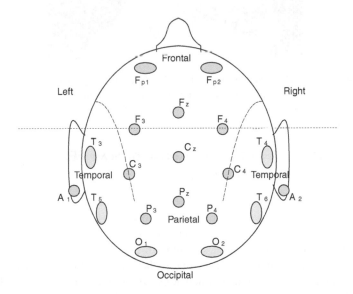

FIGURE 4.39 A top view of the head showing the standard electrode placements for the international 10-20 EEG electrode array.

Neurophysiologists, wishing to further localize the sources of EEG activity in the cortex, have gone to larger arrays of electrodes than in the standard 10–20 array. Such arrays can contain 32, 64, 128 and even 256 individual electrodes. They are used for medical diagnosis, research in physiological psychology, and biofeedback applications such as the EEG-controlled computer mouse. Figure 4.40 illustrates a subject wearing an Electrical Geodesics, Inc. Geodesic Sensor Net© EEG 128 electrode array. Other companies that make multielectrode EEG arrays are Teledyne Electronic Technologies (32 channels), and SAM Technology, Inc., with its "helmet" with up to 128 electrodes.

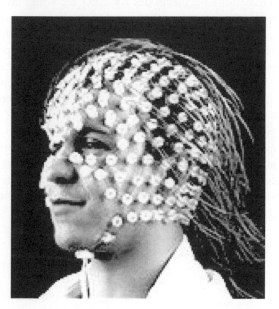

FIGURE 4.40 A Geodesic Sensor Net© EEG 128-electrode array, made by EGI, Inc. (Photo with permission of Electrical Geodesics, Inc. The Geodesic Sensor Net is a patented technology for sampling the surface of the head with a regular polygonal geometry (www.egi.com).)

4.6.4 Two-Dimensional Spatial Sampling of Scalp EEG Potentials by Electrode Arrays

The *sampling theorem,* as originally derived, deals with the analog reconstructability of periodically sampled *time* signals by ideal low-pass filtering. The sampling theorem is easily extended to the periodic sampling of one-dimensional signals in space (x-dimension), the periodic spatial sampling of 2-D, spatial signals (e.g., pictures) in Cartesian x and x-dimensions, and finally, the spatial sampling of 2-D signals on the surface of a sphere (θ and ϕ dimensions). At a given point in time, the scalp-recorded EEG can be treated as a 2-D signal mapped on the surface of an idealized *hemisphere* (the scalp). Clearly, evenly spaced electrodes on the scalp can be thought of as representing a spatial voltage-sampling array on the surface of a hemisphere. Figure 4.41 illustrates one quadrant of the hemisphere with the potential at time t_o at a point, $V(t_o,\rho,\theta,\phi)$, shown. What we are interested in is the maximum spacing (hence minimum number) of electrodes on the hemisphere surface required to accurately estimate a continuous analog distribution of the EEG voltage, $V(t_o,\rho,\theta,\phi)$.

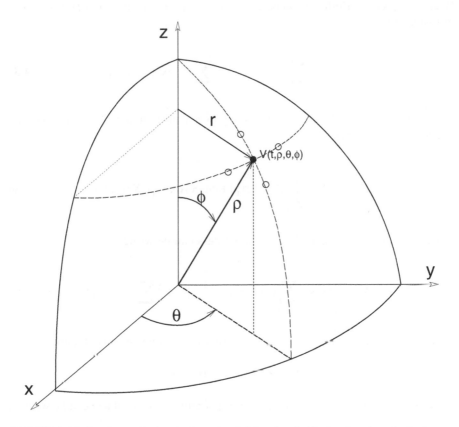

FIGURE 4.41 Quadrant of a hemisphere (model for the skull) showing the spherical coordinate system used to define the spatial distribution of electrical activity on the scalp at any time t. ρ = R in this simplified model (R is the hemisphere radius).

To begin, we will review the sampling theorem in 1-D linear space. Assume an analog voltage, V(x) exists. This voltage is periodically sampled along the x-axis, forming a number sequence, V*(x). The sampling process can be thought of as mathematically as being *impulse modulation* of the continuous signal. That is, V(x) is multiplied by a train of unit impulses along the x-axis:

$$V*(x) = V(x) \cdot P_T(x) = V(x) \sum_{n=-\infty}^{n=\infty} \delta\big(x - nX_s\big)$$ 4.83

Where X_s is the spatial sampling period, i.e., the spacing between the unit impulses. In the spatial frequency domain, this multiplication is equivalent to complex convolution. $F\{\bullet\}$ is the Fourier transform operator.

$$F\{V*(x)\} = V*(ju) = V(ju) \otimes P_T(ju)$$ 4.84

Because $P_T(x)$ is periodic, it can be expressed as an exponential form *Fourier series* in distance x:

$$P_T(x) = \sum_{n=-\infty}^{n=\infty} \delta(x - nX_s) = \sum_{n=-\infty}^{n=\infty} C_n \exp(-jnu_s x) \qquad 4.85$$

Where u_s in the spatial sampling frequency in radians/mm. $u_s \equiv 2\pi/X_s.$ The Fourier coeficient, C_n, is given by:

$$C_n = (1/X_s) \int_{-X_s/2}^{X_s/2} P_T(x) \exp(+jnu_s x)\, dx = (1/X_s), \text{all n.} \qquad 4.86$$

Thus the output of the spatial sampling process can be written:

$$V*(x) = V(x) \cdot \left[(1/X_s) \sum_{n=-\infty}^{n=\infty} \exp(-jnu_s x) \right] = (1/X_s) \sum_{n=-\infty}^{n=\infty} V(x) \exp(-jnu_s x) \quad 4.87$$

Finally, we use the Fourier transform theorem for complex exponentiation:

$$\mathbf{F}\{y(x)\, e^{-jax}\} \equiv Y(ju - ja) \qquad 4.88$$

Now, in the *spatial frequency domain,* the spatially sampled voltage can be written:

$$\mathbf{F}\{V*(x)\} = \mathbf{V}*(ju) = (1/X_s) \sum_{n=-\infty}^{n=\infty} V(ju - jnu_s) \qquad 4.89$$

Equation 4.89 is called the *Poisson sum* form of the spatially sampled signal. Figure 4.42A shows the spatial frequency spectrum of $\mathbf{V}*(x)$ when the *baseband spectrum,* $V(ju)$, contains no spatial frequencies in excess of the *spatial Nyquist frequency,* defined as: $u_N \equiv u_s/2 = \pi/X_s$. Theoretically, V(x) can be recovered from $\mathbf{V}*(ju)$ by ideal spatial low-pass filtering. In Figure 4.42(B), V(ju) contains frequencies in excess of $u_s/2$, and the overall repeating spectrum $\mathbf{V}*(ju)$ is said to be *aliased.* There is overlap between the upper and lower portions of adjacent repeated spectral components, which creates lost information when $\mathbf{V}*(ju)$ is ideal low-passed filtered in an attempt to recover V(x).

Thus, to avoid aliasing and lost information in sampling the EEG distribution, $V(t_0,\rho,\theta,\phi)$, on the scalp "hemisphere," the electrodes that constitute a spatial sampling array should be spaced closely enough together so that the highest spatial frequencies in $\mathbf{F}\{V(\theta,\phi)\}$ are less than the spatial Nyquist frequencies, π/Θ_s and π/Φ_s radians/radian, where Θ_s is the electrode spacing in radians in the θ dimension, and Φ_s is the electrode spacing in radians in the ϕ dimension. Normally, Θ_s is made equal

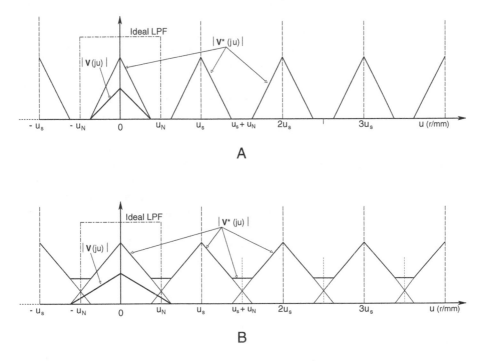

FIGURE 4.42 Illustration of spatial aliasing in a 1-D distribution of voltage in x. u is the spatial frequency of the signal V(x) and its spatially sampled array, V*(nX_s), where X_s is the distance between samples and u has the dimensions of radians/cm. In A, the bandwidth of V(ju) is low enough to prevent aliasing; all of the information in V*(ju) can be recovered. When the bandwith of V*(ju) is increased so that its maximum spatial frequency exceeds the spatial Nyquist frequency, $u_N = \pi/X_s$ r/cm, then aliasing occurs, as shown in B.

to Φ_s for ease in constructing the array. Note that, in the hemispheric head model, the radius ρ is considered constant.

It is easy to meet the *temporal* Nyquist criterion for the EEG signals at all the N electrodes when they are sampled and digitized for computer input. Each of the N, V(t,ρ,θ,φ) signals is passed through a temporal sharp cut-off low-pass anti-aliasing filter, and then sampled (digitized) at a rate at least 2.5 times the filter's −60 dB frequency. For practical purposes with the EEG, the time sampling frequency is generally made ca. 300 s/sec.

Justification for the large (e.g., N = 128 electrode) array is found in a key paper by Srinivasan et al. (1998), entitled "Estimating the Spatial Nyquist [frequency] of the EEG." In this paper, the authors consider the head to be part of a sphere with about a 9-cm radius. They examine visual event-related EEG potentials (ERPs) using the International 10-20 Electrode System (19 electrodes on the scalp and a reference on an earlobe), and also the 32, 64, and 128 geodesic electrode arrays (a geodesic is the shortest distance between two points on the surface of a sphere). Thus, the electrodes are equidistant in geodesic arrays on the head; spaced less than 5 cm on centers in a hexagonal pattern in the 32 array, less than 4 cm for a 64 array, and slightly less than 3 cm for the 128 array (Srinavasan et al., 1998).

Srinanvasan et al. defined spatial frequencies on the sphere in terms of the *orthogonal basis functions* for spherical surfaces, the spherical harmonics $Y_{mn}(\theta, \phi)$. They consider the $Y_{mn}(\theta, \phi)$ to be analogous to the sine and cosine basis functions used in the Fourier time series representation of EEG signals. They state: "Just as any time series of EEG signal can be described by its power spectrum (coefficients applied to each of a the (sic) series of sine waves), any potential field defined on a sphere can be represented as a weighted sum of spherical harmonics."

The same authors concluded that the 128-electrode geodesic electrode array was capable of resolving spherical harmonics up to degree n = 7 without aliasing. They concluded: "... we found that spherical harmonics of degree n = 9 are visibly distorted. With 64, 32, and the 19 (scalp) electrodes corresponding to the International 10-20 System, the highest spherical harmonics that can be sampled without (spatial) aliasing are n = 6, 4 and 3, respectively."

A heuristic way to visualize the n = 8 "cycles" is to consider the circumference of the sphere at its "equator" being divided into eight equal cycles of sinusoidal potential activity. These waves are shown in Figure 4.43, where we are looking down at the top of the head. The equation describing these waves is:

$$V_8(\theta, \phi) = V_8(\theta, \pi/2) = V_{o8} \sin(\theta/8) \qquad 4.90$$

θ is measured in radians, and V_8 is shown as a radial displacement from the circle's circumference The angular period of the V_8 equatorial wave is $\Theta = 2\pi/8$ radians, and its spherical spatial frequency is 8 radians/radian. Note that the electrode spacing for the 128-electrode array is ca. 2.9 cm, which subtends an angle of $\theta = \tan^{-1}(2.9/9) = 0.312$ radians. The angular period of the n = 8 spherical harmonic is 0.785 radians. The spatial Nyquist period for the n = 8 wave is 0.393 radians, so, while theoretically not aliased, the reconstruction fidelity of the n = 8 spherical sinewave is poor, giving credibility to the authors' observation that the n = 9 spherical harmonic was badly aliased.

Srinavasan et al. point out that the four-volume conductor layers formed by the meninges, the cerebrospinal fluid, the skull and the scalp, act as a spatial low-pass filter to spatial waveforms present on the surface of the cortex (the electrocortico-gram). This low-pass filter has an approximately Gaussian shape. Its transfer function magnitude is down to ca. 50% of the attenuation at the first spherical harmonic at the second spherical harmonic (n = 2), and is down to 5% of the first harmonic attenuation at n = 6. For n ≥ 7, the spatial filter transmission is < 5%. Thus, the four head layers act as a built-in spatial anti-aliasing filter with gradual high spatial frequency attenuation.

The 128-electrode scalp array allows a 2-D computer interpolation and recon-struction of the EEG potentials at all points on the head. This allows researchers to localize sites of activity (or inactivity) on the underlying cerebral cortex that are task- or situation-specific. It should make the localization of CNS pathologies easier.

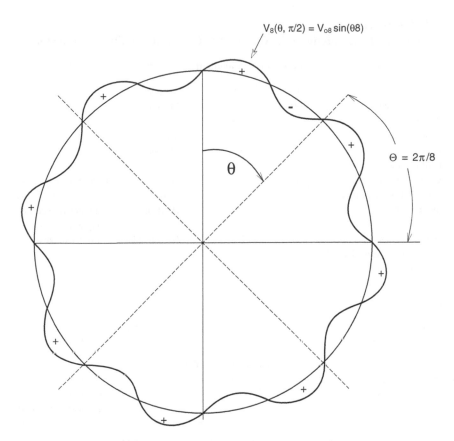

FIGURE 4.43 A spatial sinusoidal distribution of voltage shown on the "equator" of the head hemisphere model. Instead of x, we use the angular coordinate θ.

4.6.5 EEG AMPLIFIERS, INTERFACES AND SIGNAL PROCESSING

Modern EEG signal conditioners used on human subjects generally use very high-gain, low-noise, and high-input impedance RC amplifiers that have adjustable high-pass and low-pass filters to define the system bandpass. For example, the signal conditioners in the Teledyne Electronic Technologies TET-MD S3200 32-electrode EEG system have the following properties:

The EGI Net Amps® intended for use with the Geodesic Net® EEG electrode system have the following properties: input impedance, 200 Megohm; bandwidth, 0.01 Hz to 400 Hz; gain, 10^4; wide-band noise, < 1 μVrms; CMRR, 100 dB; IMR, 120 dB. Sample and hold for each channel permits synchronous sampling of all 128 channels. An eight-pole elliptical LPF is electronically adjustable from 0 to 400 Hz. The system uses opto-isolation; breakdown voltage is 1.5 kVac continuous and 2.5 kVac for 10 minutes. (DC bias current is not given.)

TABLE 4.6.5.1
Properties of the Teledyne 32-Channel EEG Signal Conditioning System

Parameter	Minimum	Maximum	Units	Notes
Dynamic range	2.0	5,000	μV ppk	
DC input impedance	100		Megohms	
Electrode dc offset		400	mV	
Input dc bias current		10	nA	
Input voltage noise		3	μV ppk	
Input resolution	0.25		μV	
Amplifier CMRR	90		dB	@ 60 Hz
Saturation recovery time		7	seconds	
Low-pass filter		75	Hz (fixed)	6th order Bessel (no ringing)
High-pass filter	0.3	0,5	Hz (variable)	1st order passive
Programmable gain/channel:		10^4, 5,000, 10^3, 902		
Number of channels:		32		
ADC				
Resolution		16 bit		
Sampling rate:		250	Samples/sec.	
Sample and hold		32		One per channel
Communication Port:				
RS485 protocol	0.5	1.0	Mbps	Baud rate
Double isolation		4,000	Vac	System with primary isolation transformer

Researchers and clinicians recording multi-electrode EEG responses have traditionally examined raw data in the time domain, much the same as cardiologists view multi-trace ECG records. However, the prospect of dealing with 128 individual traces in the time domain is daunting. Using a computer, 128-electrode spontaneous EEG data can be color mapped onto the surface of a sphere or phantom head by various MATLAB® routines developed by EGI. Colors can be chosen so deep red represents areas having high positive instantaneous EEG voltage, orange is for less positive scalp voltage, through yellow, green, blue to purple for high negative voltage. Two-dimensional time-frequency analysis can also be done in which a 2-D discrete root power density spectrum is calculated from the spatio-temporal sampled EEG, $V(t, \theta, \phi)$, i.e., $\sqrt{S_v(t, u, v)}$ rmsV/$\sqrt{rad/rad}$. Also, simple 1-D cross-correlation, cross-power spectra and coherence functions can be calculated from signals from pairs of electrodes to demonstrate functional connectivity between different parts of the brain.

It is also theoretically possible to calculate a *vector EEG* (analogous to a vector ECG) by adding the potentials recorded at each electrode vectorially. Here, $\mathbf{i}_k$ is a unit vector projecting from the center (origin) of the equivalent head hemisphere to the kth electrode site on the hemisphere surface at $\{\theta_k, \phi_k\}$. Altogether, there are N = 128 equally spaced electrode sites on the hemisphere's surface. Thus, the net EEG (dipole) vector can be written:

$$V_v\left(t, \rho, \theta, \phi\right) = \sum_{k=1}^{N} i_k V\left(t, \theta_k, \phi_k\right)$$ 4.91

The positive tip of vector $V_v(t, \rho, \theta, \phi)$ is scaled to appear inside the sphere as a point of light at some radial distance $\rho = |V_v|$ from the origin. As the EEG changes in time, the point of light will move around inside the sphere, its distance from the origin will be proportional to its magnitude, and its direction from the origin will point toward the region of maximum surface positivity. Unfortunately, unlike the heart, the EEG is composed from the superposition of the electrical activity of millions of pyramidal cells distributed evenly over the volume cerebral cortex. The cortex itself is convoluted and folded. Only a fraction of the pyramidal cells are oriented radially toward the inside of the skull. Pooling all of this diverse activity in one vector sum loses all the detail unique to cortical electrical activity. A vector EEG is probably a bad idea; in this case, it is a misapplication of reductionism. A brain is not as simple electrophysiologically as a heart.

Another approach to interpretive viewing of the EEG is to use the 128-electrode array to plot the electroencephalographic *energy density surface* on the surface of the skull hemisphere. First, 2-D splines or another interpolation algorithm are used to find an algebraic approximation to $V(t, \theta, \phi)$ on the hemisphere. Next, the computer calculates an effective, *charge density* surface, $\rho(t, \theta, \phi)$, at time t from Poisson's equation (Sears, 1953, Ch. 3):

$$\rho\left(t, \theta, \phi\right) = -\varepsilon_o \nabla^2 V\left(t, \theta, \phi\right) = -\varepsilon_o \left[\frac{\partial^2 V}{\partial \theta^2} + \frac{\partial^2 V}{\partial \phi^2}\right]$$ 4.92

ε_o is the permittivity of space (8.854×10^{-12}). Now the product of $\rho(t, \theta, \phi)$ and $V(t, \theta, \phi)$ is the desired *EEG energy density surface*, Ψ:

$$\Psi(t, \theta, \phi) = \rho(t, \theta, \phi) V(t, \theta, \phi) \text{ joules/m}^2$$ 4.93

In recording (averaged) evoked, event related potentials from the scalp, it was found by Montgomery et al. (1997) that energy-density ERPs showed larger differences between target and non-target ERPs in a one-out-of-four discrimination task. They also found that the energy density display modality showed better definition of peak activation than a simple time-averaged EEG. Of course, $\Psi(t, \theta, \phi)$ can be calculated over the hemisphere for any type of EEG voltage distribution, but then, so can the 2-D Fourier transform of $V(t, \theta, \phi)$. Perhaps 2-D T-F analysis will prove useful in interpreting EEGs as well.

4.6.6 EVENT RELATED POTENTIALS AND SIGNAL AVERAGING

Another diagnostic and scientific tool in physiological psychology is the evoked transient EEG response to periodic sensory stimulation. The stimulation can be *visual* (periodic flashes of light or presentation of a figure), *auditory* (periodic clicks or tones), or *tactile* (transient pressure applied periodically to body parts). Other sensory modalities can also be used (pain, heat, cold, odor). Such periodically applied transient stimuli evoke transient electrical activity from the brain; initially from the sensory nerve input nucleii, then from the brainstem, and, finally, from the sensory cortex. These EEG transients, also called event-related potentials (ERPs), are generally small, often around 1µV peak. Thus, ERPs are usually of the same order of magnitude as amplifier noise and noise from muscles (EMGs) picked up by the EEG electrodes. Also, ERP voltages are generally smaller than other unrelated EEG activity seen at the same electrode.

Synchronous signal averaging is used to extract the ERP transient out of its additive noise environment. In synchronous averaging, every time the stimulus is given a short record of ERP plus noise is periodically digitized and each sample is stored in an array of memory registers. Let us assume that k = M = 2048 samples are taken following each input stimulus. As each successive stimulus is given, the sampling process is repeated, and corresponding new samples are added to the summed contents of each array element. This process continues until N stimuli have been given, and N records have been sampled. Then the sum in each of the M registers is divided by N, creating an average in the array. The sample mean for the kth sample of ERP + noise is simply:

$$m_N(k) = (1/N)\sum_{j=1}^{N}\left[e_k + n_k\right]_j = (1/N)\sum_{j=1}^{N}e_{kj} + (1/N)\sum_{j=1}^{N}n_{kj} \quad (k = 1...M) \quad 4.94$$

Now we assume that the noise has zero mean and some ms value, sic:

$$E\{n_{kj}\} \equiv 0 \qquad\qquad\qquad 4.95A$$

$$E\{n_{kj}^2\} \equiv \sigma_{nk}^2 \text{ , (the noise is nonstationary).} \qquad\qquad 4.95B$$

Also, the signal is characterized by:

$$E\{s_{kj}\} \equiv \overline{s_k} \qquad\qquad\qquad 4.96A$$

$$E\{s_{kj}^2\} \equiv \sigma_{sk}^2 + \left(\overline{s_k}\right)^2 \qquad\qquad\qquad 4.96B$$

Equations 4.96A and B tell us that the ERP differs slightly from stimulus to stimulus. We are now interested in the improvement in SNR ratio between the averager's output and its input. The mean-squared (ms) SNR at the averager input is:

$$SNR_{in} = \frac{\text{ms Signal}}{\text{ms Noise}} = \frac{\sigma_{sk}^2 + \overline{s_k}^2}{\sigma_{nk}^2}, \quad k = 1...M \qquad\qquad 4.97$$

It is easy to show that the *ms Signal output* is:

$$S_o = \sigma_{sk}^2/N + \overline{s_k^2} \quad \text{mean - squared volts} \qquad 4.98$$

The *MS Noise output* can be shown to be:

$$N_o = [\sigma_{sk}{}^2 + \sigma_{nk}{}^2]/N \quad \text{mean-squared volts} \qquad 4.99$$

Thus, the ms output SNR is:

$$\text{SNR}_{out} = \frac{\sigma_{sk}^2/N + \overline{s_k^2}}{\left[\sigma_{sk}^2 + \sigma_{nk}^2\right]/N} = \frac{\sigma_{sk}^2 + N\,\overline{s_k^2}}{\left[\sigma_{sk}^2 + \sigma_{nk}^2\right]} \qquad 4.100$$

Also, if the signal is deterministic, $\sigma_{sk}^2 \to 0$, and the msSNR$_{out}$ increases linearly with N. But life is not that easy. All signal averagers have some inherent built-in noise that we can assume appears at their output such that $N_o = [\sigma_{sk}^2 + \sigma_{nk}^2]/N + \sigma_A^2$. With averager noise present, the best SNR$_{out} \to \overline{s_k}^2/\sigma_A^2$ as $N \to \infty$.

Figure 4.44 illustrates an ERP recorded using a vertex scalp electrode such as P$_z$ (reference on ear?). An auditory cognition task was used in which a subject was asked to count 2 kHz tone bursts that ocurred infrequently (15% of tones presented) and to ignore 500 Hz tones presented 85% of the time. The tones were binaurally presented at random times at 85 dB for 50 ms. The large ERP at ca. 300 ms was evoked by the two kHz tones to be counted, and the 500 Hz tones gave rise to the lower peak at ca. 250 ms. (It is not known how many responses were averaged.)

ERPs are frequently used in evaluating the effects of psychotropic drugs on the parts of the brain giving rise to the ERPs. That is, ERPs are averaged from each of the electrodes in the array for a normal patient, then for the same patient taking the drug, and comparisons are made. Data can be given as individual ERP time waveforms, or as a 2-D, color-coded, voltage map on the surface of the hemisphere model of the skull. (For a number of examples of color voltage maps, see the Forenap website: www.forenap.asso.fr/forenap.htm).

4.6.7 DISCUSSION

In this section, we have seen that the EEG is an indirect sign of brain activity. The amplitude and frequency of spontaneous EEG changes with the state of consciousness of the subject. By recording EEG over the entire head with a dense electrode array, it is possible to have a computer make a spatial map of the continuous instantaneous EEG over an hemispherical model of the scalp. The spatial EEG map is generally coded by color, e.g., large positive regions are deep red, with decreasing positive amplitudes becoming orange, then yellow. White is zero. Negative potentials range from light green through blue to purple for large negative potentials. These colors provide a heuristic three- to four-bit quantization of the EEG potentials on the scalp surface.

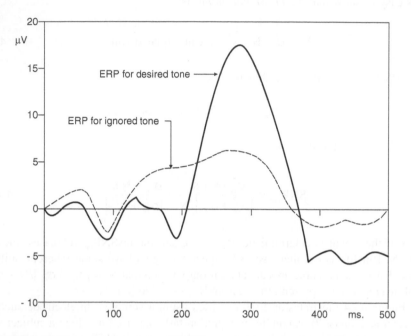

FIGURE 4.44 Example of an averaged ERP recorded from the vertex. The dark trace with the peak at 300 ms. is evoked by the tone to be noted; the lighter trace with the smaller peak is evoked by the tone to be ignored. Random presentation was used.

Event-related potentials provide a useful tool for the investigation of the brain's processing of sensory information. Signal averaging must be used to extract the ERP from the random background noise recorded with it. ERPs are used to test neonates' hearing and vision noninvasively.

Other display modalities for EEG signals are also finding favor. The energy-density plot over the skull surface vs. time is one such mode. Another is the use of time-frequency analysis on individual electrode signals. Pairs of EEG signals can be cross-correlated, and the FFT can be used to calculate their cross-power spectrum and coherence to identify causal connections (Ding et al., 2000). EEGs cannot be used to construct a unique map of brain activity (the inverse problem), because many internal patterns of neural activity can give rise to the same scalp surface potentials (functional ambiguity).

A whole laundry list of diseases and conditions can be diagnosed noninvasively by recording ERPs and spontaneous EEG signals. Some of these include: epilepsy (grand mal, petite mal and temporal lobe), abscesses, tumors, vascular lesions (cerebral infarcts and intracranial hemorrhages), sleep disorders, ingestion of psychoactive drugs, depth of anesthesia. ERPs can be specifically used to investigate how workload affects attention and task performance in the human operator (Goldman, 1987).

4.7 OTHER BODY SURFACE POTENTIALS

4.7.1 INTRODUCTION

The functioning of both nervous tissue and muscle is accompanied by electrical phenomena involving both the generation of electric potentials and the existence of current density in the surrounding volume conductors. The current density is due to the movement of mobile low-molecular-weight ions such as Cl^-, K^+, Na^+, Ca^{++} and Mg^{++} in electric fields and concentration gradients. Electrons, in general, are not involved. The physical and biochemical origins of bioelectric phenomena are more complex than can be covered here. However, it is safe to assert that nerves and muscles exhibit electric (and magnetic) behavior because of the controlled selective passage of ions through gating proteins in cell membranes. The control of trans-membrane ionic currents can be chemical, physical, or electrical in nature. In addition, all nerve and muscle cells possess ion "pumps," which are specialized trans-membrane proteins that expend metabolic energy to transfer specific ions through cell membranes (either in or out, as the case may be) against electric field forces or concentration gradients. In the steady state, the pumps establish resting, steady-state ion concentration gradients across the membrane and some electric potential difference as well. The insides of resting nerve and muscle cells are always negative with respect to the outside of these cells. The action potentials that electrophysiologists record are caused by gated transient transmembrane ion currents (ions moving in response to local electric fields and concentration gradients). The transmembrane currents and pump currents give rise to the observed extracellular current densities and electric fields.

Here we will discuss the sources, medical significance, and measurement of the *electrooculogram* (EOG), *electroretinogram* (ERG), and *electrocochleogram* (ECoG).

4.7.2 THE ELECTROOCULOGRAM

The EOG is used to test the integrity of the retinal epithelium at the back of the retina, as well as certain mid-retinal layers. Active ion transport in the retinal pigment epithelium creates a net dc potential (an effective dipole) from the cornea to the pigment layer; the cornea is normally positive. The EOG is on the order of single mV, and so can be measured with a standard ECG amplifier with gain of 10^3, and bandwidth of 0.1 to 30 Hz. (Actually, what is measured is not the dc potential, but the *change in potential* caused by having the eyes move laterally rapidly from center to left and right.) Special small AgCl electrodes located at the corners of the eye being studied (nasal and lateral *canthi*) are used. A reference (ground) electrode is attached to some remote site such as the forehead or an earlobe (see Figure 4.45). The differential voltage between the corners of the eye follows the approximate rule:

$$V_{EOG} \cong V_o \sin(\theta), \qquad 4.101$$

where θ is the lateral gaze angle measured from the eye's centered position. V_o depends on the state of adaptation of the eye to dark and light, and to the light level.

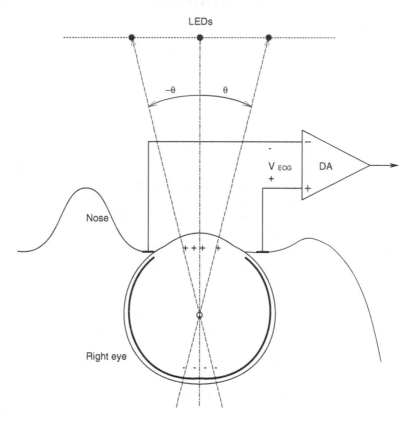

FIGURE 4.45 Schematic coronal section through the right eye and skull showing electrode placement for EOG recording.

The patient is asked to generate gaze saccades of ±30° in response to fixation LEDs that are switched (C, L, R, L, R, etc.) every 1 to 2.5 seconds. The EOG waveform appears as a rounded square wave.

Clinical EOG data can be presented in two forms: 1) The *Arden ratio* (ratio of light peak to dark trough); and 2) *Ratio of light peak to dark-adapted baseline*. The *light peak* is the peak-to-peak EOG waveform for L → R → L saccades with a light-adapted eye given a general uniform background illumination of 35 to 75 lux. The *dark trough* is the peak-to-peak EOG amplitude in response to the same amplitude saccades recorded in the dark for an eye that has been in the dark for 15 minutes. The *dark-adapted baseline* is the saccadic EOG measured for an eye that has been dark-adapted at least 40 minutes. The International Society for Clinical Electrophysiology of Vision (ISCEV) sets the standards for EOG measurement (see http://sun11. uk1.unifreiburg.de/aug/iscev/standards/eog.html).

Figure 4.46 illustrates a record of EOG peak-to-peak amplitudes for dark adaptation and then return to light by using ± 30° saccades. The responses of a typical normal eye are shown by the open circles. The values used to compute the Arden ratio are circled. The dark circles illustrate the typical responses of an eye with severe inherited retinal dystrophy. EOG can also be used in the diagnosis of toxicity affecting vision; substances such as methanol, ethanol, toluene, ethambutol and phenothiazine can be causal in retinal dysfunction.

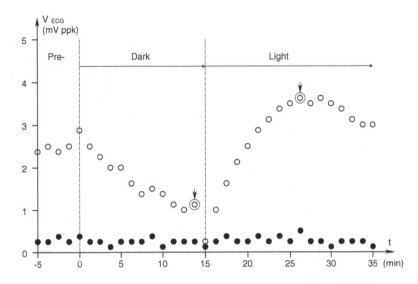

FIGURE 4.46 Record of EOG peak-to-peak amplitudes as a function of time during light- and dark-adaptation. Circles, normal eye; dots, eye with severe retinal dystrophy.

A major disadvantage of the EOG is that the test takes so long (30 minutes to an hour). The ERG, which measures the eye's transient electrical response to flashes of light with no eye movements involved, can often provide more detailed diagnostic information in far less time.

4.7.3 THE ELECTRORETINOGRAM

Figure 4.47 illustrates a horizontal section through the right eye showing how the ERG-recording electrodes are applied. The positive electrode is held on the corneal surface by a saline-filled contact lens. It can be made of a noble metal such as gold or platinum, or be a small, flat AgCl electrode. An AgCl reference electrode is placed on the side of the head near the stimulated eye. A ground electrode is attached to the ear or forehead. In ERG recording, the gaze is fixed to avoid picking up EMG artifacts from the extraocular muscles that move the eyeball. The stimulus is switched on and off (typically on for 5 ms, off for various intervals depending on the test) and the ERG voltage is recorded using a reactively coupled (AC) amplifier. Use of a DC amplifier is indicated if long flashes are used and long-term ERG behavior is of interest. (Direct coupling means that the amplifier will be subject to long-term dc drift and is unnecessary when using short flashes.) Generally, the pupil is dilated with mydriatic eye drops, and parameters such as the flash intensity, wavelength (if

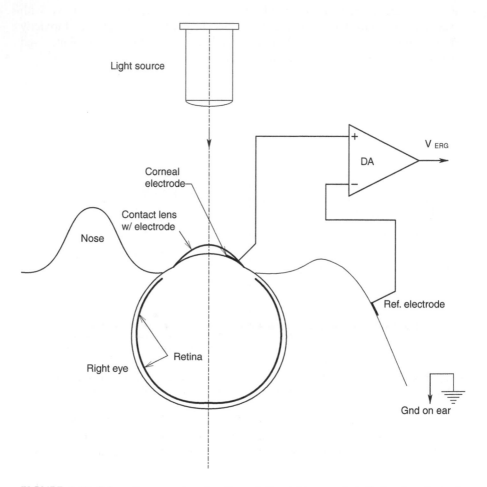

FIGURE 4.47 Schematic coronal section through the right eye and skull showing electrode placement for ERG recording.

cones are being tested), and the state of the dark- or light-adaptation of the eye are varied. The ISCEV gives standards for five types of ERG test:

1. Rod receptor response in dark-adapted eye. (The eyes are considered dark-adapted after 30 minutes in total darkness.)
2. Maximal response of the dark-adapted eye.
3. Oscillatory potentials (in a dark-adapted eye given a short, 5 ms flash).
4. Cone receptor response in light-adapted eye.
5. Flicker fusion response to periodic stimuli (5ms flashes at 30/second).

The ISCEV also gives standards for electrodes and illumination levels. They also recommend that the minimum recording amplifier bandpass be 0.3 to 300 Hz, and be adjustable for oscillatory potential recordings and special requirements; the amplifier's input resistance should be in excess of 10 MΩ. When recording very low amplitude ERG waveforms, dynamic signal averaging is recommended; the average ERG is displayed to the operator as it is collected.

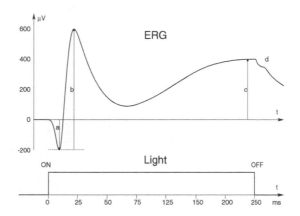

FIGURE 4.48 Typical normal ERG waveform recorded in response to 250 ms flash.

A representative 7000° K, white-light, whole-retina, dc-recorded ERG is shown in Figure 4.48. In reality, there would be noise on the recorded waveform; also, a long-duration (250 ms) flash is shown here. Note that, like the ECG, the ERG waveform has labeled segments that can be related to distinct electrophysiological events among various classes of retinal neurons. The peak-to-peak amplitude of the ERG is lower than the EOG, typically 400 to 500 µV. The fast cornea-negative *a-wave* of the ERG is probably due to the mass hyperpolarization response of the rods and cones to the test flash of light. The a-response is measured from the baseline to the first (negative) peak of the ERG. The positive *b-wave* amplitude is due to the activity of second-order retinal neurons in the middle of the retina, and involves the ionic currents around the Müller (glial) cells. The b-wave amplitude is measured from the negative a-peak to the positive b-peak. The b-wave time to peak is measured from the beginning of a flask to the b-peak. Small *oscillatory potentials* are sometimes seen on the rising edge of the b-wave. Oscillatory potentials most likely originate from the *amacrine cells* for stimulus conditions (mesopic) that elicit both rod and cone responses (Niemeyer, 1995). Parameters used in making clinical evaluations of vision from ERG tests include the a- and b-amplitudes and the b time to peak. When recording oscillatory potentials, the eye is generally dark-adapted. The amplifier band-pass is reset to 75 to 100 Hz at the low end (high-pass filter), and 300 to 1,000 Hz at the high end (low-pass filter). The ISCEV recommends that flashes be given every 15 seconds to dark-adapted eyes and 1.5 seconds apart for light-adapted eyes when studying oscillatory ERG potentials. Peak oscillatory potentials are generally less than 25 µV ppk, so signal averaging can be useful. Flicker fusion studies are usually done on light-adapted eyes at 30 flashes/sec.

To test *macular cones* for areas of dysfunction, such as from laser damage, infection, parasites, or Best's juvenile vitelliform macular dystrophy (Best's disease), a *multifocal ERG* is conducted by flashing a spot a few microns in diameter on and around the macula (e.g., from a laser) in several hundred contiguous locations, and recording the ERG at each location. Signal averaging must be used because of the very small amplitude of the multifocal ERG responses. The responses from the multifocal ERG are used to make a retinal contour map of ERG performance (see Figures 4.49 and 4.50). The high density of normal cones at the center of the macula gives a peak in the averaged response surface, and a pit at the center of a macula damaged by toxoplasmosis (Verdon, 2000).

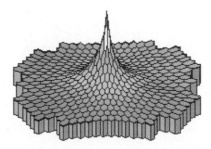

FIGURE 4.49 Contour map of averaged peak ERG responses to a flash of a spot of light from a laser directed at the macula of the retina. The spot is a few microns in diameter. The peak response at the center of the macula is from the high density of cones there.

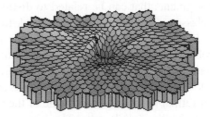

FIGURE 4.50 Contour map of averaged, peak ERG responses to a flash of a spot of light from a laser directed at the macula of the retina. The lack of response at the macula is from retinal damage from toxoplasmosis, a sporozoan intracellular parasite.

It should be stressed that the ERG and EOG do not test vision, they are used as a measure of the functional integrity of the cells in the layers of the retina being illuminated. Some of the retinal diseases that give abnormal ERG results are retinitis pigmentosa, achromatopsia, cone (Best's) dystrophy, cone-rod dystrophies, and congenital amaurosis and night blindness.

4.7.4 THE ELECTROCOCHLEOGRAM

ECoG is a noninvasive electrophysiological test of cochlear function that is used in the diagnosis of Menière's disease, endolymphatic hydrops, and in the differential diagnosis of eighth-nerve neuroma. The ECoG is a transient electrical potential produced by neurons in the cochlea in response to a repeated audio-click stimulus.

The "click" can be a short high-frequency sinusoidal tone burst of about 5 ms in duration; different frequencies are used from 1 kHz or above. For example, a 5 ms burst at 2 kHz will contain 10 cycles. Another way to produce clicks is to stimulate the transducer (usually a miniature headphone) with a narrow dc pulse. The sound produced follows the headphone's electromechanical impulse response; it is a damped sinusoid at the resonant frequency of the headphone. If the pulse polarity is such that the initial displacement of the transducer's diaphragm is toward the head, a *condensation* or compression wave stimulus is said to be produced. A *rarefaction* stimulus occurs when the initial diaphragm movement is away from the head. The ECoG responses are slightly different for each type of stimulus, as shown in Figure 4.51 (Ferraro and Tibbils, 1999). These averaged wave-forms were from a patient with Menière's disease.

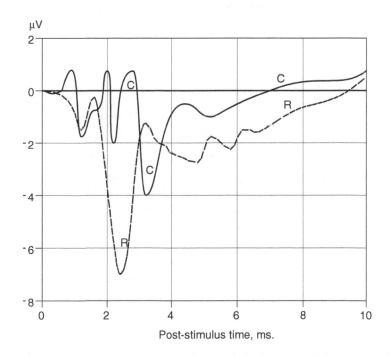

FIGURE 4.51 Averaged electrocochleograms. C is the ECoG resulting from a click that starts with a condensation or compression of sound. R is the ECoG that results when the click starts with a rarefaction. (Ferrara and Tibbils, 1999. Courtesy of *Am. J. Audiology*).

The positive electrode for recording the ECoG can be a small spherical electrode of silver or a noble metal (i.e., Pt or Au) inserted down the ear canal to gently contact the edge of the tympanal membrane (TM). In some ECoG procedures, a fine wire is inserted through the TM and middle ear space to make contact with the round window membrane of the cochlea. Certainly the electrode that touches the outer surface of the TM is less invasive and carries far less risk of infection. The ECoG signal is weaker at the TM than at the round window, however. The AgCl negative electrode is placed on the skin at the back of the ipsilateral pinna, and the ground electrode is placed on the forehead. See Figure 4.52 for a vertical section through the outer, middle, and inner ear, and the recording electrode positions.

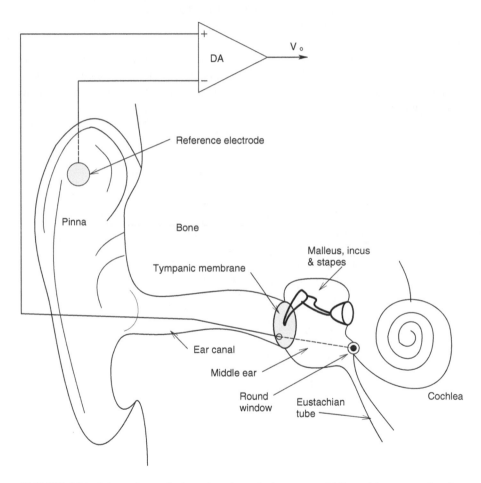

FIGURE 4.52 Schematic vertical section through the outer, middle and inner ear, showing position of ECoG recording electrodes.

The normal ECoG amplitude recorded from the TM is about 5 μV ppk, so signal averaging is required to enhance the ECoG above uncorrelated amplifier and source noise. The ECoG amplifier is reactively coupled (RC) and typically has a mid-band gain of 10^4. The −3 dB frequencies are typically 5 Hz and 3 kHz; 12 dB/octave (two pole) filters are used (Ferraro and Tibbils, 1999). Figure 4.53 illustrates the key parameters used in evaluating the ECoG in the time domain. Perhaps a Fourier transform approach, including Time-Frequency Analysis, might offer some new features that would aid diagnosis.

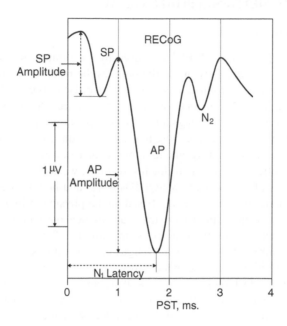

FIGURE 4.53 Key ECoG wave-form parameters used in evaluating the ECoG response.

4.7.5 DISCUSSION

That the eyes exhibit both a dc potential from the cornea to the rear of the eyeball under steady-state conditions of illumination, and transient potential changes for ON and OFF of illumination is not surprising, considering the density of retinal neurons and their physical alignment in the retinal neuropile. The dc or steady-state potential is difficult to measure accurately because of drift in the electrodes' half-cell potentials. Also, the dc potential varies with the state of light- or dark-adaptation, and the intensity of the average illumination. To avoid the problem of dc drift, the dc potential is square wave-modulated by having the subject make precise, saccadic eye movements. This allows the measurement of a square-wave EOG. Thus, a reactively coupled (RC) amplifier can be used.

In the measurement of the ERG, the gaze is fixed, and the transient potential changes in response to flashes of light are recorded with an RC amplifier. Both EOG and ERG are used to detect and quantify diseases of the retina.

The ECoG is another transient potential recorded with an RC amplifier from electrodes on the eardrum and the pinna. Caused by the acoustic stimulation of sensory neurons (hair cells) in the cochlea, the peak ECoG is in the range of single microvolts, and, like cortical-evoked responses, signal averaging must be used to visualize it. It is used primarily in the diagnosis of endolymphatic hydrops or Menière's disease. By recording the acoustic evoked cortical potential at the same time, it is possible to separate the diagnosis of Menière's or other cochlear disease from problems with the eighth nerve or brain.

4.8 THE MAGNETOENCEPHALOGRAM

4.8.1 INTRODUCTION

The magnetoencephalogram (MEG) is caused by the minute magnetic fields produced when ionic currents flow inside the brain as the result of neural activity. The potential differences that produce these currents give rise to the EEG recorded from electrodes on the scalp. Magnetoencephalography, is a true "no-touch" noninvasive recording method because the magnetic sensors used do not physically contact the head. They do, however, need to be close to it. Arrays of ultrasensitive magnetometers called *SQUIDs* (superconducting quantum interference devices) are used to measure the brain's magnetic fields. In the following sections, we will describe the physical and neural origins of the MEG, how SQUIDs work, and how they are used.

All biomagnetic measurements are based on the physical principle that moving charges generate a magnetic field. Classical mathematical derivations of the magnetic field intensity generally assume some constant current, I, flowing in a long, straight wire. Current is simply the number of charges per second passing a plane through the wire's cross-sectional area. In metal wires, current is carried by mobile conduction-band electrons. In biological systems, there are no wires, and current is best thought of as current density, $J(\rho,\theta,\phi)$, in amps/meter^2. Current density is a vector quantity whose direction is the same as the velocity of the $\oplus$ ions drifting in an electric field or responding to a concentration gradient by movement from high- to low-concentration volumes. Current density is also related to the electric field distribution in the volume conductor: $J = \sigma E$, where σ is the effective conductivity of the biological medium (e.g., the brain). In biological tissues, conductivity is also a function of position, i.e., $\sigma(\rho,\theta,\phi)$ Siemens/m.

The major ions that contribute to extracellular current density around active neurons are chloride (Cl^-), sodium (Na^+) and potassium (K^+). To a lesser degree, other mobile ions such as calcium (Ca^{++}) and magnesium (Mg^{++}) can also contribute to a net ionic current density. In densely packed neural tissues such as the cerebral cortex or the retina, when a volume of interneurons is activated by chemical synaptic inputs, the interneurons may be excited or inhibited. Both types of inputs cause certain ions to flow into or out of the post-synaptic neuron's dendrites or cell body wherever the synapses make contact. The passage of these ions through the post-synaptic membranes causes local concentration differences in those ions in the extracellular fluid, and consequent electrical potential changes. These local potential changes and concentration gradients cause the $\oplus$ ions to move en masse in the same general direction, forming a volume current density, $J(\rho,\theta,\phi)$ (in spherical coordinates). Thus, the local current density surrounding groups of active neurons is generally normal to the surface of the cortex (i.e., parallel to the axons of the pyramidal cells), and may have either sign. It is strongest in the neighborhood of the stimulated cells, and tapers off with distance from them. Note that there are about 10^7 neurons under each cm^2 of cortical surface, and two thirds to three quarters of them are perpendicular to the surface (Nunez, 1981a). Note also that the surface of the cortex is convoluted, so that in certain areas the pyramidal cell axes are perpendicular to a tangent plane to the skull; in other areas, their axes are oriented parallel to the plane, and in still other areas, their axes are at various angles to the plane over them. The magnetic field source geometry is very complex.

Refer to Figure 4.54 to examine the geometry of magnetic field production by a solid "tube" (not a wire) of moving charges. We will assume that the charges are chloride, potassium and sodium ions. The net current in the tube can be written:

$$I = A \sum_{j=1}^{N} n_j q_j v_j \qquad \text{4.102}$$

Where: A is the cross-sectional area of the tube, n_j is the number of moving ions of species j per unit volume, q_j is the charge on each of the ions of species j, and v_j is the mean drift velocity of ions of species j. Note that for Cl⁻, both q and v are negative. Also, the current density is just J = I/A. v_j varies for each type of ion.

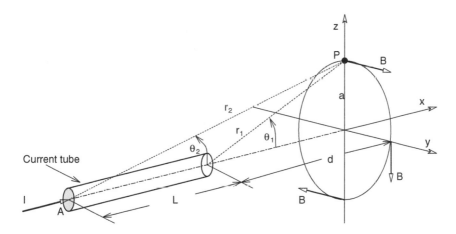

FIGURE 4.54 Diagram of the vectors relevant to calculating the magnetic flux density, **B**, at point P by a finite length current tube.

A differential volume element of the tube is dV = Adx. Using the *Biot-Savart law*, we can write an expression for elements of the magnetic field intensity, dB, produced by dVs of moving charge (Sears, 1953). Refer to the geometry in Figure 4.54.

$$dB = \frac{\mu_o \left[\Sigma \, n_j \, q_j \, v_j \right] Adx \sin(\theta)}{4 \, \pi \, r^2} \qquad \text{4.103}$$

Note that x = a/tan(θ), so dx = $-$ a csc²(θ) dθ = $-$ a dθ/sin²(θ), and sin(θ) = a/r, so r = a/sin(θ). Making substitutions for r and dx, we can finally write:

$$dB = \frac{\mu_o \left[\Sigma\, n_j\, q_j\, v_j\, A \right] \sin(\theta)\, d\theta}{4\, \pi\, a} \qquad\qquad 4.104$$

Integrating, we find the total magnetic field at point P is given by:

$$B = \frac{\mu_o \left[\Sigma\, n_j\, q_j\, v_j\, A \right]}{4\, \pi\, a} \left[\cos(\theta) \right] \Big|_{\theta_1}^{\theta_2} = \frac{\mu_o [I]}{4\, \pi\, a} \left[\cos(\theta_2) - \cos(\theta_1) \right]. \qquad 4.105$$

Note that the tube of current density, **J**, is surrounded by concentric tubes of constant B. **B** at some point P near the current tube is always at right angles to a radial line drawn $\perp$ to the tube's axis to P; its direction is given by the right-hand rule (the thumb points in the direction of **J**, and the fingers curl in the direction of **B**).

It will be obvious to the reader that, by Kirchoff's current law, current cannot flow in the tube and just stop; there must be a closed circuit. What we assume in the derivation above is that the current is concentrated in the tube (i.e., it has a high **J**), and that at the ends it fans out in all directions and disperses in volumes of very low **J**. Thus, the field at a point P is largely due to the high **J** in the finite-length tube.

As an example, let us calculate **B** at point P given the dimensions: L = 2 mm = 0.002 m, d = a = 1 cm = 0.01 m, I = 100 nA. The angles are: $\theta_1 = 45°$, $\theta_2 = \tan^{-1}(0.01/0.012) = 39.81°$. Now

$$B = \frac{4\pi \times 10^{-7} \times 100 \times 10^{-9}}{4\pi \times 0.01} \underset{0.06111}{\left[\underset{0.7682}{\cos(39.81°)} - \underset{0.7071}{\cos(45°)} \right]} = 61.1 \times 10^{-15} \qquad 4.106$$

$$= 61.1 \text{ femto Tessla}$$

Now let us calculate B at a radius a = 1 cm = 0.01 m from the center of the current tube. Now $\theta_2 = \tan^{-1}(0.01/0.001) = 84.289°$, $\theta_1 = (180° - 84.289°) = 85.711°$. Thus B = 1.99×10^{-13} T $\cong$ 200 fT. SQUIDs can resolve time varying magnetic fields on the order of 10 fT.

4.8.2 THE SQUID AND SQUID ARRAYS

A SQUID is basically a low-noise ultra-high sensitivity magnetic field-to-voltage transducer. Figure 4.55A illustrates a basic dc SQUID. The SQUID is the most sensitive sensor for magnetic fields known, being noise-limited by broadband magnetic input noise equivalent to about 5 fT rms/$\sqrt{\text{Hz}}$. At the heart of a low-temperature SQUID is a ring made from niobium (Nb), a period V_B metal that is superconducting at the 4.2° K temperature of boiling liquid helium. One property of superconductors is that they have zero resistance below their critical temperature. Hence, once a current starts to flow around a superconducting circuit, it will continue to flow if left alone.

The ring's inductance is in the nanoHenry range; its two halves are joined with two *Josephson junctions*. Physically, a Josephson junction (JJ) is a very thin (< 3 nm)

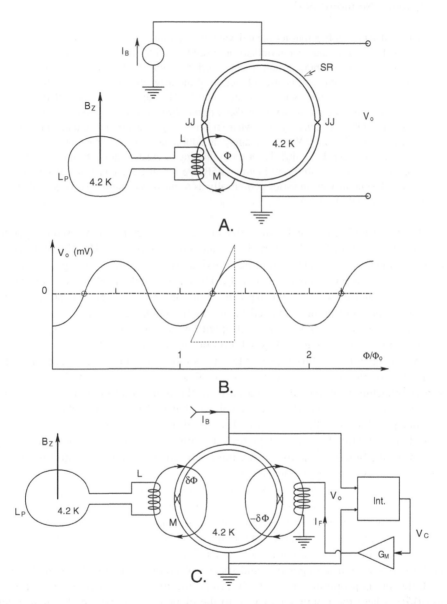

FIGURE 4.55 **(A)** Schematic of a basic SQUID. **(B)** Plot of a SQUID's output voltage at constant input current showing the periodicity as a function of the ratio of the applied flux to the flux quantum, Φ_0. **(C)** A flux-locked SQUID that uses feedback to stabilize its operating point.

film of metal oxide (e.g., Al_2O_3) insulator sandwiched between two superconducting conductors. A JJ is a quantum effect device. Current flowing in the superconductor is carried by *Cooper pairs* of electrons; the Cooper pairs pass through the JJ by *tunneling* (strangely, a dc current can flow through the JJ with zero potential difference across it).

Quoting Northrop, 1997:

"The SQUID is really a four-terminal device; two terminals are used to input a dc bias current, I_B, and the same two terminals are used to monitor the output voltage, V_o. V_o remains zero until the bias current reaches a critical value, I_o. Then the output voltage increases with current, and is also a function of the magnetic flux linking the SQUID ring. The dc bias current is made greater than I_o. The superconducting SQUID ring circuit undergoes the phenomenon of *fluxoid quantization* in which the magnetic flux linking the SQUID is given by $n\Phi_o$, where n is an integer, and Φ_o is the flux quantum, equal to $h/2q = 2 \times 10^{-15}$ Wb. If we apply an additional flux, Φ_i, through the SQUID ring, a supercurrent, $I_S = -\Phi_i/L$ is set up in the ring to create a flux which cancels Φ_i. In other words, $LI_S = -\Phi_i$. From Figure 4.55B, we see that at a constant bias current, the SQUID output voltage varies periodically as a function of Φ/Φ_o." (L is the inductance of the SQUID ring.)

In Figure 4.55C, we see that an active dc feedback current can be used to operate the SQUID as a null-flux detector, also called a *flux-locked SQUID*. The SQUID dc output voltage is integrated, amplified, and used to control a voltage-controlled current source with transconductance, G_M. The current in the feedback coil produces a flux equal and opposite to the input flux, Φ_i, nullifying V_o. By adjusting I_B, the SQUID's operating point is located at one of the open circles in the V_o vs. Φ/Φ_o plot. By using a feedback null mode of operation, the SQUID is given a large linear dynamic range; the flux-locked SQUID output is now $V_C = K\Phi_i$.

A second type of flux-locked SQUID, shown in Figure 4.56, uses a high-frequency oscillator to superimpose an ac flux on top of the net dc flux in its superconducting ring. Any dc deviation from the null operating point produces an ac component in the SQUID's output voltage that is detected by a phase-sensitive rectifier plus low-pass filter (i.e., a lock-in amplifier). The dc output of the lock-in amplifier is integrated, and the integrator's dc output, V_o, is used to set the dc feedback current to the SQUID. The use of the integrator creates a Type 1 control loop that has zero steady-state error (Ogata, 1970).

Note that all SQUIDs are operated with a superconducting pickup coil/transformer circuit that couples the flux from the $\mathbf{B_z}$ source to the SQUID ring. SQUIDs with first- and second-derivative gradiometer pickup coils (also superconducting) are shown in Figure 4.57. Gradiometer coils allow the SQUID pickup to discriminate against flux linkages common to both coils. The *first-order gradiometer* uses two pickup coils wound in opposition and spaced δz apart so that the Φ coupled to the SQUID ring is proportional to $\delta \mathbf{B_z}$. In effect, the first-order gradiometer responds to $\partial B/\partial z$, where the $\mathbf{i_z}$ unit vector is $\perp$ to the plane of the pickup coils. First-order gradients from a magnetic dipole fall off as $1/r^4$, so the first-order gradiometer coils discriminate against distant sources of interference in favor of local dipoles in the brain surface. It also responds more weakly to deep brain current dipoles. Figure 4.58 illustrates schematically how a first-order gradiometer input SQUID can sense the B field from a "current dipole" in the brain. The circle of constant B of radius a provides more flux to the gradiometer coil closest to the skull, hence produces a SQUID output. Flux cutting both coils equally, such as from the Earth's magnetic

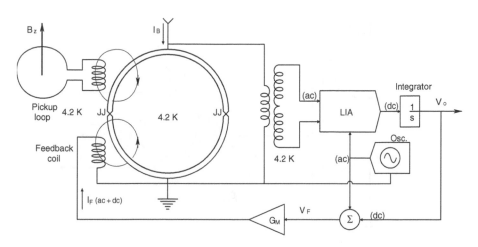

FIGURE 4.56 AC-modulated flux-locked SQUID.

field, produces no output. A three-coil gradiometer responds to $\partial^2 B/\partial z^2$, and is even better at discriminating against non-brain B noise. Note that there can be millions of current dipoles active at once, and because of the way the cortex is folded, some can be parallel to the surface of the skull, such as shown in the figure, and others may be directed radially. The B from the radial dipoles will only be sensed weakly with SQUID coils that are parallel to the skull surface.

To study the MEG in detail, a large array of SQUIDs and their pickup coils, all cooled by liquid helium, are configured in a helmet-like structure that closely surrounds the subject's head. For example, at Forenap, in the Hospital Center of Rouffach, France, a 148-sensor MEG system is used. The Forenap system was made by BTi (Biomagnetic Technologies Inc. (US)). The system is used in a magnetically shielded room supplied by IMEDCO (Swiss) and made from layers of mu-metal and aluminum. There is a −94 dB attenuation of 10 Hz external magnetic interference. The Forenap SQUIDs use simple pickup coils oriented parallel to the head surface (not gradiometers) to record deep brain activity. These coils respond to radial, B_r, from the brain. The average noise level, which sets the resolution of the SQUIDs, is 5 fT/$\sqrt{Hz}$.

The Forenap system claims software that is able to localize source current dipoles to voxels (volume sample cells) a few millimeters on a side. Event-related magnetic field responses are stimulus-induced transient changes in the MEG in a certain brain volume that are seen as a result of averaging MEGs. The Forenap system can only respond to the radial component of the brain's magnetic dipoles (www.forenap.asso.fr/meg1.htm).

A MEG system is being developed at Los Alamos National Laboratory that will use 155 SQUID sensors. They use photolithographically integrated SQUID first-order gradiometer magnetometers with a baselength distance (δz) of ca. 2 cm. The sensor bandwidth is dc to ca. 5 kHz, with 22-bit ADC resolution. The prototype system was tested with a phantom head containing 1.59 mm radius magnetic dipole

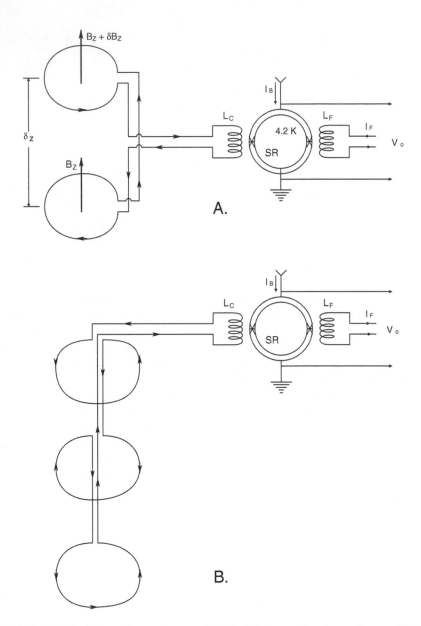

FIGURE 4.57(A) A first-order gradiometer SQUID. (B) A second-order gradiometer SQUID.

coils at various locations and orientations throughout the phantom head volume. The system had SQUID sensitivities better than 10 fT/√Hz (Krauss et al., 1999).

BioMag, the Low Temperature Laboratory at the Helsinki University of Technology has developed a MEG system using 61 dual-channel planar gradiometer SQUIDs having a 16.5 mm baselength (δz) (see: www.biomag.Helsinki.fi/meg.html).

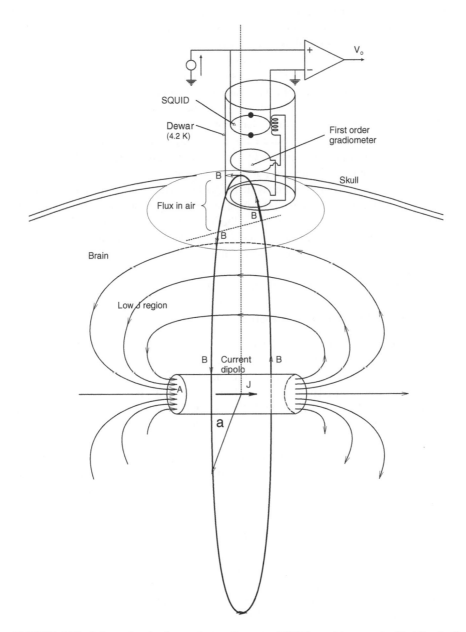

FIGURE 4.58 Schematic of a first-order gradiometer SQUID used to measure **B** at the skull surface.

This system is being used to detect the onset of epilepsy not visible via scalp EEG, as well as a host of other brain studies.

Many university centers and research hospitals around the world (e.g., U.S., U.K., Japan, Korea, Germany, Switzerland, etc.) are developing SQUID MEG array systems — too many to describe here. Three major goals of this research are: Reduce the cost, reduce the noise, and increase the voxel (volume) resolution.

Some of the problems with SQUID arrays for MEG studies is that they are very expensive (> 1 million USD, typically), and they are large, so generally not portable. A SQUID array can consume up to 3 liters of liquid helium per hour, and the patient must be thermally insulated from this cold. The thickness of this insulation forces the SQUIDs' input coils to be set back from the head, decreasing sensitivity. A SQUID MEG system also requires electronics to bias the SQUIDs, operate them under flux-locked conditions, convert the analog signals to digital form, and then process them by powerful computers for display and storage. SQUID MEG systems are not USFDA approved; they are, at the present time, experimental.

An advantage of MEG recording with a SQUID array is that it is truly a noninvasive measurement. Because the data is presented as a shifting color map of neural activity on either spherical surface approximating the head, or as a color volume display in 3-D, interpretation is arty, requiring clinical experience and, generally, simultaneous EEG recording for correlation. As a closing note, the largest experimental whole-head SQUID array for MEG research uses 256 sensors. It was developed by the Japanese Superconducting Sensor Laboratory in 1994 (cf. ITRI, 1998).

4.8.3 OTHER BIOMAGNETIC MEASUREMENTS

While the focus of biomagnetic SQUID research has been the MEG, many other biomagnetic phenomena in the body have also been studied. These include the heart (the MCG), peripheral nerves (MNG), muscles (MMG), the retina, and the smooth muscle of the intestines. The peak B field in the MCG is about 150 pT, about 1000 times larger than the MEG. The fetal MCG is smaller, no more than 12 pT. Skeletal muscles produce about 50 pT when they contract, and the retina of the human eye radiates ca. 5 pT.

While the low level of the MEG requires recording in a magnetically shielded room, the relatively larger amplitude of the MCG often permits its recording without shielding, using a first-order gradiometer in which the farther pickup coil is located on the back over the heart, and the near coil is placed over the heart on the chest. Both coils and the SQUID are bathed in liquid helium. The economy of not using a shielded room is paid for by a background magnetic noise level that requires signal averaging (presumably synchronized with the ECG QRS spike) to obtain a "clean" MCG waveform. Multiple gradiometer SQUIDS can be used to visualize a vector MCG.

Work on the development of a portable high-critical-temperature (Hi-T_c) MCG system is under way at The University of Twente, Dept. of Applied Physics, The Netherlands. An LN_2-cooled second-order gradiometer is being developed to study the fetal MCG using minimum shielding (Rijpma et al., 1999). Another Hi-T_c, SQUID gradiometer was described by workers at Friedrich Schiller University, Jena. In the Hi-T_c SQUID, made from YBCO ceramic and cooled by a four-valve pulse tube refrigerator, rather than LN_2, the gradiometer coils are mounted on a solid sapphire plate, used for a cold heat exchanger. Other non-metallic materials are used in the construction of the measurement head (e.g., hardened paper) to eliminate magnetic artifacts. Results showed an MCG plot of dB/dx in pT/cm, with the QRS spike about 14 pT/cm; 231 averages were used to reduce noise (Gerster et al., 1998).

A research group in China has also reported success in the development of a Hi-T_c YBCO film first-order gradiometer SQUID for MCG application. This gradiometer was planar, i.e., both coils lay in the same 10×5 mm plane. The group recorded the MCG with the sensor about 10 cm above the chest. After 200 averaging cycles, a relatively clean MCG wave was obtained, showing a very small P peak, no Q peak, strong R and S peaks, and a large T-wave (Tian et al., 1999). Finally, we mention the success of a Korean research group in recording the MCG using a novel Hi-T_c SQUID system. This group developed a Double Relaxation Oscillation SQUID (DROS) in the form of a two-coil, planar gradiometer. The overall chip size was 3×4 cm; the coils were square, multiturn, 1 cm on a side, and 3 cm on centers. The DROS had a high voltage transfer coefficient of 3 mV/Φ_0, and unusually low, equivalent-field gradient noise: 2.6 (fT/cm)/$\sqrt{Hz}$ in the white region, and 4.4 (fT/cm)/$\sqrt{Hz}$ at 1 Hz. An MCG recorded with that DROS system is shown in Figure 4.59. Note that only 64 averaging cycles were used to obtain a very clean MCG that closely resembles a conventional Lead I ECG. For details, the interested reader should visit the web site of the Superconductivity Group at the Korea Research Institute of Standards and Science.

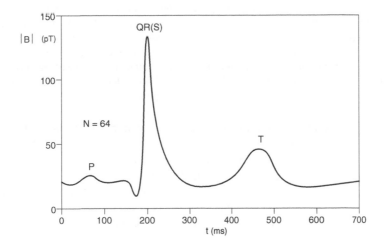

FIGURE 4.59 A typical magnetocardiogram (MCG) recorded with a double relaxation oscillation SQUID. Note the wave-form has the PQR and T features, but is missing the S peak. 64 averages were done.

4.8.4 DISCUSSION

Biomagnetic recording with SQUID arrays is an active area of research around the world. It is a particularly attractive noninvasive diagnostic modality because it is truly "no-touch." The voxel resolution of present MEG array systems is a few mm on a side at the cortex, but decreases to the order of cm in deep brain structures such as the thalamus. Loss of resolution with distance is inherent in the mode of measurement, and although deep resolution will no doubt improve with time, the measurement of the MEG with SQUID arrays is ideally suited for the study of cortical (brain surface) magnetic activity.

In the past few years, the physical size of SQUID gradiometers has decreased, and Hi-T$_c$ SQUID arrays have been developed that work at 77 K temperatures, either with LN$_2$ or special refrigeration units. To eliminate the need for magnetic shield rooms, researchers have made extensive use of first- and second-order gradiometer SQUIDs in recording MCGs. The company CES, of Springfield, Massachusetts, offers a nine-channel MCG3906, system for MCG research that plots 2-D normalized color contour maps of instantaneous cardiac magnetic activity that are useful for diagnosing cardiac muscle ischemia, for example (CES, 1999). Diagnosis from a shifting pattern of colors can be creative, to say the least. CES has developed AI software to approach this problem. Software can reconstruct an equivalent magnetic dipole in the heart and display it, as well. There is great hope for future application of SQUID sensors in MCG. To quote CES:

"One, possibly important, application will be a quick, noninvasive screening of patients coming into a doctor's office or hospital with a complaint of chest pains. Is it the heart, or something else (muscle pain, nerves, stomach)? This is an important problem. Apart from the obvious benefit to a patient, the quick, noninvasive MCG measurement can save thousands of dollars in costs per patient. Indeed, presently chest pains or accompanying symptoms (tightness in the chest, heaviness of the left arm, etc.) are treated as an impending heart attack. No stress test is possible at this point, while the rest ECG is insensitive and cannot be trusted. As a result, such a patient is likely to spend a few days in an intensive care unit of a hospital, attached to a heart monitor, with needles in the veins of both arms, before the definitive diagnosis is made. This is a billion dollar per year problem for insurance companies in the USA."

The CES scenario represents a worst-case situation. Often the ECG or VCG reveals the nature of the problem right away. The acquisition cost for a VCG system is probably one fiftieth the cost of a MCG system. The time required for diagnosis is about the same, however. While ventricular ischemia may be simple to spot on a 2-D color MCG, there are other electrical problems with the heart such as bundle block or pacemaker dysfunction that can often be resolved with ECG and VCG. How easily can they be identified with an MCG system?

4.9 SUMMARY

In this chapter, we have first addressed skin surface electrodes, which are generally of the wet silver or silver chloride type, giving a C-G-R circuit model. Amplifiers are described by their terminal properties, i.e., their input and output circuits; internal electronic circuit details are avoided. Differential (instrumentation) amplifiers and the common-mode rejection ratio are presented, as well as the fact that source impedance unbalance can drastically improve or degrade the amplifier's CMRR.

Also discussed are sources of noise in amplifiers, and how to calculate amplifier noise figure and output SNR. Low noise amplifier design is discussed.

Of all the electrical potentials recordable from the body's surface, the ECG is probably the most widely used because of its effectiveness in diagnosing heart pathologies. The ECG is simply obtained at low cost, as is the EEG. We have illustrated how departure from the simple time-domain ECG display modality to the vector cardiogram in three planes can often aid the diagnostician in locating a specific cardiac pathology.

The SQUID and its use in measuring the minute magnetic fields produced by nerve action currents in the brain are treated in Section 4.8. SQUID measurements of the MEG are generally noise limited, and researchers typically record event-related magnetic field events from the brain by repetitive averaging to improve SNR. Also, the surface of the cerebral cortex is folded in convolutions, hence the neural action currents in the cortex have different directions, causing a complex and often ambiguous vector summation of the B-fields sensed by the SQUIDS. There is probably more information to be realized about the neural activity of the brain from a large EEG electrode array than from a much smaller SQUID array. The magnetoencephalogram, recorded with large arrays of SQUIDs surrounding the head will probably find little clinical diagnostic application. SQUIDs are expensive to run because of the requirement for liquid helium for their superconductors, magnetic shielding, and the difficulty in interpreting their output signals. However, a SQUID system, such as used for MEF and MCG recording, is truly a no-touch instrumentation modality.

5 Noninvasive Measurement of Blood Pressure

5.1 INTRODUCTION

The gold standard for blood pressure (BP) measurement is the *invasive measurement* done by inserting a large-bore hypodermic needle into the desired artery or vein, then coupling this needle with a saline-filled catheter to a physiological blood pressure sensor, generally of the unbonded strain gauge type. Alternately, in a large blood vessel, a catheter can be inserted with a BP sensor in its tip. In this chapter, unless otherwise noted, blood pressure will be synonymous with arterial pressure.

During surgery, recovery, intensive care, emergency procedures, pregnancy, childbirth, etc., it is important to know a patient's blood pressure to detect *hypotension* from excessive blood loss, shock, heart failure, etc., or *hypertension* from head trauma, post-surgical release of renin by the kidneys, preeclampsia, etc. Blood pressure monitoring under clinical circumstances can either be by catheter/ transducer, or noninvasively be performed by a caregiver using a *sphygmomanometer* and stethoscope, or by a calibrated plethysmographic device.

The *brachial artery* in the upper arm is generally used for NI sphygmomanometer measurements of BP. The brachial arterial pressure follows the pumping action of the heart, reaching a peak during systole (contraction of the ventricles), and then falling to a minimum, called the *diastolic pressure*, before it begins to rise again during systole. BP is generally given as two numbers — the systolic (peak) pressure "over" the diastolic (minimum) pressure. BP units are generally given in units of mm Hg, a holdover from the use of mercury manometers to measure physiological pressures in the 19th century. The level of the blood pressure depends on the location of the artery in the body in which it is measured. Generally, the farther from the heart, the lower the arterial pressure. Normal BP is also a function of sex and age. In men, the mean systolic brachial artery pressure is 120 mm Hg at 15 years of age, rising to 140 mm Hg at 65; the mean diastolic pressure rises from 75 mm Hg at 15 years to 85 at 65. In women, the mean systolic brachial artery pressure rises from 118 mm Hg at 15 to 143 mm Hg at 65 years of age; the mean diastolic pressure is c. 72 mm Hg at 15 years and increases to c. 82 at age 65 (Webster, Section 7.29, 1992). A typical brachial BP for a young adult male might be 125/75 mm Hg.

BP is sometimes given as mean arterial pressure (MAP), which is simply the time average of BP(t) measured with a sensor. If BP(t) can be approximated by a triangular waveform with peak at P_{syst} and minimum at P_{dias}, then it is easy to show that $MAP \cong (P_{syst} + P_{dias})/2$.

Because we are interested only in noninvasive BP measurements, we will not cover catheter sensors here. In the following sections we describe how the sphygmomanometer works, and how finger plethysmographs can be used to continuously monitor BP.

5.2 THE CUFF SPHYGMOMANOMETER

More than 100 years ago, in 1896, Italian pediatrician Scipione Riva-Rocci, described his invention of the air cuff sphygmomanometer. Figure 5.1 illustrates schematically how the cuff is wrapped around the upper arm just above the elbow. When the rubber bladder inside the cuff is inflated, it exerts pressure inwardly on the soft tissues of the upper arm. The outer surface of the cuff is restrained by a thick, inelastic, fabric cover. The air pressure inside the bladder and cuff is assumed to be the internal pressure of the tissues under the center of the cuff, surrounding the brachial artery. The veins and arteries are the most compressible and elastic of the arm tissues, because blood can be squeezed axially out of them, allowing them to collapse and not conduct blood at high applied cuff pressure. The cuff's air pressure is measured with either: 1) a mercury manometer; 2) an aneroid pressure gauge; or 3) an electronic pressure sensor. The air is pumped into the cuff by either a rubber bulb pump with a check valve, or, in the case of automatic BP measurement, a regulated air supply. To make a BP measurement, the cuff pressure is slowly released by bleeding air out of a needle valve (manual or automatic).

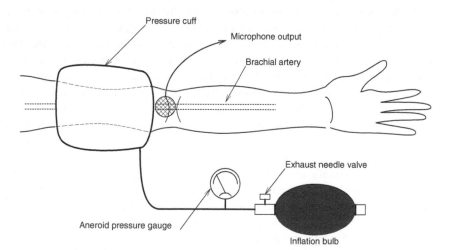

FIGURE 5.1 A sphygmomanometer cuff and Korotkow sound sensor on a left arm. Simple, and state of the art.

Besides the cuff and pressure gauge, the third essential component of a sphygmomanometer system is a listening device to sense the *Korotkow sounds*. This device can be as simple as a conventional acoustic stethoscope or a microphone connected to an amplifier, the output of which causes an LED to flash at every Korotkow sound above a fixed threshold. Still another modification of the cuff method is to place two ultrasound transducers under the cuff facing the artery; a transmitter and a receiver. The ultrasound system is operated in the CW Doppler mode (see Sections 15.2 and 15.3 of this text). The sudden pulsatile opening of the artery at systole causes a large high-velocity transient displacement of the artery's diameter, which is easily sensed as a Doppler frequency shift in the return signal.

The procedure for measuring BP with a sphygmomanometer is to pump up the air pressure to well above that required to collapse the brachial artery under the cuff. The air pressure is then slowly released at c. 2 mm Hg/sec. When it reaches the systolic BP, the BP in the upper artery forces the artery open momentarily, allowing a bolus of blood to flow. This event is characterized by a thump sound in the stethoscope, the first of the Korotkow sounds, which are caused by turbulence and the vibration of the elastic artery walls. The thumps occur at successive systolic peaks, gradually becoming softer and more muffled as the cuff pressure falls. Finally, the muffled sounds disappear, marking the transition to normal blood flow in the artery. The cuff pressure just before this transition occurs is generally taken as the diastolic BP. Because the systolic peaks are periodic transient events, and the cuff pressure is released smoothly, it is possible to miss the exact pressures where the first and last Korotkow sounds occur. Thus, the systolic pressure may be underestimated by 5–15 mm Hg, and the diastolic pressure overestimated by 10–20 mmHg. Also, errors can occur if too small a cuff is used on a large arm. The internal pressure in the arm in such a case is not distributed evenly over a significant length of artery; it is concentrated around one spot. The cuff width should be greater than 0.4 × the limb circumference.

Another approach to BP measurement with the pressure cuff that avoids listening for Korotkow sounds is *oscillometry*. In oscillometry, we make use of the small pulsatile artery transients superimposed on the cuff pressure during deflation. These transient increases in cuff pressure come from the volume of each bolus of blood that passes through the brachial artery pushing against the (almost) static pressure of the cuff. The pressure transients are sensed by a piezo-electric pressure transducer attached to the cuff. This type of transducer produces an output voltage proportional to changes in pressure (dp/dt). The overall cuff pressure and the transducer output are shown in Figure 5.2. The transducer output is amplified and low-pass filtered to remove noise, and then rectified to preserve the positive peaks. The average cuff pressure is also sensed by another dc-reading transducer. Both the average pressure and the positive pulses are sampled and digitized by a microcomputer. The computer measures the largest pulse in the record having voltage, V_m. It then finds the first pulse in the sequence with amplitude $V_s \geq 0.85 V_m$. The pressure when this pulse is found is the systolic pressure. The program then locates the last pulse in the sequence with amplitude $V_d \geq 0.55 V_m$; the pressure when this pulse occurs is the diastolic BP. In the opinion of the author, an experienced clinician is probably just as accurate as the computerized oscillometry system.

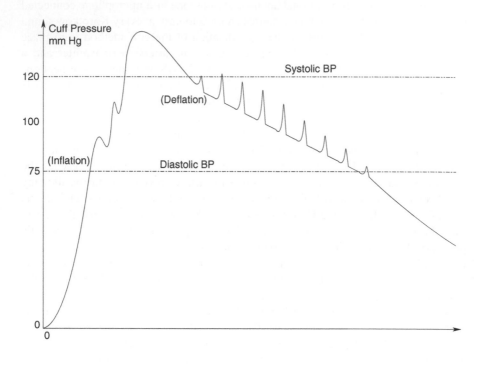

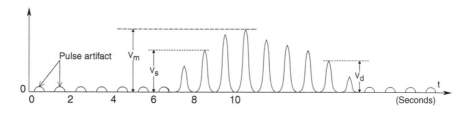

FIGURE 5.2 Upper trace: Sphygmomanometer cuff air pressure showing superimposed pressure oscillations from the brachial artery. Lower trace: Plot of the half-wave rectified derivative of the cuff pressure. The pulses are used instead of the sounds to estimate the systolic and diastolic blood pressure.

5.3 OTHER MEANS OF ESTIMATING BLOOD PRESSURE NONINVASIVELY

A problem with sphygmomanometer measurement is that it does not read the BP in a beat-by-beat manner. It takes a few seconds to inflate the cuff to, say, 160 mm Hg, and then, when in the measuring mode, it takes 50 seconds to bleed its pressure back to 60 mm Hg at 2 mm Hg/sec. Thus, a complete BP measurement can be made in around 1 minute. Continuously using the cuff blocks venous return from the lower arm, which will affect the accuracy of succeeding BP measurements made on that arm.

One way to obtain a beat-by-beat estimate of the systolic BP is to use a finger plethysmograph. In one version of this device, a patient's fingertip is inserted into the finger of a latex glove. The latex-covered fingertip is inserted into a water-filled chamber with zero compliance. The static water pressure is adjusted to some pressure well below the expected diastolic pressure of the patient. Now, as blood flows into the fingertip at systole, its volume increases. This creates a pressure acting on the compliance of the water pressure sensor. The output of the pressure sensor is a voltage proportional to the static water pressure plus a pulsatile component that follows the peripheral BP forcing blood into the finger tip. The fingertip plethysmograph is thus an inexpensive, NI means of measuring the heart rate and the peripheral BP. Since the peripheral BP in the finger is proportional to the brachial artery BP, a simple one-point calibration with a sphygmomanometer allows the fingertip plethysmograph to yield beat-by-beat quantitative BP measurement. Calibration is only valid, however, if the finger position remains fixed in the plethysmograph chamber.

5.4 SUMMARY

Sphygmomanometry is the only effective, accurate, noninvasive means of measuring blood pressure. The only refinement in the procedure, first developed by Riva-Rocci in 1896, is to have a computer automatically inflate the cuff to just above the last known systolic pressure and then release the cuff air pressure at a uniform rate by a servo-controlled valve. The Korotkow sounds are analyzed by a microphone built-in to the cuff. As soon as the last sound occurs, the cuff is rapidly deflated to restore circulation. After a preset pause, the process is repeated. The pressures are stored with times of measurement.

A continuous, noninvasive estimate of BP can also be obtained with a finger cuff plethysmometer. Such devices must be individually calibrated, and are not that accurate. They are more useful for measuring heart rate.

6 Body Temperature Measurements

6.1 INTRODUCTION

The determination of body temperature is generally a noninvasive measurement; a thermometer can be inserted in the rectum, mouth, under the armpit, or in the ear canal. Normal oral body temperature is 98.6° F (37° C), although this value can vary over a 24-hour period due to the person's metabolic state, the degree of exercise being engaged in, and the environmental temperature. Rectal temperature is about 1° higher than the orally measured value. Normal rectal temperatures can vary from 97° F due to prolonged cold exposure to 104° F as a result of strenuous exercise under hot environmental conditions. The body has several adaptive mechanisms (autonomic and behavioral) by which it maintains a relatively constant core temperature. To warm itself and conserve heat, the body may involuntarily shiver, voluntarily engage in aerobic exercise, and control heat loss by regulating blood flow to the extremities. To bring excess core temperature down, peripheral circulation can be increased to act as a radiator (this is effective only when the body temperature exceeds the air temperature), the body sweats, giving evaporative cooling, and the person ceases exercise and seeks shade. If the body cannot compensate for heat loss or gain, life is threatened. For example, prolonged immersion in cold water can result in profound hypothermia leading to death. However, the core temperature can drop to less than 75° F and the patient can still be revived. Prolonged temperatures over 105° F can produce heat stroke and brain lesions, and death is almost certain for temperatures over 110° F (Guyton, 1991).

Elevated body temperature, or fever, is one of the basic diagnostic signs of a severe viral or bacterial infection. A fever normally causes the body temperature to rise to between 100 and 104° F. *Pyrogens* are chemicals that act on thermoregulatory neurons in the hypothalamus to the intrinsic thermoregulatory setpoint of the body, thereby allowing the core temperature to increase. Two strong pyrogens are interleukin-1β (IL-1β) and interleukin-6 (IL-6). IL-1β is released by monocytes/macrophages when they are fighting an infection, notably during antigen presentation to T-cells. IL-1β is a *pleiotropic cytokine*, that is, it has many other diverse stimulatory effects on the immune system besides inducing fever (Northrop, 2000). IL-6 is produced by activated macrophages, T and B cells, endo- and epithelial cells and fibroblasts. It, too, has a pleiotropic role in the inflammation process in infection, and also serves to induce fever. Prostaglandin E_2 (PGE$_2$) is another pyrogen produced in response to IL1 and IL6 in the hypothalamus. Aspirin and other nonsteroidal anti-inflammatory drugs (NSAIDs) inhibit the enzymes that convert arachidonic acid to

PGE_2, and thus reduce fever. PGE_2 may be the substance directly responsible for inducing fever.

Probably the most common means of measuring body temperature is the traditional "shake down" mercury-filled-glass fever thermometer. Two versions exist, one for oral (sublingual) use, and the other for rectal use. An oral thermometer generally has an elongated cylindrical mercury reservoir; a rectal thermometer has a shorter, fatter, Hg reservoir that is mechanically more robust. Both types of thermometers require 1.5 to 2.5 minutes to reach thermal equilibrium with their surround. They are easy to read, and hold their reading until their mercury column is shaken down to below the expected body temperature. Because their principal disadvantage is their slow response time, many electronic thermometers with faster response times and digital readouts have been developed. The sale of mercury fever thermometers is being phased out in many states because of the fear of mercury poisoning if they break.

In the first class of electronic thermometer, temperature is sensed by a change in resistance using a Wheatstone bridge or an active electronic circuit. $\Delta R(T)$ responding devices include both positive- and negative-temperature coefficient thermistors and platinum resistance elements. Themistors have large nonlinear resistance tempcos, and must be linearized over the range of interest, which is from 92° F to 112° F in most clinical applications. Platinum resistance thermometers have smaller, positive-resistance tempcos that are linear enough to not require linearization over the 20° F range in question. Thermistors can be made in small bead configurations, and thus have low thermal mass and heat quickly to the body temperature being measured. (The tempco of a resistor is defined as $\alpha(T) \equiv (\Delta R/\Delta T)/R_o$. Where $\Delta T \equiv T - T_o$. α of metals such as platinum or nichrome is positive; α itself generally varies with T.)

All-electronic, IC, temperature sensors can also be used to measure body temperature. The Analog Devices, AD590 and AD592 temperature transducers are two-terminal current sources that produce 1 μA/ °K outputs given 4 to 15 volts across its body. The current is normally converted to voltage proportional to °C or °F by an op amp transresistor. Although these devices normally come packaged in metal cans or plastic packs, they can be obtained in chip form for custom mounting in a low-heat-capacity enclosure. National Semiconductor also makes an IC temperature transducer; the National LX5600, the op amp is on board, and the voltage output is 10 mV/°K.

6.2 CONDUCTIVE HEAT TRANSFER AND THERMOMETER RESPONSE TIME

A major problem encountered with the classical glass/mercury fever thermometer is the relatively long time required for a steady-state reading. Ideally, to save clinical staff time, a temperature reading should be stable in no more than 5 seconds; 2 is preferable. To gain an appreciation of the physical factors that contribute to limiting conductive heat flow from the body (rectum, mouth) to the actual sensing element (Hg, thermistor, IC) we will examine the dynamics of heat flow from an electrical analog circuit viewpoint.

Heat flows from a warmer mass to a colder mass until the system reaches a thermal equilibrium. In the case of a thermometer, the temperature of the sensor rises until it equals the temperature of the external medium (body temperature, T_b). It is the time course of the rise of the sensor's temperature that we will examine. Intuitively, we know that if the sensor is covered with a thick layer of thermal insulation, such as plastic, it will take longer for the sensor to reach T_b than if a thin layer of a good heat conductor, such as a metal, covers the sensor. Also, if the sensor has a large mass, it will take longer for its temperature to rise to T_b. It is obviously impractical to cover a sensor with metal directly; an electrical sensor would be short-circuited, and, in an expansion-type liquid such as Hg or colored alcohol, the liquid could not be seen. An obvious compromise is to cover the sensor with a thin layer of a chemically inert electrical insulator such as glass or plastic. Thus, the heat from the body must flow through this coating before entering the sensor mass and causing its temperature to rise.

In discussing the physics of heat transfer, we first must examine the units and parameters involved. *Heat* has the units of *energy* or *work,* and can be given in mks Joules, cgs Ergs, gramcalories, kilogram Calories, British thermal units, etc. Note that 1 gm calorie = 4.186 Joules and 1 kg Calorie = 4,186 Joules. The *specific heat capacity* of a material is the amount of heat that must be supplied to a unit mass of the material to raise its temperature 1° C. The specific heat capacity, c, = heat capacity/mass has the units of cal./(gm °C). For example, c for Hg is 0.033 cal./(gm °C) and c for glass is 0.199 cal./(gm °C).

If heat is delivered to an object such as a heat sink at a constant rate, P_i, (note that Joules/second has the dimensions of *power*) its temperature will rise above the ambient temperature until the combined heat loss rates from the object through conduction, radiation, and convection equal the input rate. This steady-state temperature rise ΔT can be written as:

$$\Delta T = P_i \, \Theta \qquad\qquad 6.1$$

In direct analogy to Ohm's law, ΔT is analogous to voltage drop, the heat flow rate, P_i, is analogous to current, and the *thermal resistance,* Θ, is analogous to electrical resistance. The units of Θ are °C/Watt. The thermal analog to electrical capacitance is heat capacity, C_H. In the electrical case,

$$v = (1/C) \int i \, dt. \qquad\qquad 6.2$$

In the thermal case:

$$\Delta T = (1/C_H) \int P_i \, dt \qquad\qquad 6.3$$

If we differentiate Equation 6.3, we can write:

$$P_i = C_H \dot{\Delta T} \qquad\qquad 6.4$$

C_H has the units of (Joules/sec)/(°K/sec) = Joules/°K. Note that C_H = mc, where m is the mass of the object and c is its specific heat capacity. Curiously, there is no thermal analog for electrical inductance, hence thermal systems can be modeled by electrical RC circuits.

In a glass/mercury fever thermometer, the mercury volume expands with increasing temperature at a greater rate than the glass, forcing it into the capillary tube in the thermometer body. When a thermometer at ambient (room) temperature, T_a, is placed under the tongue in saliva at body temperature, T_b, heat immediately flows into the glass and thence to the mercury, causing its temperature to rise toward T_b. After about 2 minutes, the mercury in the bulb has reached T_b, and the reading is stable. In this case, the glass acts as a thermal resistance, Θ_g °C/Watt. We assume that the mercury has a negligible heat loss, and that it has a thermal capacitance, C_m Joules/°C. Thus, placing the thermometer in the mouth at constant body temperature is analogous to a step of voltage applied to a resistance in series with the capacitance of the Hg bulb. The equivalent circuit is shown in Figure 6.1. The temperature of the mercury is analogous to the voltage on the capacitance. This simple series RC circuit has the well-known step response:

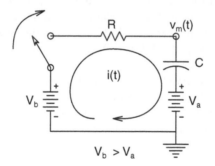

FIGURE 6.1 A simple RC analog circuit describing heat transfer in a glass/mercury fever thermometer. The switch closes when the thermometer is inserted into the body. Voltages are analogous to temperatures.

$$v_c(t) = V_a + (V_b - V_a)[1 - \exp(-t/RC)] \qquad 6.5$$

Note that the voltage source, V_a, in series with C, is necessary to model the mercury being at ambient temperature initially. By analogy, the mercury temperature is given by:

$$T_m(t) = T_a + (T_b - T_a)[1 - \exp(-t/\Theta_g C_m)] \qquad 6.6$$

$(\Theta_g C_m)$ is the thermal time constant of the system. It takes four or five time constants for the mercury to reach $\approx T_b$. Thus, $(\Theta_g C_m)$ is on the order of 20 to 25 seconds for a typical oral glass/mercury fever thermometer. Similar dynamics apply to glass-coated thermistor bead temperature sensors, however. Because the bead has a much lower mass than the Hg and its glass coating is thin, the thermistor thermometer will, in general, respond much faster than the glass/mercury thermometer. Its time constant is on the order of single seconds.

In the case of electronic IC thermosensors, there may be two time constants involved. The heat first must pass through a plastic or epoxy protective coating, and then raise the temperature of the chip substrate, which, in turn, heats the transistors that sense the temperature. Time constants here are typically longer than the thermistor bead but shorter than the glass/mercury thermometer.

In the following section, we examine the theory underlying the operation of no-touch, radiation thermometers that use a pyroelectric sensor to measure surface temperature by using the surface's blackbody radiation. The generic design of this type of radiation thermometer is also given.

6.3 THE LIR BLACKBODY THERMOMETER

6.3.1 INTRODUCTION

The long-wave infrared (LIR) thermometer is an NI instrument that comes very close to being an ideal diagnostic medical instrument. It is completely passive, and requires minimum contact with the body surface for a very short time (about 1–2 seconds) to obtain a reading. Its operating principle is based on the same technology used by IR intruder alarms and light switches. That is, when a sensitive *pyroelectic material* (PYM) is exposed to a surface having a temperature different from its ambient temperature, a minute electric current is generated by the PYM as it absorbs or loses heat to this surface by radiation. The current is converted to a voltage that is a nonlinear function of the temperature difference between the PYM and the surface. In the following sections, we describe the physics of radiation heat transfer, the behavior of PYMs, the electronic circuits required to condition their output signals, and the basic design of the Braun Thermoscan™ LIR ear thermometers.

6.3.2 THE PHYSICS OF BLACKBODY RADIATION

All objects at temperatures above absolute zero radiate heat energy as electromagnetic (EM) radiation. The maximum energy that can be radiated from an object is called *blackbody radiation*. A blackbody (BB) is a theoretical ideal object that is a perfect absorber and emitter of EM radiation. When an object is in thermal equilibrium with its environment, the total energy per unit time (power) radiated by it is equal to the power absorbed. This equality is called *Kirchoff's radiation law*. In general, many objects radiate and absorb more poorly than an ideal BB, such objects are characterized by an emissivity constant, ε, and an absorptivity constant, α. In general, both ε and α can be functions of wavelength λ. Kirchoff's radiation law tells us that $\varepsilon \equiv \alpha$, and $0 < \varepsilon(\lambda) \leq 1$. $\varepsilon = 1$ for an ideal BB; 0.92 for granular pigment (any color); a rough carbon plate = 0.75; oxidized steel = 0.7; polished copper = 0.15. When a beam of EM radiation strikes a transparent object, a fraction is absorbed, a fraction, α_t, is transmitted, and a fraction, α_r, is reflected back. For this situation, Kirchoff's radiation law yields (Barnes, 1983):

$$\varepsilon + \alpha_t + \alpha_r = 1 \qquad\qquad 6.7$$

The distribution of blackbody radiation as a function of object temperature and wavelength has a well-known form derived from quantum theory. *Planck's radiation law* equation is:

$$W_\lambda = \frac{2\pi hc^2}{\lambda^5 \left[\exp(hc/\lambda kT) - 1\right]} \quad \left(\text{Watts}/\text{m}^2\right)/(\text{meter wavelength}) \qquad 6.8$$

Note that W_λ's units are mks, and it is called a *spectral emittance*. In Equation 6.8, λ is the EM radiation wavelength in meters, c = speed of light (3×10^8 m/s), k = Boltzmann's constant (1.3806×10^{-23} Joule/°K), h = Planck's constant (6.6262×10^{-34} Joule sec.), T is in °Kelvin. W_λ is sometimes put in the form:

$$W_\lambda = \frac{c_1}{\lambda^5 \left[\exp(c_2/\lambda T) - 1\right]} \qquad\qquad 6.9$$

Where $c_1 = 2\pi hc^2$, and $c_2 = hc/k$. For mks units, $c_1 = 3.742 \times 10^{-16}$, and $c_2 = 1.439 \times 10^{-2}$. Often, workers use "hybrid" or mixed units for W_λ, e.g., (milliwatts/cm²)/(μm wavelength). The only advantage to using mixed units is that the W_λ scale units at physiological temperatures are simple integers. When these units are used, the constants c_1 and c_2 must be appropriately scaled: $c_1 = 3.742 \times 10^4$ and $c_2 = 1.438 \times 10^4$.

Figure 6.2 illustrates a log–log plot of a family of Planck's distribution curves for ideal BB radiation at different temperatures. Note that, as the BB object's temperature increases, the peaks of the W_λ curves shift toward shorter wavelengths. This shift is called the *Wien displacement law*; it can be derived formally by setting $dW_\lambda/d\lambda = 0$. The peak occurs at

$$\lambda_{pk} = 2897.1/T°K \; \mu m \qquad\qquad 6.10$$

Thus, for a human body at 310 °K, the peak W_λ is at 9.35 μm, in the LIR range.

We can find the total *radiant emittance*, W_{bb}, from a BB in Watts/m² by integrating $W_v \, dv = W_\lambda \, d\lambda$, where $c = v\lambda$. If this is done, we find:

$$W_{bb} = \frac{2\pi^5 k^4}{15\, c^2 h^3} T^4 = \sigma\, T^4 \quad W/m^2 \qquad\qquad 6.11$$

Where $\sigma = 5.662 \times 10^{-8}$, the mks Stefan-Boltzmann constant.

In the LIR thermometer, heat is transferred by radiation from the object whose temperature is being measured (e.g., an eardrum) to the internal pyroelectric sensor element at ambient temperature, T_a. The eardrum may be considered to be at constant temperature because it is well supplied with blood at body temperature, and the middle ear behind it is also at T_b. Thus, any heat lost by radiation from the eardrum to the PYM does not change the eardrum temperature.

Relative spectral emission of a blackbody

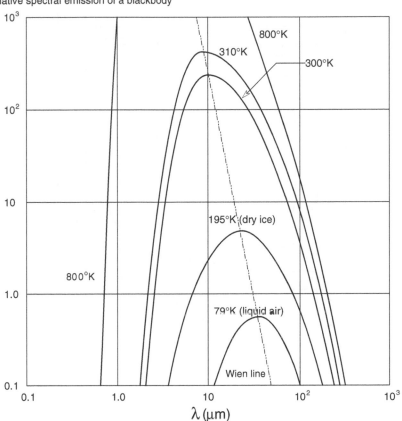

FIGURE 6.2 Log–log plots of the relative spectral emission of a blackbody at different temperatures.

Consider an ideal heat exchange system as shown in Figure 6.3. The surface on the right is the eardrum at temperature T_b. On the left is the PYM at ambient temperature T_a. The conduction lines represent the heat transfer processes taking place at the surfaces and in the space between them. Let H_a be the total *irradiance* from the PYM surface directed at the eardrum. A fraction $a_b H_a$ is absorbed by the eardrum at temperature T_b, and a fraction $(1 - a_b)H_a$ is reflected from the eardrum and returned to the PYM. The *radiant emittance* from the eardrum is $e_b W_b$, so the net irradiance, H_b, to the PYM is (note that $r_b = 1 - e_b$, and $a_b = e_b$, etc.):

$$H_b = (1 - e_b)H_a + e_b W_b \qquad 6.12$$

Congruent reasoning yields:

$$H_a = (1 - e_a)H_b + e_a W_a \qquad 6.13$$

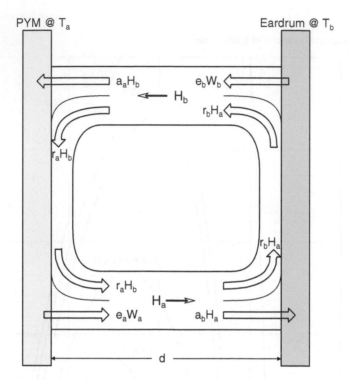

FIGURE 6.3 Heat flow balance between an eardrum and a pyroelectric temperature sensor. Emitted, reflected and absorbed irradiances are shown.

Using Cramer's rule, we solve these equations for the irradiances H_a and H_b:

$$H_a = \frac{W_a/e_b + (1-e_a)W_b/e_a}{(1/e_a + 1/e_b - 1)} \qquad\qquad 6.14$$

$$H_b = \frac{W_b/e_a + (1-e_b)W_a/e_b}{(1/e_a + 1/e_b - 1)} \qquad\qquad 6.15$$

Thus, the net radiant flux into the PYM can be found from:

$$\Delta H = H_b - H_a = \frac{W_b - W_a}{(1/e_a + 1/e_b - 1)} = \frac{\sigma(T_b^4 - T_a^4)}{(1/e_a + 1/e_b - 1)} \quad \text{Watts}/\text{m}^2 \qquad 6.16$$

The net electromagnetic power flux into the PYM is simply $P_i = A\,\Delta H$ Watts. (A is the effective PYM area receiving radiation.) A constant P_i will cause the PYM temperature to rise. However, the BB thermometer is operated with a shutter that allows P_i to reach the PYM for less than a second, so the PYM returns quickly to its ambient temperature, T_a, and is ready for the next measurement in about 8 seconds.

6.3.3 TEMPERATURE MEASUREMENT WITH PYROELECTRIC MATERIALS

Pyroelectric materials are crystalline or polymer substances that generate internal electrical charge transfer in response to internal *heat flow*. The charge transfer can be sensed as a current or voltage change, depending on the kind of electronic signal conditioning associated with the PYM. In general, PYM materials are also piezo-electric; i.e., they also respond to applied mechanical stress by internal charge transfer. PYM sensors include the polymers polyvinylidine fluoride (PVDF) and polyvinyl fluoride (PVF); and the crystalline substances lithium tantalate (LiTaO$_3$), strontium and barium niobate; triglycine sulfate (TGS); Rochelle salt; KDP (KH$_2$PO$_4$); ADP (NH$_4$H$_2$PO$_4$); Barium titanate (BaTiO$_3$); LZT, etc.

PYM sensors are fabricated by taking a thin rectangle or disc of the material and coating both sides with a very thin layer of vapor-deposited metal such as gold, silver or aluminum. Electrical contact is made with silver epoxied wires or pressure contacts. The side of the sensor that is to receive radiation is often given an extra thin rough heat-absorbing coating such as platinum black. This coating maximizes the ratio of absorptivity to reflectivity for the PYM sensor. Because the original Thermoscan™ LIR thermometers were designed with PVDF sensors, we will focus our attention on this material in the following developments.

First, it will be seen that PYM sensors respond only to *change* in temperature. In the thermal steady-state, there is no net internal charge transfer, and no voltage across their electrodes. Thus if a constant input radiation power, P_i, is applied, the sensor's temperature rises to an equilibrium value, $T_a' > T_a$, where radiation and conduction heat losses equal the input power. In general, we can write a heat balance differential equation for the PYM sensor:

$$P_i(t) = C_T \frac{d(T_a' - T_a)}{dt} + \frac{(T_a' - T_a)}{\Theta} = C_T \frac{d\Delta T}{dt} + \frac{\Delta T}{\Theta} \qquad 6.17$$

Where: C_T is the PYM material's heat capacity in Joules/°K, Θ is its *thermal resistance* in °K/Watt, and $\Delta T = T_a' - T_a$. T_a is the starting, steady-state, ambient temperature of the PYM and T_a' is the temperature it rises (or falls) to as a result of absorbing (radiating) P_i over some time T_s. Θ depends on the PYM material used, its configuration, and even how it is mounted. (Θ can be reduced by direct thermal conduction (heatsinking) and by air convection.) C_T is given by:

$$C_T = c \, A \, h \qquad 6.18$$

Where c is the PYM's specific heat in Joules/(cm^3 °K), A is the absorbing surface area in cm^2, and h is the PYM thickness in cm.

If $\Delta T/T$ is small, we can assume that P_i remains constant over T_s. The differential equation 6.17 can be Laplace transformed and written as a transfer function:

$$\frac{\Delta T}{P_i}(s) = \frac{\Theta}{s\,\Theta\,C_T + 1} \qquad 6.19$$

Now the short-circuit current from the irradiated PYM is given by:

$$i_p(t) = K_p A \dot{\Delta T} \qquad 6.20$$

Laplace transforming:

$$I_p(s) = K_p A\, s\, \Delta T(s) \qquad 6.21$$

When Equation 6.21 for $I_p(s)$ is substituted into Equation 6.19, we can finally write the transfer function:

$$\frac{I_p}{P_i}(S) = \frac{s\, K_p A\Theta}{s\Theta C_T + 1} \qquad 6.22$$

K_p is the PYM's pyroelectric constant in Coulombs/(m² °K). Table 7.3.1 gives the important constants of certain common PYMs (note units).

TABLE 6.3.1
Physical Properties of Certain PYMs

Pyroelectric Material	Pyroelectric Coefficient K_p in μCb/(m² °K)	Dielectric Constant $\kappa = \varepsilon/\varepsilon o$	Thermal Resistance Θ °K/Watt	Specific Heat c in J/(cm³ °K)
Triglycine sulfate (TGS)	350	3.5	2.5×10^{-3}	2.5
Lithium tantalate (LiTaO₃)	200	46	2.38×10^{-4}	3.19
Barium titanate (BaTiO₃)	400	500	3.33×10^{-4}	2.34
PVDF film	40	12	7.69×10^{-3}	2.4

Source: Data from Fraden, 1993b; Pállas-Areny and Webster, 1991.

Assume the PYM sensor is at thermal equilibrium at temperature T_a. The radiation-blocking shutter is opened, permitting a *step* of radiation from the warm object at constant temperature T_b to reach the sensor. The short-circuit current is given by Equation 6.22:

$$I_p(s) = \frac{P_{io}}{s}\frac{s\,K_p A\Theta}{(s\Theta C_T + 1)} = P_{io}\frac{K_p A/C_T}{\left[s + 1/(\Theta C_T)\right]} \qquad 6.23$$

In the time domain, this is simply an exponential decay waveform:

$$i_p(t) = (P_{io} \, K_p A/C_T) \exp[-t/(\Theta C_T)] \qquad\qquad 6.24$$

$\Theta \, C_T$ is the sensor's *thermal time constant* that is material- and dimensionally dependent. P_{io} is assumed constant and is given by:

$$P_{io} = A\Delta H = K_s\left(T_b^4 - T_a^4\right) \qquad\qquad 6.25$$

$$K_s = A \, \sigma/(1/e_a + 1/e_b - 1) \qquad\qquad 6.26$$

Now examine the circuit in Figure 6.4. The PY sensor is connected to an op amp as a transimpedance. Note that the equivalent circuit for the PYM can be configured as an *ideal current source*, $i_p(t)$, in parallel with the sensor's electrical leakage conductance, G_p, and its electrical self-capacitance, C_p. $i_p(t)$ is given by Equation 6.24 for a step input of IR power. Let us first neglect the op amp's feedback capacitor, C_F. The output voltage of the op amp is given y (note the direction of i_p):

$$V_o(t) = R_F \, i_p(t) = R_F \, (P_{io} \, K_p \, A/C_T) \exp[-t/(\Theta C_T)] \geq 0 \qquad\qquad 6.27$$

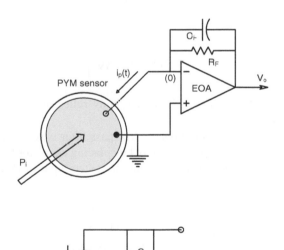

FIGURE 6.4 Top: Current to voltage op amp circuit responsive to PYM sensor short-circuit current. Bottom: Equivalent circuit of a PYM sensor alone. See Equation 6.23 for an expression for the short-circuit current.

The peak $V_o(t)$ is $V_{opk} = R_F \, (P_{io} \, K_p \, A/C_T)$ volts, hence we can calculate the temperature T_b of the warm object from V_{opk} and a knowledge of the system's constants.

$$T_b = \left[T_a^4 + \frac{V_{opk} C_T}{R_F K_p A K_s}\right]^{1/4} = \left[T_a^4 + V_{opk} K_{sys}\right]^{1/4} \qquad 6.28$$

The problem with this approach is that, while V_{opk} is measured fairly accurately, the system's constants and T_a are generally not that accurately known; hence a known BB temperature source at T_{cal} can be used to find the lumped constant K_{sys}.

$$K_{sys} = \left(T_{cal}^4 - T_a^4\right) / V_{ocal} \qquad 6.29$$

Such a BB reference source can be built into the transient radiation thermometer, or be an external BB source, such as the Mikron™ Model 310 blackbody radiation calibration source made by Kernco Instruments, Inc.

Another approach to self-calibration is to keep the PYM at a known T_a, then expose it to T_{cal} and measure the peak V_{ocal}, then expose it to T_b and measure V_{opk}. The computer subtracts V_{opk} from V_{ocal} to form ΔV_o:

$$\Delta V_o = \left(1/K_{sys}\right)\left[T_{cal}^4 - T_b^4\right] \qquad 6.30$$

Solving for T_b:

$$T_b = \left[T_{cal}^4 - K_{sys}\Delta V_o\right]^{1/4} \qquad 6.31$$

Thus, we see that the calculated T_b of the body relies on measurement of ΔV_o, K_{sys}, and known T_{cal}.

To counteract measurement noise, a low-pass filter was added to the current-to-voltage conversion op amp in Figure 6.4 by placing capacitor C_F in the feedback path. With C_F in place, the system response to a step input of IR radiative power, P_i, is:

$$V_o(s) = P_{io} \frac{K_p A / \left(C_F C_T\right)}{\left[s + 1/\left(C_F R_F\right)\right]\left[s + 1/\left(C_T \Theta\right)\right]} \qquad 6.32$$

The inverse Laplace transform of Equation 6.32 can be shown to be:

$$v_o(t) = \frac{P_{io} K_p A}{\left(C_F R_F - C_T \Theta\right)} \frac{R_p \Theta}{} \left\{\exp\left[-t/\left(C_F R_F\right)\right] - \exp\left[-t/C_T \Theta\right]\right\} \qquad 6.33$$

This is a positive waveform that rises with an initial time constant $C_T \Theta$, and falls more slowly with time constant $R_F C_F$. Its peak is proportional to P_{io}. The measurement noise comes from:

- Unwanted mechanical vibration of the PYM sensor which is piezoelectric
- Electronic noise from the op amp
- Thermal (Johnson) noise from the PYM's Norton conductance and from R_F.

The $v_o(t)$ transient that occurs when the shutter is opened, exposing the T_b BB is sampled and A/D converted. The thermometer's resident microcomputer finds the peak $v_o(t)$ and stores it in memory. Similarly, $v_o(t)$ resulting from the calibration source at T_{cal}, is digitized and the peak is found and stored. The microcomputer can then use Equation 6.31 to find T_b.

6.3.4 THE THERMOSCAN™ LIR THERMOMETERS

The original non-contact LIR thermometer design using the transient method of exposing the PYM sensor to the BB surface whose temperature is being measured was patented by Fraden (1989a, 1989b, 1993a, 1994). A full product line of this type of thermometer is currently offered by Braun/ThermoScan™, division of the Gillette Co. of Boston, MA. Figure 6.5 illustrates schematically the basic design of a ThermoScan-type LIR thermometer. The shutter is electromechanical. Accelerating the mass of the shutter vane and stopping it when opening creates mechanical vibrations that are sensed by the piezoelectric PYM, producing an initial artifact output voltage. However, these initial glitches in $v_o(t)$ are ignored by the resident microcomputer, which is programmed to find the peak of the $V_o(t)$ transient some hundred milliseconds after the shutter opens. The peak $v_o(t)$ is less than, but proportional to, V_{opk} as given by Equation 6.27.

In one version of the thermometer, the shutter has three positions: closed, open to the eardrum at T_b, and open to a calibration source at T_{cal}.

Fraden (1993b) shows how the dimensions of the eardrum and LIR thermometer earpiece and PYM sensor affect the BB radiation power from the eardrum absorbed by the PYM. An eardrum is a flat, oval structure with area A_b m^2 maintained at body core temperature, T_b. As a BB, it radiates a total IR power into a solid angle of 4π steradians given by:

$$P_e = A_b \varepsilon_b \sigma \left(T_b^4 - T_a^4 \right) \quad \text{Watts} \tag{.34}$$

Here we assume the surrounding space has an absorptivity of 1, and the eardrum an emissivity of ε_b. Assume that the BB radiation from the eardrum is distributed uniformly on the surface of a (hypothetical) hemisphere of radius R. Thus the irradiance on the surface of the hemisphere is:

$$H = A_b \varepsilon_b \sigma \left(T_b^4 - T_a^4 \right) / \left(2\pi R^2 \right) \quad \text{Watts}/\text{m}^2 \tag{6.35}$$

Assume that the end aperture of the otoscope-shaped thermometer probe is R m from the eardrum. Its opening has an area of A_T m^2. Thus, the thermal power entering the probe is $P_p = A_T H$ watts. Because the internal surface of the probe is polished

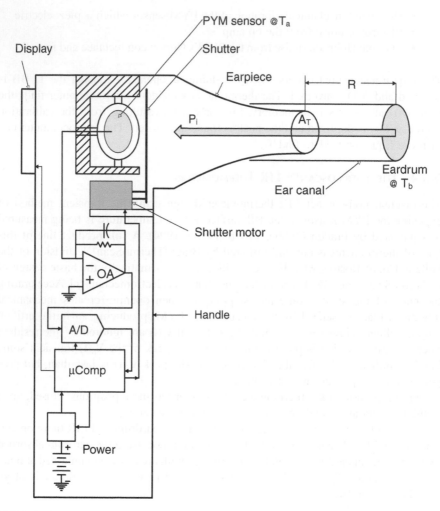

FIGURE 6.5 Simplified schematic of a hand-held pyroelectric thermometer such as that invented by Fraden.

and highly reflective to LIR, we can assume that nearly all the LIR power entering the probe impinges on the PYM sensor.

Thus, the power absorbed by the sensor is:

$$P_i \cong \varepsilon_s \, A_T \, H \text{ Watts} \qquad\qquad 6.36$$

$\varepsilon_s = \alpha_s$ is the emissivity = absorbtivity of the PYM sensor. Fraden (1993) makes the assumptions that $(1 + T_b/T_a) \cong 2$ and $(1 + T_b^2/T_a^2) \cong 2$ to obtain the final approximation:

$$P_i \cong 2\varepsilon_b \varepsilon_s \, A_T A_b \, \sigma \, T_a^3 \, \Delta T / (\pi R^2) \quad \text{Watts} \qquad\qquad 6.37$$

Where $\Delta T = (T_b - T_a)$. It takes about 8 seconds for the PYM sensor in the Thermoscan Model EZ HM3 LIR thermometer to return to T_a and be ready for the next measurement.

Not all of the Braun/Thermoscan LIR thermometers use pyroelectric LIR radiation sensors; the Models PRO 3000 and IRT 3520 use *thermopile sensors* (thermopiles are many dc thermocouples in series) that take 8 readings in 1 second and display the highest reading. They are ready for the next reading in 2 seconds.

The PVDF PYM sensors offer several advantages over thermopiles: they are less expensive, can have large detector areas, are robust mechanically, and are insensitive to moisture. The pyroelectric constant of PVDF is about one tenth of other crystalline PYMs, but for most applications, this is not a problem, certainly not for ear LIR thermometers. Some ear LIR thermometers use polyethelene Fresnel lenses to concentrate the input LIR radiation on the sensor.

6.3.5 DISCUSSION

We have seen that LIR radiation thermometers are complex devices based on a simple principle, that is, infrared blackbody radiation from the hotter eardrum causes a net heat flux to the cooler pyroelectric sensor, which warms slightly. When the sensor warms, a current is generated in proportion to he difference of the two surface temperatures raised to the 4th power. The chief advantage of the LIR radiation thermometer is that it is fast, accurate, and has a digital readout. It certainly is more expensive than a simple glass/mercury fever thermometer, but carries no risk to the patient as does a conventional thermometer if it breaks (broken glass and metallic mercury).

6.4 SUMMARY

Body temperature measurements are really concerned with the core temperature. Body temperature is important in diagnosing fever from infection or heatstroke, or hypothermia from immersion in cold water. It is also useful in predicting the time of ovulation.

Traditionally, core temperature is approximated by use of a glass fever thermometer inserted into the mouth under the tongue, or into the anus. Only in the past ten years has a no-touch radiation thermometer been developed to the point of clinical acceptance. The Thermoscan™ series of instruments was described in Section 6.3. These instruments measure the LIR blackbody radiation from the eardrum, which is richly supplied with arterial blood at core temperature. A Thermoscan instrument's probe (like an otoscope cone) is inserted into the ear canal. Otherwise, there is no contact with the body. Response time of a Thermoscan LIR thermometer is in seconds, vs. minutes for a glass/mercury fever thermometer. There is little chance for error in reading an LIR thermometer because of its digital readout, and no hazard from mercury or broken glass if the thermometer tip should break.

Thermisters and platinum RTD elements are also used to measure body temperature. Like the glass/mercury thermometer, these devices require intimate body contact, but are faster than glass thermometers and slower than LIR radiation thermometers in their response. They, too, have digital readouts. Resistance thermometers are generally less expensive than LIR radiation thermometers because of simpler electronics.

7 Nonvasive Blood Gas Sensing with Electrodes

7.1 INTRODUCTION

The metabolism of all living cells in the body requires oxygen and an energy substrate, generally glucose. As the result of oxidative metabolism, heat and CO_2 are produced as well as regulated molecular byproducts, and O_2 in the blood is consumed. The lungs are the organ in which the external atmosphere interfaces with the body's blood supply; O_2 is taken in and CO_2 is exhaled. The partial pressure of oxygen (pO_2) in an alveolus is typically 104 mmHg. Venous blood entering a capillary in the alveous wall has a pO_2 of c. 40 mmHg. Thus, an initial pressure gradient of $104 - 40 = 64$ mmHg causes O_2 gas to diffuse into the capillary, combine with hemoglobin in red blood cells (RBCs) and be dissolved in the water in the blood. The blood exiting the capillary contains c. 104 mmHg pO_2. All the oxygenated alveolar blood mixes with venous blood from the non-oxygenating tissues of the lungs, bringing the pO_2 down to about 95 mmHg. This is the pO_2 of arterial blood pumped to the body from the left ventricle.

In the peripheral systemic capillaries, oxygen diffuses into the interstitial fluid, which has a pO_2 of c. 40 mmHg. Thus, venous blood returned to the heart and lungs has a pO_2 of c. 40 mmHg. The average pO_2 in the systemic capillaries is about 70 mmHg (blood enters with a pO_2 of 95 and exits with 40 mmHg).

Normally, about 97% of the O_2 carried in arterial blood is combined with hemoglobin molecules inside red blood cells (erythrocytes), and the remainder of the O_2 is dissolved in the plasma. In terms of partial pressures, 92.2 mmHg is carried as oxyhemoglobin (HbO), and 2.8 mmHg O_2 is carried dissolved in arterial blood. The venous blood sent to the lungs under resting (basal metabolic) conditions has about 75% HbO, and a pO_2 of 40 mmHg. Under conditions of intense exercise, the venous HbO can drop to as low as 19% saturation; the interstitial fluid (and venous) pO_2 drops to c. 15 mmHg (Guyton, 1991, Ch. 40).

Any disease or condition that interferes with the normal exchange of gases in the alveoli, the transport of O_2 to the systemic capillaries, the return of CO_2 to the lungs, and the exchange of O_2 and CO_2 in the systemic micro-circulation will give rise to life-threatening hypoxia or acidosis. Section 7.2 describes noninvasive chemical means of monitoring pO_2 in the body. (Note also that Section 15.8 covers *pulse oximetry*, a noninvasive optical technique of measuring the percent O_2 saturation (sO_2) of hemoglobin in the peripheral circulation.)

Also considered in this chapter is the NI transcutaneous measurement of pCO_2 in the peripheral blood, $tcpCO_2$. High blood $tcpCO_2$ is a sign of metabolic acidosis, which can have several causes, including damaged alveoli in the lungs. (Damaged alveoli will also give low tcpO$_2$ readings.) Normal blood pH is c. 7.4. If the pH decreases for any reason, the rate of breathing increases automatically to exhale CO$_2$ at a greater rate, and the kidneys also compensate for elevated acidity in the extracellular fluid by actively excreting hydrogen ions at an increased rate. Thus, another cause of high pCO$_2$ can be kidney failure, in which the tubular epithelial cells actively transport H$^+$ ions from their interiors into the collecting tubes for excretion in urine at a reduced rate. Low blood flow to the kidneys or damaged tubular cells can decrease this normal mechanism for blood pH regulation. High pCO$_2$ can occur normally in exercise, but it drops in minutes due to increased breathing effort and H$^+$ elimination by the kidneys. Acidosis can also result from gluconeogenesis in diabetes mellitus. Here, low intracellular glucose concentration causes liver cells to break down fatty acids to acetoacetic acid and acetyl-Co-A. Acetyl-Co-A is used as an energy source, and acetoacetic acid enters the blood, causing the pH to fall. Although CO$_2$ is not involved directly, the lower pH causes the ratio of pCO$_2$ to [HCO$_3^-$] to increase. Loss of intestinal bicarbonate in severe diarrhea can also cause acidosis, and an elevated pCO$_2$ to [HCO$_3^-$] ratio (Guyton, 1991, Ch. 30).

7.2 TRANSCUTANEOUS O$_2$ SENSING

7.2.1 INTRODUCTION: THE CLARK ELECTRODE

Several methods, given *direct contact* with a blood sample, can accurately measure the pO$_2$ of blood. For a description of these invasive instrumental means, see Webster (1992). In this text, however, we are devoted to examining noninvasive medical instruments, and there is presently only one effective means of transcutaneously measuring peripheral tissue blood pO$_2$. This system is based on the electrochemical *Clark electrode*, first described in 1956 (Hahn, 1998).

The basic Clark electrode can measure pO$_2$ in gases or liquids. It is an electrochemical, polarographic system in which a fixed potential is maintained across the electrodes through which a dc current flows that is proportional to the concentration of the rate-limiting reagent, O$_2$, which participates in oxidation/reduction reactions that take place at the electrode surfaces (oxidation takes place at the anode; reduction occurs at the cathode). A plastic membrane porous to O$_2$ separates the *sample compartment* from the *reaction compartment* (around the electrodes). The reaction compartment is filled with an aqueous buffer solution (at about pH 7), containing chloride ions (which can be from KCl). The O$_2$ that reacts at the electrode surfaces must diffuse in through the membrane from the sample compartment. Figure 7.1 illustrates a cross section through the basic Clark cell. The anode (+ electrode) is a AgCl-coated Ag ring or "washer;" the cathode (− electrode) is the small exposed tip (12 to 25 μm diameter) of an insulated platinum wire. The membrane is typically 25 μm polyethelene or polypropylene. The chemical reactions that occur at the Pt cathode are reductions (Hahn, 1998):

$$O_2 + H_2O + 2e^- \rightarrow HO_2^- + OH^- \qquad\qquad 7.1$$

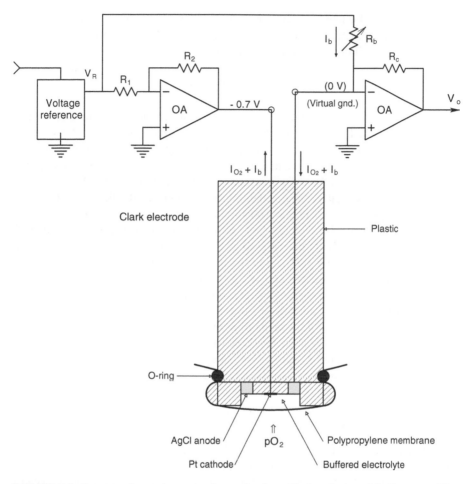

FIGURE 7.1 Cross-section and support electronics for a Clark polarographic O_2 sensor. The left-hand op amp and reference source supply the 0.7 V bias voltage for the cell. The right-hand op amp serves as a current-to-voltage converter. R_b sets dc current I_b to cancel out the zero-oxygen current of the Clark cell.

$$HO_2^- + H_2O + 2e^- \rightarrow 3OH^- \qquad\qquad 7.2$$

$$HO_2^- \xrightarrow{\text{catalytic decomposition}} \tfrac{1}{2}O_2 + OH^- \qquad\qquad 7.3$$

or, as a net reaction:

$$O_2 + 2H_2O + 4e^- \xrightarrow{\text{direct}} 4OH^- \qquad\qquad 7.4$$

The OH$^-$ ions are buffered to maintain neutral pH, and the chloride ions carry charge to the AgCl anode. Four electrons flow for every diatomic oxygen molecule reacted; thus, the Clark cell current at a given temperature is given by:

$$I_C = I_b + K_C \, pO_2 \hspace{4cm} 7.5$$

By U.S. convention, in metal wires, current flows in the opposite direction to electrons. The Clark cell is generally operated at a fixed potential of 0.7 volts; its current is linearly proportional to the pO_2 in the measurement compartment. A small dc *background current*, I_b, flows at $pO_2 = 0$, which is due to ion drift in the electric field between the electrodes. The current vs. pO_2 graph taken with $V_{cell} = 0.70$ V and pH 6.8 is essentially linear, enabling a two-point calibration of a Clark O_2 electrode (at $pO_2 = 0$ and $pO_2 = 160$ mmHg (atmospheric)). The left op amp in Figure 7.1 acts as a 0.7 V voltage source; the right op amp is a low-dc drift FET-input type with very low I_B that is used as a current-to-voltage converter (transimpedance). Its output, after subtracting the background current, I_b, is $V_o = K_C \, pO_2$. The normal tempco of a Clark cell is 2% per degree Celsius, and the linearity is better than 1% over the physiological pO_2 range (Hahn, 1998).

The response time of a Clark cell to a step change in measured pO_2 is largely governed by the thickness of the membrane, but also depends on O_2 and ion diffusion times in the electrolyte. Typical Clark cell response time (time to reach half the steady-state value) is on the order of tens of seconds. For a theoretical treatment of Clark cell response dynamics, see Hahn (1998). Because of the low-pass characteristic of the Clark cell's response, it responds to a smoothed, or time-averaged pO_2.

7.2.2 THE TRANSCUTANEOUS TCPO$_2$ SENSOR

The transcutaneous tcpO$_2$ sensor uses a Clark cell that is internally heated and temperature regulated to operate at a temperature of 40° to 45° C, ± 0.1° when on the skin. The elevated temperature of the Clark cell membrane is necessary to cause vasodilation and reddening of the skin under the sensor. A thin layer of an isotonic aqueous contact gel is placed between the skin and the heated sensor's membrane to facilitate outward diffusion of O_2 from the skin through the membrane. The sensor has built-in thermistors to monitor the Clark cell's electrolyte temperature and the skin temperature under the membrane. The thermistor outputs are used to control the power supplied to a heater coil surrounding the cell.

Initially, transcutaneous operation of the heated Clark cell was found to be effective in babies and small children because of their thinner skin. Unfortunately, because of the delicate skin of infants, prolonged application of a heated sensor can cause second-degree (blister) burns, unless the sensor is moved every hour or so. There is a time × temperature product that must be observed to avoid skin damage. The heated Clark sensor must be given a two-point calibration at its chosen operating temperature before use.

Heated transcutaneous pO_2 sensor systems (the TCM instrument series), made by Radiometer Copenhagen, are sold worldwide. They are used for such applications as monitoring neonatal pO_2 to sense apnea, respiratory distress, etc. They are now also used in adults for applications in hyperbaric medicine, vascular surgery, wound care, and in reconstructive plastic surgery to monitor angiogenesis.

7.3 TRANSCUTANEOUS CO_2 SENSING

7.3.1 INTRODUCTION: THE STOW-SEVERINGHAUS ELECTRODE

The basis for transcutaneous pCO_2 sensing is the Stow-Severinghaus (S-S) electrode, developed in 1957–1958 (Hahn, 1998). At the heart, literally, of an S-S electrode is the glass pH electrode half cell, as shown in Figure 7.2. The half-cell EMF of the glass pH electrode is really two half-cell potentials in series: an EMF is developed across the special tip glass envelope that is proportional to the pH, and the EMF of the internal, AgCl coupling electrode immersed in the 0.1 N HCl internal filling solution. In general,

$$E_{GL} = E_{GL}^0 + (2.3026\ RT/F)[pH] \qquad\qquad 7.6$$

Where pH is defined as $-\log_{10}(a_{H^+}) \cong -\log_{10}([H^+])$, R is the gas constant = 8.3147 joule/(mole °K), T is the Kelvin temperature, F is the Faraday number = 96,496, and 2.3026 comes from converting natural logs to $\log_{10}$. At 25° C, $(2.3026\ RT/F)$ = 0.059156 V.

Interestingly, the pH of the 5 to 20 mM bicarbonate solution surrounding the glass pH electrode is proportional to the negative logarithm of the partial pressure of the CO_2 in the external solution over the range of 10 to 90 mmHg (Webster, 1992, Ch. 10]. First, CO_2 must diffuse from the external test solution into the bicarbonate solution through the Teflon membrane, where the following equilibria occur:

$$CO_2 + H_2O \Longleftrightarrow H_2CO_3 \Longleftrightarrow H^+ + HCO_3^- \qquad\qquad 7.7A$$

$$HCO_3^- \Longleftrightarrow H^+ + CO_3^- \qquad\qquad 7.7B$$

$$NaHCO_3 \Longleftrightarrow Na^+ + HCO_3^- \qquad\qquad 7.7C$$

Adding the equations, we find:

$$CO_2 + \overset{xs}{H_2}O + \overset{Solid}{NaHCO_3} \Longleftrightarrow 2H^+ + CO_3^= + HCO_3^- + \overset{Constant}{N_a^+} \qquad 7.8$$

Note that the constant, a, relating the equivalent concentration of CO_2 gas dissolved in blood to the partial pressure is found from:

$$a = \frac{[CO_2]}{pCO_2} \qquad\qquad 7.9$$

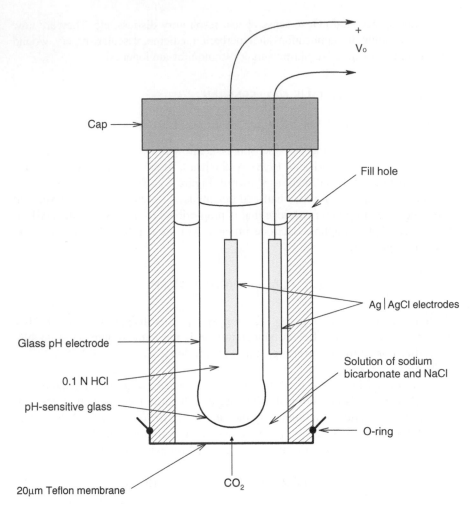

FIGURE 7.2 A Stow-Severinghaus electrode to sense pCO_2. A glass pH electrode responds to the pH of the inner solution, which is shown to be a function of $\log_{10}(pCO_2)$ in Equation 7.14.

a for blood is c. 0.03 (mmol/liter)/mmHg pCO_2. At chemical equilibrium we have:

$$K\{a(pCO_2)\} = [H^+]^2[CO_3^=][HCO_3^-][Na^+] \qquad 7.10$$

K is the equilibrium constant for reaction 7.8. Also, from Equation 7.7B at equilibrium:

$$K' = \frac{[H^+][CO_3^=]}{[HCO_3^-]} \rightarrow [CO_3^=] = K'[HCO_3^-]/[H^+] \qquad 7.11$$

Substituting Equation 7.11 into Equation 7.10, we can write:

$$Ka(pCO_2) = [H^+][HCO_3^-]^2[Na^+]K'$$
  7.12

Taking the logarithm$_{10}$ of terms in Equation 7.12, and noting that pH is defined by $pH \equiv -\log_{10}[H^+]$,

$$\log(Ka) + \log(pCO_2) = -pH + 2\log[CO_3^=] + \log[Na^+] + \log(K')$$
  7.13

or

$$pH = -\log(pCO_2) - \log(Ka/K') + 2\log[HCO_3^-] + \log[Na^+]$$
  7.14

which is of the form

$$pH = -\log(pCO_2) + A$$
  7.15

because Ka/K', [HCO$_3^-$] and [Na$^+$] are constant. Thus a Stow-Severinghaus pCO$_2$ meter computes the pCO$_2$ by exponentiating (pH − A), sic:

$$pCO_2 = B10^{(-k(pH-A))}$$
  7.16

The constants B and k are for display scaling.

Because the pH electrode and the chemical dissociation reactions involved are all temperature sensitive, any application of the Stow-Severinghaus pCO$_2$ sensor *in vivo, in vitro* (with blood), or transcutaneously requires precise temperature regulation to maintain calibration.

7.3.2 TRANSCUTANEOUS TCPCO$_2$ SENSING

The tcpCO$_2$ sensor can be combined with a tcpO$_2$ sensor in the same housing. Such units are described by Hahn (1998) and Webster (1992) and Radiometer Copenhagen offers their model TCM™/3, combined tcpCO$_2$ and tcpO$_2$ monitor. The combined sensor can use the same 0.1 N bicarbonate buffer used in the Stow-Severinghaus pCO$_2$ sensor with the addition of NaCl for the Clark cell electrolyte. Figure 7.3 illustrates the author's version of a combined tcpO$_2$ + tcpCO$_2$ sensor. Note that it uses a common electrolyte and membrane. The entire cell is heated and thermostatically regulated (not shown in figure). The elevated (c. 44° C) temperature causes vasodilation under the sensor and increases upward diffusion of O$_2$ and CO$_2$ through the *stratum corneum* of the skin to the sensor's membrane. The electrometer amplifier used to amplify the pH electrode voltage has an ultra-low bias current (in 10s of fA), and super-high input resistance (c. 10^{14} Ω). Thus, its bias current will be c. 10^{-14} A, which is negligible compared with the 10^{-8} A Clark cell current. OA-2 thus can serve as a virtual ground

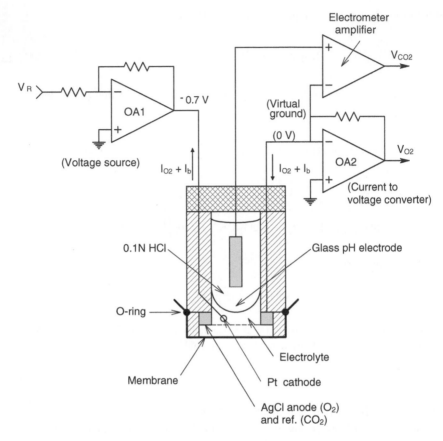

FIGURE 7.3 A proposed combined pO_2 and pCO_2 electrode. OA2 outputs a voltage proportional to pO_2, and the electrometer amplifier outputs a voltage $V_{CO2} \propto -\log_{10}(pCO_2) + A$.

for both the Clark cell and the Severinghaus electrode; its voltage output depends only on the Clark cell current.

7.4 SUMMARY

There are several reliable chemical gas sensors that work well when immersed in blood, *in vitro* or *in vivo,* but only two, as we have seen above, have been adapted to reliable approved nonvasive percutaneous operation.

A wide variety of other sensors work well to sense pO_2 and pCO_2 in the gas phase. O_2 has been sensed by using the fact that it is weakly paramagnetic, i.e., O_2 gas molecules are attracted by a magnetic field, and thus can be separated from N_2, Ar and CO_2 in air. Oxygen's magnetic susceptibility is the basis for several commercial gaseous oxygen meters: The thermomagnetic O_2 "bridge," the Hartmann & Braun Magnos 7G, the differential pressure "bridge," the Siemens Oxymat 5M, the Datex OM-101 differential pressure fast-response O_2 sensor, and the Servomex 1111

Faraday balance type O2 sensor (Moseley et al., 1991). O_2 also can be the rate-limiting reactant in a fuel cell so output voltage is proportional to pO_2, or in a polarographic chemical reaction (e.g., the Clark cell). The speed of sound in O_2 at a given pressure and temperature is different from other gases, and this property has been used to sense the pO_2 in air (Hong and Northrop, 1991). The fact that O_2 absorbs light at 760 nm is the basis for another optical pO_2 sensor using the airpath absorption of light at 760 nm and at another wavelength where O_2 does not absorb, and Beer's law.

A major means of sensing atmospheric (and respiratory gas) pCO_2 makes use of the IR absorption of the CO_2 molecule. Again, two wavelengths are used, one where CO_2 absorbs (e.g., at 4.2 μm) and the other where it doesn't (e.g., at 3.5 μm). Water vapor interferes in some CO_2 IR absorption bands, so CO_2 sensing in respiratory gases requires the gas input to the IR cell to be dried; the drying can be done chemically, or by heating the gas.

Fiber optic (FO) optical sensors have been used to sense pH through the use of a pH-sensitive indicator dye, such a phenol red bound to the surface of 5–10 μm diameter polyacrylamide microspheres mixed with 1 μm diameter polystyrene microspheres for light scattering. The dye and microspheres are enclosed in a small plastic tube permeable only to H^+ ions. One end of the microtube is sealed; the other is joined to two optical fibers (input and output). Phenol red in aqueous solution has an isobestic wavelength at c. 480 nm (wavelength where reflectance is independent of pH). The wavelength at which maximum change in reflectance vs. pH occurs is c. 560 nm. By using these two wavelengths to illuminate the indicator dye and computing the difference in reflected intensities over their sum, pH from 6.1 to 7.6 can be measured (Wolfbeis, 1991). This type of sensor is called an *optrode*. Note that, if this sensor is surrounded by a bicarbonate solution that is separated from the skin by a CO_2-permeable membrane, this pH sensor should be usable to measure $tcpCO_2$. Other indicator dyes have also been used in similar pH optrode sensors. These include, but are not limited to: sulfo-phenolphthalein, bromthymol blue, and bromphenol blue (Wolfbeis, 1991).

Another optrode strategy to measure pH (and possibly pCO_2) makes use of light-induced fluorescence, which is pH-sensitive. In one system, immobilized 8-hydroxy-1,3,6-pyrenetrisulfonate (HPTS) is excited by pulses of 455 nm light. The fluorescence response at 520 nm becomes stronger as the pH goes from 5 to 8. HPTS also has a fluorescence isobestic excitation wavelength at 435 nm. The response here is also at 520 nm, but its intensity does not change with pH. The 99% response time of the HPTS sensor was about 1.7 minutes (to a step change of pH; 6 → 8 → 6, etc.), and its accuracy was c. ± 0.1 pH unit. Other fluorescent pH indicators have also been used: aminofluorescein and 7-hydroxycoumarin-3-carboxylic acid (HCC) (Wolfbeis, 1991). Again, an H^+ permeable membrane serves to isolate the immobilized fluorescent chemical. This type of sensor, too, has the potential for measuring $tcpCO_2$.

It is possible that certain solid-state pH sensors can be adapted to $tcpCO_2$ operation. It is known that silicon oxynitride is pH-sensitive over a large pH range when used as a coating for the gate of a chemically sensitive field-effect transistor

(CHEMFET) (Kelly et al., 1991). A heated membrane would still be required over the skin, but the analyte gas would diffuse into a low-volume bicarbonate solution-filled measurement compartment with which the coated gate of the CHEMFET was in contact.

8 Tests on Naturally Voided Body Fluids

8.1 INTRODUCTION

Naturally voided body fluids obtained noninvasively include urine, saliva, sweat, pus draining from wounds, serum draining from burns, and, for purposes of continuity, feces (arguably not normally a fluid except in the stomach and part of the small intestine). The chemical composition of these substances provides important information that is used in diagnosis of infections, cancer, hormonal diseases (e.g., diabetes mellitus, thyroid diseases, diseases of the adrenal glands, gastrointestinal disorders, liver cirrhosis, etc.). Much diagnostic information can also be obtained from the blood, but unless it is taken from a hemorrhaging wound, its collection is certainly invasive, and therefore its consideration in this chapter is proscribed.

Section 8.2 will describe various instrumental means used in laboratory medicine to measure the concentrations of physiologically important ions used in medical diagnosis. These include, but are not limited to: Li^+, Na^+, K^+, Ca^{++}, Mg^{++}, Zn^{++}, Cu^{++}, Hg^{++}, Cd^+, HCO_3^-· Cl^-, HCO_3^-, phosphates, etc. In addition, in the diagnostic process it is often required to sense molecules such as glucose, urea, specific antibodies, certain steroid hormones, peptide hormones, enzymes, bilirubin, bile, occult blood (from internal bleeding), certain drugs (or their metabolites) used in therapy (e.g., methotrexate, used in cancer chemotherapy, and theophylline used to treat asthma), and drugs used in substance abuse. Specific bacteria can also be sensed by *in vitro* antibody tests, or by surface plasmon resonance antibody reactions (See Section 8.2.4).

Most tests for disorders of blood electrolytes also have counterparts in the noninvasive measurement of ions in the urine and urine flow rate. The kidneys, the loops of Henle and the collecting ducts serve as hormonally controlled regulators for blood volume, blood osmotic pressure (blood sodium ion concentration), blood potassium ion concentration, and blood calcium ion concentration. Thus, the urine volume and its ionic concentrations reflect the selective filtering actions of the kidneys. Section 8.3 describes necessary (but not sufficient) diagnostic signs based on measurement of urine electrolytes, glucose, proteins, enzymes, etc. Analysis of the feces, described in Section 8.4, aids the diagnosis of GI bleeding, endoparasites, gallstones, etc. Section 8.5 deals with what can be learned from the ionic concentration of saliva, and finally, in Section 8.6, we consider analysis of gases in the breath to detect diseases such as diabetes mellitus, lung infections (possibly cancer), throat infections, sinus infections, gum disease (gingivitis), stomach ulcers, etc. Most breath analysis is by the physician's nose, but modern analytical techniques such as surface plasmon resonance and gas chromatography can provide more-objective measurements and diagnoses.

8.2 INSTRUMENTAL METHODS

8.2.1 INTRODUCTION

In this section we will describe some of the analytical instruments used in laboratory medicine to measure the concentration of physiologically important ions in body fluids, as well as small- and large-molecular weight proteins and other molecules (enzymes, hormones, antibodies, bilirubin, urobilinogen, stercobilins, etc.), as well as bacteria and viruses. Some of the instruments used are exquisitely sensitive and correspondingly expensive (spectrophotometers, gas chromatographs, mass spectrometers), others are amazingly simple (e.g., specific ion electrodes, flame photometry, surface plasmon resonance) and can be adapted for field use.

We begin the description of instrumental methods used in medical laboratory analysis with consideration of dispersive spectroscopy, in which the substance being measured (the analyte) absorbs, reflects, or transmits light at different wavelengths with a characteristic signature.

8.2.2 DISPERSIVE SPECTROPHOTOMETRY

A *dispersive spectrophotometer* has a *monochromator*, which is an optical system that acts as a narrow-band-pass filter for a broadband light source. A monochromator can be made from a prism, a diffraction grating, or two diffraction gratings. The output of a monochromator is a beam of nearly monochromatic light. In an analogy to a tuned RLC circuit, the "Q" of a monochromator can be defined as the ratio of the wavelength at its peak intensity to the wavelength difference defining the points where its intensity is one half the peak. For example, a certain grating monochromator may produce an output beam centered at 600 nm, with a 6 nm half-power width, giving it a "Q" = 100.

At the heart of dispersive spectrophotometry is the interesting property that molecules in solution, (or in the solid or gas states) absorb transmitted light more at certain wavelengths than at others. This phenomenon is the basis for spectrographic quantification of many important biological molecules found in blood, serum, urine, saliva, breath, etc. Dispersive spectrophotometry is used to detect the presence of particular molecules and ions, and also to estimate their concentrations. At the heart of spectrophotometry is the fact that molecules have a total energy that is the sum of several components:

$$E_{tot} = E_{translational} + E_{electronic} + E_{rotational} + E_{vibrational} + E_{other} \qquad 8.1$$

When light at a particular wavelength is passed through a solution of an analyte, the energy from a photon can be absorbed to increase the energy of a molecule in one of its several components. Which component is increased depends on the frequency of the light, ν, in Hz. In general, the energy increase of the molecule is given by:

$$\Delta E = h\nu \text{ joules} \qquad 8.2$$

Where h is Planck's constant: 6.624×10^{-34} joule seconds. Note that the light wavelength is $\lambda = c/\nu$ meters. In the visible region, λ is usually given in nanometers (nm), while in the infrared, its dimensions are customarily in micrometers (μm). Often, molecular transmittance spectra are plotted vs. *wavenumber*, $\xi = \lambda^{-1}$, instead of wavelength. In the IR region, the wavenumber is related to the wavelength by:

$$\text{Wavenumber in cm}^{-1} = 10^4/(\lambda \text{ in } \mu m) = 1/(\lambda \text{ in cm}) \qquad 8.3$$

Table 8.2.2.1 illustrates the ranges of wavelength over which certain forms of photon absorption occur by molecules, and the energy absorption mechanism.

The energy absorbed from photons by molecules can be re-radiated as radio waves, heat (IR), or photons (fluorescence). This re-radiation also provides a molecular signature; however, our concern here is in the details of photon absorption.

Most photon absorption by molecules follows the *Beer-Lambert law,* or simply, *Beer's law.* Lambert observed that each unit length of an analyte through which monochromatic light passes absorbs the same fraction of the entering light power (or intensity). Beer extended Lambert's observation to solutions of an analyte at concentration, C. Stated mathematically, this is:

$$dI = -k C I dl \qquad 8.4$$

Rearranging terms we can write:

$$\frac{dI}{I} = -k C dl \qquad 8.5$$

Integrating, we find:

$$\int_{I_{in}}^{I_{out}} (dI/I) = -kC \int_0^L dl \qquad 8.6$$

$$\downarrow$$

$$\ln (I_{out}/I_{in}) = -kCL \text{ or } \log_{10} (I_{out}/I_{in}) = -(k/2.303) C L \qquad 8.7$$

In describing spectrophotometric spectra, various measures are used: The *transmittance* is defined as $T \equiv I_{out}/I_{in} = 10^{-kCL/(2.303)} = \exp(-kCL)$. T ranges from 0 to 1. Often the *% transmittance* is used; $\%T \equiv 100T$. The *absorbance* is defined as $A \equiv \log_{10}(I_{in}/I_{out}) = -\log_{10}(T) = \varepsilon CL$, where L is the total optical path length through the solution, C is the molar concentration of the analyte, and $\varepsilon = (k/2.303)$ is the *molar extinction coefficient* for the solution. What makes spectrophotometry possible is the fact that ε is a function of λ; it is dependent on atomic bond resonances that are peculiar to the structure of each species of analyte molecule. A is also called the *optical density;* it also can be written as: $A = 2 - \log_{10}(\%T)$.

TABLE 8.2.2.1
Wavelength and Energy Levels in Spectrophotometric Absorption (after Reilley and Sawyer, 1961)

λ range	100–10 cm	10–1 cm	1–0.1 cm	100–10 μm	10–1 μm	10^3–100 nm	100–10 nm	10–1 nm	1–0.1 nm	< 0.1 nm
Type of radiation	radio	μ wave	μwv, FIR	Mid-IR	Near-IR	Visible/UV	Vacuum UV	Vac UV/Xrays	Xrays	γrays
Energy transition	Spin orientation	Molection rotations	Molection rotations	Molection vibrations	Molection vibrations	Valence electron xitions	Valence electron xitions	Inner-shell e⁻ xitions	Inner-shell e⁻ xitions	Nuclear xitions
Photon energy range	1.987 E-25–E-24 J	1.987 E-24–E-23 J	1.987 E-23–E-22 J	1.987 E-22–E-21 J	1.987 E-21–E-20 J	1.987 E-20–E-19 J	1.987 E-19–E-18 J	1.987 E-18–E-17 J	1.987 E-17–E-16 J	> 1.987 E-16 J
Frequency range	0.3–3 GHz	3–30 GHz	30–300 GHz	3–30×10^{12} Hz	30–300×10^{12} Hz	0.3–3×10^{15} Hz	3–30×10^{15} Hz	30–300×10^{15} Hz	0.3–3×10^{18} Hz	$> 3 \times 10^{18}$ Hz

A general-purpose spectrophotometer used for chemical analysis employs a monochromator to generate nearly monochromatic light over a wide range of wavelengths. Early monochromators used a glass prism to break white light into its spectral components and selected the output band with an exit slit. Now, they use one or two *diffraction gratings* to disperse the input source light into its spectral components. The desired narrow range of wavelengths is selected by adjusting the grating angle with respect to the input beam of white light and passing the input and output beams through narrow slits. By adjusting the grating angle and the slits, the spectrum can be scanned from ultraviolet (UV) through the far infrared (IR). Special gratings, glasses and mirror surfaces must be present in monochromators used for far-IR (FIR), mid-IR, and UV. As we have discussed, the quantum physical mechanisms of photon energy absorption by molecules in the UV, visible and IR ranges are different. Thus, depending on the application, different types of spectrophotometers are used. These are generally subdivided into instruments that cover the NIR to FIR wavelengths, and instruments that cover the visible spectrum and UV.

Figure 8.1 shows the architecture of a dual-beam IR spectrophotometer. Note that beam forming is done with gold-plated front-surface mirrors rather than expensive IR lenses. The power from the broadband IR source is divided equally and passed through a reference cuvette and a sample cuvette containing the analyte(s). Emerging power is next chopped by a chopper wheel having alternate mirror, window, and absorbing segments. The chopped IR is then passed through a monochromator that scans through the desired range of wavelengths. The single photosensor thus receives alternating pulses of light, first from the reference path, then from the sample, and finally a "dark" pulse. The spectrophotometer's electronic components store and average each like series of pulses and use this information to compute %T (or A) vs. λ (or wavenumber). An alternate configuration of the dual-beam instrument places the monochromator directly in front of the broadband photon source; two matched photosensors are used. The performance is the same, however. Note that the dual-beam architecture is used for IR, as well as vis/UV applications.

Figure 8.2 illustrates a simple *single-beam spectrophotometer* designed to be used with visible light/near UV. Often, such simple instruments will measure a single analyte using only two wavelengths, rather than examining the whole transmission or absorption spectrum. One wavelength, λ_i, is chosen to be at the *isobestic point*, where the transmission of the sample is the same regardless of the presence of the analyte, and a second wavelength is chosen where the analyte has a strong absorption peak given by Beer's law.

A third and very important category of spectrophotometer is the *Fourier Transform Infrared* (FTIR) *System*. As shown in Figure 8.3, a BB IR source such as a Globar rod is used to generate a continuous broadband IR spectrum given by Planck's radiation law. Collimated radiation from this source is the input to a time-modulate, *Michelson Interferometer*. The interferometer's mirror is periodically displaced by an amount, $\delta(t)$, around a center position, L_2. To understand what happens at the interferometer's output, we must first consider what happens to a *monochromatic input ray* with wavelength λ_1. Assume that the distances L_1 and L_2 are chosen such that there is maximum *constructive interference* at the interferometer output. Thus, neglecting interfacial losses, the output intensity, I_o, equals the input intensity, I_{in}.

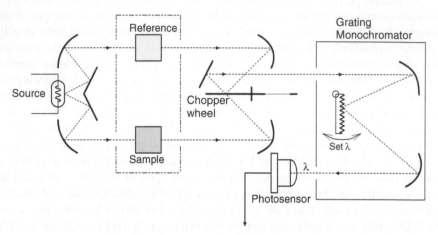

FIGURE 8.1 Schematic top view of a dual-beam spectrophotometer. A single grating monochromator disperses the light before the photodetector; the slits are not shown.

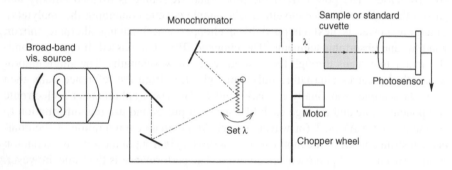

FIGURE 8.2 A schematic top view of a single-beam spectrophotometer. In this design, the light is dispersed and chopped before passing through the sample.

Now let the mirror move $\delta = \lambda/4$ away from the beam-splitter. The light must now travel a total distance of $\lambda/2$ μm more to return to the beam-splitter, where there is now *destructive interference*, and the output intensity has a null. This extra length the light must travel is called the *retardation distance*, ρ. In general, $\rho = 2\delta$. We can write an empirical expression for the output intensity as a function of the wave retardation, ρ, around L_2:

$$I_o(\rho, \lambda_1) = I_{in}(\tfrac{1}{2})\left[1 + \cos(2\pi\rho\lambda_1)\right] \quad \text{Watts} \qquad 8.8$$

In terms of wavenumber, $\xi_1 \equiv \lambda_1^{-1}$, I_o can also be written:

$$I_o(\rho, \xi_1) = I_{in}(\tfrac{1}{2})\left[1 + \cos(2\pi\xi_1\rho)\right] \quad \text{Watts} \qquad 8.9$$

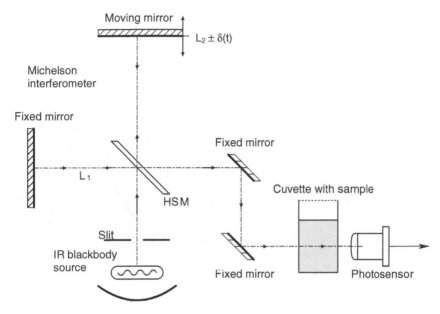

FIGURE 8.3 Schematic of the optical system of a Fourier transform IR spectrophotometer. A Michelson interferometer is used to modulate the transmitted light.

Note that $I_o(\rho, \xi_1)$ is an even function in $\rho\xi_1$. When two other beams having wavenumbers ξ_2 and ξ_3 are added to the beam of wavenumber ξ_1, then the output of the time-modulated Michelson interferometer can be written:

$$I_o(\rho) = \sum_{k=1}^{3} I_{ink}\left(\tfrac{1}{2}\right)\left[1 + \cos\left(2\pi\xi_k\rho\right)\right] \quad \text{Watts, at a given retardation.} \qquad 8.10$$

When this even interferogram function is plotted vs. ρ, we see a strong peak at the origin surrounded by ripple, as shown in Figure 8.4. In the more general case, when the source intensity input to the interferometer is described by a *continuous density distribution* in terms of wavenumber ξ, the interferogram intensity is given by the *inverse cosine Fourier transform*:

$$I_o(\rho) = \int_{-\infty}^{\infty} W_B(\xi)\left(\tfrac{1}{2}\right)\left[1 + \cos\left(2\pi\xi\rho\right)\right] d\xi = I_{Wo} + \int_{-\infty}^{\infty} W_B(\xi)\left(\tfrac{1}{2}\right)\cos\left(2\pi\xi\rho\right) d\xi \qquad 8.11$$

Where $W_B(\xi)$ is assumed to be even in ξ, so $W_B(\xi) = W_B(-\xi)$. Thus:

$$I_{Wo} = \int_{0}^{\infty} W_B(\xi)\, d\xi \qquad 8.12$$

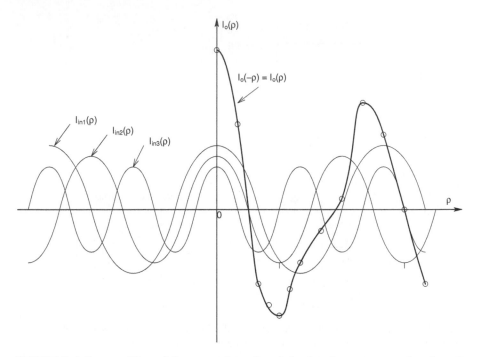

FIGURE 8.4 Superposition of the output intensity of the interferometer as a function of wavenumber and retardation distance, ρ, which is time-modulated. Note that with just three discrete wavenumbers, a peak in the interferogram grows around $\rho = 0$.

The cosine integral can be considered to be the real *inverse* Fourier transform of $W_B(\xi)$.

$$\mathbf{I}_o(\rho) = (\tfrac{1}{2})\mathbf{F}^{-1}\{W_B(\xi)\} \qquad\qquad 8.13$$

Note that, by the Euler relation, $e^{-j\omega t} = \cos(\omega t) - j\sin(\omega t)$, and one definition of the continuous Fourier transform (CFT) is:

$$\mathbf{F}(\omega) = R(\omega) + jX(\omega) \equiv \int_{-\infty}^{\infty} f(t)[\cos(\omega t) - j\sin(\omega t)]\, dt \qquad\qquad 8.14$$

When f(t) is real and even, then

$$\mathbf{F}(\omega) \equiv \int_{-\infty}^{\infty} f(t)\cos(\omega t)\, dt \qquad\qquad 8.15$$

and the continuous inverse FT is:

$$f(t) \equiv (2\pi)^{-1} \int\limits_{-\infty}^{\infty} F(\omega)\cos(\omega t)\, d\omega \qquad\qquad 8.16$$

Where ω is in radians/sec, and $X(\omega) = 0$. Note that we have defined the blackbody radiation density, $W_B(\xi)$ watts/cm^{-1} as an even function in wavenumber ξ. Let ξ be analogous to frequency in Hz, and the retardation distance, ρ, be analogous to time in Equation 8.15. Thus, $F(\omega/2\pi) \to W_B(\xi)$. We see that modulation of the source light's spectral distribution, $W_B(\xi)$, by the Michelson interferometer generates an even, inverse Fourier (intensity) function of $W_B(\xi)$, $I_o(\rho)$, at its output. Sic:

$$I_o(\rho) = \int\limits_{0}^{-\infty} W_B(\xi)\cos(2\pi\xi\rho)\, d\xi \qquad\qquad 8.17$$

Now, if we sample the IFT, $I_o(\rho)$, at intervals $\Delta\rho$, and take its DFT, we recover an estimate of the input BB intensity distribution, $W_B(\xi)$, as shown in Figure 8.5. This $W_B(\xi)$ estimate is stored in the FTIR system's computer memory. (See Section 7.3.2 for a more thorough discussion of BBR.) Figure 8.6 illustrates a typical interferogram as a function of the retardation, ρ.

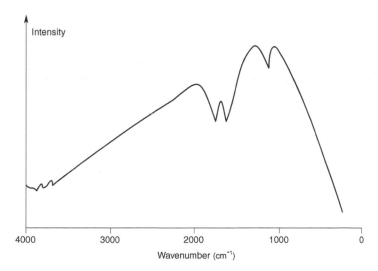

FIGURE 8.5 Plot of the blackbody source's intensity spectrum vs. wavenumber, as determined by taking the Fourier transform of $I_o(\rho)$ given by Equation 8.17.

The next step in the operation of an FTIR spectrometer is to pass the interferometer-modulated IR source radiation through the sample where selective absorption (attenuation) in certain wavenumber bands occurs. Again, as in Equation 8.9, let us look at one particular wavenumber, ξ_1. The intensity of the light emerging from the sample, $I_e(\rho, \xi_1)$ is given by:

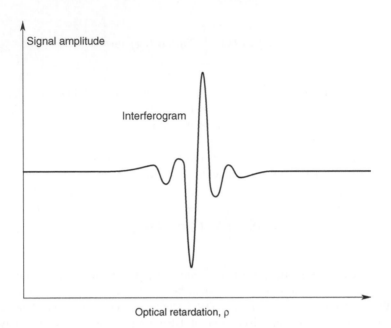

FIGURE 8.6 A typical, continuous interferogram output of the photosensor.

$$I_e(\rho, \xi_1) = I_{in}(\xi_1) T_s(\xi_1) (\tfrac{1}{2})\left[1 + \cos(2\pi\xi_1\rho)\right] \qquad 8.18$$

Where $T_s(\xi_1)$ is the wavenumber-dependent $(0 \Leftrightarrow 1)$ transmittance of the analyte and sample, and $I_{in}(\xi_1)$ is the input intensity at $\xi = \xi_1$. If the input is replaced by the BB distribution, $W_B(\xi)$, we can write:

$$I_e(\rho) = (\tfrac{1}{2}) \int_{-\infty}^{\infty} W_B(\xi) T_s(\xi)\left[1 + \cos(2\pi\xi\rho)\right] d\xi \;=\; I_{ewo} +$$

$$8.19$$

$$(\tfrac{1}{2}) \int_{-\infty}^{\infty} W_B(\xi) \cos(2\pi\xi\rho)\, d\xi$$

Clearly, the "dc" term is,

$$I_{ewo} = \int_{0}^{\infty} W_B(\xi) T_s(\xi)\, d\xi \qquad 8.20$$

and the integral is the *inverse* FT of the frequency-domain product $W_B(\xi)\, T_s(\xi)$. When the output interferogram, $I_e(\rho)$, is DFTd at intervals, $\Delta\rho$, we obtain an estimate of the output spectrum,

$$S_{Sa}(\xi) = (\tfrac{1}{2})W_B(\xi)T_S(\xi) \qquad\qquad 8.21$$

Since we already know $W_B(\xi)$, the desired sample transmittance is easily found by the relation:

$$T_S(\xi) = \frac{2\,S_{Sa}(\xi)}{W_B(\xi)} \qquad\qquad 8.22$$

A high-speed computer capable of calculating DFTs and generating plots of $T_s(\xi)$ and absorbance $A(\xi)$ is a necessary component of an FTIR spectrometer.

We have seen that all spectrophotometers pass light through a cuvette holding the analyte in solution. In some designs, the light is broadband ('white'), and the emergent light from the sample is passed through a monochromator to examine the transmittance or absorbance at particular wavelengths. In other designs, monochromatic light is passed through the sample. In nearly all cases, the light beam is chopped so that phase-sensitive demodulation can be used (equivalent to a lockin amplifier) to improve sensitivity and reject noise. In the FTIR spectrophotometer, the modulation is provided by the Michelson interferometer.

Another mode of operation of conventional spectrophotometers is to measure the wavelength-dependent absorption of back-scattered light from superficial tissue (skin, dermis, capillaries, etc.). This approach is commonly used to measure the percentage of oxygen saturation of capillary blood hemoglobin, and may find application in measuring other blood constituents such as glucose, cholesterol, alcohol, heroin (diacetyl morphine) etc. The measurement of the absorption of back-scattered light is greatly facilitated by the use of an *attenuated total reflection* (ATR) prism, as shown in Figure 8.7. The input light enters the ATR prism and is directed through its bottom surface into the skin (or absorbing sample). The light that is back-scattered from the tissue reenters the ATR prism, and is totally reflected from its top surface, being directed again into the tissue where it is again back-scattered, etc. The repeated reentry and back-scattering of the beam from the tissue increases the sensitivity of the spectrophotometric process by effectively increasing L in Beer's law. Increases in sensitivity of a factor of 20 can sometimes be obtained.

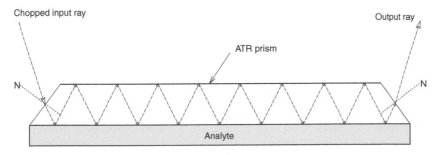

FIGURE 8.7 Side view of an ATR prism or plate. Each time the traversing ray reflects off the interface between the ATR and the analyte, there is selective absorption by analyte molecules in the interface layer.

All sorts of medically important molecules from body fluids can be quantified by spectrophotometry. These include, but are not limited to: cholesterol, steroid hormones, thyroxine, theophylline, opiates, opioids, tranquilizers, etc. Knowledge of a drug concentration in blood or urine can be used clinically to adjust the dosage, and also to detect drug abuse.

8.2.3 Nondispersive Spectroscopy

Nondispersive spectroscopy (NDS) is a chemical analytical method that avoids using an expensive monochromator to quantify a specific analyte. Instead of plotting percent $T(\lambda)$ or $A(\lambda)$ for a sample, and using the resulting peaks and valleys to quantify the analyte, an NDS instrument selects a narrow range of wavelength, $\Delta\lambda$, in which the analyte has a unique peak and valley in its percent $T(\lambda)$ curve. The $\Delta\lambda$ band is generated by passing broadband light through a band-pass filter made from one or more *interference filters*. Figure 8.8 illustrates a basic NDS system that uses manual nulling. Light in the band, $\Delta\lambda$, is first chopped, then passed through a half-silvered, beamsplitter mirror. The direct beam passes through the sample cuvette, thence to a photosensor (PS_1). The reference beam passes through an adjustable calibrated neutral density wedge (NDW), and thence to photosensor PS_2. The outputs of the photosensors are conditioned to remove dc, then amplified by a difference amplifier (DA). The DA output is a square wave at chopper frequency whose amplitude an phase ($0°$ or $180°$) is determined by the relative intensities at PS_1 and PS_2. In calibration, with no analyte present, the NDW is manually adjusted to null the dc signal, V_o, to compensate for reflection and absorption by the sample cuvette. With the analyte present, more light in $\Delta\lambda$ is absorbed and the intensity at PS_1, I_A, is reduced. Now the NDW must be advanced further to renull V_o. The additional neutral density required to renull the system can be shown to be proportional to the analyte concentration.

A further refinement of the NDS system is to make it self-nulling. This design is shown in Figure 8.9. Now V_o is integrated to make a type 1 control system with zero steady-state error, and the integrator output, V_o', is conditioned to drive a linear positioning system that moves the NDW. Now it can be shown that the difference in the voltage V_o' with no analyte, and V_o' with analyte is proportional to the (linear) change in ND, hence in the analyte concentration.

We now demonstrate mathematically how an NDS system works. Assume that the output of the interference filter is a rectangular spectrum of width, $\Delta\lambda$. After being split by the half-silvered mirror (HSM), both source spectrums still have width $\Delta\lambda$, and equal magnitudes, $S_1(\lambda)$ watts/nm. The reflected reference spectrum is attenuated by the NDW's transmittance, T_{ND}. In general, $T_{ND} \equiv (I_{out}/I_{in}) \equiv 10^{-\beta x}$, where x is the displacement of the wedge from 0 on the linear x scale, and β is the NDW's attenuation constant ($ND \equiv \beta x$). Note that an ND of 1 means the input light is attenuated by a factor of 0.1, or $I_{out} = I_{in}/10$. Thus, the intensity at the reference photosensor is:

$$I_R = S_1 \, \Delta\lambda T_{ND} \quad \text{Watts.} \qquad 8.23$$

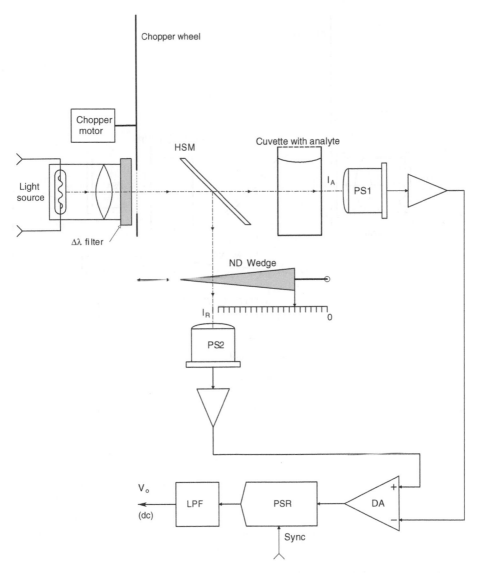

FIGURE 8.8 Schematic of a manually nulled, nondispersive spectrophotometer. A phase-sensitive rectifier (PSR) and low-pass filter (LPF) are used to change the square wave output of the DA to a dc error signal, V_o. V_o is nulled by adjusting the ND wedge so that the matched photosensors each have the same total intensity input over the $\Delta\lambda$ filter passband. The passband also contains a wavelength where the analyte absorbs.

The spectrum that passes through the HSM also passes through the walls of the sample cuvette twice (in and out) and also through the test solution with analyte. The input spectrum is attenuated by passing through the cuvette by a factor $T_{cuv} < 1$, and also by the test solution independent of the analyte by a factor $T_{sol} < 1$. We assume that in a narrow band, $\delta\lambda$, around λ_o, the analyte has a strong absorption.

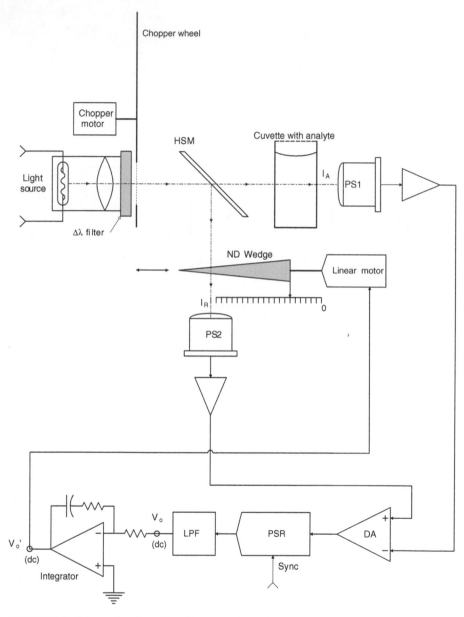

FIGURE 8.9 Schematic of a self-nulling, nondispersive spectrophotometer. V_o is integrated and the integrator output drives a linear actuator that advances the wedge to automatically null the system.

Hence the spectrum exiting the cuvette, $S_{1A}(\lambda)$, has a reduced total intensity as shown in Figure 8.10. Using Beer's law, the intensity of $S_{1A}(\lambda)$ is simply:

$$I_A = S_1 \; \Delta\lambda \; T_c T_{solv} - S_1 \; \delta\lambda T_c T_{solv} \, (1 - T_A) \qquad\qquad 8.24$$

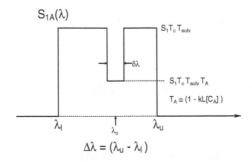

FIGURE 8.10 Idealized spectral band after passing through the analyte. The notch is from spectral energy that the analyte has absorbed.

The transmittance minimum of the analyte is given by Beer's law:

$$T_A = \exp(-kL[A]) \cong 1 - kL[A] \qquad\qquad 8.25$$

Here we have assumed that $kL[A] \ll 1$. $[A]$ is the concentration of the analyte, and the value of k is both wavelength- and concentration-dependent. Thus, after some algebra, we can write the intensity of the light exiting the cuvette as:

$$I_A = S_1 \Delta\lambda\, T_c T_{solv} \{1 - (\delta\lambda/\Delta\lambda)kL[A]\} \text{ Watts} \qquad\qquad 8.26$$

If there is no analyte in the cuvette, the V_0 null occurs when $I_A = I_R$. That is, when:

$$S_1 \Delta\lambda T_{NDo} = S_1 \Delta\lambda T_c T_{solv} \qquad\qquad 8.27$$

or,

$$T_{NDo} = T_c T_{solv} = 10^{-\beta x} \cong (1 - 2.303\beta x_o) \qquad\qquad 8.28$$

With analyte present, the wedge is advanced until again, $I_R = I_A$, and $V_0 = 0$. Thus at null we have:

$$S_1 \Delta\lambda T_{ND} = S_1 T_c T_{solv} \Delta\lambda\{1 - (\delta\lambda/\Delta\lambda)kL[A]\} \qquad\qquad 8.29$$

So

$$T_{ND} = T_c T_{solv} \{1 - (\delta\lambda/\Delta\lambda)kL[A]\}$$

$$\downarrow$$

$$(1 - 2.3\beta x) \cong (1 - 2.3\beta x_o)\{1 - (\delta\lambda/\Delta\lambda)kL[A]\}$$

$\downarrow$

$$1 - 2.3\beta x \cong 1 - 2.3\beta x_o - (1 - 2.3\beta x_o) (\delta\lambda/\Delta\lambda)kL[A]$$

$\downarrow$

$$2.3\beta(x - x_o) \cong (T_cT_{solv})(\delta\lambda/\Delta\lambda)kL[A]$$

$\downarrow$

$$\Delta x \cong (T_cT_{solv}/\beta 2.303)(\delta\lambda/\Delta\lambda)kL[A] \qquad\qquad 8.30$$

Thus the additional displacement of the NDW by Δx to renull the NDS when an analyte is present is simply proportional to the analyte's concentration, [A], assuming Beer's law holds, and the NDW's ND is given by $10^{-\beta x}$, where $\beta x \ll 1$. The 2.3 factor comes from approximating $10^{-\beta x}$ by the use of $e^{-\epsilon} \cong 1 - \epsilon$. Note that $\log_{10}(a) = \ln(a)/2.303$.

The reader should note that other system configurations for NDS systems have been used, as shown in Figure 8.11. (The choppers for these three systems are not shown.) System A in the figure is basically the one described above, except a blank cuvette filled with solvent is used so that, in the absence of analyte in the sample, ND = 0. System B is more sophisticated in that a reference concentration of analyte is used in the input cuvette. System configuration C is a *bad configuration* in which the sample and the reference cuvettes have been interchanged. Analysis of system B is given below.

In system B, the spectrum $S_2(\lambda)$ exiting the reference cuvette containing a known, reference concentration of analyte, $[A_o]$, has intensity I_2, given by:

$$I_2 = S_1T_cT_{solv}\,\Delta\lambda\{1 - (\delta\lambda/\Delta\lambda)kL[A_o]\} \qquad\qquad 8.31$$

This intensity is divided by 2 at the HSM. The reference beam passes through the NDW, and thence to a blank cuvette. The intensity I_R is thus:

$$I_R = \int_0^\infty S_4(\lambda)\,d\lambda \qquad\qquad 8.32$$

$$I_R = \tfrac{1}{2}S_1\Delta\lambda T_c^2T_{solv}^2 T_{ND} - \delta\lambda\left[\tfrac{1}{2}S_1T_c^2T_{solv}^2 T_{ND} - \tfrac{1}{2}S_1T_c^2T_{solv}^2 T_{ND}T_{Ao}\right]$$
$$\qquad\qquad 8.33$$
$$I_R = \tfrac{1}{2}S_1T_c^2T_{solv}^2 T_{ND}\left[\Delta\lambda - \delta\lambda + \delta\lambda T_{Ao}\right]$$

The intensity I_A is given by:

$$I_A = \int_0^\infty S_3(\lambda)\,d\lambda \qquad\qquad 8.34$$

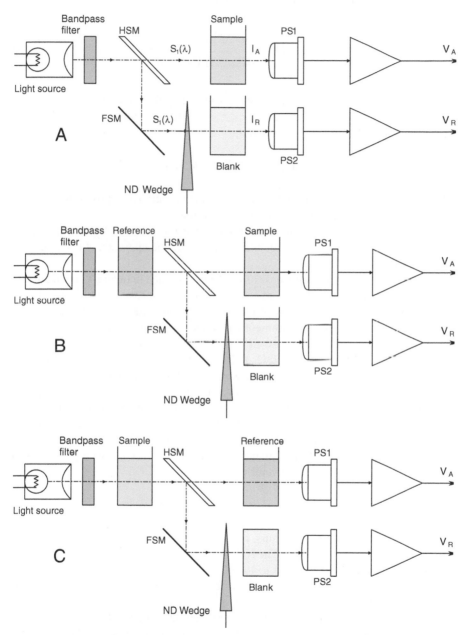

FIGURE 8.11 Three possible architectures for nondispersive spectrophotometers. The choppers are not shown. It can be shown that configuration C will not work.

$$I_A = \tfrac{1}{2} S_1 \Delta\lambda T_c^2 T_{solv}^2 - \delta\lambda \left[\tfrac{1}{2} S_1 T_c^2 T_{solv}^2 - \tfrac{1}{2} S_1 T_c^2 T_{solv}^2 T_{Ao} T_A \right]$$

$$I_A = \tfrac{1}{2} S_1 T_c^2 T_{solv}^2 \left[\Delta\lambda - \delta\lambda + \delta\lambda T_{Ao} T_A \right]$$

8.35

Now, when the instrument is nulled, $I_A = I_R$, so we can write:

$$T_{ND} = \frac{\left[1 - (\delta\lambda/\Delta\lambda)(1 - T_{Ao}T_A)\right]}{\left[1 - (\delta\lambda/\Delta\lambda)(1 - T_{Ao})\right]} \qquad 8.36$$

Recall that the transmittances can be approximated by the relation, $e^{-\varepsilon} \cong 1 - \varepsilon$, $\varepsilon \ll 1$, and also, $1/(1 - \varepsilon) \cong 1 + \varepsilon$, and $\varepsilon^2 \ll \varepsilon \ll 1$. If these relations are substituted into Equation 3.36, we can finally write:

$$T_{ND} \cong 1 - (\delta\lambda/\Delta\lambda)kL[A] \qquad 8.37$$

Thus, the null setting for the NDW (at low concentrations) is proportional to the concentration of the analyte in the sample solution.

It is left as an exercise for the reader to demonstrate why the NDS configuration in Figure 8.11C is a faulty architecture. (Hint: using the approach above, solve for T_{ND} at null.)

To demonstrate the effectiveness of the NDS approach in quantifying an analyte, Fellows (1997) designed, built and tested an NDS to measure oxyhemoglobin *in vitro*. Percutaneous measurement of the percent O_2 saturation of RBC hemoglobin (Hb) is an established NI measurement technique. The pulse oximeter (described in detail in Section 15.8) makes use of the differential absorption of red and near infrared (NIR) light by Hb vs. HbO. Pulse oximeters use a red and an NIR light-emitting diode (LED) (not a laser) as a 2-λ source to make the measurement. Fellows' NDS system was developed as a proof-of-concept design, rather than a competing instrument for the very simple pulse oximeter. Her system architecture closely followed the design shown in Figure 8.11(B), except, instead of a linear neutral density wedge, she used a rotating screen as a variable ND attenuator. Unlike the linear wedge, the screen's transmittance is a function of its angle with respect to the beam being attenuated, and is given by:

$$T_{SC} = (1 - 2r/d)[1 - (2r/d)\sec(\theta)] \qquad 8.38$$

Each wire in the screen has a radius, r, and d is the center-to-center spacing of the wires; a square mesh is assumed. The ND screen was rotated by a servo-galvanometer whose angle, θ, was proportional to its dc input voltage.

Fellows used a filter that passed light in a 650 to 750 nm band. 1 cm cuvettes were used for the test solution, the standard and the compensation. Sigma® freeze-dried human hemoglobin was made up at a concentration of 12 g/L in water buffered to pH 7.4. To make either HbO or Hb, either O_2 gas or CO_2 gas was bubbled through the sample and reference cuvettes, respectively.

Fellows' servo-nulling NDS system was able to measure HbO, but was difficult to calibrate because of the very nonlinear ND relation. A linear wedge or ND disk would have simplified the operation of her system.

A logical application of the NDS system would be to attempt to noninvasively and percutaneously measure (tissue) blood glucose in the far infrared (FIR) range. Glucose has three absorption peaks in the FIR: One at 10.97 μm, one at 11.98 μm, and one at 12.95 μm. If the LIR bandpass filter passed from 10.5 to 11.5 μm, the peak at 10.97 μm could be used. Figure 8.12 illustrates a basic FIR NDS system that might use a finger web or ear lobe (always with constant L). The FIR beam is defined by an IR bandpass filter, chopped, and the null is detected using a phase-sensitive rectifier. A light-tight box excludes stray IR from the pyroelectric photo-sensors (e.g., PVDF). Such a system would be easy to build, but its accurate use would depend on individual calibration with a standard blood glucose test and the absence of other tissue and blood substances that might overwhelm the glucose absorption peaks.

8.2.4 Chemical Analysis by Surface Plasmon Resonance

Surface plasmon resonance (SPR) sensors are a relatively new analytical tool. They allow rapid specific determination of the concentration of a variety of medically and biologically important analytes. For example, specific bacteria, antibodies, theophyl-line, caffeine, NO_2, pesticides, explosives, controlled substances (opioid drugs), etc., have been sensed with SPR. Threshold sensitivities for certain analytes have been reported as low as 0.05 ppb (10^{-11}). SPR technology is relatively simple and inex-pensive to implement, compared with analytical systems such as HPLC, mass spec-trometry, IR spectrometry, and gas chromatography, and it lends itself well to field measurements. Since this text is about noninvasive medical instruments, the analytes are presumably derived from urine or saliva, or smears from mucous membranes, etc. There is no reason, however, that SPR sensors cannot be used on gases or blood to look for any analyte (chemical, antibody, bacteria, etc.) therein.

SPR is a *quantum* phenomenon that occurs when a beam of monochromatic linear polarized light (LPL) is reflected off a thin metal film, vapor-deposited on one side of a glass prism, or when a beam of LPL is incident at a critical angle on a gold-coated diffraction grating. For illustrative purposes, we will examine in detail the prism SPR system using the so-called *Kretschmann geometry*. This system is shown schematically in Figure 8.13. A thin (c. 50 nm) film of conducting metal such as gold or silver is vapor-deposited on one face of a prism, or on the flat face of a half-round rod. A beam of LPL of a known wavelength is directed into the prism or rod so that it strikes the gold film face at an angle of incidence, θ_i. The incident beam's **E** vector must lie in the plane of incidence (be in the TM mode) for SPR to occur. In intimate contact with the other side of the gold film is a thin film of the analyte having a permittivity of ε_a. It has been experimentally observed that when the incoming beam's wavelength and angle of incidence have unique critical values, the intensity of the reflected beam reaches a *minimum*. The depth of the null in the output beam intensity is a function of how much energy from the input LPL beam is coupled into the generation of surface plasmons in the metal film. The degree of coupling is a function of λ, θ_i, and, most importantly, the dielectric constant of the analyte material.

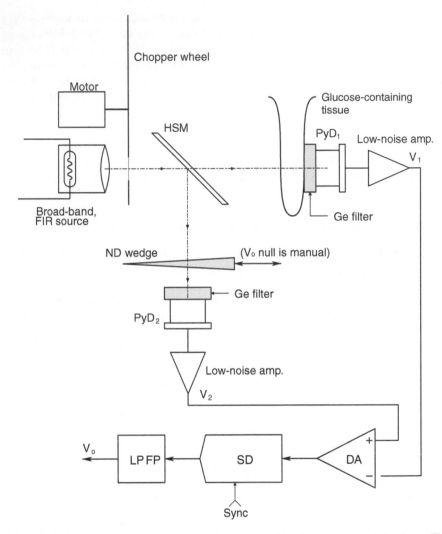

FIGURE 8.12 A proposed IR NDS applied to measure blood glucose in earlobe tissue. The $\Delta\lambda$ passband might span from 11.5 to 12.5 μm to include the 12 μm glucose absorption peak. A pyroelectric IR sensor could be used in the $\Delta\lambda$ range specified. Such an instrument would have to be individually calibrated against the patient's blood glucose with a fuel-cell type blood glucometer.

Surface plasmons can be thought of as induced wave-like fluctuations in the density of conduction-band electrons in the thin metal film. These fluctuations exist in both space and time, i.e., they can be thought of as traveling waves induced by the incident TM, LPL. The basis for using SPR as an analytical chemical tool is based on the conditions required for resonance. Under conditions of non-SP resonance, the incident beam of LPL reflects off the metalized surface of the prism, and exits the prism to a photosensor. The metal film effectively forms a conducting mirror surface, and conventional refraction and reflection optical laws apply.

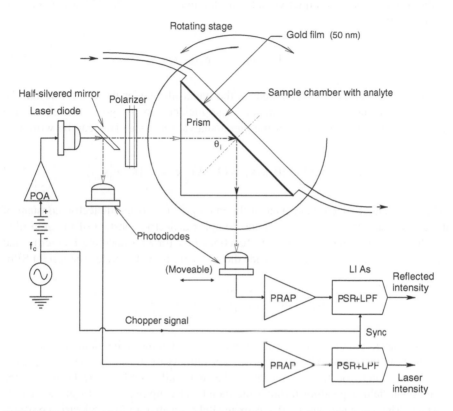

FIGURE 8.13 A surface plasmon resonance (SPR) system of the Kretschmann geometry. Resonance is reached by varying the angle θ of the monochromatic polarized light incident on the gold film.

The velocity of light *in vacuo* is $c = 2.998 \times 10^8$ m/sec. In transparent liquids or glass, light travels more slowly; the ratio of the speed if light *in vacuo* to the speed of light in the medium is defined as the *refractive index* of that medium, n_m. That is, $n_m \equiv c/v_m$. From electromagnetic (EM) theory, $c \equiv 1/\sqrt{\varepsilon_o \mu_o}$ and $v_m = 1/\sqrt{\kappa_m \varepsilon_o \mu_m}$ However, in non-magnetic materials, the magnetic permeability $\mu_m \cong \mu_o$. Thus, we can write the refractive index as:

$$n_m \cong \sqrt{\kappa_m} \qquad\qquad 8.39$$

v_m (and n) are generally functions of frequency. An EM wave in a medium or free space such as light, or surface plasmon waves, which basically exist in two dimensions, can be described by their *wave vector*, **k**. **k** is directed along the direction of wave propagation, and its magnitude *in vacuo* for EM waves is:

$$k_o = \omega/c = 2\pi v/c = 2\pi/\lambda \qquad\qquad 8.40$$

In the prism glass with refractive index n_1, the magnitude of the EM wave vector is (Krauss, 1953):

$$k_1 = \omega/v_1 = \omega\sqrt{\kappa_1}/c \qquad 8.41$$

Surface plasmons are generated on the metal film under the condition that the magnitude of the wave vector in the glass incident on the gold film equals the magnitude of the wave vector at the metal/analyte interface. This can be written:

$$k_i = (2\pi/\lambda)\sin(\theta_i)\sqrt{\kappa_1} = (2\pi/\lambda)\sqrt{\kappa_a|\kappa_m|/(\kappa_a + |\kappa_m|)} \qquad 8.42$$

Where κ_1 is the dielectric constant of the glass prism, κ_a is the dielectric constant of the analyte, and $\kappa_m = \kappa_m' + j\kappa_m''$ is the complex dielectric constant of the gold film. All dielectric constants are generally functions of v (or λ). Canceling like terms and solving for the angle of incidence inside the prism, we have the angle criterion for SPR:

$$\theta_{iR} \cong \sin^{-1}\left\{\sqrt{(\kappa_a\kappa_m)/[(\kappa_a + \kappa_m)\kappa_1]}\right\} \qquad 8.43$$

The resonance condition is due to momentum matching of incident photons with plasmons in the metal. The fact that the permittivity of the analyte layer (typically c. 250 nm thick) on the other side of the metal affects SPR may be due to the evanescent field expanding through the metal and coupling into SPs at the analyte surface. The resonance angle, θ_{iR}, is exquisitely sensitive to the dielectric constants of the metal and the analyte in contact with it. Thus, any chemical reaction that takes place at the metal surface, such as binding of antibodies to metal-bound antigens, will affect ε_a and the value of θ_{iR}. Thus, surface reactions of analyte can be used to sense antibodies, or if the antibodies are bound to the metal, it can sense antigen molecules such as those on bacterial and viral surfaces, or analyte molecules in solution or suspension.

Figure 8.14 illustrates typical SPR curves for a Kretschmann prism system receiving monochromatic light. Note that when the analyte index of refraction increases due to antibody bonding at the metal–analyte surface, κ_a also increases to κ_a', and the SPR curve as a function of incidence angle shifts to the right and broadens. (Note that $n_a \cong \sqrt{\kappa_a}$) Thus, the intensity measured at angle θ_{im} increases, while the intensity minimum moves to θ_{iR}'. Both shifts, either taken together in a formula or as separate phenomena, can be used to quantify the extent of the binding reaction at the metal surface. The depth of the null at SPR depends in part on the thickness of the metal film (Foster, 1996).

Another way of using the Kretschmann system is to set the incidence angle at the SPR null for some standard source λ. The source λ is then varied by a monochromator, and the output intensity is plotted as a function of λ as a surface reaction takes place. Typical intensity vs. λ curves is illustrated in Figure 8.15. Because the permittivities of the glass, metal film and analyte are functions of λ, we again see

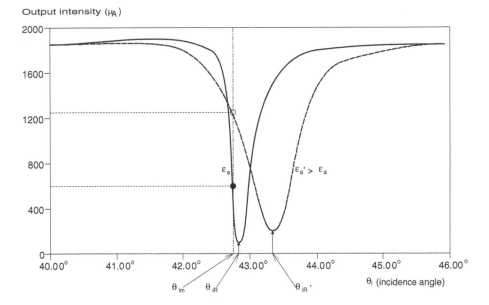

FIGURE 8.14 Reflected light intensity as a function of incidence angle for the Kretschmann SPR system. The solid curve is the system response in the absence of analyte; the dotted curve is obtained with analyte in intimate contact with the gold film.

a shifting and broadening of the SPR intensity curves with λ as antibody binding at the metal surface takes place. While varying the source λ can yield good analytical results, it makes the SPR system more expensive because of the need for a precision monochromator.

The design of SPR devices for chemical analysis is a rapidly growing field. One alternative configuration of an SPR sensor places the analyte solution over the surface of a plastic diffraction grating whose surface has been vapor deposited with gold, silver or aluminum (gold is generally preferred). The plastic top of the grating acts as an attenuated total reflection (ATR) prism, where light reflected from the grating where the beam strikes it initially is reflected back many times to the grating surface. Such a grating SPR design was proposed by Simon (1998). Figure 8.16 shows a side view of Simon's "long range" SPR grating system. SPR occurs at a critical beam input angle, θ_i, giving a minimum of output light intensity when the coupling component of the monochromatic TM-polarized input beam wave vector satisfies the relation:

$$\left(2\pi/\lambda\right)\sin\left(\theta_i\right)+\left(2\pi/b\right)=\left(2\pi/\lambda\right)\sqrt{\left(\kappa_a\kappa_m\right)/\left(\kappa_a+\kappa_m\right)} \qquad 8.44$$

Here, b is the grating constant, κ_a is the dielectric constant of the analyte, and κ_m is the magnitude of the complex dielectric constant of the metal film. A very thin layer of antigen with high affinity to the antibody to be detected is chemically

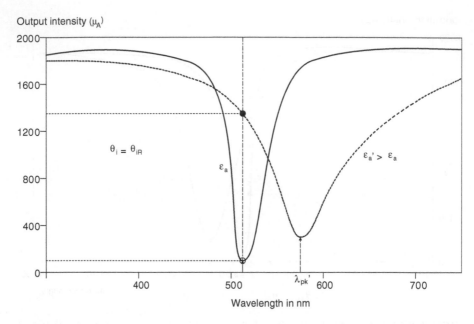

FIGURE 8.15 Reflected light intensity as a function of the wavelength of the incident polarized beam in a Kretschmann SPR system. The dotted curve is obtained with analyte in intimate contact with the gold film.

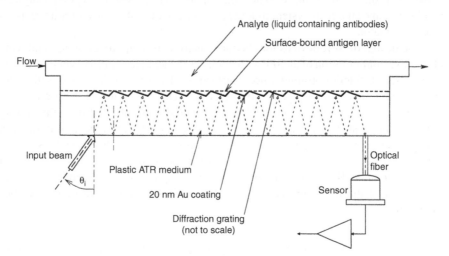

FIGURE 8.16 An SPR system that uses a metal film-covered, plastic diffraction grating. The analyte is in intimate contact with the metal film, as in the Kretschmann SPR system. The multiple light reflections in the grating body are reminiscent of the ATR prism. SPR systems have been operated with both liquid and gas phase analytes.

bound to the 20 nm gold film over the grating surface. Antibodies in the analyte liquid bind to the protruding antigen molecules, changing κ_a at the gold–solution interface. This change of dielectric constant changes the interfacial refractive index and "retunes" the SPR to a new input angle, θ_i. Either by changing θ_i to reattain a minimal light output, or by measuring the increase in light output due to $\Delta\kappa_a$, the number or density of bound antibodies can be quantified. A possible disadvantage of Simon's grating SPR configuration is the formation of bubbles on the grating surface, and, because the measurement is a "one-shot" event; a virgin antigen surface must be reapplied to the gold film and the output nulled again before another antibody assay can be done. Simon (1998) claims that the output signal from the ATR layer increases by approximately fivefold when about 2 nm of antigen-antibody complex forms at the gold surface. Also, a refractive index change in the analyte of less than 1% causes a 0.5° shift in θ_i to renull the system.

Other embodiments of the grating SPR system place the analyte over the gold-film-covered grating; the monochromatic TM-polarized light is directed through a thin layer of analyte onto the grating. Jory et al. (1995) reported on an exquisitely sensitive grating SPR system in which an acousto-optical tunable filter (AOTF) element was used to control the wavelength of the incident beam to a precision of 0.0005 nm. They used their system to measure the concentration of NO_2 gas in N_2 (a gas phase analyte). By depositing a thin layer of phthalocynanine over the gold coating, a wavelength shift of -0.004 nm renulled the system from zero concentration when 0.01 ppm NO_2 in N_2 was applied. They claimed that the sensitivity of their system allowed detection of changes in the refractive index of the gas of 1×10^{-6}. The fact that very small concentrations of gas are detectable suggests that the grating SPR technology might be developed in the future to detect medical gas concentrations, or even trace gases emanating from controlled drugs and explosives. (At this writing, trained dogs have the best record for detecting explosives and controlled drugs.)

The potential application of SPR sensors in medical diagnosis is enormous, and is just beginning to be realized. As we have seen, both gas and liquid-phase sensing are possible. Practically any analyte that can react with a reactant bound to the gold film surface on a prism or grating with a strong affinity can be sensed by SPR. The reaction must cause a change in the refractive index or the permittivity at the gold surface to affect the SPR conditions (λ or θ_i). SPR antigen-antibody reactions can be used to sense specific antibodies, bacteria, viruses, proteins, hormones, cytokines, etc. Note that specific monoclonal antibodies can also be bound to the gold film to sense any protein or molecule for which they can be made specific.

The problem of quick, efficient, SPR sensor regeneration remains to be solved, however. Once the bound surface reactant has combined with the analyte, the analyte must be totally removed before the next measurement without affecting the bound reactant, or the complex must be removed and the surface reactant layer must be renewed or rejuvenated.

8.2.5 Ion Selective Electrodes

One important analytical tool for measuring the concentrations of electrolyte ions in plasma, urine, saliva, etc. is the *ion selective electrode* (ISE). Ion selective electrodes include the well known glass hydrogen ion-selective electrode used to measure the pH of a solution. All ion-selective electrodes are used with a *reference electrode* (RE). In electrochemistry, each electrode is known as a *half cell*; the ISE and the RE together compose a whole cell, or EMF battery. The half-cell EMF of the RE is generally a constant regardless of the analyte ion's concentration. The half-cell EMF of the ISE is proportional to the logarithm of the analyte ion's *electrochemical activity*, *a*. *a* is very nearly equal to the ion's molar concentration at low concentrations.

The EMFs of both the ISE and RE vary with temperature, so all pH and ion measurements must be done at a constant temperature following calibration with a standard solution, or an automatic electronic temperature correction can be made by the instrument by continuously measuring the test solution's temperature.

The net cell potential of the RE and ISE electrodes in the analyte solution is measured under conditions of negligible current flow through the cell. Negligible current flow is required to avoid polarization at the electrodes' surfaces, overvoltages, and ohmic voltage drops (a typical glass pH electrode has an equivalent dc resistance of c. 5×10^9 ohms). To meet this condition, the cell's EMF is measured with a direct-coupled differential *electrometer amplifier* having bias currents on the order of 10 fA or less and an input resistance on the order of 10^{13} ohms.

As a first example of an ISE application, we consider the glass pH electrode shown in Figure 8.17. This electrode has a thin glass membrane at its end. It is filled internally with a solution of 0.1 N hydrochloric acid. Internally, a silver│silver chloride electrode makes contact with the HCl. The Ag│AgCl electrode's half cell potential is a logarithmic function of the Cl⁻ concentration, which is the same as the HCL's H⁺ concentration. The typical reference half-cell for pH measurement is the calomel electrode, also illustrated in Figure 8.17. Thus, the pH measurement system has three half-cells — calomel, glass, and Ag│AgCl. This cell can be written in electrochemical notation: Ag│AgCl(s), 0.1 N HCl│Glass│Solution(pH = x)│Calomel. The definition of pH is: $pH \equiv -\log_{10} a_{H+} \cong -\log_{10}[H^+]$. a_{H+} is the activity of hydrogen ions in the solution under measurement and [H⁺] is their concentration. The half-cell EMF of the glass electrode plus the Ag│AgCl(s) electrode is thus:

$$E_G = E_G^0 - (RT/F)\ln(a_{H+}) = E_G^0 + (2.3026\,RT/F)\,pH \text{ volts} \qquad 8.45$$

Where R is the MKS gas constant [8.31 joules/(mol K)], T is the Kelvin temperature of the solution, F is the Faraday number (96,500), and 2.3026 comes from converting natural logs to $\log_{10}$. The half-cell potential of the saturated calomel electrode is:

$$E_{Cal} = 0.2415 - 7.6 \times 10^{-4}\,(t - 25°) \text{ volts} \qquad 8.46$$

where t is the Celsius temperature. Thus, the net EMF of the pH cell at 25°C is:

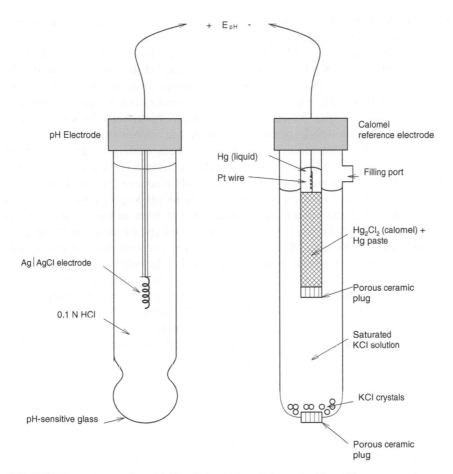

FIGURE 8.17 A glass pH and calomel electrode cell for measuring pH.

$$E_{pH} = E_G^0 + (2.3026\ RT/F)\ pH - 0.2415$$

$$= (E_G^0 - 0.2415) + 0.0591\ (pH)\ volts \qquad 8.47$$

Equation 8.47 can be solved for pH:

$$pH = \frac{E_{pH} - (E_G^0 - 0.2415)}{(2.3026\ RT/F)} = \frac{E_{pH} - \Delta E_G}{0.0591} \qquad 8.48$$

The value of ΔE_G can be determined by calibration with a pH standard solution. ΔE_G is not only a function of temperature, but is also different for each glass pH electrode. Commercial pH meters automatically compensate for test solution temperature, and, once standardization is done, subtract a dc voltage from ΔE_G so that $E_{pH} = 0.1$ (pH) volts. Thus, a voltmeter with a zero to 1,400 mV scale can be calibrated in 0 to 14 pH units. Modern pH meters have a precision of ± 0.01 pH unit, and can be read to ± 1.0 mV on an expanded (2 pH unit or 200 mV) scale.

Other ISEs are used in laboratory medicine to measure: NH_4^+, Ca^{++}, Cl^-, CN^-, I^-, Pb^{++}, NO_3^-, NO_2^-, K^+, Na^+, SCN^-, etc. Unless the ISE is combined with the RE in the same housing, each ISR requires a corresponding RE half-cell (usually calomel). All ISEs suffer what is known as *interferences* from certain other ions that may be in solution with the analyte. For example, Metrohm® ISEs offer a Cl^--responding electrode with a crystal membrane having a sensitivity range of 5×10^{-5} mol/L to 1 mol/L. This electrode develops erroneous readings in the presence of Hg^{++}, Br^-, I^-, $S^=$, CN^-, NH_3, and $S_2O_3^=$ ions. The Metrohm® Na^+ electrode (aka Ross electrode) has a glass membrane (not unlike a pH electrode) and measures in the range of 1×10^{-5} to 1 mol/L; it is interfered with by pH > (pNa + 4), Ag^+, Li^+ and K^+ ions. pH, silver and lithium are not normally a problem in biological fluids, but potassium is, and would have to be corrected for. Similarly, the Metrohm K^+ electrode is interfered with by Cs^+, NH_4^+, H^+, and Na^+. The concentrations of cesium and ammonium ions are normally negligible, the pH is relatively constant, and sodium must be compensated for in bio-samples. Some ISEs have polymer membranes, the Na^+ electrode has a glass membrane, and others use an LaF_3 crystal membrane. For example, Pb^{++} and Cl^- electrodes both use crystal membranes, but K^+ and other Cl^- electrodes use plastic membranes. In all ISEs, as in the glass pH electrode, there is an ion-selective barrier (membrane, glass, or crystal), an inner electrolyte, and an inner half-cell. The EMF of an ISE measurement system will generally be of the form:

$$E_i = \Delta E_i - (RT/F)\ln(a_i) \text{ volts} \qquad 8.49$$

where the activity on the ionic analyte is approximated by its molar concentration. If the ion is divalent, such as Ca^{++}, then F is replaced by $2F$ in Equation 8.49.

Some of the companies that make ISEs are Vernier Software & Technology, Beaverton, Oregon, 2000 Metrohm, Ltd, Herisau, Switzerland, Phoenix Electrode Co., Houston, Texas, and Beckman Coulter, Inc., Fullerton, Oregon.

8.2.6 FLAME PHOTOMETRY

The flame photometer is a relatively inexpensive instrument that is used to determine, *in vitro*, the concentration of physiologically and medically important ions in body fluids such as urine, CSF, and blood plasma. (Of course, invasive procedures are used to collect samples of blood and CSF.) There are two types of flame photometer: the *flame emission spectroscope* (FES), and the *atomic absorption spectroscope* (AAS). Both instruments are described in this section.

FES and AAS are effective in determining the concentrations of the ions of lithium, sodium, potassium, calcium, magnesium, rhubidium, copper, arsenic, cadmium, mercury, etc., in solution. FES and AAS are unresponsive to the noble gases, the halogens, hydrogen, nitrogen, oxygen, phosphorus, and sulfur (cf. http://kern.lerc.nasa.gov/techniq/faa.htm). As we saw in Section 8.1, the concentrations of

Na^+, K^+, Ca^{++}, Mg^{++} in various body fluids can be used in the diagnosis of many diseases, conditions, and hormonal disorders. Lithium (as carbonate or citrate) is medically important in the treatment of manic depressive (bipolar) mental illness. The heavy metals, As, Cd, Cu, and Hg, are toxic, and are associated with environmental poisoning.

Figure 8.18 illustrates the architecture of a typical FES instrument. A key component is the burner in which a fuel (e.g., H_2, acetylene [C_2H_2], propane, etc.) is mixed with either air or pure O_2. An aerosol of the solution containing the ion to be measured (the analyte) is injected into the base of the flame. All three flows are made constant to ensure a stable flame and a stable level of atomic emission. Table 8.2.6.1 gives the approximate flame temperatures for various fuel-oxidizer conditions. Note that the oxyacetylene flame has the highest temperature.

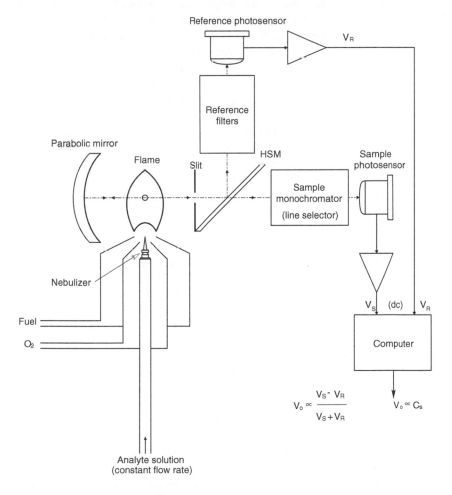

FIGURE 8.18 Schematic of a flame emission spectroscope. Two channels are used to compensate for intensity noise in the flame.

TABLE 8.2.6.1
Flame Temperatures for
Different Fuel–Oxidizer
Mixes

Oxidizer	Fuel	Flame temp., °K
Air	H_2	2000–2100
Air	C_2H_2	2100–2400
O_2	H_2	2600–2700
O_2	C_2H_2	2600–2800

The heat of the flame vaporizes the sample constituents without chemical change. The combination of high temperature and the fuel (reducing gas) decomposes and reduces the analyte ions to atomic form in vapor phase. (For example, a Na^+ ion picks up an electron.) The high temperature excites the outer shell electrons of some atoms to higher energy states. As the excited atoms rise, they cool, and the high-energy state electrons fall back into their normal orbits with the emission of photons of wavelength $\lambda = hc\Delta E$, where $\Delta E = E_e - E_g$, h is Planck's constant (6.624×10^{-34} joule sec), c is the speed of light *in vacuo* (2.998×10^8 m/sec), E_g is the ground state energy of the outer electron, E_e is the excited state energy of that electron, and λ is in meters. In the gas phase, excited elements such as Li, Na and K emit multiple unique narrow line spectra. For example, the principle emission lines of Na are at 330.2 (600), 330.3 (300), 568.26 (50), 568.82 (300), 589.00 (9,000), 589.60 (5,000); here wavelengths are in nm, and the numbers in parentheses are relative intensities. Potassium's strongest lines are at 766.50 (9,000) and 770.00 (5,000) nm. All biological fluids contain both K^+ and Na^+, so either optical interference band-pass filters or a simple grating mono-chromator can be used to select the unique strong lines for measurement.

The intensity response vs. analyte concentration is sigmoid, as shown in Figure 8.19. The reasons for this sigmoid curve are easy to understand. It has a low slope at low analyte concentration (region A) because emission is lower due to reionization of the reduced metal analyte (e.g., $K \rightarrow K^+ + e^-$). At higher concentrations, there is little reionization. The mid-region (B) is linear, with intensity proportional to concentration or the number of atoms emitting/second. Finally, at high concentrations, (region C), there is self-absorption of emitted photons by other ground-state atoms in the flame. If a sample is introduced, and the resulting line intensity exceeds I_H, usual practice is to dilute the sample a known amount to bring the resulting emission intensity back into the linear region where $I(C) = b + mC$. If the intensity is below I_L, then vacuum evaporation of the solvent can be used to increase the analyte concentration.

Other design features of the typical AES instrument include a parabolic mirror to concentrate emission line intensity, a slit to restrict beam width entering the sample monochromator that selects the analyte's principal emission line(s). The half-silvered mirror splits the beam into the sample beam and a reference beam that is passed

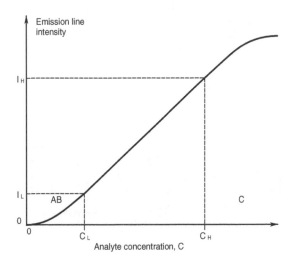

FIGURE 8.19 The flame emission intensity vs. concentration is sigmoid at a selected wavelength with a linear region.

through a filter that excludes the analyte's line(s). The reference beam is used to compensate for random fluctuations in flame intensity, as shown in Figure 8.18.

The key to flame photometer accuracy is calibration. Two concentrations of standard solutions of an analyte are used to obtain the constants b and m in the I(C) relation above. Two-point calibration must also be used with the AAS.

A diagram of a typical AAS instrument is shown in Figure 8.20. This is a more complex instrument than the FES described above. Here, the flame is used as a narrow-band Beer's law absorber of light from a special *hollow-cathode lamp* (HCL). The cathode of the HCL is a hollow cylinder with a cupped end, made from or coated with the element whose concentration is to be measured. The anode is generally a tungsten wire. The interior of the HCL is filled with He or Ar at 1–2 mm Hg pressure. A high-voltage pulse is used to make a momentary spark, which ionizes the gas. Gas ions are given velocity by the internal dc E field and strike the cathode, heating it and forming more gas ions that bombard it. The hot cathode emits the line spectra characteristic of its coating element (the same lines seen from the flame of the FES above). Along with the element's line energy, there is blackbody IR from the hot cathode, and emission lines from the gas. The HCL output beam is chopped before it reaches the flame so that a phase-sensitive detector can discriminate against the flame's intrinsic dc emission lines. The flame is made long (c. 10 cm) and narrow; the test solution is atomized into it similar to the FES instrument's flame.

The chopped beam from the HCL passes through the flame and the specific emission line(s) from the HCL interact with the ground state (un-ionized) analyte atoms. The amount of emission-line-wavelength light from the chopped HCL beam absorbed is proportional to the density of ground-state analyte atoms in the flame. At the line wavelength, the exiting beam intensity, I_s, is given by the Beer-Lambert law:

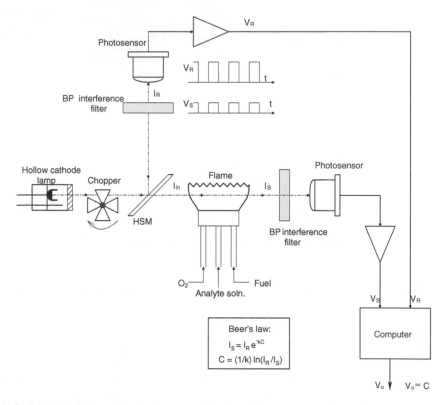

FIGURE 8.20 Schematic of a flame atomic absorption spectroscope (AAS).

$$I_s = I_{in} \exp(-k\,C) \qquad\qquad 8.50$$

where: C is the analyte concentration in the sample, and k is a constant proportional to the length the beam travels in the flame. Note that a reference beam is again used to compensate for fluctuations in the HCL output intensity as it warms up. The analyte aspirated into the flame emits the same line(s) as the HCL. However, the AAS instrument does not respond to it because it is a dc signal. Only the chopper-modulated intensity, I_s, is sensed. The AAS instrument is not as flexible as the FES because a new HCL must be used for each different analyte measured.

The detection limits for the FES and AAS instruments for certain elements are shown in Table 8.2.6.2. It should be noted that a new technique called electrothermal atomic absorption has detection limits that are about 1,000 times lower (better) than AAS and FES. .

While detection sensitivity of AAS systems to certain analytes can be very high, overall accuracy of this type of flame spectrophotometer is not high. Qi (1990) reported that the percent standard deviations for the measurement of Cu, Zn, Fe, Ca, Mg, Na, and K in human serum with a Varian "SpectrAA-40" AAS system were 2.2, 2.9, 3.9, 1.3, 1.7, 0.8 and 3.1, respectively. Ten samples of each analyte were measured. The line wavelengths used were: 324.8, 213.9, 248.3, 422.7, 202.5, 330.3,

---

TABLE 8.2.6.2
Detection Limits for
Selected Elements (in
ng/ml)

Element	AAS	FES
Ca	1	0.1
Cu	2	1
Hg	500	4×10^{-4}
Mg	0.01	5
Na	2	0.1
Pb	1	100
Zn	2	5×10^{-4}

---

and 404.5 nm, respectively. 10 ml of 1:10 diluted serum was required for each measurement.

A partial list of manufacturers of commercial AAS flame photometers includes: Buck Scientific (model 210VGP), Varian, Carl Zeiss (Analytik Jena AAS5- FL), Hitachi Scientific Instruments (Z-5000 series), Perkin-Elmer (2380 AAS), and Shimadzu (AA-6000 series AAS). Many AAS instruments have eight-lamp turrets that hold eight different HCLs to permit rapid sequential analysis of eight different analytes. FES instruments include those made by SEAC (FP10 and FP20), and Jenway (PFP7). Precision and reproducibility error for FES instruments are generally about 1%.

8.2.7 GAS CHROMATOGRAPHY

Gas chromatography (GC) is an exquisitely sensitive chemical analytical tool that is very competitive with spectrophotometry in terms of the analytes it can quantify in medically derived samples. If an analyte is stable (does not decompose) when in the gas or vapor phase at temperatures up to 400° C, it probably can be identified and quantified by GC. GC works by the simple principle that the volatile components of a sample injected as a bolus travel though the GC's column at different speeds. Each sample component is adsorbed by the column's stationary phase and then released, forming a continuous traveling wave of adsorbed component. The speed of a given traveling wave depends on many physical and chemical factors of the GC system. Of particular importance is that there is very little dispersion (broadening) of an individual analyte's peak as it propagates through the column. Thus, the time that a particular analyte exits the column is peculiar to that analyte, given identical conditions of carrier gas, carrier gas flow rate, column temperature, column length and inside diameter, and column stationary phase adsorber. Gas chromatography is well suited to separate mixtures of analytes in samples of complex composition. It can be used to identify and quantify such biochemicals as alcohol, acetone, various steroid hormones, drugs such as multiple tricyclic antidepressants, theophylline, opioids, etc. The schematic of a typical GC system is shown in Figure 8.21.

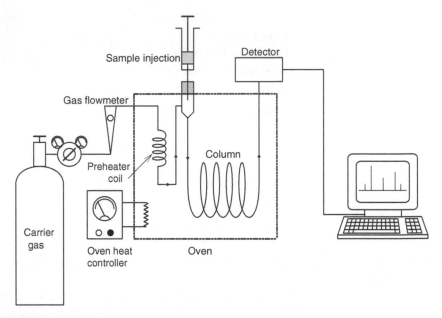

FIGURE 8.21 Schematic of a modern gas chromatograph. Many different types of eluent detectors can be used.

A basic GC has seven key components:

1. A source of *inert carrier gas*, such as dry nitrogen, helium or argon. The gas literally carries the sample and analyte through the column.
2. A sample injection port.
3. The *capillary column* is a long, thin tube of stainless steel or fused silica coated on the inside surface with polyimide resin. Column lengths can range from 10 m to 60 m, with 20 to 30 m being most typical. The resolution of a GC (ability to separate two nearly coincident eluent peaks) is proportional to the square root of the column length. Capillary column diameter is typically from 0.32 to 0.25 mm. As column diameter decreases, the retention of a given solute will increase, other factors being constant. This means that a smaller-diameter column provides better resolution (wider separation of the eluent peaks).
4. The inside of a GC column is coated with a thin layer of a thermally and chemically stable *stationary phase absorber* (SPA). The thickness of the SPA is another critical parameter affecting GC separation resolution. A thicker SPA will give greater solute retention, hence better resolution of adjacent eluent peaks. SPA thicknesses can range from 0.25 to 1 μm in capillary columns; the SPA coats the inside walls of the column. The materials used for SPAs are described below.
5. The entire column is placed inside an oven. The oven temperature can be held constant, or programmed to increase (e.g., from 80° to 280°C at

5°/min.) The temperature limits and rate of increase are set according to the particular analysis.

6. The detector senses the changes in eluent gas composition from pure carrier gas when boluses of sample constituents (and the desired analyte) exit the column. The many kinds of detectors are described in detail below. Detector sensitivities allow limits of detection ranging from 100 ppm to 100 ppb (analyte to carrier gas).

7. The detector output consists of voltage peaks of different heights and widths from sample components that exit the column at different times. A complete GC run might take from 5 to 30 minutes; GCs are not fast instruments. The GC detector output voltage is digitized, and the GC's computer integrates each peak to determine the concentration of each sample component (eluent), including the desired analyte. An analyte sample of known concentration is injected into the column for calibration purposes. The time it exits is peculiar to that analyte, and its area is proportional to the concentration, providing it is in the linear range of the column and detector.

There are many types of GC detectors. Some types of detectors respond to any analyte exiting from the column, others are specific for certain chemical classes of eluents, such as chlorinated hydrocarbon insecticides. As in many branches of measurements, the threshold detection concentration and resolution of a GC system are set primarily by noise arising in the detector and its electronic amplifiers. The *minimum detectable amount* (MDA) of an eluent is defined as the concentration or amount of analyte that will produce a minimum output peak voltage twice the RMS noise voltage. Thus, the practical lower limit of detector operation is set by its MDA. All GC detectors also have a linear dynamic range (LDR) of analyte concentration above their MDAs in which their outputs follow the linear relation: $V_o = b + m[A]$ to within ± 5%. ([A] is the analyte concentration in g/ml, or ppm.) Table 8.2.7.1 lists the names and characteristics of some GC detectors.

We will examine the operating mechanisms of two of these detectors in detail. The *TCD*, one of the simplest general-purpose GC detectors, is generally used with helium carrier gas. Figure 8.22 illustrates the circuit of this detector. Note that it is a simple Wheatstone bridge; the resistors of two opposite arms are surrounded with carrier plus eluent gases at temperature T_C, the other two arms are surrounded with pure He at column temperature, T_C. The resistors are platinum or nichrome. Current is passed through the bridge arms so they heat to a temperature, T_B, above T_C. The moving helium gas surrounding the resistors conducts heat away from them, lowering their temperature toward T_C. (Helium is unique in that it has a very high heat conductivity.) The drop in resistor temperature is given by the relation:

$$(T_B - T_R) = \Delta T = P_R \, \Theta_R > 0, \; T_B < T_R < T_C \qquad 8.51$$

Where T_R is the actual equilibrium resistor temperature in moving He, T_B is the reference temperature, P_R is the electrical power dissipated in each resistor, and Θ_R

TABLE 8.2.7.1
Summary Characteristics of the Major Detectors Used in Gas Chromatography

Detector Type	MDA (g/ml)	LDR (decades)	Comments
Thermal Conductivity Detector (TCD)	10^{-7}	c. 5	A general detector used with He carrier gas. Temp. differences on Wheatstone bridge resistor arms due to analyte sensed.
Flame Ionization Detector (FID)	10^{-12}	5 to 7	A mass-sensitive detector for C-H bonds. H_2 is burned, creating ions from analytes.
Photoionization Detector (PID)	10^{-12}	5 to 6	Sensitive to aromatics and olefins. Uses 10.2 eV UV lamp to ionize analytes.
Electron Capture Detector (ECD)	10^{-14}	3 to 4	Uses radioisotopes to ionize halogens, quinones, peroxides and nitro groups. Used for insecticides and PCBs.
Flame Photometric Detector (FPD)	10^{-11}	3 to 5	Used for S- or P-containing analytes. H_2 flame causes atomic emission of S @ 394 nm & P @ 526 nm. A PMT is used.
Electrical Conductivity Detector (ELCD)	5–10 pg (halogens) 10–20 pg (S) 10–20 pg (N)	5 to 6 4 to 4 3 to 4	Eluents react at high T with reaction gas. Products dissolved in solven, are passed through electrical conductivity cell.
Mass Spectrometry (MS)	1–10 pg (selected ion monitoring mode)	5 to 6	A mass spectrometer replaces detector. The MS measures the mass/charge ratio of ions fragmented at high T by e⁻ bombardment.
Nitrogen-Phosphorus Detector (NPD)	1–10 pg	4 to 6	Similar to FID except uses *rhubidium bead* to enhance sensitivity to N compounds by X50 and P compounds by X500.

is the thermal resistance seen by a resistor in moving He. In general, $\Theta_R = \Theta_{Ro} + \beta[A]$. That is, the eluent analyte gas decreases the ability of the pure He to conduct heat away from the two R_A resistors. Θ_{Ro} and β are positive constants, and [A] is the eluent analyte concentration in the He carrier gas. A metal resistor has a *positive tempco*, that is, its resistance increases as its temperature increases. This property can be approximated by the relation:

$$R(\Delta T) \cong R_o (1 + \alpha \Delta T), \alpha > 0 \qquad 8.52$$

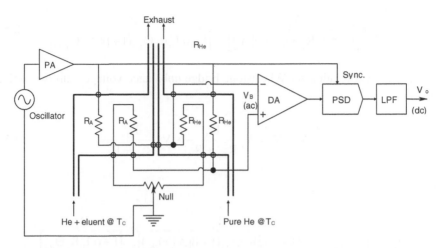

FIGURE 8.22 Schematic of a Wheatstone bridge, thermal conductivity detector and associated circuitry.

R_o is the resistance at the reference temperature, T_B. If we combine relations 8.51 and 8.52, we can write:

$$\Delta T = I_B^2 R_o (1 + \alpha \Delta T) \Theta_R \qquad\qquad 8.53$$

Solving for the equilibrium ΔT, we find:

$$\Delta T = \frac{I_B^2 R_o \Theta_R}{\left(1 - \alpha\, I_B^2 R_o \Theta_R\right)} \qquad\qquad 8.54$$

I_B^2 is the mean-squared ac current through each resistor (assumed constant). $I_B \cong V_s/2R_{He}$. Knowing the temperature drop, we can find the resistance from relation TC above:

$$R(\Delta T) = \frac{R_o}{\left(1 - \alpha I_B^2 R_o \Theta_R\right)} \qquad\qquad 8.55$$

For pure He:

$$R_{He} = \frac{R_o}{\left(1 - \alpha I_B^2 R_o \Theta_{Ro}\right)} \qquad\qquad 8.56$$

When an eluent analyte is present, Equation 8.55 becomes:

$$R_A = \frac{R_o}{\left[1 - \alpha I_B^2 R_o \left(\Theta_{Ro} + \beta[A]\right)\right]} = \frac{R_o}{\left[1 - \alpha I_B^2 R_o \Theta_{Ro} \left(1 + \beta[A]/\Theta_{Ro}\right)\right]} \qquad 8.57$$

Now the general relation for Wheatstone bridge unbalance voltage with two active arms is:

$$V_B = V_1 - V_2 = V_s \frac{R_A}{R_{He} + R_A} - V_s \frac{R_{He}}{R_{He} + R_A} \qquad 8.58$$

So

$$\frac{V_B}{V_s} = \frac{R_A - R_{He}}{R_A + R_{He}} = \frac{\dfrac{R_o}{\left[1 - \alpha I_B^2 R_o \Theta_{Ro} \left(1 + \beta[A]/\Theta_{Ro}\right)\right]} - \dfrac{R_o}{\left[1 - \alpha I_B^2 R_o \Theta_{Ro}\right]}}{\dfrac{R_o}{\left[1 - \alpha I_B^2 R_o \Theta_{Ro} \left(1 + \beta[A]/\Theta_{Ro}\right)\right]} - \dfrac{R_o}{\left[1 - \alpha I_B^2 R_o \Theta_{Ro}\right]}} \qquad 8.59$$

After some algebra, Equation 8.59 reduces to:

$$\frac{V_B}{V_s} \cong \left(R_{He}/2\right) \alpha I_B^2 \beta[A] \qquad 8.60$$

That is, the balanced bridge output is zero, and any eluent gas mixed with He will reduce the cooling (increase Θ_R), allowing the two R_A resistors to warm slightly, raising their resistance, unbalancing the bridge, and producing an output. An advantage of the TCD is that no chemical change occurs in the eluents. Thus, they can be individually captured by condensation in nearly pure form, or passed on to another type of detector for more detailed analysis, such as a mass spectrometer.

The *electron capture detector* (ECD) is an exquisitely sensitive means of detecting chlorinated pesticide residues and PCBs in and on foods, and in humans and animals. Mass sensitivities to halogenated hydrocarbons of from 0.1 to 10 pg are possible with the ECD. Figure 8.23 illustrates a schematic cross-section of an ECD. Ionization is caused by beta-emitting isotopes of either tritium (^{3}H) or nickle (^{63}Ni) foil. The electrons are accelerated to and captured by the anode electrode. Chlorinated hydrocarbon molecules in the detector chamber capture some of the radio-electrons and reduce the net anode current, signifying the presence of the analyte. The ECD is insensitive to amines, alcohols and hydrocarbons. The carrier gases used with ECD are N_2 or Ar/CH_4; gas temperature ranges from 300 to 400° C.

As shown in Table 8.2.7.1, many other application-specific detectors exist. The interested reader should consult http://myhome.shinbiro.com/~yb9080/index.html for an excellent description of GC technology and GC detectors.

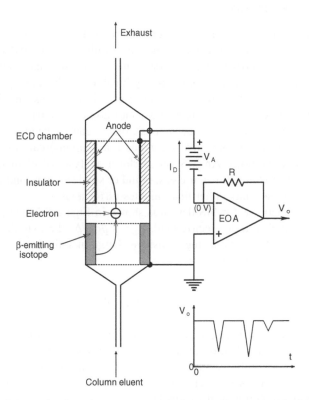

FIGURE 8.23 Schematic of an electron capture detector used to sense chlorinated hydrocarbon eluents.

Common stationary-phase GC column coatings (or fillings) range from the mundane zeolite particles ("kitty litter"), to styrene beads, aluminum oxide particles, or a host of thermally stable liquid polymers such as the various polysiloxanes and polyethene glycols used with capillary columns. The solid-phase, porous open layer tubular (PLOT) columns are very retentive, and are used to separate analytes whose peaks would be nearly coincident if using a conventional capillary column. The Lawrence-Livermore National Laboratory described a spiral capillary GC column micromachined on a silicon wafer. The object of the instrument development was to create a field-portable GC with rapid response time (c. 2 minutes) to sense environmental pollutants (see www-cms.llnl.gov/haas_dvlpmnt/gas_chrom.html).

Commercial GCs are generally heavy bench-top instruments because of their ovens, gas supplies, and associated computers. The columns and detectors are relatively compact, however. GC manufacturers and vendors include: The ThermoQuest Corp. (CE Instruments, Finnigan Corp.), Hewlett-Packard, Varian Associates, Tremetics, Tracor, Gow Mac, Chromatographic Instruments Company (build custom GCs), Gilson, Inc., Beckman-Coulter, SRI Instruments, Burdick & Jackson Div. of Baxter Healthcare Corp., and, of course, Shinbiro.

8.2.8 Mass Spectrometry

The mass spectrometer (MS) is another important analytical instrument used in medical diagnosis. While instruments like spectrophotometers and gas chromatographs allow investigators to examine intact molecules, the flame photometer and the MS gain their analytical information by breaking molecules apart. In an MS, the sample molecules are bombarded with energetic electrons, moving atoms, or photons from a laser beam to break them into component parts; some parts are positively charged (positive ions or cations), others can be neutral (i.e., have zero charge; they are lost), and negatively charged ions (anions) can also be produced under the right conditions. An MS can perform analysis of elements (isotopes), compounds, and mixtures. It can use gas, liquid or solid samples, and is fairly rapid, yielding results in seconds rather than minutes as for a GC.

A basic magnetic sector MS design is shown in Figure 8.24. The positive ions are first accelerated in a dc electric field, $E_1 = V_1/d_1$. At the exit slit, S_2, it can be shown that the positive ions having a positive charge magnitude of one electron (q) and a mass m will have a velocity

$$v_1 = \sqrt{2q\,V_1/m_1}\quad \text{m/s} \qquad\qquad 8.61$$

That is, the velocity is inversely proportional to the square root of the ion's mass. Positive ions with a distribution of velocities determined by their masses next enter a *velocity filter* formed by two electrodes parallel to the velocities of the entering ions. The positive ions are attracted to the cathode by a force $\mathbf{F_e} = \mathbf{E_2}q = (V_2/d_2)q\mathbf{i}$. ($\mathbf{i}$ is a unit vector pointing at the cathode.)

Because there is a $\mathbf{B}$ field perpendicular to the velocity (into page), the moving ions also experience a magnetic Lorenz force, $\mathbf{F_m} = q(\mathbf{v} \times \mathbf{B})$, the direction of which is given by the *right-hand screw rule*. That is, $\mathbf{F_m}$ points in the direction that a normal right-hand screw would advance if rotated in the direction of rotating $\mathbf{v}$ into $\mathbf{B}$. Thus $\mathbf{F_m}$ is opposite to $\mathbf{F_e}$. Because of the narrow separation (d_2) of the velocity filter's electrodes only positive ions with velocities such that $F_m \cong F_e$ emerge through slit S_3. This selected velocity can be shown to be:

$$v_o \cong V_2/(d_2\,B)\quad \text{m/s} \qquad\qquad 8.62$$

Again, the ions with velocity v_o are acted on by the Lorenz force in the $\mathbf{E}$ field-free chamber of the MS. Because $\mathbf{B}$ is perpendicular to v_o, the ion trajectories are semicircular. The ions strike the detector electrodes at a distance $D = 2R$ from S_3. Elementary physics (Sears, 1953) tells us that:

$$D = 2R = \left(2\,v_o\,m\right)/(q\,B) = (m/q)\frac{2V_2}{d_2 B^2}\quad \text{meters} \qquad\qquad 8.63$$

Thus, the distance D at which the ion beam strikes the collector is proportional to the ratio of mass to charge of the ion exiting the velocity filter. The + ion beam at

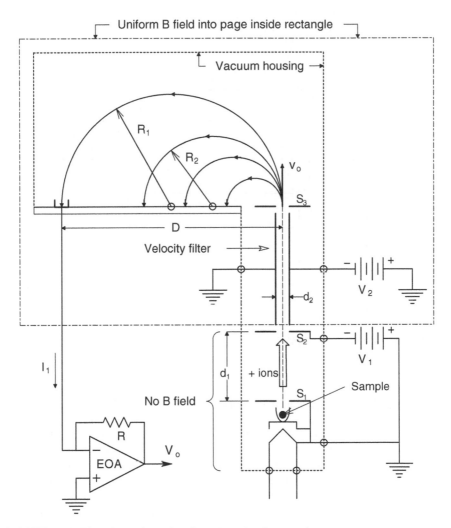

FIGURE 8.24 Plan view schematic of a conventional magnetic mass spectrometer.

D can be collected by an electrode (Faraday cup), and the resulting electron current, I_1, converted to a voltage, V_o, by an electrometer op amp connected as a transresistor.

Compound identification and quantification can also be carried out on analytes with mass ranges less than 10^3 Daltons by *negative ion mass spectrosopy* (NIMS). Negative ions are created in a sample by *resonance electron capture,* or direct ionization by low energy electron bombardment of the sample through a buffer gas such as methane. The methane gas slows down the electrons and stabilizes the resultant anions. Now the anions are accelerated through an electric field toward an anode, thence a velocity filter, thence into the magnet chamber. The anions bend to the right, however, because the Lorenz force has the opposite sign.

Unless the investigator has an *a priori* knowledge that a certain compound is present in a sample, identification of a molecular species from its mass fragment

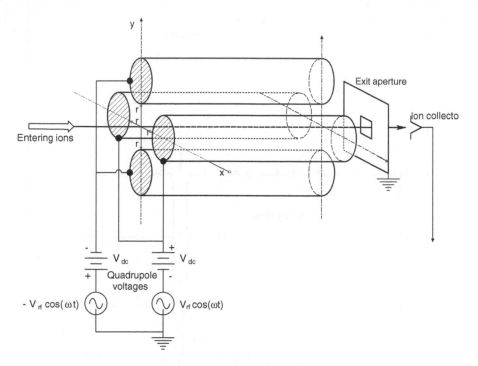

FIGURE 8.26 View of a quadrupole mass spectrometer. No magnetic field is used.

peaks can often be challenging. Table 8.2.8.1 illustrates commonly lost mass fragments that lack + charges and thus cannot produce peaks (they cannot be accelerated).

Figure 8.25 Shows some common stable mass fragment cations (Young 1996b).

In the analysis of biochemical and drug molecules from respiratory gases, urine, stool, blood, and tissue samples, the investigator often knows what molecules to expect, and thus, an MS system can be setup or "tuned" for a specific molecule in terms of the ionization method, and the expected Ds for the expected group of anions. A given analyte molecule can produce as many as 10 or more anions when fragmented and ionized. As in GC, the integral of a peak's area is proportional to the amount of an ion present.

General-purpose MS instruments, with few exceptions, are generally large, heavy and fixed. Smaller portable MS systems have been designed to measure respiratory gases such as O_2, CO_2, N_2, Halothane, etc. Ion ambiguities exist so that O_2 and CO_2 cannot be measured when ether ($C_4H_{10}O$) or N_2O is present (Webster, 1992). N_2 and carbon monoxide also have the same mass number (28).

The *quadrupole MS* (QPMS) was developed in the mid-1950s by Wolfgang Paul and associates at the University of Bonn. The QPMS is a lighter, more portable instrument than conventional MSs because its ion selectivity does not depend on a magnetic field (or the need for heavy magnets). Instead, ion selectivity depends entirely on the interaction of moving ions with combined ac and dc electric fields

TABLE 8.2.8.1
Commonly Lost Mass Fragments
(Young, 1996b)

Approximate Mass	Fragment
15	$-CH_3$
17	$-OH$
26	$-CN$
28	$H_2C=CH_2$
29	$-CH_2CH_3$, $-CHO$
31	$-OCH_3$
35	$-Cl$
43	$CH_3C=O$
45	$-OCH_2CH_3$
91	Benzine-CH_2

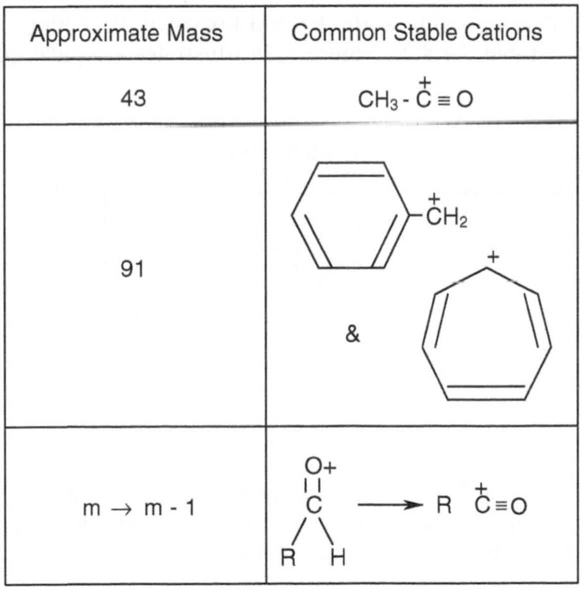

Approximate Mass	Common Stable Cations
43	$CH_3 - \overset{+}{C} \equiv O$
91	$\overset{+}{C}H_2$ (benzyl) & (tropylium cation)
$m \to m-1$	$\overset{O+}{\underset{R\ \ H}{C}} \longrightarrow R\ \overset{+}{C} \equiv O$

FIGURE 8.25 Some common stable mass fragments encountered in mass spectrometry. (Based on data from Young, 1996b.)

maintained between four cylindrical electrodes, as shown in Figure 8.26. The voltage applied to the two electrode pairs is the sum of a dc potential and an ac RF voltage; $V_+ = V_{dc} + V_{rf} \cos(\omega t)$, and $V_- = -[V_{dc} + V_{rf} \cos(\omega t)]$. The QPMS is "tuned" for specific m/q values by linearly increasing the V_{dc} voltage between 0 and 300 V while simultaneously increasing the peak RF voltage, V_{rf}, from 0 to

1.5 kV. It can be shown that the complex electric field between the tubes causes the entering ions to effectively "run the gauntlet." If an ion has an inappropriate mass/charge ratio, it will collide with an attracting tube and lose its $\oplus$ charge. Such non-charged molecular fragments are pumped out by the vacuum system. An ion with the "tuned" mass/charge will describe a spiral or corkscrew path between the electrodes, emerging through the exit window and striking the ion collector; its charge contributes to the collector current. The voltages on the QPMS's electrodes are increased linearly in time, providing a swept tuning of the mass/charge. As the voltages increase, larger and larger mass ions can pass through the quadrupole electrodes without collision. Thus, by plotting current peaks from the detector vs. the electrode sweep voltage, one can obtain a rapid mass spectrogram. The computer plots relative ion current vs. m/z. The advantages of QPMSs is that they are relatively inexpensive, smaller and faster (a scan completed in milliseconds) than conventional electrostatic/magnetic sector MS systems. They also give relative mass readings and have good reproducibility, but do not have the resolution of conventional MSs. Like gas chromatographs, QPMS machines must be calibrated with standard samples. Figure 8.27 shows a spectrogram for a methanol sample. Note that the molecular ion has the highest (32) m/z ratio. Relative abundances of the fragments are peculiar to the ionization method used. The very small peaks are due to the natural presence of isotopes of C, H and O in methanol (see Table 8.2.8.2). Figure 8.28 illustrates a typical QPMS spectrum of exhaled air.

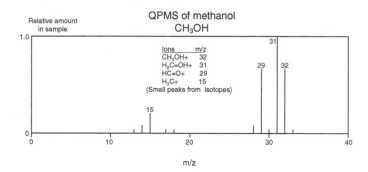

FIGURE 8.27 A quadrupole mass spectrogram for methanol. Peaks are from various + charged mass fragments, as well as from the same fragments containing stable element isotopes, giving the fragments slightly different masses.

The table, for example, shows that, for every 100 ^{12}C atoms, there will be 1.11 ^{13}C atoms, while, for every 100 ^{79}Br atoms, there are 98 ^{81}Br atoms, a surprisingly large ratio. Thus, a mass spectrogram of a compound containing a bromine atom will exhibit curious double peaks of almost the same size for those ions containing Br.

Several other types of MS exist in addition to the QPMS and magnetic sector MS described above. These include: The Time-of Flight MS, the Ion Cyclotron Resonance MS, and the Fourier Transform Ion Cyclotron Resonance (FTICR) MS.

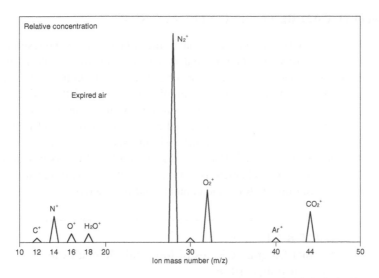

FIGURE 8.28 A representative quadrupole mass spectrogram of exhaled air. Note that the absolute value of O_2 and CO_2 can be determined on-line, as well as anesthetic gas (not shown).

TABLE 8.2.8.2
Relative Abundance of Some Naturally Occurring Non-Radioactive Isotopes

Natural Isotope at 100%	Isotope & Rel. Abundance	Isotope & Rel. Abundance
Carbon: ^{12}C	^{13}C: 1.11	
Hydrogen: ^1H	^2H: 0.16	
Nitrogen: ^{14}N	^{15}N: 0.38	
Oxygen: ^{16}O	^{17}O: 0.04	^{18}O: 0.20
Sulfur: ^{32}S	^{33}S: 0.78	^{34}S: 4.40
Chlorine: ^{35}Cl		^{37}Cl: 32.5
Bromine: ^{79}Br		^{81}Br: 98.0

In summary, we see that compound separation and identification using an MS can be a considerable challenge. An MS gives the total number of each constituent atom in a compound (the empirical formula), but can seldom provide clues about molecular structure that can be given, for example, by an optical spectrophotometer. Often, a molecular formula is found by trial and error from the ion mass peaks, using information from isotope abundance as well. Because gas chromatographs separate pure compounds in time as they traverse the column, feeding the column output into an MS simplifies the analysis of an unknown sample under the assumption that the MS will be analyzing one pure eluent compound at a time. Hence the popularity of GC/QPMS systems.

8.3 WHAT CAN BE LEARNED FROM URINE

Urine is derived from the glomerular filtrate of the kidneys, and is the result of many active and passive exchanges of ions and molecules with the filtrate as it passes through the loops of Henle and the collecting ducts of the kidneys. It is not our purpose here to describe in detail the complex functions of the kidneys in the production of urine, but to describe how substances in the urine can aid in the diagnosis of disease. Urine is either collected noninvasively by a midstream catch, or clinically by a sterile catheter (a "moderately invasive" procedure).

"Normal" parameters for substances and ions in a healthy person's urine have statistical ranges that can be characterized by means and standard deviations. Table 8.3.1 lists the ± 1 SD ranges for urine contents and parameters.

TABLE 8.3.1
Normal Clearance Rates of Ions and Molecules in Urine (Collins, 1968)

Substance	Normal Clearance Range or Concentration
Acetone	0
pH	5.5–7.5
Albumin	0
Ammonia	0.5–1.0 g/24 h.
Amylase	2,200 – 3,000 Somogyi units/24 h.
Bilirubin	0
Ca^{++}	100 – 150 mg/24 h. (4.8 mEq/l)*
Cl^-	119 mEq/24 h. (134 mEq/l)
Creatine	< 100 mg/24 h.
Creatinine	1.5–2.0 g/24 h. adult males (196 mEq/l)
	0.8–1.5 g/24 h. adult females
Erythrocytes	< 5.E5 cells/24 h.
Glucose	0.5–0.75 g/24 h. (0)
Leucocytes	1–2. E6/24 h. (1.–4.E3 cells/ml)
K^+	25–100 mEq/24 h. (60 mEq/l)
Na^+	111 mEq/24 h. (128 mEq/l)
Urea nitrogen	20–35 g/24 h. (1,820 mEq/l)
Urobilinogen	0–4 mg/24 h.
Mg^{++}	(15 mEq/l)
$H_2PO_4^- + HPO_4^=$	(50 mEq/l)

* Concentrations in parentheses are from Table 27.1 in Guyton (1991). They are based on a urine production of 1.44 liters/24 h.
Note: These rates and concentrations can vary widely even under normal conditions, and will differ from tabular source to source.

One of the most basic diagnostic tests that can be done on urine is for *glucose*. Normally, plasma glucose that is lost from the blood in glomerular filtrate is actively reabsorbed in the tubules and returned to the blood. However, this active reabsorption process can handle only about 320 mg/min. (the transport maximum). If the blood glucose rises above c. 160 mg/dl, then glucose begins to appear in the urine. When blood glucose exceeds c. 260 mg/dl, then the glucose concentration in the urine rises linearly with the blood glucose concentration. This phenomenon is illustrated in Figure 8.29. High blood glucose can be the result of untreated diabetes mellitus. It can also be elevated in renal glycosuria, Cushing's syndrome, pancreatitis, acromegaly, and hyperthyroidism. Urine glucose concentration can be estimated with glucose-sensitive indicator paper or chemical color tests, or quantitated with a glucose-specific (fuel-cell) electrode.

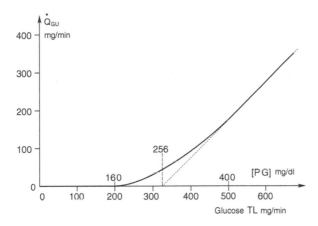

FIGURE 8.29 The well known curve for glucose loss rate in urine when the blood glucose concentration exceeds the level at which the kidneys can reabsorb glucose from the glomerular filtrate. Under nomoglycemic conditions, 500 to 750 mg glucose is lost over 24 hours, or about 0.5 mg/min on the average.

In cirrhosis of the liver and viral hepatitis, the concentration of urine *urobilinogen* can increase. Carcinoma of the head of the pancreas and gallstones both cause a decrease in urine urobilinogen (Collins ,1968).

The urine concentration of Na^+ and K^+, and the pH and volume of urine can be correlated with a number of diseases and physiological conditions. The concentration of Na^+, K^+ can be measured with a flame photometer or specific ion electrodes; pH is measured with a special glass pH electrode. Table 8.3.2 summarizes some of these correlations.

Tests to determine the concentrations of certain hormones in the urine can also aid in the diagnosis of hormonal regulatory disorders. Table 8.3.3, derived from data in Collins, 1968, illustrates the diseases and conditions associated with imbalances of urine *17-hydroxycortico-steroids, 17-ketosteroids, aldosterone* and *gonadotropins.* At least 13 steroid hormones are made in the adrenal cortex; it is a busy place. The 17-hydroxycorticosteroids are produced from cholesterol in response to ACTH secreted by the anterior pituitary gland; they include the glucocorticoids hormones *progesterone* and *cortisol.* The 17-ketosteroids include the androgenic hormones

TABLE 8.3.2
How Disorders of Blood Electrolytes Affect Na+, K+, pH and Volume of Urine (Collins, 1968)

Disease or Condition	Na+	K+	pH	Volume
Dehydration	↑	↑	↓	↓
Starvation	N or ↑	N or ↑	↓	↑ with ketones
Malabsorption syndrome (e.g., sprue)	↓	↓	↓	N
Congestive heart failure	↓	N	N	↓
Pyloric obstruction	↓	N	↑	↓
Diarrhea	↓	N or ↓	↓	↓
Diaphoresis w/ water replacement	↓	N	N	N
Acute renal failure	↓	↓	N or ↑	↓
Pulmonary emphysema	↓	N	↓	N
Salicylate toxicity*	↑	N or ↑	↑	N
Adrenal cortical insufficiency	↑	N or ↓	N or ↑	N or ↓
Diabetes insipidus (↓ ADH)	N	N	N	↑↑
Primary aldosteronism	↓	↓	N or ↓	↑
Chlorothiazide diuretics	↑	↑	N or ↑	↑
Hereditary renal tubular acidosis	↑	↑	↑	↑
Chronic renal failure	↑	↑	↑	variable ↑
Diabetic acidosis	↑	↑	↓	↑ w/ ketones

* Same symptoms with fever, head trauma, high altitude, and hyperventilation syndrome.

dehydroepiandosterone (DEA), and *testosterone* (made in the testicles). The mineral corticoid, *aldosterone,* is also synthesized in the adrenal cortex (West, 1985). Its principle role is in the regulation of plasma potassium ions (Northrop, 2000). Human anterior pituitary *gonadotropin hormones* include the glycoproteins, *follicle-stimulating hormone* and *luteinizing hormone.*

Means of measuring hormones, proteins, and ions in the urine include chemically treated dipsticks, electrophoresis, high-precision liquid chromatography, gas chromatography, electrophoresis, immune methods including immunoelectrophoresis, radioimmunoassays, antibody-based surface plasmon resonance, and specific ion electrodes and flame photometry (for Na+, K+, Ca++, etc.).

For example, certain urine protein (*proteinuria*) dipsticks respond to as little as 0.5 to 2.0 mg/ml albumin, the predominant protein found in most renal diseases, but are less sensitive to globulins and mucoproteins. Albumin in the urine is due to increased permeability of glomerular capillaries or reduced reabsorption of filtered proteins by the tubules. These changes can be due to infection, physical damage (due to injury from jogging, boxing, a fall, etc.), or a neoplasm.

Glucose dipsticks respond with a color change to urine glucose concentrations from about 100 mg/dl to over 1 g/dl. A urine glucose concentration of 100 mg/dl signifies a blood glucose of c. 350 mg/dl, well above normal. Glucose in the urine is called *glucosuria.*

TABLE 8.3.3
Responses of Urine Hormone Levels to Hormone Disorders
(from data in Collins, 1968)

Disease or Condition	17-hydroxy-corticosteroids	17-ketosteroids	Aldosterone	Gonadotropins
Acromegaly	N	N	N	N
Basophilic adenoma of the pituitary	↑	↑	N	N
Panhypopituitarism	↓	↓	N	↓
Pituitary hypogonadism	N	↓	N	↓
Hyperthyroidism	N	N	N	N
Subacute thyroiditis	N	N	N	N
Myxedema	N	N	N	N
Addison's disease	↓	↓	↓	N
Primary aldosteronism	N	N	↑	N
Cushing's syndrome	↑	↑	N	N
Adrenogential syndrome	N	↑	N	N
Turner's syndrome	N	N	N	↑
Polycystic ovaries	N	↑	N	N
Menopausal syndrome	N	N	N	↑
Pregnancy	↑	N	N	↑
Chorionepithelioma	N	N	N	↑
Seminoma	N	N	N	↑
Klinefelter's syndrome	N	N or ↓	N	↑

Other urine dipsticks are color sensitive to acetoacetic acid and acetone, both of which are found in the urine of persons with *ketonuria.* Ketonuria is present in uncontrolled diabetes mellitus, starvation, and, occasionally, in ethanol intoxication. *Hematuria,* or hemoglobin in the urine, can also be sensed by a dipstick color test. Hematuria is symptomatic of acute renal failure. In *nitrituria,* the dipstick responds to the conversion of nitrate from dietary metabolites to nitrite by certain bacteria in the urine. Normally, no nitrite is present. Thus a positive nitrituria test is seen in about 80% of bladder infections (*bacteriuria*). The urine with nitrate needs to incubate in the bladder in the presence of the bacteria at least 4 hours. Urinary pH is also measured with a color dipstick responsive in the range from 5 to 9. Knowledge of the urine pH helps to identify crystals (e.g., oxalate, phosphate, urate) that may be found on microscopic examination. All dipstick color tests are of low accuracy, three-bit (one part in eight) at the most.

Microscopic examination of the urine sediment after centrifuging a specimen allows the clinician to observe the presence of crystals (see above), casts (cylindrical masses of mucoprotein in which cellular elements, fat droplets, or other proteins may be trapped), leucocytes (WBCs), erythrocytes (RBCs), and occasional bacteria. Over 10 WBCs/μL is diagnostic for urinary tract infection.

Gas chromatography or mass spectrometry is used to screen urine samples for drugs such as cocaine, marijuana (tetrahydrocannabinol = THC), amphetamines, and the opiates codeine and morphine. Cocaine use is detected by measuring the concentration of the cocaine metabolite, *benzoylecgonine*, in urine. Benzoylecgonine (BZG) concentration in the urine reaches a maximum from 4 to 10 hours after cocaine use, and persists for 2 to 3 days. After the peak, the BZG concentration decays with a $T_{1/2}$ of c. 6 hours thereafter. The THC metabolite in urine is 11-nor-9-carboxy-delta-9-THC. When a marijuana cigarette containing c. 33.8 mg of THC was smoked, the peak concentration of 11-nor-9-carboxy-delta-9-THC appeared at a mean time of 13.5 hours. The peak concentrations ranged from 29.9 to 355.2 ng/ml (153.5 ng/ml mean) for six individuals. Many over-the-counter drugs give positive urine tests for amphetamines; these include ephedrine, pseudoephedrine (for sinuses), L-methamphetamine (in Vick's inhaler) and phenylpropanolamine. However, they can be separated from amphetamine and D-methamphetamine by correctly executed GC/MS tests. The opiates codeine and morphine appear in the urine as morphine. Eating foods with poppy seeds can also produce morphine in the urine. As much as 10 µg/ml morphine has been measured in the urine after a subject ate food with poppy seeds (cf. www.dome-research.com/urinalysis.html).

Of final diagnostic interest is the relatively rare family of diseases called *porphyrias*. Any hereditary deficiency in the biosynthesis of one (or more) of the enzymes involved in heme synthesis causes a porphyria disease in which several metabolic precursors to heme are over-produced (e.g., porphyrins, porphobilinogen (PBG), and δ-aminolevulinic *acid* (ALA)). There are three major categories of porphyria: *Acute intermittent porphyria* (AIP), *Porphyria cutanea tarda* (PCT), and *Erythropoietic protoporphyria* (EPP) (Merk, 2000). The latter two porphryias affect the skin, causing rashes, blistering and lesions. AIP is the result of low levels of the enzyme *PGB deaminase*. AIP does not affect the skin, but rather the central and peripheral nervous systems, causing acute abdominal and organ pain. Tachycardia, muscle weakness, damage to motor and cranial nerves, tremors, seizures, and psychiatric symptoms can occur in individuals with severe AIP.

A key diagnostic symptom of AIP is that porphobilinogen (PBG) and ALA appear in the urine at high levels (PBG @ 50–200 mg/day; ALA @ 20–100 mg/day; normal PBG @ 0–4 mg/day; normal ALA @ 0–7 mg/dal). PBG spontaneously forms *uroporphyrin,* and also breaks down into substances called *porphobilins*. The ALA that is overproduced in the liver may be metabolized to porphyrins in other cells. PBG and ALA are initially colorless, but soon oxidize to a reddish purple-to-brown color (the name porphyria comes from the Greek word for purple). Uroporphyins fluoresce under UV illumination, and all porphyrins have unique IR absorption spectra.

In PCT, the deficient enzyme is *uroporphyrinogen decarboxylase.* In EPP, the deficient enzyme is *ferrochelatase,* which places Fe^{++} in the heme ring. In EPP there is a build-up of *protoporphyrin IX* in bone marrow and erythrocytes. This excess protoporphyrin enters the plasma and is excreted by the liver into bile and feces.

8.4 WHAT CAN BE LEARNED FROM THE FECES

Direct observation of a stool sample under the microscope can lead to the detection of various endoparasites (from their bodies, eggs or cysts) including Giardia, tapeworms, round worms (ascarids), etc. Infestations of these parasites are often accompanied by cramps, bloating, diarrhea, and bleeding.

Chemical analysis of stool samples can detect whole blood from internal bleeding; this blood can be from stomach ulcers, parasites, colorectal cancer, bacterial toxins, Krohn's disease, etc. The tetramethyl benzidine reagent test and the guaiac test are commonly used to detect occult blood in urine or feces (Collins, 1968). They use the principle that heme proteins act as peroxidases, catalyzing the reduction of H_2O_2 to water, giving a color reaction as the indicator substance is oxidized in the reaction. False positive chemical tests may occur if the patient's diet has recently included foods rich in peroxidases such as brassicas (cauliflower, broccoli, etc.), radishes and cantaloupe. A false negative can occur if vitamin C in excess of 250 mg/day is taken (vitamin C is an antioxidant). A more sensitive and specific test for occult blood is the F.O.B. Rapydtest®, which uses monoclonal antibodies to human hemoglobin. In this test, two colored bands appear on a test strip when a positive result occurs.

Bilirubin is a normal by-product of hemoglobin metabolism. Red blood cells, or erythrocytes, have a mean life span of about 120 days. The cell membranes of old erythrocytes rupture, releasing hemoglobin molecules. Special macrophages, the reticuloendothelial cells of the liver, spleen and bone marrow, take up the free hemoglobin and break the protein globin from the heme ring. Normally, 7 to 8 grams of hemoglobin are broken down daily by cells of the reticulo-endiothelial system. The heme ring is opened enzymatically and the free iron is taken up by the enzyme transferrin for recycling; the heme is formed into a straight chain of four linked pyrrole nuclcii. The tetrapyrrole molecules are first converted to *biliverdin,* then reduced to bilirubin, which is released by the reticuloendothelial cells. Once in the blood, the free bilirubin combines strongly with the plasma albumin. It is transported as this stable complex in the blood. The complex is taken up by liver cells (hepatocytes), in which the tetrapyrrole molecule is split from the albumin, and then made water-soluble by conjugation with glucuronic to form bilirubin mono- and diglucuronide (c. 80%), also, bilirubin sulfate (c. 10%) and other bilirubin salts (c. 10%) are formed. It is these water-soluble bilirubin forms that are secreted into the bile, which is injected into the small intestine as part of the process of digestion (Guyton, 1991).

The action of certain bacteria in the intestines converts the bilirubin salts to the compounds, *urobilinogen* and *stercobilinogen.* In 24 hours, from 50 to 300 mg of bilirubin are secreted as stercobilinogen in a normal adult. This mass is derived from the normal breakdown of from 7 to 8 g of hemoglobin, plus that derived from myoglobins, cytochromes and catalases. Outside the body, stercobilinogen is further oxidized to *stercobilin.* Some of the intestinal urobilinogen, which is quite soluble, is reabsorbed by the intestinal mucosa, and finds its way back to the liver and the kidneys. Normally, about 4 mg of urobilinogen in 24 hours appears in the urine.

Jaundice is a condition where the skin, mucous membranes, whites of the eye, etc. turn yellow because of an excess of bilirubin in the blood. The presence of jaundice can signal one of two conditions: 1) The rate of red cell destruction is sufficiently above normal (*hemolytic jaundice*) so that the normal hepatocytes cannot keep up with the conversion of the bilirubin-albumin complex in the blood to bilirubin, thence to bile. 2) In *obstructive jaundice,* there may be damage to the hepatocytes from some form of hepatitis (viral, chemical), or the bile ducts may be blocked by bile stones or a cancer. Because of the blockage, bile ducts may rupture, and the circulating bilirubin is now of the conjugated form. In the disease malaria, jaundice can be from both damaged hepatocytes and ruptured erythrocytes.

The concentration of urobilinogen in the stool is thus greatly reduced when a gallstone blocks the bile duct (there is also acute pain, which needs no laboratory analysis). Stool urobilinogen is also moderately reduced in viral hepatitis, cancer of the pancreatic head, and in chemical hepatitis.

Celiac disease, or *non-tropical sprue (NTS)*, is one of several intestinal malabsorption syndromes that can be partially diagnosed from analysis of the stool. Its incidence in the United States is about 1:5,000. Celiac disease is a genetically based autoimmune disease that destroys the microvilli lining the small intestine, preventing the normal absorption of dietary fats as well as a host of other substances including the fat-soluble vitamins A, D and K, as well as vitamin B_{12} and folic acid. In severe NTS, there is malabsorption of calcium, iron, protein and carbohydrates. Other symptoms presented in NTS include bone demineralization, anemia, failure of blood to clot, and the general symptoms of starvation, although the diet is normal. NTS is caused by the *gliadin* fraction of *gluten* in wheat, rye, barley and oats, which are eaten as bread, cereal, etc. Ingested gliadin forms an immune complex in the intestinal mucosa, and the patient's immune system responds with an aggregation of macrophages and killer lymphocytes that generate inflammation and systematically destroy the celiac microvilli through which nutrients are absorbed (Merk, Sect. 3, Ch. 30, 2000; Guyton, 1991).

In NTS, the feces contain an abnormally high content of fats (steatorrhea). They are pale, greasy, and float on water. Generally, stool fat over 6 g/24 h, given 100g per day fat in the diet, is diagnostic for NTS. Stool fat can be identified nonquantitatively by staining a smear with the dye Sudan III.

A patient with NTS must be put onto a gluten-free diet. Gluten is also found as a food additive in hot dogs, ice cream, soups, etc., so it can be difficult to eliminate it from the diet. Recovery is accelerated by administering vitamins and minerals to treat the starvation symptoms. Oral corticosteroids (e.g., prednisone) may be given in severe cases to reduce bowel inflammation.

Tropical sprue (TS) is an ideopathic version of NTS. TS can be caused by an unknown parasite, bacteria or virus infection, or a bacterial toxin from spoiled food. It has similar symptoms, including steatorrhea. The treatment of choice for TS is the antibiotic tetracycline, which may be administered for as long as 6 months. As in NTS, vitamins and folic acid are also given.

8.5 WHAT CAN BE LEARNED FROM SALIVA

Saliva is a complex exocrine secretion of the three pairs of salivary glands; the *parotids,* the *submandibulars,* and the *sublinguals.* The parotid salivary glands are the largest. The net out-put of the salivary glands when a person is chewing is about 2.5 ml/min, but the secretion rate can vary with the sensed flavor and aroma of the food being eaten. Saliva contains two major components, a fluid part containing ions and small molecules, and proteins that come from secretory vesicles in the gland cells. Apparently, control of the fluid component is by parasympathetic nerve stimulation; sympathetic nerve stimulation causes the release of the proteins. The formation of saliva is a complex, active process; the interested reader should see the website (www.umds.ac.uk/physiology/rbm/saliva.htm) for details.

Some of the proteins and enzymes in saliva include the following: albumin, β-glucuronidase, cystatins, esterases, gustin, antibodies (IgA, IgG, IgM), lactoferrin, lactic dehydrogenase, mucins, parotid aggregins, phosphatases, ribonucleases, vitamin-binding proteins, α-amylase, epidermal growth factor, fibronectin, histatins, kallikrein, lipase, lysozyme, nerve growth factor, peptidases, salivary peroxidases, etc. Also, the low molecular weight molecules: glucose, creatinine, lipids, sialic acid, uric acid, urea, etc. The secreted ions include: Na^+, K^+, Ca^{++}, Mg^{++}, Cl^-, I^-, F^-, $SO_4^=$, HCO_3^-, $HPO_4^=$, $H_2PO_4^-$, SCN^-, etc.; see (www.cybermedical.com/salagen.dir/oral.dir/oral.html).

Of medical diagnostic significance is the presence in saliva of the bacteria *Heliobacter pylori* (which normally is not present), signifying possible peptic ulcers, gastritis or stomach cancer. Saliva has also been used in the detection of all forms of hepatitis. Marijuana (THC), cocaine, codeine, nicotine and alcohol appear in it and can be detected using the same techniques used with urine. One of the more important noninvasive diagnostic uses of saliva is in the estimation of blood (plasma) glucose concentration (BG).

Reports in the literature have made a variety of claims, ranging from the glucose concentration in saliva's being poorly correlated with blood glucose concentration (BG) and cannot be used to manage diabetes (Forbat, et al., 1981), to the fact that salivary glucose, properly collected, is highly correlated with (BG] (with a time delay) and shows promise for an input for a glucoregulation algorithm (Yamaguchi et al.., 1998, Andersson, et al., 1998). In a pilot study, Yamaguchi, et al. gave six healthy young men 75g oral glucose-tolerance tests (OGTTs). They measured salivary glucose (SG) and (BG) with an enzymatic glucose electrode. Figure 8.30 illustrates the broad range of responses from the six subjects. Note that individual (BG) responses to the test differ significantly, as do the (SG) levels. Figure 8.31 shows the averaged regression lines between (BG) and (SG) for the six subjects. The correlation coefficients for subjects A through F were 0.89, 0.71, 0.65, 0.80, 0.82 and 0.66, respectively. Time lags (t_{bs}) between the first (BG) peak in the OGTT and the first peak in the (SG) curve were incredibly variable, and, in some cases, the means were positive (a phase lead). For subjects A through F, the lags were: -16 ± 4, -3 ± 4, $+1 \pm 5$, $+6 \pm 11$, -20 ± 7 and $+3 \pm 1$ 4 minutes, respectively.

What the data of Yamaguchi, et al. show is that properly collected saliva samples can indeed be used to estimate (BG). However, because of individual variability in (BG)/(SG), t_{bs}, and r, a salivary (BG) estimator would have to be custom-calibrated to an individual using an OGTT. It remains to be seen whether the noninvasive salivary (BG) estimation method can prove as reliable as the finger-prick/blood drop/colorimeter test now most widely used by diabetics.

8.6 WHAT CAN BE LEARNED FROM THE BREATH

From its origin in the lungs, exhaled breath should ideally contain only water vapor, CO_2, O_2, N_2 and traces of CO, H_2 and Ar. Unfortunately, one's breath is not always

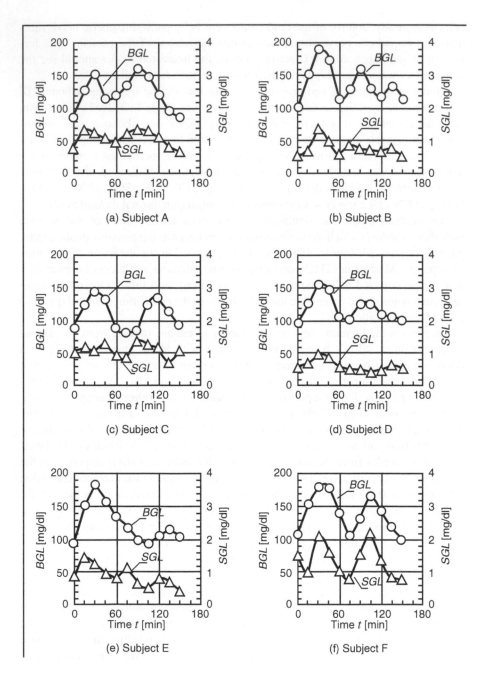

FIGURE 8.30 How saliva glucose levels track blood glucose concentration in six subjects. Figure from Yamaguchi et al, 1998. (With permission from IEEE.)

odorless. *Halitosis* is a term applied to the general phenomenon of unpleasant, malodorous, or bad breath. The offensive odors can be from several sources, and, in some cases, can be of diagnostic value to a physician or dentist.

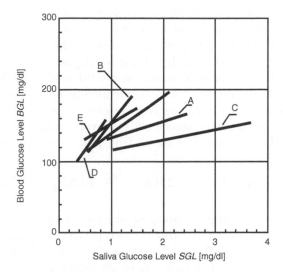

FIGURE 8.31 Averaged regression line between (BG) and (SG) for the six subjects whose data is shown in Figure 8.30. (With permission from IEEE.)

Other vapor-phase additives to exhaled breath can include volatile substances in the blood such as acetone (present in severe, untreated diabetes mellitus), volatile substances from the nasal passages, sinuses and throat (e.g., from nasal polyps, nasal infection, sinusitis or throat bacterial infection), and substances from the mouth (gum disease, rotting food between the teeth, bacteria on the tongue). Many of the odors of halitosis that come from the bacterial breakdown of food trapped between the teeth (and between the teeth and gums) are due to sulfur compounds. Some of the more obnoxious odorants from the mouth include hydrogen sulfide, methyl mercaptan, dimethyl disulphide, putrescene, cadaverine, skatole and indole; (see the website: www.quality.dentistry.com/dental/halitosis/myths.html).

Other bad breath odors might be associated with internal organ diseases which could include the lungs, the stomach, gallbladder dysfunction, and kidney failure. Various carcinomas are reported to cause malodor, as well. Perhaps in the future, a noninvasive screening test for lung cancer can be developed that relies on the enormous sensitivity of FTIR spectroscopy or GC/QPMS to quantify a specific odorant associated with this disease. It is reasonable to expect that if a relatively insensitive human olfactory system can smell an odor, a modern analytical instrument can also measure it.

One of the more successful NI diagnostic measurements (relative sensitivity = 97.6%, relative specificity = 94.1%) that can be made using exhaled breath is the test for the bacterium that is largely responsible for stomach ulcers, *Helicobacter pylori*. *H. pylori* was discovered by Warren and Marshall in 1982 (cf. www.prometheus-labs.com/patients/ulcer.htm]; it is a spiral or corkscrew-shaped bacterium that lives in the stomach in the interface between the mucous gel and the gastric epithelial cells. Technically, it is outside of the body, and difficult for immune system cells to attack. *H. pylori* is highly correlated with *antral gastritis,* and with duodenal and gastric ulcers. Its presence is also strongly correlated with the incidence of stomach cancer (there is a sixfold increase in the incidence of stomach cancer in patients carrying *H. pylori* (pharminfo,1996). The presence of *H. pylori* in the stomach can be definitively determined invasively by taking a biopsy from an ulcer with a gastroscope. A blood antibody test also is fairly accurate in identifying an *H. pylori* infection. The accurate noninvasive "urea breath test" for the bacterium makes use of the fact that *H. pylori* survives on the stomach lining by secreting the enzyme *urease*, which breaks urea in the stomach contents down to ammonia and carbon dioxide. The ammonia forms ammonium hydroxide, which neutralizes stomach hydrochloric acid in the vicinity of the bacteria, protecting them. The reaction is:

$$2\,H_2N\left(^{13}CO\right)NH_2 + 2\,H_2O \xrightarrow{\text{urease}} 4\,NH_3 + 2\,^{13}CO_2 \qquad 8.64$$

In the ^{13}C test, the patient is asked to swallow 75 mg of urea containing the nonradioactive carbon isotope ^{13}C. If *H. pylori* is present, it rapidly breaks down the ^{13}C-urea to NH_3 and $^{13}CO_2$. The $^{13}CO_2$ goes rapidly into the blood and thence to the lungs, where most of it is exhaled in the breath, enriching the normal fraction of $^{13}CO_2/^{12}CO_2$ to well above 1.11/100. The ratio of $^{13}CO_2/^{12}CO_2$ is sensed with a mass spectrometer. Two breath samples are taken at 0 minutes, and two more at 30 minutes. A $\geq 4\%$ increase in the $^{13}CO_2/^{12}CO_2$ ratio is considered evidence that *H. pylori* is present in the stomach. The very small amount of ^{13}C-urea ingested is considered innocuous.

An alternate isotope test for *H. pylori* uses ^{14}C-urea. Carbon-14 is a radioisotope that emits 156 keV β particles (electrons) with a half-life of 5,730 years! (It is better known for its use in dating organic archeological samples.) One microCurie of ^{14}C-urea is administered to the patient. Again, if *H. pylori* is present, it rapidly breaks down the ^{14}C-urea to ammonia and $^{14}CO_2$. The $^{14}CO_2$ is rapidly passed into the blood and most is exhaled. The β radioactivity of breath samples taken at 0, 6, 12, and 20 minutes is counted, and this data is used to assess the presence of *H. pylori*. The ^{14}C-urea test is not given to pregnant women, possibly because, in both tests, some CO_2 becomes bicarbonate and can end up in the bones or other biomolecules. ^{13}C is innocuous, but the long-term presence of even pC amounts of ^{14}C in the body carries some risk of cell damage.

Another breath test that uses a mass spectrometer or a gas chromatograph with a molecular seive is the *hydrogen test* used in the diagnosis of the genetic condition of *lactase deficiency,* otherwise known as lactose (milk sugar) intolerance. In the normal digestive process, the disaccharide lactose is broken apart by the enzyme lactase to form *galactose* and *glucose*. (Lactase is normally found in the brush borders of epithelial cells lining the small intestine. Galactose is also converted to glucose enzymatically.) As a result of this cleavage, the plasma glucose concentration rises. In lactase-deficient individuals, plasma glucose does not significantly rise. The undigested lactose is fermented in the colon by bacteria. Lactose fermentation by-products include hydrogen gas (H_2), which is absorbed into the blood and released through the lungs in exhaled breath. About 21% of H_2 produced in the colon exits the body through the lungs (Di Palma, 2000).

In the hydrogen breath test, 10 to 50g of lactose in solution is ingested, followed by periodically monitoring the H_2 gas partial pressure in the exhaled breath by a mass spectrometer or gas chromatograph. Normally, there is very little H_2 in the exhaled breath; however, it rises in cases of lactase deficiency to over 20 ppm above the baseline pH_2, given a 50g lactose oral input. Other sugars in the gut (e.g., fructose, d-xylose, sucrose) also can ferment to raise the breath H_2 concentration, giving a false positive reading, so before a patient is given the hydrogen breath test, the preceding day's diet must be low in carbohydrates and free of sweets (especially lactose) and antibiotics (Di Palma, 2000).

Because CO_2 is another byproduct of the metabolic breakdown of sugars, radio-active ^{14}C-d-xylose and ^{14}C-glycochocolate can also be used in enzyme-deficiency breath tests. In this case, $^{14}CO_2$ is assayed in the breath by counting β emissions with a Geiger counter (Perkins, 1999). There is no reason that ^{13}C-sugars could not also be used (as in the case of the *H. pylori* urea test), and the $^{13}CO_2/^{12}CO_2$ ratio can be measured with a mass spectrometer.

Lee, Majkowski and Perry (1991) reported on an exquisitely sensitive tunable IR diode laser spectrometer that could resolve $^{12}C^{16}O$ vs. $^{13}C^{16}O$ (carbon monoxide) in exhaled breath in sub-ppm concentrations. They suggested that their prototype instrument could find application in studies of the catabolism of the heme protein. One molecule of CO is produced along with every bilirubin molecule. Other bio-chemical applications of their IR diode spectrophotometer could lie in studies of heme formation and its abnormalities such as the porphyrias. They also noted that other molecules with IR signatures such as CO_2, NH_3, formaldehyde, H_2O_2, etc., can be quantified in breath by their instrument.

In summary, we see that there are established noninvasive tests using breath gases. At present, the presence of the bacterium *H. pylori* can be detected, and a variety of digestive enzyme disorders involving sugar metabolism can be verified. Gas chromatographs, mass spectrometers and Geiger counters are used for these purposes. Other gases in the breath resulting from infections, cancers, etc., will probably be identified, and may eventually be used in diagnostic screening tests. FTIR spectrometers, gas chromatographs, mass spectrometers, and surface plasmon resonance systems have the requisite sensitivities, if correctly applied. These are avenues of research that should be pursued.

8.7 SUMMARY

In this chapter, we have seen that modern analytical instruments can quantify nano-mole quantities of analytes in noninvasively obtained body fluids, including saliva, urine, the breath and the feces. It appears that certain kinds of bacteria, other pathogens, and cancers emit characteristic molecules into their surrounding milieus. These range from DNA from mitochondria to various metabolites, including hydro-gen gas. All of the instrumental methods described in Section 8.2 are well established in laboratory medicine, with the exception of surface plasmon resonance (SPR). In the future, expect to see SPR used to quantify specific bacterial antigens or antibodies in body fluids, as well as to identify other biomolecules. SPR devices will be miniaturized, and perhaps even incorporated into biochips as a readout modality.

Obviously, no one instrumental method is good for all analytical tests. In most cases, at least two modalities can be used on the same analyte. Not every instrumental method was covered in this chapter; for example, liquid and electrophoretic chromatography were not covered — not because I consider them unimportant, but because they have little engineering complexity to justify including them in a text on instrumentation.

Photonics in the form of fluorescence, spectrophotometry, SPR, Raman, etc. will dominate laboratory medicine and noninvasive nonimaging diagnostic procedures.

9 Plethysmography

9.1 INTRODUCTION

Plethysmography is a term for a set of noninvasive techniques for measuring volume changes in parts of the body, or even the whole body. The more frequently measured volume changes are those caused by breathing (lung and chest expansion), those due to blood's being forced into arteries, veins and capillaries of the legs, arms, hands and feet by the pumping of the heart, and the volume change of the heart itself as it pumps. It is also possible to measure local volume changes in arms and legs as muscles contract.

The two main techniques used today for plethysmography are volume displacement using air or water outside the body, and the measurement of the electrical impedance or admittance of the body part being studied. In the latter method, as you will see, volume changes translate into impedance changes. Volume changes can also be estimated by ultrasonic and X-ray imaging. Imaging is described in Chapter 16 of this text.

9.2 VOLUME DISPLACEMENT PLETHYSMOGRAPHY

Many techniques have been developed to measure volume changes in the body. One of the simplest, used on arms and legs, is the pneumatic sphygmomanometer cuff. The cuff is placed around a limb, e.g., the calf, and is inflated to a pressure, P_o, well below the patient's diastolic blood pressure. Some known air volume, V_o, is required to reach this pressure. The outside of the cuff has little compliance due to the stiff fabric material over the rubber bladder. From elementary physics, we know that $P_o V_o = nRT$, or $P_o = nRT/V_o$. Now, if the limb expands against the compliant bladder by some ΔV, the pressure can be written as:

$$P = nRT/\left(V_o - \Delta V\right) = \frac{nRT}{V_o\left(1 - \Delta V/V_o\right)} \cong \frac{nRT}{V_o}\left(1 + \Delta V/V_o\right) = P_o\left(1 + \Delta V/V_o\right) \quad 9.1$$

By measuring $\Delta P = P_o\left(\Delta V/V_o\right)$, we can calculate ΔV of the limb. Constant temperature is assumed.

Another direct means of measuring the ΔV of a limb is to enclose it with a water-filled bladder, the outside of which is non-compliant. (Water displacement is probably the oldest mode of plethysmography.) Because water is not compressible, any positive ΔV of the limb will force water up a capillary tube calibrated in volume.

The height of the water in the capillary tube can be converted to an electrical output signal photoelectrically.

A pneumatic whole-body plethysmograph can be used to estimate the functional residual capacity (FRC) of the lungs (West, 1985). The subject sits in a hermetically sealed box of volume V_B. The subject's body volume is V_S, measured by positive water displacement. Thus, the air volume in the box with the patient in it is $V_o = V_B - V_S$. The air in the box is at atmospheric pressure, P_o. The subject is asked to blow into a sealed tube containing a pressure transducer, which creates a pressure, $P_2 > P_o$. This exhalation effort compresses the gas in the subject's lungs so that the lung volume decreases slightly by ΔV. Thus, the box volume increases by ΔV, causing the pressure in the box to drop slightly to $P_3 < P_o$. We apply Boyle's law to both the box and the lungs. For the lungs:

$$P_o V_L = P_2 (V_L - \Delta V), \text{ so } V_L = P_2 \Delta V/(P_2 - P_o) \qquad 9.2$$

For the box:

$$P_o V_o = P_3(V_o - \Delta V), \text{ so } \Delta V = V_o(P_o/P_3 - 1) \qquad 9.3$$

ΔV estimates the amount the FRC space in the lungs is compressed by the exhalation effort against the closed tube. Once found, ΔV can be used in Equation 9.2 to find V_L, the initial lung volume.

9.3 IMPEDANCE PLETHYSMOGRAPHY

9.3.1 INTRODUCTION

Yet another way to measure the volume changes in body tissues is by measuring the electrical impedance of the body part being studied. As the heart forces blood through arteries, veins and capillaries, the impedance is modulated. When used in conjunction with an external air pressure cuff that can gradually constrict blood flow, impedance plethysmography (IP) can provide noninvasive diagnostic signs about abnormal venous and arterial blood flow. Also, by measuring the impedance of the chest, the relative depth and rate of a patient's breathing can be monitored noninvasively. As the lungs inflate and the chest expands, the impedance magnitude of the chest increases; air is clearly a poorer conductor than tissues and blood.

IP is often carried out using, for safety's sake, a controlled ac current source of fixed frequency. The peak current is generally kept less than 1 mA, and the frequency used typically is between 30 to 75 kHz. The high frequency is used because the human susceptibility to electroshock, and the physiological effects on nerves and muscles from ac decreases with increasing frequency (Webster, 1992). The electrical impedance is measured indirectly by measuring the ac voltage between two skin surface electrodes (generally ECG- or EEG-type, AgCl + conductive gel) placed between the two current electrodes. Thus, four electrodes are generally used, although the same two electrodes used for current injection can also be connected to the high-input-impedance ac differential amplifier that measures the output voltage, V_o. By Ohm's law, $V_o = I_s Z_t = I_s [R_t + j B_t]$.

At a fixed frequency, the tissue impedance can be modeled by a single conductance in parallel with a capacitor. Thus, it is algebraically simpler to consider the tissue *admittance*, $Y_t = Z_t^{-1} = G_t + j\omega C_t$. Both G_t and C_t change as blood periodically flows into the tissue under measurement. The imposed ac current is carried in the tissue by moving ions rather than electrons. Ions such as Cl^-, HCO_3^-, K^+, Na^+, etc., that drift in the applied electric field (caused by the current-regulated source), have three major pathways: a resistive path in the extracellular fluid electrolyte, a resistive path in blood, and a capacitive path caused by ions that charge the membranes of closely packed body cells. Ions can penetrate cell membranes and move inside cells, but not with the ease that they can travel in extracellular fluid space, and in blood. Of course, there are many, many cells effectively in series and parallel between the current electrodes. C_t represents the net equivalent capacitance of all the cell membranes. Each species of ion in solution has a different mobility. The mobility of an ion in solution, $\mu \equiv v/E$, where v is the mean drift velocity of the ion in a surrounding uniform electric field, E. Ionic mobility also depends on the ionic concentration, and the other ions in solution. Ionic mobility has the units of $m^2 sec^{-1} volt^{-1}$. Returning to Ohm's law, we can write in phasor notation:

$$V_o = I_s/Y_t = I_s \frac{G_t - j\omega C_t}{G_t^2 + \omega^2 C_t^2} = I_s\left[\text{Re}\{Z_t\} - j\,\text{Im}\{Z_t\}\right] \qquad 9.4$$

Where $\text{Re}\{Z_t\}$ is the real part of the tissue impedance = $G_t/(G_t^2 + \omega^2 C_t^2)$, and $\text{Im}\{Z_t\}$ is the imaginary part of the tissue impedance, $B_t = -\omega C_t/(G_t^2 + \omega^2 C_t^2)$. Note that both $\text{Re}\{Z_t\}$ and $\text{Im}\{Z_t\}$ are frequency-dependent. Note that V_o lags I_s.

There are several ways of measuring tissue Z_t, both magnitude and angle. In the first method, described in detail below, an ac voltage, V_s, is applied to the tissue. The amplitude is adjusted so that the resultant current, I_o, remains less than 1 mA. I_o is converted to a proportional voltage, V_o, by an op amp current-to-voltage converter circuit. In general, V_o and V_s differ in phase and magnitude. A self-nulling circuit operates on V_o and V_s. At null, its output voltage, V_z, is proportional to $|Z_t|$. A second method uses the ac current source excitation, I_s, and the output voltage described above, V_o, is fed into a servo-tracking, two-phase, lock-in amplifier which produces an output voltage, $V_z \propto |Z_t|$, and another voltage, $V_\theta \propto \angle Z_t$.

9.3.2 Self-Balancing Impedance Plethysmographs

A self-nulling plethysmograph designed by the author is illustrated in Figure 9.1. A 75 kHz, sinusoidal voltage, V_s, is applied to a chest electrode. A current, I_o, flows through the chest, and is given by Ohm's law:

$$I_o = V_s [G_t + j\omega C_t] \qquad 9.5$$

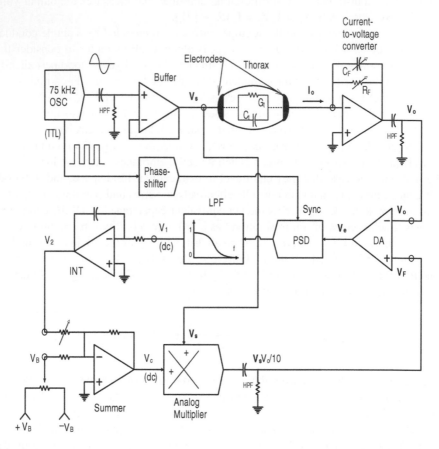

FIGURE 9.1   Block diagram of a self-nulling impedance plethysmograph designed by the author.

This current is converted to ac voltage, $\mathbf{V}_o$, by the current-to-voltage op amp:

$$\mathbf{V}_o = -\mathbf{I}_o \frac{G_F - j\omega C_F}{G_F^2 + \omega^2 C_F^2} = -\mathbf{V}_s \left[G_t + j\omega C_t\right] \frac{G_F - j\omega C_F}{G_F^2 + \omega^2 C_F^2} \qquad 9.6$$

$$\downarrow$$

$$\mathbf{V}_o = -\mathbf{V}_s \frac{G_t G_F - j\omega C_F G_t + j\omega C_t C_F + \omega^2 C_t C_F}{G_F^2 + \omega^2 C_F^2} \qquad 9.7$$

With the patient exhaled and holding his breath, C_F is adjusted so that $\mathbf{V}_o$ is in phase with $\mathbf{V}_s$. That is, C_F is set so that the imaginary terms in Equation 9.7 $\rightarrow 0$. That is,

$$C_F = C_{to}/(R_F G_{to}).$$ 9.8

Then we have:

$$V_o = -V_s \frac{G_{to}G_F + \omega^2 C_{to}C_F}{G_F^2 + \omega^2 C_F^2} \rightarrow -V_s R_F G_t$$ 9.9

Now, when the patient inhales, the lungs expand and the air displaces conductive tissue, causing the parallel conductance of the chest, G_t, to decrease from G_{to}. Let us substitute $G_t = G_{to} + \delta G_t$ and $C_t = C_{to} + \delta C_t$ into Equation 9.7, and also let $R_F C_F = C_{to}/G_{to}$ from the initial phase nulling. After a considerable amount of algebra, we find:

$$\frac{V_o}{V_s}(j\omega) = \frac{-R_F}{\left[1 + \omega^2 \left(R_F C_F\right)^2\right]} \left[G_{to}\left(1 + \delta G_t/G_{to}\right)\right.$$

$$\left. + \omega^2 \left(R_F C_F\right)^2 G_{to}\left(1 + \delta C_t/C_{to}\right) + j\omega C_{to}\left(\delta C_t/C_{to} - \delta G_t/G_{to}\right)\right]$$ 9.10

This relation reduces to Equation 9.9 for $\delta C_t = \delta G_t \rightarrow 0$. If we assume that $\delta C_t \rightarrow 0$ only, then Equation 9.10 can be written:

$$\frac{V_o + \delta V_o}{V_s}(j\omega) \cong -R_F G_{to} - \frac{\delta G_t R_F}{\left[1 + \omega^2 \left(R_F C_F\right)^2\right]}$$ 9.11

Note that $\delta G_t < 0$ for an inhaled breath.

Figure 9.2 illustrates a systems block diagram for the author's self-balancing plethysmograph, configured for the condition where $\delta C_t \rightarrow 0$. The three, RC high-pass filters are used to block unwanted dc components from V_s, V_o and V_F. In the first case, we also let $\delta G_t \rightarrow 0$. In the steady-state, $V_e \rightarrow 0$, so:

$$V_s V_c/10 = -V_s R_F G_{to}$$ 9.12

Thus

$$V_c = -10 R_F G_{to} = -(V_B + \beta V_2),$$ 9.13

and the integrator output is proportional to G_{to}:

$$V_2 = (10 R_F G_{to} - V_B)/\beta$$ 9.14

V_B, G_{to}, and V_s do not change in time, so the steady-state analysis above is valid. Using superposition, we can examine the system's response to a time-varying δG_t. The transfer function, $\delta V_2/\delta G_t$ can be written:

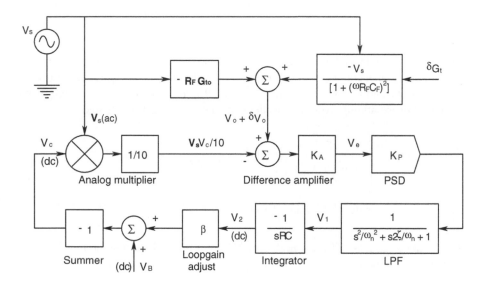

FIGURE 9.2 Systems block diagram of the self-nulling plethysmograph of Figure 9.1, showing system dynamics.

$$\frac{\delta V_2}{\delta G_t}(s) = \frac{V_s K_A K_p \Big/ \Big\{ RC \big[1 + (\omega R_F C_F)^2 \big] \Big\}}{s\big(s^2/\omega_n^2 + s2\zeta/\omega_n + 1\big) + V_s \beta K_A K_p /(10RC)} \qquad 9.15$$

The damping of the cubic closed-loop system is adjusted with the attenuation, β. The steady-state incremental gain is:

$$\frac{\delta V_2}{\delta G_t} = \frac{10}{\Big[\big(1 + (\omega R_F C_F)^2\big)\Big]\beta} \quad \text{volts/Siemen} \qquad 9.16$$

A prototype of this system was run at 75 kHz and tested on the chests of several volunteers after informed consent was obtained. Both $\delta V_2 \propto \delta G_t$ and $V_1 \propto \dot{\delta} G_t$ were recorded. System outputs followed the subjects' respiratory volumes, as expected.

A second type of IP makes use of a novel self-balancing two-phase lock-in amplifier (LIA) developed by McDonald (1992) and McDonald and Northrop (1993). A lock-in amplifier is basically nothing more than a synchronous or phase-controlled full-wave rectifier followed by a low-pass filter. Its input is generally a noisy amplitude-modulated, or double-sideband-suppressed carrier ac signal. The LIA output is a dc voltage proportional to the peak height of the input signal; the low-pass filter averages out the noise and any other zero-mean output component of the rectifier. Signal buried in as much as 60 dB of noise can be recovered by an appropriately set-up LIA.

Figure 9.3 illustrates how the LIA is connected to the voltage across the tissue, $\mathbf{V_o}$, where $\mathbf{V_o} = \mathbf{I_s} (R_t + jB_t)$, $(B_t = -1/\omega C_t)$. Note that, if the angle of $\mathbf{I_s}$ is taken as zero (reference), then the angle of $\mathbf{V_o}$ is $\theta_s = \tan^{-1}(B_t/R_t)$. The ac reference voltage, $\mathbf{V_r}$, in phase with $\mathbf{I_s}$ is used to control the LIA's synchronous rectifier. $\mathbf{V_r}$ also allows us to monitor $\mathbf{I_s}$ because $\mathbf{V_r} = \mathbf{I_s} R_P$. Figure 9.4 shows a block diagram of McDonald's two-phase servo LIA.

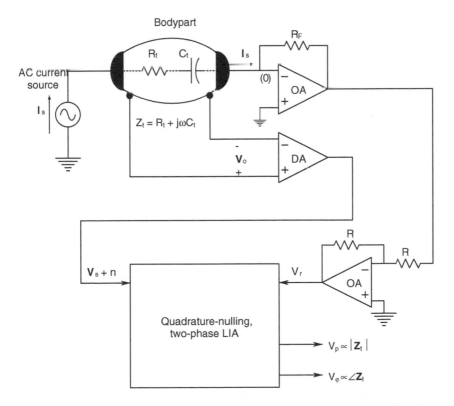

FIGURE 9.3 The two-phase self-balancing lock-in amplifier developed by McDonald and Northrop (1993) used as an impedance plethysmograph. The SBLIA gives voltage outputs proportional to the body part's admittance magnitude and admittance angle.

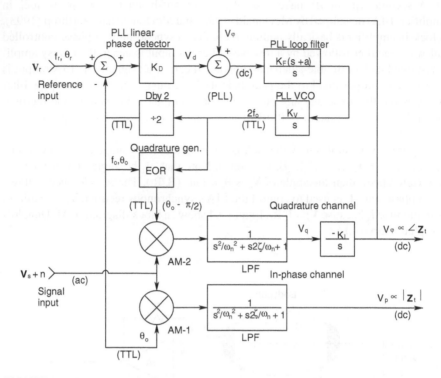

FIGURE 9.4 Systems block diagram of the SBLIA of McDonald and Northrop (1993).

At the heart of a basic LIA is a synchronous rectifier, one basic form of which is a pure analog multiplier (AM), or mixer. Assume one input to the multiplier is a reference signal, $v_r(t) = V_R \cos(\omega_o t + \theta_r)$, the other is a signal whose amplitude we wish to measure; $v_s(t) = V_s \cdot \cos(\omega_o t + \theta_s)$. By trig identity,

$$v_p(t) = v_r(t)\, v_s(t) = (V_R V_s/2)[\cos(2\omega_o t + \theta_r + \theta_s) + \cos(\theta_r - \theta_s)] \qquad 9.17$$

When the multiplier output, $v_p(t)$, is run through a low-pass filter, the double frequency term is removed (seriously attenuated), and only the dc component of the product appears at its output:

$$\overline{v_p(t)} = (V_R V_s/2)\cos(\theta_r - \theta_s) \qquad 9.18$$

If the phase and frequency of the signal and reference are the same, $\overline{v_p(t)} = (V_R V_s/2)$. That is, the output voltage of the LPF is proportional to V_S. (V_R is constant.)

In McDonald's design, the reference signal is phase-shifted by $-90°$ to detect any quadrature component of $v_s(t)$. Two analog multipliers are used with two low-pass filters, one for the in-phase component and the other for the quadrature component of V_S. A phase-locked loop (PLL) is used as a voltage-controlled phase shifter in a feedback loop that automatically adjusts the reference phase to null the quadrature output, i.e., force $V_q \rightarrow 0$. By nulling V_q, we simultaneously maximize V_p, the in-phase output. To see how V_φ can set the phase of the PLL's VCO, we note that the PLL is a type II feedback system in which in the steady-state, $V_d + V_\varphi = 0$. Note that $V_d = K_D(\theta_r - \theta_o)$. Thus, we can write:

$$\theta_o = \theta_r + V_\varphi/K_D \qquad\qquad 9.19$$

Where: θ_o is the VCO phase, θ_r is the reference phase, K_D is the phase detector's gain in volts/radian, and V_φ is the dc signal used to adjust θ_o. To generate quadrature phase, the PLL's VCO is forced to run at $2f_r = 2f_o$, and a flip-flop is used to halve its frequency before phase comparison. By inputting $2f_o$ and f_o to an exclusive OR gate, we generate an output TTL signal of frequency f_o and phase $(\theta_o - \pi/2)$. In the steady-state, the servo- PLL makes $\theta_o = \theta_s$. $(\theta_r - \pi/2)$ is the quadrature phase reference used in the nulling loop. The reference inputs to the analog multipliers are TTL signals given zero mean by passing through simple RC, high-pass filters (not shown in Figure 9.4). To simplify analysis, we consider the zero mean TTL signals to be represented by their sinusoidal first harmonic components of the Fourier series for the square waves. Thus the output of the quadrature multiplier channel before low-pass filtering is:

$$V_q' = V_R \sin(\omega_o t + \theta_r)\, V_s \cos(\omega_n t + \theta_s)$$

$$= (V_R V_s/2)[\sin(2\omega_o t + \theta_r + \theta_s) + \sin(\theta_r - \theta_s)] \qquad 9.20$$

After low-pass filtering, the double-frequency term drops out and we have:

$$V_q = (V_R V_s/2)\,\sin(\theta_r - \theta_s) \qquad\qquad 9.21$$

In the steady-state, the negative feedback forces $V_q \rightarrow 0$, so V_φ assumes a value so that $\theta_r = \theta_s$ and $V_q \rightarrow 0$. Also under this condition, $V_d = V_\varphi$, from which we obtain:

$$V_\varphi = K_D(\theta_s - \theta_r) \qquad\qquad 9.22$$

In words, V_φ is proportional to the phase difference between the I_s reference phase and V_o measured across the tissue under study. Because the steady-state θ_o is forced to be θ_s, the output voltage of the in-phase channel is proportional to $|Z_t|$. Thus the McDonald self-nulling quadrature PLL outputs a dc voltage V_φ proportional to the phase difference between I_s and V_o, and a dc voltage V_p proportional to the magnitude of the impedance, $|Z_t|$, of the tissue under study. V_p and V_φ follow the slow physiological variations in Z_t caused by blood flow or breathing. The modulation of R_t and B_t by pulsatile blood flow or lung inflation can have diagnostic significance.

9.3.3 Applications of Impedance Plethysmography

A major application of impedance plethysmography (IP) is in *occlusive impedance phlebography* (OIP). This procedure is used to detect venous blood clots in deep leg veins. IP can also be used to detect blood clots in the lungs. Note that most blood clots in lung vessels are complications of clots in deep leg veins. Also, there are many other signs of clots in the legs and lungs that can be used to verify IP results.

In OIP, an inflatable cuff is placed around the mid-thigh or just below the knee; this is the low-pressure cuff used to block venous return. A high-pressure cuff is placed just above the ankle to occlude both veins and arteries. The IP electrodes are placed high and low on the dorsal (rear) surface of the calf, or on the sides of the calf. When the thigh cuff is inflated, normal venous return is blocked, but not arterial blood flow into the lower leg. Restricting venous flow causes blood to pool in the calf veins, and, consequently, $|\mathbf{Y}_t|$ increases. The thigh cuff pressure is released suddenly, allowing the pooled venous blood to return to the heart. If one or more venous clots are present, it takes longer for $|\mathbf{Y}_t|$ to drop to its original value than for normal venous circulation. The OIP test is generally done on both legs for comparison purposes. OIP can also be effectively applied to detect thromboses in proximal (thigh) veins (femoro-popliteal). According to one source (Chin and McGrath, 1998), OIP is highly sensitive (a 92% detection rate) and specific (95%) when used on patients exhibiting symptomatic proximal deep vein thromboses (DVT). The sensitivity of OIP is low in calf vein thromboses (20%) and in screening for DVT in asymptomatic postoperative high-risk patients (22%). There are several other NI, diagnostic modalities used in detecting and quantifying DVTs. These include color Doppler ultrasound imaging, magnetic resonance venography, and the iodine-125 fibrinogen scan. Of these NI modalities, OIP is the least expensive.

A multichannel IP investigation of pulsatile blood flow in leg arteries was done by Jossinet et al., 1995. A sinusoidal current of 3 mArms at 64 kHz was injected into the legs through a pair of standard ECG electrodes, one placed on each foot. Sixteen pairs of sensing electrodes were used to record voltages at various sites on the legs. Recording-electrode pair spacing was 45 mm on centers. Signal processing of each electrode pair's voltage gave an output voltage proportional to dZ/dt. This information was used to examine the arterial pulse wave velocity in various locations in the legs. This technique may have usefulness in diagnosing asymetrical problems with arterial circulation in the legs such as might be caused by injury, infection or embolism.

IP is also used to monitor breathing (and also heart beats) in intensive care and neonatal applications. When used as an impedance pneumograph, electrodes are generally placed on the sides of the chest. Modulations of the peak output voltage are proportional to lung expansion by inhaled air; failure of lung expansion can signify central apnea, and, in some cases, extreme obstructive apnea. Since the shape changes of the beating heart are also correlated with expansion and contraction of the aorta, vena cava and pulmonary vessels, the transthoracic $\mathbf{Z}_t$ is also modulated at heart rate frequency. In adults, the heart rate is normally higher than the respiration rate, and the two waveforms can be partially separated by band-pass filtering so separate assessments of heart rate, respiration rate and effort can be made. In infants, the respiratory rate can occasionally approach the heart rate, so instead of demodulating the IP voltage for both respiratory and heart rate signals, an ECG amplifier preceded by a pair of low-pass filters can be connected to the IP output electrodes to directly record the ECG signal. The low-pass filters are set to attenuate the c. 60

kHz IP modulation signal by at least −120 dB. Often, a third modality is used for infant apnea monitoring, e.g., a pulse oximeter, to measure the percent O_2 saturation of hemoglobin (see Section 15.8).

Impedance pneumograph-cardiotachometers used for neonatal and ICU applications have an alarm system that measures a sudden increase in measured impedance such as would be caused by electrodes' drying out, coming detached or falling off the chest. They are also set to alarm for respiration effort or rate, and heart rate under or over preset limits. Many medical-instrument manufacturers make ICU and pediatric care monitors that incorporate impedance pneumograph functions. For example, the Sechrist Co. makes an enhanced infant ventilator system (SAVI&trade ©) that is designed to operate a synchronized inhalation and exhalation on-demand assist system from signals derived from an impedance pneumograph.

9.3.4 DISCUSSION

Impedance plethysmography was seen to have two major applications as a noninvasive, diagnostic method: 1) To measure blood flow (or obstruction) in veins and arteries of the legs, and 2) to measure respiratory effort and rate in ICU and neonatal monitoring applications. The injected ac current is physically and physiologically innocuous because of its low peak value and high frequency.

9.4 PHOTO-PLETHYSMOGRAPHY

A fingertip photo-plethysmograph can be used to measure heart rate, and to estimate blood pressure when individually calibrated. This device fits over the tip of a finger, (or on an earlobe in another incarnation). Modulated light from a red or NIR LED is shone into the tissue, and a silicon photodiode senses the back-scattered light. Its signal is demodulated by a phase-sensitive rectifier (PSR) plus low-pass filter. The PSR ensures that only light from the LED is used to derive the pulse rate signal. As blood is forced into the tissue's blood vessels, they expand and the level of back-scattered light changes. This heart-rate change appears as a signal at the output of the LPF. In 1980, a photo-plethysmographic pulse-rate monitor integrated circuit (HLSS-0533D) was available from Hughes Solid State Products that interfaced the NIR LED and photo-diode to a heart-rate display. The 0.9 μm LED was pulsed at 73 Hz in the Hughes system.

Once the back-scattered modulated NIR light is demodulated, a periodic analog voltage waveform is available for further processing. This analog waveform is passed through a comparator to derive a heart-rate logic signal. The rising edges of this signal trigger a one-shot multivibrator that makes a train of narrow pulses at the heart rate. The heart rate can be found in analog form by low-pass filtering the one-shot's output pulses and subtracting out the dc offset of the logic LO voltage. To find the heart rate in digital form, the narrow one-shot output pulses are used to start and stop a fast clock input (e.g., 1 MHz) to a counter. When the leading edge of the second pulse of a pair of output pulses arrives, the counting is stopped and the counter reading (total number of microseconds) is downloaded in parallel to an arithmetic unit that takes its reciprocal. The falling edge of the second pulse resets the counter and starts the counting process again, etc. The reciprocal of the count is proportional to the *instantaneous frequency* (IF) of the heart. Several consecutive instantaneous frequency outputs can be averaged to minimize the normal variation in heart rate caused by cardioregulatory action. The appropriately scaled, averaged IF output drives a digital heart-rate display.

A pulse oximeter is a more elaborate incarnation of a fingertip plethysmograph. The oximeter uses two LEDs of different wavelength to measure the percent of blood hemoglobin saturation with oxygen. However, it is also responsive to the blood volume in the tissue on which it is used, and thus can give pulse rate information as well as SpO_2. (Section 15.8 gives a thorough description of pulse oximeters.)

9.5 CHAPTER SUMMARY

We have seen that plethysmography is a relatively simple noninvasive means of measuring local changes in body volume, generally occurring as the result of respiration, blood flow or muscle contraction. A device as simple as a blood pressure cuff can be used on a limb to measure volume changes caused by either blood flow or muscle contraction. Using Equation 9.1, an electronic pressure sensor attached to the cuff can measure $\Delta P = P_o(\Delta V/V_o)$. That is, the change in air pressure, ΔP, is proportional to the increase in limb volume, ΔV. P_o is easily measured, and V_o can be determined by filling the cuff with a known volume of air at P_o.

Because impedance changes are generally small compared with the overall impedance, it is feasible to use a closed-loop self-nulling bridge type of circuit to sense the desired $|\Delta Z|$ as a ΔV_o. It appears that many of the applications of plethysmography are in physiological research, rather than in diagnosis.

10 Pulmonary Function Tests

10.1 INTRODUCTION

The function of the vertebrate respiratory system is to keep the arterial blood supplied with oxygen, and to allow the absorption and dissipation of the metabolic by-product, carbon dioxide, in the exhaled breath. The biochemistry of the respiratory process is complex, and will not be reviewed here. Rather, we will focus our attention on the physical side of the respiratory process — that is, the mechanics of breathing and the gas exchange processes taking place at alveolar capillaries.

Factors that restrict normal breathing and gas exchange are medically important and have a variety of causes, ranging from heart failure to allergy, infection, cancer, emphysema, and hereditary disease. When patients complain to their physicians that they are "out of breath," the first step in finding out why and how to cure or mitigate this condition is to quantitatively measure the mechanical parameters of the respiratory system by *spirometry* and to compare them with those of "normal" persons of similar sex, age, body mass and height, etc. Deviations from the norm in these tests are only the first step in complete diagnosis, which can also involve CAT scans, MRI, blood-gas tests, etc.

The volume-displacement spirometer was invented c. 1846 by Hutchison, an English anatomist (West, 1985). Spirometers basically measure respiratory volumes, or, in the case of modern units, respiratory volume flow rate, which is integrated to determine volume. Some of the common parameters used in spirometry are:

- **FVC** (forced vital capacity): This is the total volume of air a patient can exhale after a maximum effort inspiration. Patients with *restrictive lung disease* (RLD) have a lower FVC than do patients with *obstructive lung disease* (OLD).
- **FEV1** (forced expiratory volume in 1 second) (also, FEV1/2): The volume of air expired in the first second following the beginning of maximum expiratory effort. FEV1 is reduced from normal in both obstructive and restrictive lung diseases, but for different reasons; increased airway resistance in OLD, and decreased vital capacity in RLD.
- **FEV1/FVC**: This ratio is about 0.7 in healthy subjects. It can be as low as 0.2 to 0.3 in patients with OLD. Patients with RLD have near normal ratios.
- **FEF(25-75%)**: (forced mid-expiratory flow rate): The average rate of flow during the middle of the FVC maneuver. Reduced in both OLD and RLD.

- **DLCO** (diffusion capacity of the lung for carbon monoxide): The poison gas CO can be used to measure the diffusion capacity of the alveoli. The diffusion capacity of the lung is decreased in parenchymal diseases such as emphysema. It is normal in asthma. (Other gases can be used.)
- **FRC** (functional residual capacity): The volume of air remaining in the lungs and trachea after an exhalation in normal breathing.
- **RV** (residual volume): The volume of air left in the lungs after a maximum FVC exhale. It is the "dead space" of the respiratory system, mostly combined trachea and bronchial tube volumes. It cannot be measured directly.
- **TV** (tidal volume): The volume exchanged in normal relaxed breathing.
- **AV** (alveolar volume): Total volume of all the minute alveoli in the lung parenchyma.

Note that all spirometric tests are NI and require a high degree of patient cooperation. If a patient is unconscious or paralyzed, they cannot be used. The physician must then rely on imaging or sound transmission tests such as described in Sections 3.4, 15.2, and 15.4.

Figure 10.1 illustrates the graphical significance of the parameters FVC, TV, FRC, and RV from a volume spirometer kymograph record. FEV1 is illustrated in Figure 10.2. Computer-generated flow/volume (F/V) curves are generally made from the outputs of pneumotach flow meters. Typical F/V curves are shown in Figure 10.3. Note that extensive databases have been compiled to enable the physician or respiratory therapist to compare a patient's volumes and FEV performance with norms for a given age, height, weight and sex. Such tables can be found at the Spirometry website (Pierce and Johns, 1995) and also in the form of nomographs from W.E. Collins Co.

10.2 SPIROMETERS AND RELATED EQUIPMENT

All spirometers can be classified as positive-displacement types of instruments using pneumotachs. An example of the positive displacement spirometer is the classic W.E. Collins Model P-600 recording vitalometer (cf. Figure 10.4), which uses a water-sealed, counter-weighted, rigid bell chamber to measure patient air volumes at near atmospheric pressure. Other types of positive displacement spirometers use a bellows, or a giant piston in a cylinder.

The trend now is not to use a bulky volume spirometer that requires sterilization of its connecting tubes for each patient, but rather a small hand-held *pneumotachometer* (pneumotach). There are three different types of pneumotach (PT):

1. In the *flow resistance type*, a fine screen or a parallel cluster of capillary tubes forms a pneumatic "resistor." The pressure differential across the resistance is proportional to the volume flow in liters/sec (in analogy to Ohm's law for electric circuits). The resistance made from many parallel capillary tubes is known as the *Fleisch type PT* (see Figure 10.5). Because condensed water vapor from the breath can clog the tubes or screens and

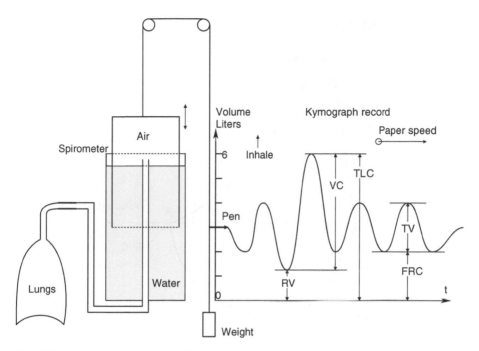

FIGURE 10.1 Schematic of a volume spirometer, showing some critical volumes and capacities.

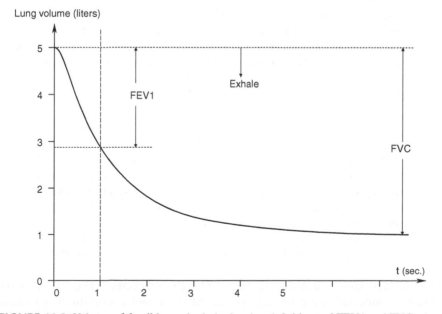

FIGURE 10.2 Volume of forcibly expired air showing definitions of FEV1 and FVC.

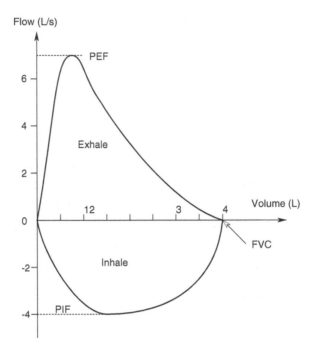

FIGURE 10.3 A representative computer-generated flow-volume curve; the patient blows into a pneumotach.

raise the PT resistance, causing it to lose calibration, the screens or tubes are often heated to prevent condensation.

2. The second type of PT uses a light plastic *turbine fan* mounted in the mouthpiece housing with its axis of rotation in the center of the housing. The fan rotates at an angular velocity proportional to the volume flow rate through the PT. The angular velocity is measured photoelectrically or magnetically without contact with the turbine fan. In both schemes, the pulse frequency is proportional to turbine rpm, which is proportional to volume flow rate.

3. A third type of PT uses a *hot-wire anemometer*. This is a nonlinear flow rate sensor in which a fine wire is heated by passing electric current through it. In still air, it reaches a certain temperature $T_o > T_a$ (ambient temperature) and has a certain resistance, $R_o(T_o)$, which is measured. Air flowing past the hot wire cools it and its temperature drops, lowering its resistance. A feedback circuit senses this lowered resistance and passes more current through the hot wire, reheating it to T_o and R_o. After some nonlinear compensation circuitry, the hot wire anemometer circuit outputs a voltage proportional to the air volume flow rate (Northrop, 1997).

Most modern spirometers use the heated Fleisch architecture. The PT's pressure sensor is connected to a computer's digital interface, and a specialized spirometry software package computes and stores the test parameters described above, and also

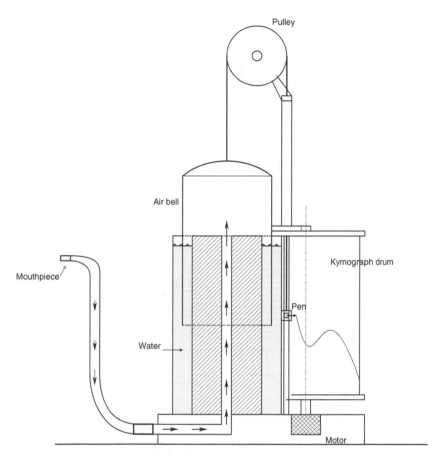

FIGURE 10.4 A water-sealed volume-displacement spirometer. The "bell" is counterbalanced so its weight exerts negligible pressure on the trapped gas.

compares patient performance with the normal entries in its database. Note that the Fleisch PT's output is a voltage proportional to pressure. The pressure is the difference across the pneumatic resistance, which, in turn, is proportional to flow rate in liters/sec. Thus, the computer must integrate the differential pressure sensor output signal to determine lung volumes.

10.3 TESTS WITH SPIROMETERS

In this section, we will describe the uses of gas dilution to measure certain respiratory parameters. For example, helium dilution can be used to measure RV and FRC. A known concentration of helium in air is put into a positive displacement spirometer. The subject exhales, then breathes the mixture in and out several times. Helium is almost insoluble in blood, so that, after a few breaths, the helium is diluted by the amount of air in the FRC volume. The initial concentration of helium is C_1 in a total spirometer volume, V_1. So C_1V_1 is the initial amount of He at STP. This amount of

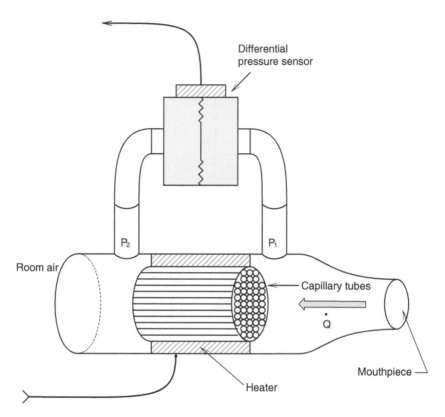

FIGURE 10.5 Schematic of a Fleisch-type pneumotach.

He does not change because a negligible amount of He is absorbed in the lungs, so we can write:

$$C_1 V_1 = C_2 (V_1 + FRC) \qquad\qquad 10.1$$

Solving for FRC:

$$FRC = \frac{V_1 (C_1 - C_2)}{C_2} \qquad\qquad 10.2$$

where V_1 is the initial spirometer volume, C_1 is the initial He concentration, and C_2 is the He concentration after several mixing breaths. C_1 and C_2 can be measured by a mass spectometer tuned for He, or by measuring the change in sound velocity in the He–air mixture (for details on this latter method see Section 8.6).

A less accurate means of measuring FRC is by "open-circuit nitrogen washout" (West, 1985). In this method, patients start in the exhaled condition in which there is 80% N_2 in their lungs. They then take many breaths of pure O_2 from a source, and their exhales are directed into an "empty" large-capacity spirometer. After about

5 to 7 minutes, all of the N_2 in the FRC or RV of the lungs has been replaced by pure O_2, and this original N_2 is now in the spirometer along with exhaled O_2, CO_2 and water vapor. (The CO_2 and water vapor can be absorbed, if desired.) The concentration of N_2, C_{N2} in the final spirometer volume, V_2, is measured. FRC or RV is calculated from:

$$C_{N1}RV = C_{N2} V_2 \qquad\qquad 10.3$$

This method assumes that all of the N_2 in the lungs is washed out, which may not be the case in certain types of OLD.

Still another method of estimating FRC and RV makes use of a *whole-body plethysmograph*. The patient sits in a hermetically sealed coffin-like box. The internal pressure of the box (with patient) can be measured very accurately. Initially, the pressure in the box with the patient is made atmospheric, P_a, before it is sealed. Patients are asked to make a strong respiratory exhalation, starting at FRC, against a closed mouthpiece containing a pressure sensor. As they compress the gas in their lungs from P_1 to P_2, the lung and chest volume decrease slightly by ΔV, causing the gas volume of the box to increase slightly by the same amount. Because the amount of gas in the box (outside of the patient) has not changed, the gas pressure in the box decreases from P_a to $P_3 < P_a$. Using Boyle's gas law ($P_1 V_1 = P_2 V_2$ @ constant temperature and amount of gas), we can write for each patient:

$$P_a \text{ FRC} = P_2(\text{FRC} - \Delta V) \qquad\qquad 10.4$$

Thus, FRC is given by:

$$\text{FRC} = \frac{P_2 \Delta V}{(P_2 - P_a)} \text{ liters} \qquad\qquad 10.5$$

Now ΔV can be found from Boyle's law applied to the box. Initially the box is at P_a, so:

$$P_a V_{BP} = P_3(V_{BP} + \Delta V) \qquad\qquad 10.6$$

The increase in box volume caused by the patient's blocked exhalation effort causes the box pressure to fall by $P_3 < P_a$. V_{BP} is the gas volume of the sealed box with patient inside, resting.

$$\Delta V = V_{BP}(P_a/P_3 - 1) \qquad\qquad 10.7$$

When this relation for ΔV is substituted into Equation 10.5, we obtain finally:

$$\text{FRC} = \frac{P_2 V_{BP}\left[(P_a/P_3) - 1\right]}{(P_2 - P_a)} \text{ liters} \qquad\qquad 10.8$$

P_a, P_2 and P_3 are all directly measured pressures; V_{BP} needs to be determined. One way of measuring V_{BP} with Boyle's law is to include in the box during the above measurements a completely evacuated, thin-walled gas tank of volume V_T. With the box sealed, the patient opens the tank's valve and lets it fill with box air. The box pressure drops to a measured P_4. This maneuver effectively increases the box volume by a known V_T. Thus, by Boyle's law:

$$P_a V_{BP} = P_4(V_{BP} + V_T)$$

$$\downarrow$$

$$V_{BP} = V_T P_4/(P_a - P_4) \qquad 10.9$$

Equation 10.9 is substituted into Equation 10.8 above for a complete solution to FRC from known or measured parameters.

> West (1985) observes: "It should be noted that the body plethysmograph and the gas dilution (or washout) method(s) may measure different volumes. The body plethysmograph measures the total volume of gas in the lungs, including any which is trapped behind closed airways and which therefore does not communicate with the mouth. By contrast, the helium dilution and nitrogen washout methods measure only communicating gas, or ventilated lung volume. In young normal subjects these volumes are virtually the same, but in patients with lung disease the ventilated volume may be considerably less than the total volume because of gas trapped behind obstructed airways."

Another important respiratory parameter is *alveolar ventilation* (AV). If a person's tidal volume (TV) (the volume breathed out in a normal breathing cycle) is 0.6 liter, and there are 14 breaths/minute, then the total volume leaving the nose each minute is $0.6 \times 14 = 8.4$ liters/minute. This number is known as the person's *minute volume.* The volume of air entering the nose is slightly greater, because more O_2 is taken in than CO_2 is given off. Significantly, not all of the air taken in reaches the alveoli, where the actual O_2/CO_2 gas exchange takes place. Of each 0.6 liter inhaled, c. 180 ml remains behind in the *anatomical dead space*. Thus, the AV is $(600 - 180) \times 14 = 5,880$ ml/min. The AV is an important parameter in evaluating the health of a person's respiratory system. It represents the actual amount of fresh air available for gas exchange.

The calculation of alveolar ventilation depends on measurement of the anatomical dead space (ADS), which is basically the volume of the gas conducting airways (the trachea, the bronchial tubes, and various types of bronchioles), and is sex-, weight-, height- and posture-dependent. The anatomical dead space can be measured by Fowler's method (West, 1985). A subject breathes normal air (80% N_2, 20% O_2), then takes a maximum inhale of pure O_2, and then exhales fully into a spirometer that records the exhaled volume. At the same time, a fast mass spectrometer-type N_2 analyzer measures the N_2 in the exhaled breath at the mouth. First, pure O_2 comes out from the upper airways, then, as the exhalation continues, the N_2 concentration rises to a plateau whose value is the N_2 concentration in the alveolar gas. Graphs of the typical concentration of N_2 vs. time and N_2 vs. exhaled volume are shown in Figure 10.6. The ADS is estimated by drawing a vertical line on Figure 10.7 so that the areas A_1 and A_2 are equal (West, 1985).

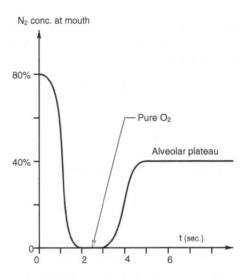

FIGURE 10.6 Representative graph of exhaled N_2 vs. time in the Fowler test to measure anatomical dead space (ADS) in the lungs. The exhaled N_2 concentration is measured with a quadrupole mass spectrometer.

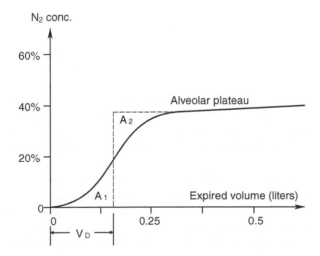

FIGURE 10.7 Detail of measuring the ADS.

Another means of estimating dead space was described by Bohr (1891) (cited by West). Bohr's technique measures *physiological dead space* (PDS), which is different from ADS. It is obvious that respiratory CO_2 emission comes from the alveoli, and not the PDS. Thus, we can write:

$$TV \; C_{ECO2} = AV \; C_{ACO2} \qquad\qquad 10.10$$

Where AV is the total alveolar gas volume, C_{ECO2} is the concentration of CO_2 in the expired breath, and C_{ACO2} is the concentration of CO_2 in the alveoli just before expiration. It is well known that:

$$TV = AV + PDS \qquad\qquad 10.11$$

Hence,

$$AV = TV - PDS \qquad\qquad 10.12$$

Substituting AV from Equation 10.10, we can write:

$$\frac{PDS}{TV} = \frac{C_{ACO2} - C_{ECO2}}{C_{ACO2}} \qquad\qquad 10.13$$

Two more assumptions are made: 1) The partial pressure of a gas is proportional to its concentration. 2) The P_{CO2} of alveolar gas is nearly equal to the P_{CO2} of arterial blood, P_{aCO2}. Finally, we have the *Bohr equation*:

$$\frac{PDS}{TV} = \frac{P_{aCO2} - P_{ECO2}}{P_{aCO2}} \qquad\qquad 10.14$$

West (1985) states:

> "The normal ratio of dead space to tidal volume is in the range of 0.2 to 0.35 during resting breathing. The ratio decreases on exercise but increases with age.
> Bohr's method measures the volume of the lung which does not eliminate CO_2. Because this is a functional measurement, the volume is called the physiological dead space."

Note that, in Equation 10.14, TV is directly measured by spirometry, and the partial CO_2 pressures are measured with sensors — in the expired gas by an infrared absorption sensor, and in an arterial blood sample by a Severinghaus P_{CO2} electrode (Webster, 1992). (The Severinghaus P_{CO2} sensor is described in detail in Section 7.3 of this text.)

It is also of interest in a medical evaluation of the respiratory system to noninvasively measure the alveolar capillary blood flow. One means of measuring the *instantaneous pulmonary blood flow* is to have the subject again sit in the hermetically sealed full-body plethysmograph chamber in which there is a collapsible gas bag containing a mixture of 21% O_2 and 79% nitrous oxide (N_2O) at atmospheric pressure. The air inside the chamber is initially at atmospheric pressure, P_o. The subject breathes the gas mixture. N_2O is taken up by the capillary circulation very rapidly; absorption by alveolar capillaries being almost complete in c. 100 ms. The transfer of N_2O into the pulmonary capillary blood is said to be *perfusion limited*. Because the N_2O volume "disappears" by solution into the pulmonary blood flow, the net gas volume in the chamber increases as the N_2O is absorbed. By Boyle's law,

$$(P_o + \Delta P) = K/(V_o + \Delta V) = (K/V_o)[1 - \Delta V/V_o] \qquad 10.15$$

The decrement in pressure in the chamber is related to the increase in chamber volume.

$$\Delta P = \frac{K\Delta V}{V_o^2} \qquad 10.16$$

The chamber pressure thus drops in a slow stepwise manner, with the steps synchronized with the heartbeat. ΔP is measured, ΔV (of N_2O) is calculated, and, from the known solubility of N_2O in blood at atmospheric pressure, it is possible to calculate the blood volume per heartbeat through the alveolar capillaries (West, 1985).

10.4 SUMMARY

Physical pulmonary function tests are an important NI means of diagnosing obstructive lung diseases. In general, they do require patient cooperation. Modern turbine-type or Fleisch pneumotachs interfaced with a PC enable clinicians to acquire and store patient data and recall past performance records for clinical comparison. The effectiveness of a bronchodilator can be evaluated in one patient visit. Emphysema only gets worse with time; it is important to be able to quantitatively track the progress of this debilitating condition.

Physiological tests of the ability of the alveolar tissues to exchange gases can also be performed by having the patient breath O_2 + a tracer gas such as He or N_2O. How readily the tracer gas is taken up or dissipated (once a steady-state concentration in blood is reached) is an indication of alveolar blood flow and available gas-exchangeable tissue area.

Asthma and other OLDs are common in today's society. The increase of emissions from Diesel engines and power plants adds to the bad air quality in urban and industrial regions. Other chemicals such as gasoline additives contribute to the level of air contamination in spite of sealed gas tanks and catalytic mufflers. (When a car is first started, its catalytic muffler is cold and ineffective.) Simple, quick, NI pulmonary function testing as a diagnostic tool is becoming more important.

11 Measurement of Basal Metabolism

11.1 INTRODUCTION

Metabolism, in general, is the sum of all of the chemical reactions that occur in the body; both in intracellular and extracellular compartments. Because biochemistry is so complex, we generally focus our attention on certain subsets of metabolic reactions, such as mineral metabolism, further divided into subsets such as calcium, copper, iron, magnesium, potassium and sodium metabolisms, as well as carbohydrate, fat and protein metabolisms, to cite a few.

Basal metabolism is the study of *oxidative metabolism* in cells in a resting animal in which certain energy sources such as glucose are oxidized to form molecules of the ubiquitous high-energy molecule *adenosine triphosphate* (ATP). The formation of ATP molecules is accompanied by the utilization of respired oxygen, and the production of heat, carbon dioxide, and other "metabolic products." ATP is ubiquitous because the energy stored in two phosphate bonds of the molecule can be released enzymatically to drive many other endothermic biochemical reactions. For example, active ion pumps in cell membranes, including muscle, where it is required to drive the molecular engines that actively take up the calcium ions released in the process of muscle contraction, use ATP as an energy source. (Muscle cannot relax unless the Ca^{++} is taken up from the actin and myosin and stored in the membrane cells of the sarcoplasmic reticulum.)

The structural formula for ATP is shown in Figure 11.1. Each of the two high-energy phosphate bonds contains about 12 Calories/mole of ATP (12 Cal = 12,000 calories). Most intracellular ATP is formed in the mitochondria of cells in which it is used to power various biosynthetic reactions, ion pumps, etc. In the various linked biochemical pathways in which glucose is oxidized to get the energy to form ATP, a net two ATP molecules are formed in the process of *glycolysis*, in which one glucose molecule is consumed. Also produced in glycolysis are two pyruvic acid molecules per glucose molecule. The two pryuvic acid molecules are enzymatically converted to two molecules of *acetyl CoA*, one of which then enters the *citric acid cycle*, where two more ATP molecules are formed per initial glucose molecule. During glycolysis and the citric acid cycle, 24 hydrogen atoms are released. These hydrogen atoms are further oxidized to give an additional 34 ATP molecules per glucose molecule. Thus, as many as 38 ATP molecules can be synthesized from each glucose molecule. A gram mole of glucose then can produce 456 Cal. stored in the phosphate bonds of the resultant ATP. During the complete oxidation of a mole of glucose, 686 Cal. are released, giving an overall efficiency of 66%. The difference of 686 − 456 = 230 Cal., which is released as waste heat. This heat acts

265

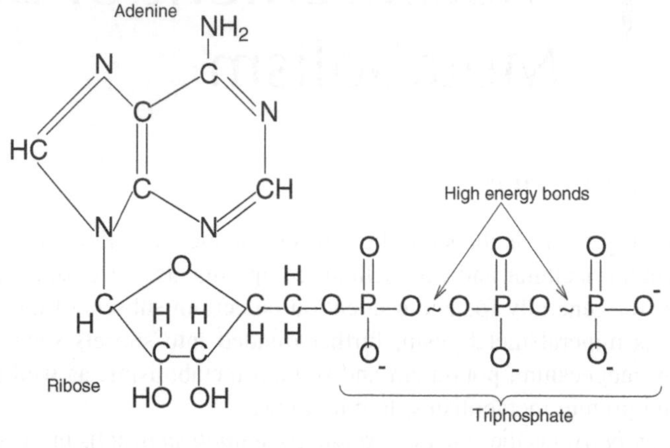

FIGURE 11.1 An adenosine triphosphate (ATP) molecule.

to raise the temperature of the cells above ambient temperature. In mammals and birds, this temperature is regulated, and the enzyme systems and metabolic pathways in the body are found to work optimally in the narrow range of regulated body temperature (Guyton, 1991).

The processes of ATP synthesis and its utilization in the various intracellular reactions are under closed-loop control by various regulatory hormones. These include thyroid hormone (thyroxine), triiodothyronine, adrenaline, and growth hormone. A disorder or disease affecting the regulation of the concentrations of these hormones affects overall cellular glucose metabolism, including the production of ATP, heat and CO_2, and the consumption of O_2. To noninvasively test for problems in the regulation of hormones that modulate metabolism, it is possible to test under standard resting (basal) conditions, the amount of glucose that is oxidized by the body. One rather elaborate test is to immerse the subject in an insulated tank of water that is just below normal body temperature. Each Calorie released by the body through the skin theoretically will raise each kilogram of water 1 degree Celsius. In a complex process, the water is chilled by a closed-loop control system that circulates cool water through the tank, keeping its temperature constant. By keeping track of the heat removed from the tank in order to keep it at a constant temperature, and knowing the patient's mass and skin area, it is then possible to obtain a measure of the basal metabolism. The isothermal water tank method may have a sound theoretical basis, but is unwieldy and expensive. Consequently, the measurement of O_2 consumption has proven to provide the same information, is less expensive, and is generally a simpler procedure to perform. The *metabolator* method of measurement of basal metabolism is described in the next section.

11.2 THE BMR TEST PROCEDURE

More than 95% of the energy expended in the body comes from oxidation reactions with respired O_2. If 1 liter of O_2 at standard temperature and pressure (STP) is used to burn an excess of glucose in a calorimeter, 5.01 Calories of energy are released. Excess starches burned with 1 liter of O_2 at STP release 5.06 Calories; protein releases 4.60, and fat 4.70 Calories. It has been found that, for the average diet, the adult human metabolism will release 4.825 Calories of heat for each liter of O_2 "burned" in the body (Guyton, 1991). To accurately measure the volume of O_2 consumed, a volumetric system called a metabolator, shown schematically in Figure 11.2, is used. The water-sealed bell is filled with a known volume of O_2 at STP. To measure basal O_2 consumption, the patient must have fasted overnight and be comfortably recumbent in a warm room with no skeletal muscle activity. The patient breathes pure O_2 and exhales a mixture of O_2, CO_2 and water vapor. One-way valves direct the exhaled gases to a canister of soda lime where the CO_2 is totally absorbed, and the exhaled O_2 and some water vapor are returned to the bell. The overnight fast is necessary because, following a meal, the blood concentration of glucose rises, falls below resting level, then returns to the resting level. The blood concentration of insulin also rises in response to eating while the concentration of the pancreatic hormone, glucagon, falls during the rise in insulin level. The perturbations in the levels of these glucoregulatory hormones also affect metabolism, as do the transients in blood glucose concentration.

The patient breathes the O_2 from the metabolator for about 1 hour, and the total volume of O_2 consumed is noted. The rate of O_2 consumption under basal conditions depends on the patient's skin surface area, age, and gender. The patient's surface area can be estimated from the formula of DuBois (West, 1985):

$$A \text{ (cm}^2\text{)} = (\text{Weight, kg})^{0.425} \times (\text{Height, cm})^{0.725} \qquad 11.1$$

For example, an 80-kg man 180 cm tall has A = 2 m^2. Let V be the total liters of O_2 at STP consumed under basal conditions. The total Calories burned is then estimated by:

$$H = 2.825 \text{ V Cal.} \qquad 11.2$$

The BMR is found by dividing H by the body area in m^2 and the time in hours taken to burn V liters of O_2. As a round figure, the BMR of a normal male adult male is ca. 35–40 Cal/m^2/hr, or, in terms of weight, ca. 1 Cal/kg/hr. Figure 11.3 illustrates the age and gender differences in human BMR. (Note the downslope beginning around age 45 for both males and females. If a corresponding decrease in total dietary caloric input does not accompany this reduction in BMR, obesity can result.)

11.3 SUMMARY

BMR is often given as a percentage above or below the average BMR for a "standard" person of a given age and gender. If the BMR is abnormally high, it may be indicative of excess circulating thyroxine, which, in turn, can be symptomatic of a thyroid tumor. Likewise, an abnormally low-percentage BMR can point to a low thyroid hormone level. The simple inexpensive BMR test thus can point to the need for

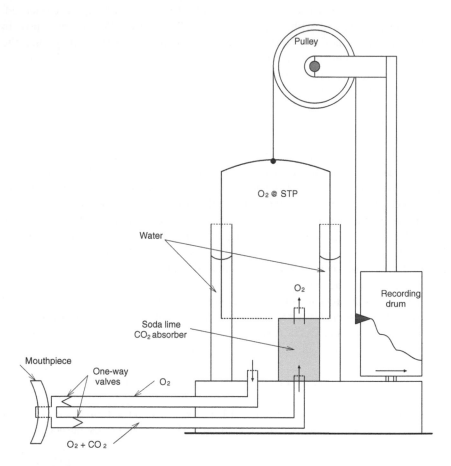

FIGURE 11.2 A metabolator. It is a modified bell spirometer.

definitive antibody blood tests for thyroid hormone, as well as other tests such as the uptake of radio-iodine (^{131}I), which is a β- and γ-ray emitter with a half-life of 8 days. Thyroid cells specifically take up iodine ions, and thus, circulating thyroxine and 3-iodotyrosine (3IT) become labeled and can be radio-assayed. The thyroid gland itself becomes radioactive and can "take its own picture" on X-ray film, providing an indication of thyroid metabolic activity. There are many other symptoms correlated with high TH level, so basal metabolism is not necessarily a definitive test for hyperthyroidism.

Other hormones can also produce high-percentage BMR readings. These include adrenaline, anabolic steroids and growth hormone, all of which stimulate metabolism. Certain neurosecretory endings in the median eminence of the hypothalamus release *thyrotropin-releasing hormone* (TRH), which stimulates the anterior pituitary to release *thyroid stimulating hormone* (TSH), which, in turn, causes the thyroid gland cells to increase their output of TH and 3IT. High titers of circulating TH and 3IT inhibit the rate of secretion of TSH, providing feedback regulation of hormone

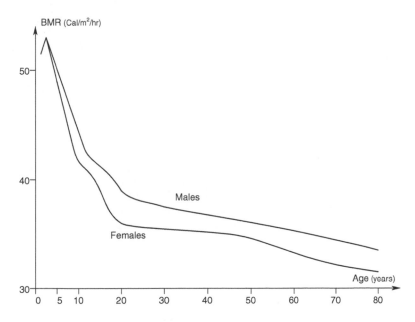

FIGURE 11.3 Normal basal metabolic rates for men and women according to age. Note the decline with age.

concentration. Brain tumors that interrupt the TRH → TSH → TH pathway can lead to low TH and low-percentage BMR.

In summary, the BRM test is simple and noninvasive, and can point to the need for more detailed tests on the metabolic endocrine system. It does require some preparation (fasting) and takes about 1 hour, however.

12 Ocular Tonometry

12.1 INTRODUCTION

Ocular tonometry is a class of noninvasive measurement that allows an ophthalmologist (and some optometrists) to estimate the internal hydraulic pressure in the eyeballs, called the *intra-ocular pressure* (IOP). The IOP is the result of the constant production (and outflow) of the liquid *aqueous humor* (AH). The AH is found around the lens and in the anterior chamber of the eye. It serves as a nutrient solution for the lens, the iris and the inside of the cornea, and its pressure helps to maintain the proper shape of the eyeball. Aqueous humor (AH) is continuously formed in a normal eye at a rate of about $\dot{Q}_{AH} = 2$ mm³/min. by the cells of the *ciliary process,* a tissue lying behind the lens having an exposed area of about 6 cm² (Guyton, 1991). AH is formed by the active metabolic "pumping" of Na^+ ions from inside ciliary process cells to the perilenticular region inside of the eyeball. There is also active transport of ascorbate and certain amino acids into the eyeball. Osmotic pressure and diffusion down concentration gradients cause water, chloride, glucose and bicarbonate ions to follow the ions pumped into the eyeball. AH contains mainly low-molecular-weight substances, including Na^+, K^+, HCO_3^-, citrate, ascorbate, urea, glucose, etc.

Clearly, in the steady state, the AH must exit the eye at the same volume flow rate that it enters. Outflow of AH is through the *Canal of Schlemm* into the episcleral veins, and thence into the main venous circulation, etc. The eyeball is slightly elastic, with most of its compliance coming from the thin clear cornea. Normal intraocular pressure (IOP) is about 16 mm Hg. If there is an increase in the outflow resistance, the normal IOP rises, and if the IOP exceeds its normal high range (about 30 mm Hg), the condition known as *glaucoma* exists. In extreme situations, the IOP can exceed 60–80 mm Hg. Such acute glaucoma sharply reduces normal arterial blood flow to the retina, causing poor oxygenation and impaired nutrition of retinal neurons and glial cells. If prolonged, glaucoma can lead to the death of retinal neurons, including the loss of retinal ganglion cells, the axons of which compose the optic nerve. Such neuron loss is irreversible, causing loss of visual field, acuity, and even total blindness. Thus, it is medically important as part of every routine eye examination to measure the IOP, especially in older patients, who are more susceptible to glaucoma.

It is important to point out that, while high IOP is not the only diagnostic sign for glaucoma; it is an important one. The retinal nerve damage ("cupping") associated with glaucoma has been observed in 50% of patients with a baseline IOP less than 21 mm Hg. Also, 50% of patients with a Goldmann tonometer-measured IOP of over 30 mm Hg never developed glaucomatous visual field loss. Fewer than 10% of patients with IOP > 21 mm Hg have field loss (Spear, 1999). Such a loose correlation between elevated IOP and glaucoma indicates that, in the diagnosis of glaucoma, the examining physician should also rely on measurements of losses of the visual field and fundoscopy of the optic nerve head and its blood vessels.

The simplest, most inaccurate and subjective means of estimating IOP is by digital (finger, not computer) manipulation of the cornea through the closed eyelid. Examining physicians rest their hands on the patient's forehead for stability, and press through the closed eyelid inward and toward the center of the eyeball with their index fingers. The perceived ocular compliance is related to extensive personal experience to arrive at an estimate of IOP that may approach 2-bit accuracy (1 part in 4, e.g., low, normal, elevated and high).

The ideal invasive means of measuring IOP would be to penetrate the eyeball with a saline-filled hypodermic needle and cannula connected to a mercury manometer or pressure sensor. Fortunately, an indirect noninvasive means of estimating IOP, called ocular tonometry, has evolved. Two major types of tonometer use the elastic property of the thin cornea: *Applanation tonometers*, such as the Goldmann (1957) type, and various air puff tonometers (APTs) based on the Forbes APT design that generate a pneumatic force that flattens a specified area of the cornea. The IOP is approximately equal to the applied force divided by the flattened area. *Impression tonometers* include the Schiøtz hand-held and electronic tonometers, and the McLean (1919) tonometer. Impression tonometers measure the amount of indentation caused by a known force on a small-diameter probe contacting the center of the cornea. All tonometers that directly touch the cornea require its anesthetization and sterile technique.

The simplified mechanics of applanation tonometry are illustrated in Figure 12.1. Here, a force, either from direct mechanical contact with the cornea or from air pressure, causes a small area of the cornea to flatten. In the figure, we assume, for simplicity, that the entire eyeball is a hollow sphere of radius R and volume $V_1 = (4/3)\pi R^3$ cm^3. Inside is the intraocular hydraulic pressure that we wish to measure — call it P_1. The external force F is increased until a known area A of the cornea is flattened. This area is $A = \pi r^2$ cm^2. As a result of this flattening, it can be shown that a volume, $\Delta V = (1/6)\pi\delta(3r^2 + \delta^2)$ cm^3 is subtracted from the original eye volume, V_1. Assume that the AH is an incompressible liquid, the eyeball is elastic, and no AH leaves the eyeball during the short period of IOP measurement so that applanation causes a small transient elevation in IOP, ΔP, and an equivalent expansion of the eyeball expressed by a net ΔR. This relation can be summarized by:

$$P_1 V_1 \cong (P_1 + \Delta P)(V_1 - \Delta V) \qquad 12.1$$

Furthermore, we assume that the applanating pressure, $F/A = (P_1 + \Delta P)$. Thus we can write:

$$P_1 V_1 = F/(\pi r^2)(V_1 - \Delta V) \qquad 12.2$$

This relation reduces to:

$$P_1 = (F/A)\left[1 - \frac{\Delta V}{V_1}\right] \qquad 12.3$$

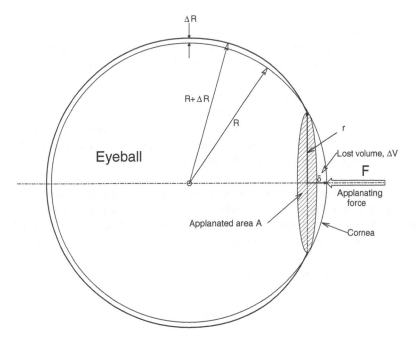

FIGURE 12.1 Simplified cross-section of an eyeball showing corneal applanation.

Using Equation 12.3, we can finally write:

$$P_{app} = (F/A) \cong IOP\left[1 + \frac{3\,r^2\delta}{8\,R^3}\right] \cong IOP \qquad\qquad 12.4$$

F and A are generally known; and from the geometry and real dimensions, $3r^2\delta/(8R^3)$ << 1, so the approximation is generally valid for the Goldmann and air-puff applanation tonometers. In the sections below, we will first examine the clever air-puff tonometer developed by Forbes, et al., (1974), and then describe the Schiøtz, McLean and Goldmann tonometers.

12.2 THE AIR-PUFF NONCONTACT APPLANATION TONOMETER

All applanation tonometers are based on the principle that if a sufficient force is applied to the cornea, it will flatten when the (force × flattened area) ≅ IOP. This simple assumption neglects the natural stiffness of the cornea. In 1974, Forbes, Pico and Grolman published the design and evaluation of a unique, innovative, no-touch tonometric system consisting of four subsystems:

1. The first is a pneumatic system that delivers a short collimated air pulse whose force increases linearly in time. The collimated air stream is

directed at the center of the cornea. Initially, the force of the air pulse on the cornea increases linearly with time.

2. The second is an electro-optical system that detects applanation (flattening) of the cornea due to a critical air pressure with microsecond resolution.
3. The third is an electro-optical system that ensures the correct alignment of the first two systems on the patient's cornea.
4. The fourth subsystem is a dedicated computer that controls the air-puff tonometer's (APT) operation, processes sensor output data, and calculates and displays the estimated IOP digitally.

The *first system* is shown schematically in Figure 12.2. A rotary solenoid is coupled by a two-arm crank to a carbon piston sealed in a polished stainless-steel cylinder. When the solenoid is energized, its rotation forces the piston into the cylinder, compressing the air so that the internal pressure rises as $P = kt^2$ at first. The small tube through the center of the alignment system lens assembly acts as a pneumatic resistance, R_t, so that the volume flow through the tube is given by:

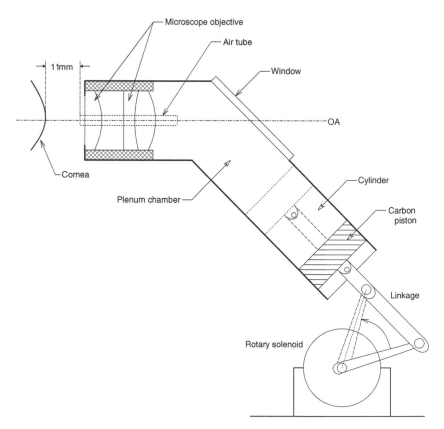

FIGURE 12.2 Simplified cross-section of an air-puff tonometer.

$$\dot{Q}_A = P(t)/R_t \quad cm^2/sec \qquad\qquad 12.5$$

Hence, the volume flow of air directed at the center of the cornea also increases $\propto$ t^2 in time. It takes about 7.5 ms for $\dot{Q}_A$ to reach its maximum square-law value from zero flow, and the entire pulse of air flow is over in about 25–30 ms, before the subject can blink. The force exerted by the air stream on the corneal apex can be given by Newton's second law: $F = ma$. The mass of the air stream (neglecting compression in the short tube) is $m = (AL\rho/g)$ grams, where A is the tube's cross sectional area, L is its length, ρ is the air density, and g is the acceleration of gravity. The acceleration of the gas in the tube can be shown to be:

$$a = \ddot{x} = \dot{Q}_A/A \quad cm/sec^2 \qquad\qquad 12.6$$

And the rate of change of volume flow can be written (Northrop, 2000):

$$\ddot{Q}_A = \dot{P}\,\pi\,r^4/(8L\eta) \quad cm^3/sec^2 \qquad\qquad 12.7$$

Here, r is the tube's radius in cm and η is the gas viscosity in Poise. Thus, the force on the cornea increases approximately linearly in time during the rising phase of the air pulse.

$$F_c = \dot{P}\left(\frac{\rho\,\pi\,r^4}{8\,g\,\eta}\right) = 2\,k\,t\left(\frac{\rho\,\pi\,r^4}{8\,g\,\eta}\right) \quad dynes \qquad\qquad 12.8$$

At the critical F_c, the cornea flattens, then becomes concave. As the air flow goes to zero, the cornea again flattens, then becomes normally convex. The orifice of the tube is held about 11 mm from the apex of the cornea.

The *second system* that detects the instant of applanation is shown schematically in Figure 12.3. A collimated low-powered NIR laser beam is directed at a point at the center of the to-be-applanated cornea. When the cornea is normally convex, the reflected laser beam is dispersed by reflection from the curved corneal surface, and the photodiode receives very low NIR light intensity When the force of the air puff causes corneal applanation, the collimated laser beam is reflected from the flat surface of the cornea directly into the telescope to the photodiode. A sharp spike of voltage that has two functions is produced: 1) It causes the power to the solenoid to be interrupted, aborting the further increase of air force on the cornea, and 2) The pulse signals the tonometer's computer the time at which applanation occurred. Because the air puff force vs. time is the same for every measurement, the applanation time can be related to IOP by previous calibration, and the fact that the force increases linearly with time.

The *third system* is a complex system of lenses and mirrors that allows the operator to align the tonometer's axis perpendicular to a plane tangent to the apex of the cornea and adjust its distance from the corneal apex.. In other words, align

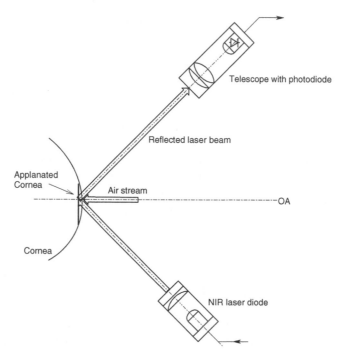

FIGURE 12.3 Schematic of the applanation-detecting optics used in the air-puff tonometer.

it along the gaze axis of the eye under measurement when the eye is fixated at a red LED fixation target. Alignment is critical because, if the air puff is directed off-center from the gaze axis, the measured IOP will be higher than seen for an on-axis measurement. The alignment system uses an LED beam reflection off the normally curved corneal apex to guarantee alignment. Different lenses can be switched into this optical pathway to compensate for near- or farsighted eyes. If the LED beam is not in registry with its sensor, the system will not generate an air puff, and the operator must realign the tonometer.

For the original calibration of the APT, Goldmann applanation tonometry was done on the same eyes as the air puff system (Forbes, et al., 1974). Five hundred and seventy different eyes were examined, with IOPs ranging from 7 to 60 mm Hg. The Goldmann tonometer was considered to be the "gold standard" (true IOP). Linear regression of a scatter diagram of APT vs. Goldmann readings showed that:

$$\text{Air Puff IOP} = 0.953 \,(\text{Goldmann IOP}) + 1.01, \; r = 0.90 \qquad 12.9$$

Thus, the accuracy of the APT is acceptable for clinical use. Its advantages are that it is quick and does not require either sterile technique or corneal anesthesia. Because it is computer-based, it can store patient data from previous exams and plot this data so that the treating physician can examine progress in the pharmacological treatment of high IOP. Disadvantages include the requirements that patients have clear, smooth corneas, be able to see the fixation target clearly, and be able to fixate.

12.3 CONTACT TONOMETERS

All contact tonometers require sterile technique and anesthetization (e.g., by 0.5% proparacaine) of the corneal surface. They all estimate IOP by exerting an inward force on the corneal surface and either measuring the amount of indentation produced, or the area flattened for some critical force that causes flattening. In the latter case, the IOP ≈ Applied force/Area flattened.

Figure 12.4 is a photograph of a modern Schiøtz and an early 20th-century McLean indentation tonometer. In both, a vertical weighted rod makes contact with the cornea through a hole in the center of a concave cup that rests on the apex of the cornea. In the Schiøtz, the end of the rod is 3.00 mm in diameter, and is slightly concave where it contacts the cornea. The McLean's rod is 2.50 mm in diameter and has a flat face. Both the tonometers' cups are about 1.0 cm in diameter. The Schiøtz instrument has a general 0–20 scale, and can have weights of 5.5, 7.5 and 10.0 grams added to the rod. It is used with a look-up table for IOP (the Friedenwald table). The McLean tonometer has a weight built into its rod, and reads IOP directly on its nonlinear scale. Protocol for use of this type of tonometer requires three successive readings from which an average is then taken.

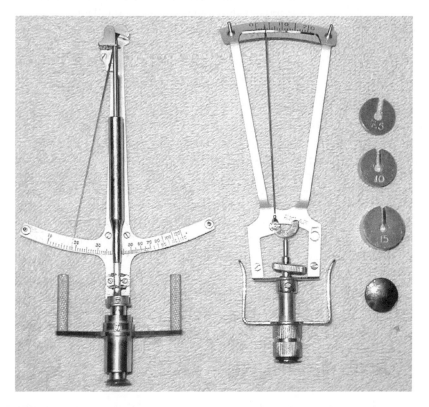

FIGURE 12.4 Two hand-held tonometers owned by the author: (left) an antique McLean indentation tonometer; (right) a modern Schiøtz tonometer with its weights.

The *Goldmann applanation tonometer* has been used as a gold standard to evaluate the performance of other types of tonometers (Forbes, et al., 1974; Wingert, et al., 1993), and is probably the most common tonometer used by modern ophthalmologists and optometrists. During its use, the patient's head is erect, resting in a three-point headrest (chin and two forehead pads) with the eyes looking straight ahead at a fixation point. A drop of saline containing the fluorescent dye *fluorescein sodium* is placed on the end of the probe. Fluorescein fluoresces yellow-green when irradiated with blue light, which is produced by the tonometer. The optical probe of the Goldmann tonometer is slowly advanced until it just touches the apex of the anesthetized cornea. This point is sensed optically. Then the probe is slowly advanced until the operator sees a particular pattern through the optical prism structure built into the probe. The pattern is caused by the probe face's flattening a circle on the cornea and forcing a ring of fluorescein to its circumference. The shape of the pattern tells the operator whether the probe is aligned correctly, and also the size of the flattened area. A hand-held Goldmann-type tonometer (the Perkins tonometer) using a prism probe is also available; it allows IOP to be measured from eyes of supine as well as seated patients.

Other electronic tonometers also measure the indentation displacement either with a constant force, or the force required to produce a given flattening area of the cornea. The former is an electronic Schiøtz instrument that uses a linear variable differential transformer (LVDT) length sensor with micron resolution. The latter is called the MacKay-Marg tonometer.

12.4   SUMMARY

Tonometry is an important NI diagnostic technique used to detect elevated intraocular pressure that could lead to the condition of glaucoma (generally a disease of the elderly) and progressive vision loss. An abnormally high IOP is a necessary, but not sufficient, condition for diagnosis of glaucoma. If high IOP is detected during a routine eye exam, it should be followed up by direct observation of the retina and tests for vision loss.

The air-puff tonometer is a truly no-touch NI diagnostic instrument, but tonometry done during eye exams is done by an electronic, Goldmann-type instrument that makes direct contact with the cornea, and thus requires corneal anesthetization and sterile technique.

13 NI Tests Involving the Input of Audible Sound Energy

13.1 INTRODUCTION

In this chapter, we will examine how low-intensity air-coupled acoustic energy in the range from 0.2–5,000 Hz can be used to characterize the health of the respiratory system (trachea, bronchial tubes, alveoli, and lung tissues) and the middle ear components of the auditory system through the measurement of *acoustic impedance*. The frequency characteristics of sound transmission through the thorax is also considered as a means of diagnosing obstructive lung diseases.

Acoustic impedance, $\mathbf{Z}_{ac}(j\omega)$, is defined in this chapter as the vector ratio of pressure (e.g., in dynes/cm^2) to volume flow (e.g., in cm^3/sec.) caused by that pressure at a given sinusoidal frequency of pressure. It is analogous to electrical impedance in that pressure is analogous to voltage, and volume flow is analogous to electrical current. The units of $\mathbf{Z}_{ac}(j\omega)$ are *CGS acoustic ohms*, and its fundamental dimensions are $ML^{-4}T^{-1}$.

Measurement of a $\mathbf{Z}_{ac}(j\omega)$ can be done with two pressure sensors or two microphones, and a pure acoustic resistance, R_{ac}. This measurement is analogous to measuring electrical impedance (magnitude) with a voltmeter, ammeter and resistance The acoustic circuit generally used is shown in Figure 13.1, drawn as its electrical analog. As you will see below, the only problem with "pure" acoustical resistances is that they develop a phase shift at high frequencies due to acoustic *inertance* (analogous to a series electrical inductance).

It is well known that various anatomical and physical changes happen to the bronchioles and alveoli of the lungs in *obstructive lung diseases* (e.g., asthma, atelactesis, byssanosis, cystic fibrosis, emphysema, pneumonia, silicosis, tuberculosis, etc.). These changes alter the acoustic impedance of the lungs as measured orally through the tracheal airway. For example, in emphysema, the walls separating adjacent alveoli break down, producing larger alveolar spaces with walls having less elasticity. In cystic fibrosis, the alveoli and bronchioles become clogged with mucus, increasing airway resistance and reducing lung volume, etc. Different physical changes in lung tissues will lead to different $\mathbf{Z}_{ac}(j\omega)$ plots. Hereafter, we will refer to the $\mathbf{Z}_{ac}$ of the respiratory system "seen" through the pharynx and trachea as $\mathbf{Z}_{rs}$.

How these impedance conditions occur can be appreciated by a consideration of the basic components making up a complex acoustical impedance. For example, a cylindrical tube whose diameter is small compared with its length, whose length

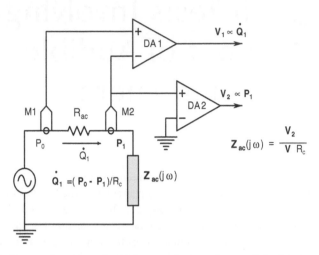

FIGURE 13.1 System for measuring the acoustic impedance of the lungs, eardrum, etc. Acoustic volume flow can be measured, in analogy to Ohm's law, by using two microphones to measure the pressure drop across a pure acoustic resistance. The driving pressure for the impedance being measured comes from microphone M2.

is small compared with the sound wavelength, and for which $r < 0.2/\sqrt{f}$ has an acoustical impedance given by (Olson, 1940):

$$\mathbf{Z}_{ac}(j\omega) = (L/\pi r^2) [(8\eta/r^2) + (4\rho\, j\omega/3)]$$ 13.1

Where L is the tube's length, r is its radius, η is the CGS viscosity coeficient of air $= 1.86 \times 10^{-4}$ poise at 20°C, and ρ is the density of air in $g/cm^3 = 1.205 \times 10^{-3}$. A narrow rectangular slit whose height is small compared with its length, and whose length is small compared with the wavelength has an acoustic impedance given by:

$$\mathbf{Z}_{ac}(j\omega) = (6L/wd)[2\eta/d^2 + j\omega\rho/5]$$ 13.2

Where L is the length of the slit in the direction of the flow in cm, w = width of slit normal to the direction of flow in cm, and d is the height of the slit in cm. ρ and η are the same as above. Note that these impedances are "inertive," characterized by a positive phase angle at high frequencies. The frequency at which the real part of $\mathbf{Z}_{ac}(j\omega)$ equals its imaginary part (ω at which $\angle\, \mathbf{Z}_{ac}(j\omega_b) = +45°$) is $\omega_b = (6\eta)/(\rho r^2)$ r/s for the tube, and $\omega_b = (10\eta)/(\rho d^2)$ r/s for the slit.

All cavities or chambers with rigid boundaries have *acoustical capacitance* C_{ac}. C_{ac} is analogous to electrical capacitance, defined by $i = C_e(dv/dt)$. As we have seen, the current is analogous to volume flow rate $\dot{Q}$, cm^3/sec, and voltage is analogous to acoustic pressure, p. Thus, C_{ac} is defined as the ratio of

$$C_{ac} \equiv \frac{\dot{Q}}{\dot{p}}$$ 13.3

Olson (1940) shows that C_{ac} of a stiff-walled chamber is given by (assuming acoustic wavelengths are large compared with the cavity's linear dimensions):

$$C_{ac} = V/(\rho c^2) \qquad 13.4$$

Where c is the speed of sound in air, and ρ is the mean air mass density in g/cm^3. Another way to realize acoustic capacitance is by using a chamber with thin elastic low-mass walls, or with a thin low-mass elastic diaphragm coupling between two ducts. In these cases, C_{ac} = (mechanical compliance of the diaphragm) × (area squared of the diaphragm). Mechanical compliance is defined as $c_m \equiv x/f_m$, where x is the displacement caused by a mechanical force, f_m. f_m is of course, (acoustic pressure) × (diaphragm area). c_m is the reciprocal of stiffness. The fundamental dimensions of acoustical capacitance are $M^{-1}L^4T^2$.

If a tube with Z_{ac}, given by Equation 13.1, is terminated in a stiff-walled cavity, the series driving-point Z_{ac} is:

$$Z_{ac}(j\omega) = (L/\pi r^2) [(8\eta/r^2) + (4\rho j\omega/3)] + (\rho c^2)/(j\omega V) \qquad 13.5$$

In electrical terms, this impedance is analogous to a series RLC circuit with the capacitor grounded. Thus, it has a resonant frequency, ω_o, at which $Z_{ac}(j\omega)$ is real and minimum. Elementary complex algebra tells us this is at:

$$\omega_o = (c\,r/2)\sqrt{(3\pi/VL)} \quad \text{r/s} \qquad 13.6$$

This type of acoustic circuit is called a *Helmholz resonator.*

The reactive terms in Equations 13.1 and 13.2 for the Z_{ac} of a tube are due to the inertance or mass of the air in the tube and slot. In an electrical inductance, we have the well-known relation:

$$v = L (di/dt) \qquad 13.7$$

In acoustic terms, this is analogous to:

$$p = M_{ac}\left(d\dot{Q}/dt\right) \qquad 13.8$$

M_{ac} is the inertance analogous to inductance, p is pressure analogous to voltage, and $\dot{Q}$ is volume flow, analogous to electric current in coulombs/sec. Olson (1940) showed that the inertance of a thin cylindrical tube is simply:

$$M_{ac} = (4L\,\rho)/(3\,\pi\,r^2) \qquad 13.9$$

Inertance has the fundamental dimensions of ML^{-4}.

The acoustic impedance of the ear canal and eardrum at audio frequencies depends on the dimensions of the auditory canal and the mechanical loading of the eardrum at its end. The eardrum drives the three ossicles that couple the sound energy from the outer ear to the cochlea, where acoustic sensory transduction takes place. The "handle" of the *malleus* ossicle is connected to the inside center of the eardrum. At the other end, the malleus is tightly bound by ligaments to the *incus* (anvil). The end of the incus articulates with the *stapes* (stirrup), the base of which moves the membrane of the oval window, transmitting sound energy to the fluid in the cochlea. Normally, the three ossicles compose a fairly compliant assembly that is efficient in coupling sound from the eardrum to the cochlea over a wide range of frequencies (20 Hz to 15 kHz). If a sudden loud sound occurs, the CNS' *auditory attenuation reflex* (AAR) causes the two small muscles in the inner ear, the *stapedius* and the *tensor tympani*, to contract after about 40–80 ms. Contraction of the tensor tympani pulls the handle of the malleus inward, and the stapedius forces the stapes outward. These opposing forces cause the ossicles to become very rigid. This rigidity has the effect of attenuating low-frequency sound (below 1 kHz) as much as 30–40 dB. This protects the cochlea from mechanically damaging low-frequency vibrations and also allows the person to screen out loud low-frequency sounds while listening to information-carrying sounds above 1 kHz. The AAR causes a change in the acoustic impedance of the eardrum as measured from the ear canal. In normal individuals, if $Z_{ac}(j\omega)$ of one ear is measured while the other ear is presented with a sudden loud low-frequency sound, the AAR will cause a simultaneous $Z_{ac}(j\omega)$ change in both ears that can be measured in one ear.

Measurement of the $Z_{rs}(j\omega)$ of the lungs or the eardrum can serve as simple NI means of screening outpatients for COLD or hearing problems. In the following sections, we will examine the history of respiratory acoustic impedance measurement (RAIMS), and a RAIMS system developed by the author and his graduate students. We will also describe auditory $Z_{ac}(j\omega)$ measurement systems, and a prototype system that measures the acoustic transfer function $H_{rs}(j\omega)$, of the thorax (including the lungs) using acoustic white noise.

13.2   ACOUSTIC IMPEDANCE MEASUREMENT OF THE RESPIRATORY SYSTEM

Figure 13.2 illustrates the acoustic and electronic components of a general system for measuring respiratory acoustic impedance. The trachea and lungs constitute a complex distributed-parameter acoustic impedance that, at a given frequency, may appear reactive capacitive, reactive inductive or even real (resistive, a resonance condition).

One of the first efforts at characterizing the acoustic impedance of the respiratory system was made by Pimmel et al., 1977. Acoustic pressure was generated by an acoustic suspension loudspeaker (Acoustic Research Corp., AR-3), and volume flow was measured as the pressure drop across a heated Silverman pneumotach (H. Rudolph Co., model 3700), which served as an acoustic resistance at low frequencies. Two Validyne model MP-45 pressure sensors were used as low-frequency microphones to measure the sound pressure at the input (loudspeaker) end of the pneumotach, P_1, and at the mouth end of the pneumotach, P_2. Because of the sinusoidal nature of P_1 and P_2, the phase between these signals (i.e., the phase of $\dot{Q}(t)$ with respect to P_2) was

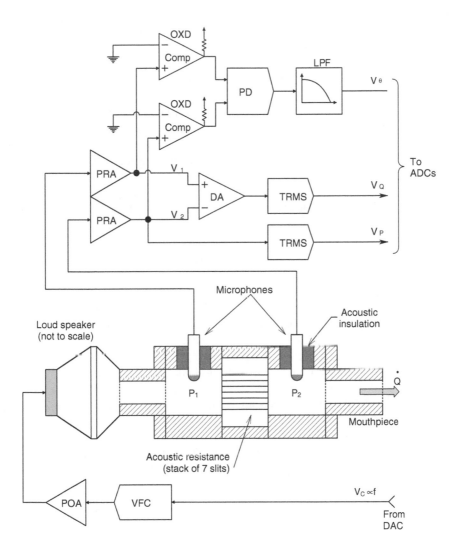

FIGURE 13.2 System designed by the author to measure the acoustic impedance of the lungs, Z_{rs}. A special low-inertance pneumotach was designed to keep the pneumotach impedance resistive to over 300 Hz. DC voltages proportional to volume flow, driving-point pressure, and the angle of Z_{rs} are provided at any frequency from 1 to 200 Hz.

measured by passing the conditioned sinusoidal output voltages from the sensors into zero-crossing comparators to make phase-coherent TTL signals, then passing the TTL signals into a digital phase detector subsystem. The flow was determined by:

$$\dot{Q}(t) = \left[P_1(t) - P_2(t) \right] / Z_{pt}(j\omega) = K_m \left[V_1(t) - V_2(t) \right] / Z_{pt}(j\omega) \qquad 13.10$$

Here, P_1 and P_2 are the actual sinusoidal pressures across the pneumotach, K_m is the sensor scaling constant, and $Z_{pt}(j\omega)$ is the acoustical impedance of the pneumotach. $Z_{pt}(j\omega)$ is generally of the form:

$$Z_{pt}(j\omega) = R_{pt} + j\omega M_{pt} \qquad 13.11$$

At low frequencies, $Z_{pt}(j\omega) \cong R_{pt}$ (real), which is what is desired. As the frequency increases, the phase angle of $Z_{pt}(j\omega)$ increases because of the inertance (M_{pt}) inherent in the pneumotach. Pimmel et al. used the frequency where there was a 2° phase in $Z_{pt}(j\omega)$ as the upper frequency of operation of their instrument. This criterion can be interpreted as:

$$\omega_H = (R_{pt}/M_{pt})\tan(2°) = 0.035\ (R_{pt}/M_{pt})\ \text{r/s} \qquad 13.12$$

or

$$f_H = (5.5578 \times 10^{-3})\ (R_{pt}/M_{pt})\ \text{Hz} \qquad 13.13$$

Pimmel et al. found $f_H = 16$ Hz in their system. They examined the $Z_{rs}(j2\pi f)$ of mongrel dogs over a frequency range of 1 to 16 Hz. The $Z_{rs}(j2\pi f)$s of normal animals were compared with those given IV physostigmine, a powerful bronchoconstrictor, at a dose of 0.025 mg/kg. The $Z_{rs}(j2\pi f)$ magnitude showed a minimum at about 5 Hz, then increased slowly with frequency. The phase of $Z_{rs}(j2\pi f)$ at 1 Hz was typically about −70°, increased smoothly to zero (resonance) at about 5 Hz, then continued to increase, ending at ca. +70° at 16 Hz. The dogs given physostigmine clearly showed a uniform increase in $|Z_{rs}(j2\pi f)|$ at all frequencies, but little change in the phase plot of $Z_{rs}(j2\pi f)$ vs. that for normal dogs. Other plots of $|Z_{rs}(j2\pi f)|$ and $\angle Z_{rs}(j2\pi f)$ for a dog who had been conditioned to replicate a heavy smoker, and a dog with a congenital tracheal hypoplasia showed pronounced increases in $|Z_{rs}(j2\pi f)|$ at all frequencies, and a steeper slope on the phase plots between 5 and 8 Hz. Clearly, the respiratory acoustical impedance measurement system (RAIMS) of Pimmel et al. could detect respiratory system anomalies. Presentation of $Z_{rs}(j2\pi f)$ data as polar plots might have given the investigators a more sensitive tool than separately plotting magnitude and angle. Also, extending the high-frequency range of measurement can provide more useful data, given a pneumotach design with low inertance.

The author realized that the design of a low-inertance pneumotach was essential in developing a prototype RAIMS that could cover at least two decades of frequency (1 to > 100 Hz). Comparison of the acoustic impedance function for screens, tubes and slits showed that slits offered an advantage over tubes and screens in terms of their R_{pt}/M_{pt} ratio:

$$\left[R_{pt}/M_{pt}\right] = \frac{10\ \eta}{\rho\ d^2} \qquad 13.14$$

Using $\eta = 1.86 \times 10^{-4}$ Poise, $\rho = 1.205 \times 10^{-3}$ g/cm^3, and d = 0.0051 cm (a value we used), the ratio is equal to 5.9345×10^4. Using Equation 13.13 for a 2° phase shift at f_H, we find $f_H = 330$ Hz. Thus the parallel slit acoustic impedance for the pneumotach appears real until the operating frequency approaches 330 Hz ($2°$ criterion). Putting seven such slits in parallel divides R_{ac} by 7, but does not affect the overall f_H of $\mathbf{Z}_{pt}$.

Figure 13.2 illustrates a prototype RAIMS system developed by the author. In general, $P_1 > P_2$, so $V_1 > V_2$ at any frequency. The sinusoidal signals V_1 and V_2 are converted to dc by true RMS converters. $V_Q = K_D(v_{1rms} - v_{2rms})$ is a dc voltage proportional to the volume flow into the lungs, $\dot{Q}$. The ratio V_P/V_Q is calculated by the system's computer after analog-to-digital conversion; it is proportional to the $|\mathbf{Z}_{rs}|$ of the respiratory system. The sinusoidal signals V_1 and V_2 are passed through comparator-zero-crossing detectors to form two TTL signals of the applied acoustic frequency that are shifted in phase relative to the respiratory system input pressure, P_2. A digital phase detector and low-pass filter generate a dc voltage, V_θ, which is proportional to the phase shift. The computer generates the dc voltage input to the voltage-to-frequency converter, V_C, which generates the variable frequency sinusoidal signal that drives the loudspeaker. The computer is able to make standard Bode dB amplitude and phase plots vs. frequency, polar plots, and $R_e\{\mathbf{Z}_{rs}\}$ and $I_m\{\mathbf{Z}_{rs}\}$ vs. f plots. The system of Figure 13.2 was tested satisfactorily on known acoustic loads and chest phantoms, and normal, consenting humans.

In *in vivo* $\mathbf{Z}_{rs}$ measurements, the state of expansion of the lungs is an important parameter. $\mathbf{Z}_{rs}$ measurements can be made with the airway at ambient atmospheric pressure, or at some mean positive pressure, P_{tr}, to ensure complete lung expansion. The applied sound pressure is then a small perturbation on top of P_{tr}. In small-signal, single-frequency $\mathbf{Z}_{rs}$ measurements, it has been noted generally that both $R_e\{\mathbf{Z}_{rs}\}$ and $I_m\{\mathbf{Z}_{rs}\}$ are frequency-dependent in a complex manner. This is because of the parallel combination of many component $\mathbf{Z}_{rs}$ s with different natural frequencies.

If a *large-amplitude* forced oscillation technique (FOT) is used, three problems can arise:

1. The pneumotach resistance, R_{pt}, used to measure $\dot{Q}$, can become nonlinear due to departure from laminar flow conditions.
2. Pneumotach inertance effects can become more pronounced at high flow rates, limiting the accuracy in the high frequency range of study.
3. The elasticity of lung tissues is no longer linear.

It should be noted that statistical techniques of estimating $\mathbf{Z}_{rs}$ have been used in which the excitation sound pressure, P_1, is pseudorandom binary noise (with zero mean), rather than a sinusoid. Cross-power spectral techniques (Northrop, 2000) are then used to extract an estimate of $\mathbf{Z}_{rs}$ (j2πf). Suki and Lutchen (1992) have demonstrated that input signals of the general form of sum of sinusoids, thus:

$$p_1(t) = \sum_{k=1}^{N} p_k \cos\left[2\pi f_k + \varphi_k\right]$$

can also be used to characterize the nonlinear respiratory system's $\mathbf{Z}_{rs}$.

In summary, it appears that the major challenge in making high-frequency measurements of the Z_{ac} (j2πf) of the respiratory system lies in the design of a pneumotach acoustic impedance that remains real over the range of frequencies of interest. Even with this limitation, Z_{rs} measurements have been used in a variety of diagnostic trials. Young et al. (1996) measured Z_{rs} in horses with heaves (analogous to asthma) using forced oscillations at 1.5, 2, 3 and 5 Hz. They examined $\left| Z_{rs} (f) \right|$ and $R_e\{Z_{rs} (f)\}$ and concluded that a significant indicator of heaves was an increase in $R_e\{Z_{rs}\}$ in the 1.5–3 Hz range (no doubt due to bronchospasm). There was no significant change in the Z_{rs} inertance.

Hall et al. (1996) used sinusoidal pressure excitation between 0.5 and 21 Hz to measure Z_{rs} of normal infants under the age of 2 years. The purpose of their study was to study how the different lung tissues (airways and parenchyma) grew in the first 2 years. Reisch et al. (1999) used the forced oscillation technique (FOT) to measure Z_{rs} of persons with obstructive sleep apnea syndrome (OSAS). In OSAS patients, pharyngeal collapses are correlated with a loss of muscle tone in the upper airway, and its consequent partial or total collapse. They concluded that the FOT is a valuable tool for assessing the degree of upper airway obstruction in patients with OSAS.

The broad applications of respiratory FOT were studied and described by Wesseling 1999. Z_{rs} was measured for a variety of pharmacologically induced and natural respiratory problems. Wesseling comments:

"… it is concluded that respiratory impedance measurements using the technique of forced oscillations can be easily performed in many different categories of patients. Unlike spirometric tests, the [FOT] measurements can be made at the low flow rates occurring during breathing at rest, thus avoiding the effects that forced respiratory manoeuvres may have on the smooth muscle tone of the respiratory system, and they do not necessitate active cooperation from the subjects. It forms a sensitive method to obtain information on the mechanical characteristics of the respiratory system in various disease entities."

13.3   ACOUSTIC IMPEDANCE MEASUREMENT OF THE EARDRUM (TYMPANOMETRY)

The auditory canal and eardrum can be modeled by a cylinder closed at its far end by a compliant (elastic) membrane, the eardrum. The degree of eardrum compliance is affected by two significant factors: 1) The difference in mean air pressure between the auditory canal (atmospheric pressure) and the air pressure in the middle ear, and 2) the mechanical loading on the eardrum imposed by the ossicles and the oval window (cf. the discussion in Section 13.1). The point of maximum compliance of the eardrum occurs in the absence of loud sound when the air pressure in the auditory canal equals the air pressure in the middle ear. If, at the point of maximum eardrum compliance, the contralateral ear is stimulated by a loud broadband sound, the reflex contraction that occurs in the muscles of the middle ear causes a stiffening of the tympanic membrane and a consequent increase in the auditory impedance measured in the ipsilateral ear. In other words, the auditory reflex causes a decrease in the compliance of the eardrum and a ca. 30 dB attenuation of sound coupled to the oval window. Measurement of the non-subjective acoustic reflex by sensing small changes in the acoustic input impedance (or admittance) of the ear canal and eardrum has diagnostic significance in both hearing and neurological problems.

In this section, we will describe two ways that have been devised to quantitatively measure the acoustic reflex. In measurement of the acoustic impedance of the respiratory system, we saw it was possible to use an acoustic resistance to measure the volume flow into the oral airway and thus calculate the acoustic impedance as the vector ratio of input pressure to volume flow, given single-frequency sinusoidal excitation. Because of the much smaller size of the ear canal, the acoustic driving point impedance, Z_a, can be more easily measured by driving the outer ear canal with a sinusoidal volume flow source (analogous in an electrical circuit to an ac current source) and measuring the resultant pressure across Z_a. Such a scheme was devised by Pinto and Dallos, (1968). Figure 13.3 illustrates their system. A volume flow source is approximated by putting the primary sinusoidal pressure source, P_1, in series with a large acoustic resistance, $Z_{LS}(j\omega)$. The effective ac volume flow source is $Q_1 \equiv P_1/ Z_{LS}$. Z_{LS} couples P_1 to Z_a in parallel with another large Z_m to the microphone. Design makes $|Z_{LS}|$ and $|Z_m| >> Z_a$ at the operating frequency. Thus $P_a = Q_1 Z_a = P_1 Z_a/Z_{LS}$. (We neglect volume flow in Z_m as being << that in Z_a.)

Using superposition, we see that the potentiometer serves as a ratiometric adder to form V_i.

$$V_i = \rho V_m + (1 - \rho)V_r, \quad 0 \leq \rho \leq 1 \qquad\qquad 13.16$$

In Figure 13.3 we see how the bridge is nulled. The ac source, V_{in} is phase shifted by θ, then its amplitude is adjusted by a factor of β to make $V_i = 0$ (null). Thus $V_r = \beta V_{in} \angle\theta$ in phasor notation. V_r is next attenuated by $(1 - \rho)$ and added to ρV_m. Note that $0 \leq \rho \leq 1$. V_m is the conditioned microphone output. V_m is given by:

$$V_m = V_{in} \frac{A_1(j\omega)L(j\omega)Z_a(j\omega)}{Z_{LS}(j\omega)}M(j\omega)A_2(j\omega) \qquad\qquad 13.17$$

Where A_1 and A_2 are amplifier voltage gains, L is the loudspeaker transfer function in (dynes/cm^2)/rms volt, M is the microphone transfer function in rms volts/(dyne/cm^2), and Z_{LS} is the high series CGS acoustic impedance between P_1 and P_a. Hence, at null:

$$V_i = 0 = \beta(1-\rho)\angle\theta + \rho\frac{A_1(j\omega)L(j\omega)Z_a(j\omega)}{Z_{LS}(j\omega)}M(j\omega)A_2(j\omega) \qquad 13.18$$

The vector acoustic impedance of the auditory canal and eardrum can thus be written:

$$Z_a(j\omega) = \frac{-\beta(1-\rho)\angle\theta}{\rho A_1(j\omega)A_2(j\omega)L(j\omega)M(j\omega)/Z_{LS}(j\omega)} \qquad\qquad 13.19$$

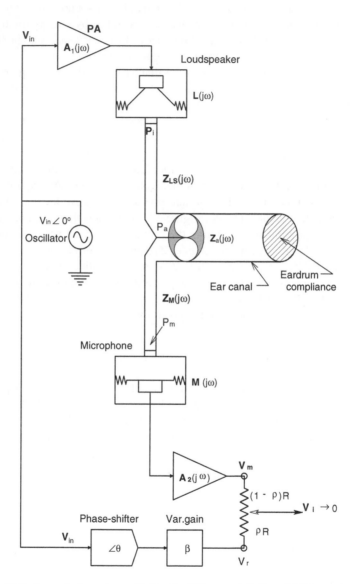

FIGURE 13.3 Acoustic impedance "bridge" of Pinto and Dallos (1968), used to measure eardrum impedance.

ρ, β and θ are set to null V_i, and the values of the vectors in the denominator at $\omega = 2\pi f$ are known by prior measurement.

In Figure 13.4, we illustrate a slightly different version of the Pinto and Dallos auditory impedance bridge, modified by the author. The ratiometric voltage divider has been replaced by a difference amplifier with gain K_D. V_i is now given by:

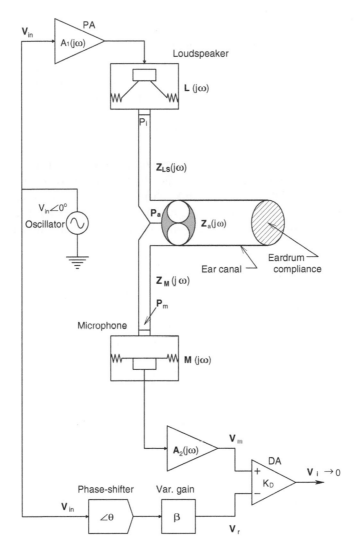

FIGURE 13.4 A modified Pinto and Dallos bridge.

$$\mathbf{V_i} = K_D(\mathbf{V_m} - \mathbf{V_r}) = K_D \, [V_{in} \, \mathbf{A_1}(j\omega) \, \mathbf{A_2}(j\omega) \, \mathbf{L}(j\omega) \, \mathbf{M}(j\omega) \, \mathbf{Y_{LS}}(j\omega) \, \mathbf{Z_a}(j\omega)$$

$$- V_{in} \, \beta\angle\theta] \qquad\qquad 13.20$$

If $\mathbf{V_i}$ is nulled under resting conditions, $\mathbf{Z_a}(j\omega)$ can be calculated from Equation 13.20. When a loud sound is applied to the contralateral ear, the acoustic reflex causes $\mathbf{Z_a}$ to increase by some $\Delta\mathbf{Z_a}$, unbalancing the null. The unbalanced $\mathbf{V_i}$ can be written:

$$\mathbf{V_i} = K_D\left[V_{in}\mathbf{A_1}(j\omega)\mathbf{A_2}(j\omega)\,\mathbf{L}(j\omega)\,\mathbf{M}(j\omega)\,\mathbf{Y_{LS}}(j\omega)\left\{\mathbf{Z_a}(j\omega) + \Delta\mathbf{Z_a}\right\} - V_{in}\beta\angle\theta\right]$$

$$= K_D\left[\begin{array}{c} V_{in}\mathbf{A_1}(j\omega)\mathbf{A_2}(j\omega)\,\mathbf{L}(j\omega)\,\mathbf{M}(j\omega)\,\mathbf{Y_{LS}}(j\omega) \\ \left\{\dfrac{\beta\angle\theta}{\mathbf{A_1}(j\omega)\mathbf{A_2}(j\omega)\,\mathbf{L}(j\omega)\,\mathbf{M}(j\omega)\,\mathbf{Y_{LS}}(j\omega)} + \Delta\mathbf{Z_a}\right\} - V_{in}\beta\angle\theta \end{array}\right]$$ 13.21

$$\mathbf{V_i} = K_D V_{in}\left[\mathbf{A_1}(j\omega)\mathbf{A_2}(j\omega)\,\mathbf{L}(j\omega)\,\mathbf{M}(j\omega)\,\mathbf{Y_{LS}}(j\omega)\right]\Delta\mathbf{Z_a}$$

Because the magnitude and phase of $\mathbf{V_i}$ are known, as are V_{in}, K_D and the five vectors, it is possible to calculate the exact $\Delta\mathbf{Z_a}$ elicited by the acoustic reflex. By using two phase-sensitive demodulators on $\mathbf{V_i}$ with $V_{in}\angle(\phi)$ and $V_{in}\angle(\phi + 90°)$ (quadrature) as references, where ϕ is the net angle of the $\mathbf{A_1}(j\omega)\,\mathbf{A_2}(j\omega)\,\mathbf{L}(j\omega)\mathbf{M}(j\omega)\,\mathbf{Y_{LS}}(j\omega)$ vector at $\omega = 2\pi f$, it is possible to resolve the vector $\Delta\mathbf{Z_a}$ into its real and imaginary values in nearly real time.

Another system for measuring the magnitude of $\mathbf{Y_a} = \mathbf{Z_a}^{-1}$ was described by Ward in U.S. Patent No. 4,009,707 (1977). Instead of using a constant volume rate flow source, Ward measured $\mathbf{P_a}$ at the entrance to the auditory meatus, and used a type 1 feedback control loop to adjust V_{in} so as to keep $\mathbf{P_a}$ constant as $\mathbf{Z_a}$ changed during the auditory reflex. Although his patent is titled *Automatic Acoustic Imped-ance Meter*, Ward's device actually has an output proportional to $\mathbf{Y_a}$: nor is it very "automatic." Ward's system is illustrated in Figure 13.5. The loudspeaker generates a sound pressure $\mathbf{P_1}$, which creates a volume flow, $\dot{Q}_1$, in the connecting tube from the loudspeaker to the ear. This tube has impedance $\mathbf{Z_t}(j\omega)$. The acoustic admittance of the auditory canal and eardrum, $\mathbf{Y_a}$, is shunted by the very small admittance of the tube to the microphone. Thus, practically all of $\dot{Q}_1$ passes into $\mathbf{Y_a}$. Because of the very small flow in the microphone tube, the pressure at the microphone is essentially the pressure at the auditory meatus, i.e., $\mathbf{P_3} \cong \mathbf{P_a}$. These conditions are illustrated in the equivalent electrical analog circuit of Figure 13.6.

To examine how the Ward system operates, we first note that in the steady state, the type 1 controller causes $V_e = 0$. Thus $V_r \equiv v_3 = K_m K_3 p_a$, where K_m is the volts/(dynes/cm^2) conversion gain of the microphone, K_3 is the amplifier gain, and p_a is the rms pressure at the auditory meatus. However, from the analog circuit,

$$\mathbf{P_3} \cong \mathbf{P_a} = \mathbf{P_1}\,\mathbf{Z_a}/(\mathbf{Z_t} + \mathbf{Z_a})$$ 13.22

$$\mathbf{P_a}\,(\mathbf{Z_t} + \mathbf{Z_a}) = \mathbf{P_1}\,\mathbf{Z_a} = \mathbf{Z_a}\,[V_s(1 + V_m)/10]\,\mathbf{L}\,K_p$$ 13.23

$$\mathbf{P_a}\,(1 + \mathbf{Y_a}\,\mathbf{Z_t}) = [V_s\,(1 + V_m)/10]\,\mathbf{L}\,K_p$$ 13.24

However, the rms $p_a = V_r/[\,|\,\mathbf{M}\,|\,K_3]$ in the steady state, so we can finally write:

$$\frac{V_r}{|\mathbf{M}|\,K_3}\left|(1 + \mathbf{Y_a}\mathbf{Z_t})\right| = v_s|\mathbf{L}|\,K_p\,(1 + V_m)/10$$ 13.25

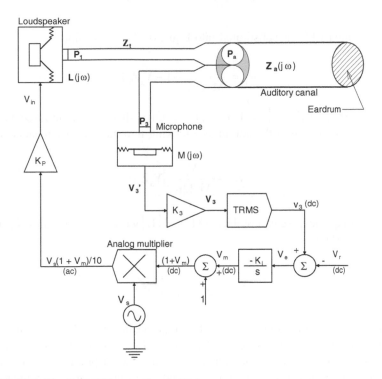

FIGURE 13.5 Ward's (1977) acoustic admittance measurement system.

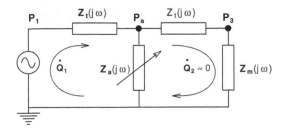

FIGURE 13.6 Lumped-parameter acoustic circuit relevant to the analysis of Ward's acoustic admittance measurement system.

v_s is the rms source voltage. The rms input to the loudspeaker is:

$$v_{in} = v_s \, K_P (1 + V_m)/10 \qquad\qquad 13.26$$

Solving for v_s, we can write:

$$v_s = v_{in}/[\ K_P(1 + V_m)/10]$$
13.27

When Equation 13.27 is substituted into Equation 13.25, we find:

$$v_{in} = \frac{V_r}{|M||L|K_3}\left|(1 + Y_a Z_t)\right|$$
13.28

Now if we make $|Y_a Z_t)| \gg 1$, the final result is that the rms loudspeaker drive voltage is proportional to the admittance looking into the auditory meatus, $Y_a(j\omega)$:

$$v_{in} \cong \frac{V_r}{|M||L|K_3}\left|Y_a Z_t\right|$$
13.29

At a fixed frequency, we can replace $|M|$ and $|L|$ with the scalar gains K_m and K_L respectively. Thus:

$$v_{in} \cong \frac{V_r}{K_m K_L K_3}\left|Y_a Z_t\right|$$
13.30

Note that unlike the nulling system of Pinto and Dallos, the Ward system does not give high sensitivity to measure the ΔY_a caused by the auditory reflex. The Ward system does, however, allow the clinician to adjust the air pressure in the ear canal to obtain maximum eardrum compliance under resting conditions. Shown in the original Ward patent is an analog sample-and-hold circuit that allows the user to measure the small differential output voltage due to ΔY_a, i.e.,

$$\Delta v_{in} \cong \frac{V_r}{K_m K_L K_3}\left\{\left|(Y_a + \Delta Y_a)Z_t\right| - \left|Y_a Z_t\right|\right.$$
13.31

In general, $|Y_a/\Delta Y_a| \ll 1$, so as a final approximation,

$$\Delta v_{in} \cong \frac{V_r}{K_m K_L K_3}\left|\Delta Y_a Z_t\right|$$
13.32

In general, the auditory reflex makes ΔY_a negative, so Δv_{in} is negative in response. Ward's system appears useful as a clinical instrument, even though it only measures the magnitudes of Y_a and ΔY_a.

Both Ward's and Pinto and Dallos' measurement systems use different approaches to the quantification of the auditory reflex. Both also require extensive acoustic and electrical calibration of their components. If Pinto and Dallos' bridge system could be made self-nulling, it would be ideal, because it would provide vector information on ΔZ_a, resulting from the auditory reflex.

13.4 TRANSTHORACIC ACOUSTIC TRANSFER FUNCTION AS A POSSIBLE MEASURE OF LUNG CONDITION

13.4.1 INTRODUCTION

As we have seen in Section 3.4, a trained clinician using a stethoscope can detect pulmonary edema from the absence of intrinsic breath sounds transmitted through the thoracic wall, or internal bubbling and gurgling sounds. Pulmonary edema can be caused by a number of factors, including: congestive heart failure; pneumonia and other infections; allergies; high-altitude syndrome; near drowning; or exposure to toxic chemical fumes or smoke. Pulmonary edema can become life threatening because it decreases active lung volume and decreases O_2/CO_2 exchange, leading to hypoxia and acidosis. X-ray and CAT scan are common NI methods of visualizing pulmonary edema and verifying diagnosis made with a stethoscope.

Another noninvasive approach to detecting and locating volumes of pulmonary edema is to introduce sound into the lungs through the trachea, or by coupling it through the thoracic wall (e.g., on the back), and to use a sensitive microphone on the front of the chest to detect differences in the sound propagation that accompany fluid-filled alveoli. Tissue changes in the lungs that go along with pulmonary emphysema, and, in the small airways, the presence of excess mucous that occurs with cystic fibrosis or asthma, can also alter the acoustic transfer function from the source, through the chest walls, through the lung tissues, to the pickup microphone.

Another medical condition that can affect transthoracic sound propagation is an excess of fluid accumulated in the pleural cavity, between the outside of the lungs and the inside of the chest wall. Factors leading to this *pleural effusion* include: blockage of the normal lymphatic drain system of the pleural cavity, heart failure, greatly reduced plasma colloid oncotic pressure, and inflammation of the pleural surfaces as caused by infection.

We first consider a model for sound transmission in the lung parenchyma. In a normal lung, the parenchyma can be considered to be a two-phase elastic continuum in which the alveolar air sacs are embedded in tissue (Rice, 1983). In general, the speed of sound in an elastic continuum is given by:

$$c = \sqrt{(B/\rho)} \quad \text{cm/sec} \qquad\qquad 13.33$$

Where B is the bulk modulus of the medium in dynes/cm^2 and ρ is its density in grams/cm^3. Let h be the volumetric fraction of the parenchyma that is tissue, and $(1 - h)$ be the fraction that is gas, the composite bulk modulus is:

$$B = \left[(1-h)B_g^{-1} + hB_t^{-1}\right]^{-1} \qquad\qquad 13.34$$

where the subscripts t and g refer to tissue and gas, respectively. The average density is easily seen to be:

$$\rho = (1 - h)\rho_g + h\rho_t \qquad\qquad 3.35$$

ρ of lung tissue is typically from 0.5 to 0.8 g/cm^3. Wodicka et al. (1989) have used $h = 0.25$ for a normal lung, based on an air volume of 2,500 cm^3, and an air-free tissue volume of 900 cm^3 in an adult male. They increased h to 0.35 to model edema in the parenchyma.

Sound is generally considered to propagate under adiabatic conditions. Thus $B_g = \gamma p_o$, where γ is the ratio of the specific heats $= C_p/C_v = 1.4$ for air, but in the lung, nearly isothermal conditions occur, so $\gamma = 1.0$ is a better value (Wodicka et al., 1989). The mean gas pressure is p_o. When the relations above are substituted into Equation 13.33, we obtain:

$$c = \left[\left(\frac{1-h}{\gamma p_o} + \frac{h}{B_t} \right) \left\{ (1-h)\rho_g + h\rho_t \right\} \right]^{-\frac{1}{2}} \quad \text{cm/sec} \qquad 13.36$$

Assuming nearly isolated alveolar gas chambers, the lung can be considered to be like gas bubbles in a fluid. When the bubbles are closely packed and their radius is << than a sound wavelength, they do not act as independent scattering centers. For example, at $c = 2,400$ cm/sec, and an alveolar radius of 150 μm (0.015 cm), the maximum frequency before the alveoli act as independent scattering centers is c. 24 kHz. For $c = 6,000$ cm/sec, $f_{max} \approx 20$ kHz. Note that in the presence of pulmonary edema, h approaches unity, and c increases.

Wodicka et al. (1989) reported on the results of a computer modeling study of sound propagation from the oral airway into the trachea and bronchioles, through the parenchyma, and thence through the chest wall to an accelerometer or microphone. They used a lumped-parameter transmission-line architecture based on acoustic parameters of the tissue structures, including the chest wall. They concluded that considerable sound energy was coupled into the parenchyma directly from the stiff walls of the large airways. Their model predicted that the decreased transmission of sound to the chest wall at high frequencies was due to thermal (resistive) losses in the parenchyma.

The introduced sound pressure can be sinusoidal or an input sound pressure of bandwidth-limited, broadband Gaussian noise. Under the assumption that the sound transmission through the lungs and chest is a linear process (i.e., it obeys superposition), linear system theory shows us that the sinusoidal frequency response function between the driving point acoustic pressure phasor and the pickup point pressure can be written as:

$$\frac{\mathbf{P_o}}{\mathbf{P_i}}(j\omega) = \mathbf{H}(j\omega) \qquad\qquad 13.37$$

$|\mathbf{H}(j\omega)|$ is generally low-pass in nature, and << 1.

When the input sound pressure is Gaussian random noise with a two-sided power density spectrum, $\Phi_{ii}(\omega)$, then it is well known (Northrop, 2000) that $\mathbf{H}(j\omega)$ can be found from the relation:

$$\mathbf{H}(j\omega) = \frac{\Phi_{io}(j\omega)}{\Phi_{ii}(\omega)}$$ 13.38

providing that the system frequency response, $\mathbf{H}$, is linear, stationary, and ergodic. The autopower spectrum, $\Phi_{ii}(\omega)$, is an even, positive-real function. $\Phi_{ii}(\omega)$ is the Fourier transform of the two-sided autocorrelation function, $\varphi_{ii}(\tau)$, of the input pressure given by:

$$\varphi_{ii}(\tau) \equiv \lim_{T\to\infty} \frac{1}{2T} \int_{-T}^{T} p_i(t)\, p_i(t+\tau)\, dt$$ 13.39

The cross-power density spectrum, $\Phi_{io}(j\omega)$, is a vector function of frequency. It is found by taking the Fourier transform of the cross-correlation function, defined by:

$$\varphi_{io}(\tau) \equiv \lim_{T\to\infty} \frac{1}{2T} \int_{-T}^{T} p_i(t)\, p_o(t+\tau)\, dt$$ 13.40

In practice, computation of $\mathbf{H}(j\omega)$ is not as simple as Equation 13.38 would suggest. The signal $p_o(t)$ contains noise from the heart's beating, and other low-frequency noises from digestion and breathing, etc. It also contains electronic noise from amplifiers. Both $v_o(t)$ and $v_i(t)$ must be bandpass filtered to minimize the effect of these noises, and the high cutoff frequency of these filters must be chosen for anti-aliasing. The filtered $v_o(t)$ and $v_i(t)$ are digitized with a finite number of samples (e.g., 4096), and the windowing and computation of the auto- and cross-power spectra and the estimate of $\mathbf{H}(j\omega)$ are done by computer using Fast Fourier transform techniques. A number of estimates, $\hat{\mathbf{H}}(j\omega)$, of $\mathbf{H}(j\omega)$ are made and then averaged to reduce the noise in the computed frequency response function.

In the sections below, we describe the perthoracic noise method of estimating $\mathbf{H}(j\omega)$ developed by Rader (1998), and the technique of Pohlmann et al. (1999) in which broadband noise sound was introduced into the oral airway.

13.4.2 TRANSTHORACIC PROPAGATION OF BROADBAND ACOUSTIC NOISE TO EVALUATE PULMONARY HEALTH

Figure 13.7 illustrates schematically the system used by Rader (1998) to investigate how sound introduced at the back propagates through the chest walls and the lungs. Because her work was the development of a prototype instrument, she used normal healthy adult volunteers in her study. The sound input subsystem consisted of a 5" acoustic suspension loudspeaker mounted in a flexible foam "box," open at the end

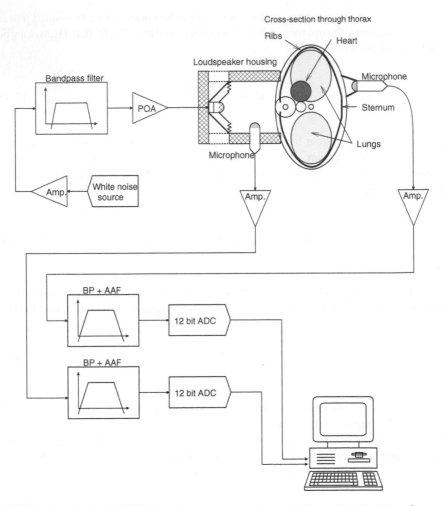

FIGURE 13.7 Rader's (1998) system to measure the acoustic transfer function of sound through the chest using broadband noise and cross-power spectral techniques.

that made contact with the subject's back. The box was pressed firmly against the subject's back to prevent acoustic leakage into the air. A B&K Model 4117 microphone was mounted through a hole in the foam box to monitor the input sound pressure in the air. Another matched B&K 4117 microphone was mounted in a 4-in.-diameter soft rubber cup to pick up sound transmitted through the wall of the front of the chest. The cup served to space the microphone about 1.5 in. from the skin surface and to shield the microphone from other sounds in the air.

A Quan-Tech Model 420 broadband analog Gaussian noise generator (flat from 0 to 100 kHz) was used as a primary noise source. Its output was amplified and bandpass-filtered (half-power frequencies of 16 Hz and 1 kHz) to define the input power density spectrum. A total of 4.5 watts noise power was delivered to the 5-in.

loudspeaker. Both piezo-microphone outputs were conditioned by charge amplifiers to preserve low-frequency signal components, then passed through band-pass filters to exclude heart sounds and their first few harmonics, and sharply attenuate any frequencies above 1000 Hz (for anti-aliasing filtering). Analog-to-digital conversion using 12 bit conversion of the filtered p_i and p_o microphone signals took place at 5,000 samples/second. The A/D conversion was under the control of the system computer. In each data epoch, 4096 samples were taken of the p_i and p_o signals; yielding a spectral resolution of 0.8192 Hz in FFT calculations. Rader investigated the suitability of using four different windowing functions on her sampled random data; rectangular (no window function), Bartlett (triangular), Blackman and Hanning. In some cases, to reduce noise, Rader averaged several like spectra taken by consecutive sampling.

Rader found that the Blackman windowing function gave the best performance in terms of minimizing the noise on the input autopower spectrum and the cross power spectrums. Figures 13.8 and 13.9 illustrate representative input-, output-, and cross-power spectrums and coherence for one of Rader's subjects. Note that data acquisition of one epoch (4096 samples) at 5 kSa/s takes 0.8192 sec, and five epochs (to average) takes a total of 4.1 seconds. Computation of $\mathbf{H}(j2\pi f)$ using Equation13.38 above takes a few more sec. once data is acquired. Rader presented only the magnitude of $\Phi_{io}(j2\pi f)$ in her dissertation. By inspecting the estimate of $\mathbf{H}(j2\pi f)$ as a polar plot, or as real and imaginary parts vs. f, it is expected that more insight into lung condition might be had.

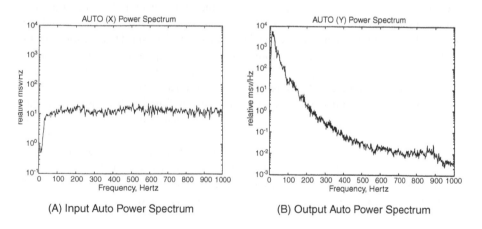

(A) Input Auto Power Spectrum   (B) Output Auto Power Spectrum

FIGURE 13.8 (A) Representative power spectra from Rader's study. Input autopower spectrum. (B) Output autopower spectrum. Note attenuation of high frequencies.

The technique developed by Rader has the advantage of being totally safe, noninvasive and rapidly repeatable. Once it has been clinically validated with patients with respiratory problems, it should be able to assess the amount of pulmonary edema in a patient and track its progress, minimizing the need for more costly CAT scans and X-rays.

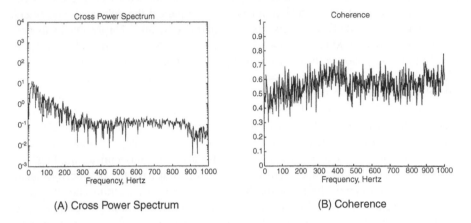

(A) Cross Power Spectrum   (B) Coherence

FIGURE 13.9(A) The calculated cross-power spectrum magnitude. There are three distinct regions. (B) System coherence.

13.4.3 THE USE OF WHITE NOISE SOUND INTRODUCED INTO THE ORAL AIRWAY TO ASSESS LUNG CONDITION

Pohlmann et al. (1999) reported on an investigation of acoustic transmission through the respiratory system. In many ways, their study was similar to that of Rader (1998) except that the sound was introduced through the oral airway. Pohlmann et al. used a noise-input spectrum with half-power frequencies of 50 and 700 Hz. Sound was recorded with microphones from the left and right, T3 and T6 positions on the posterior chest. A sampling epoch consisted of 2048 samples at a 7.5 kHz sampling frequency. Auto- and cross-power spectra were computed using standard FFT techniques; 12 consecutive epochs were averaged to reduce noise.

Pohlmann et al. found that the acoustic transfer function was both frequency and lung inflation dependent. At the lower frequencies, there was about 20 dB attenuation in $H(j2\pi f)$; attenuation increased steadily with increasing frequency. It also increased with increasing lung inflation. Lung inflation expands the parenchyma by inflating the alveoli, thus decreasing the average density of the parenchyma. Pohlmann et al. comment that the use of vibration sensors (accelerometers) directly on the skin may improve their system's signal-to-noise ratio.

13.4.5 DISCUSSION

The lungs present a complex acoustical impedance to a driving source at the mouth. They also affect the acoustic transfer function between the back and front of the chest. The extent to which obstructive lung disease changes this impedance or transfer function has been the topic of research for a number of years. At present, no clinical application of low-frequency acoustical testing of the respiratory system's acoustical impedance or transfer function has been forthcoming. Extensive clinical trials will be needed to establish a database for this simple noninvasive testing modality. If the trials are done, will this method be sensitive enough to detect various forms of obstructive lung disease before they become debilitating? Perhaps diagnosis will be more certain using conventional spirometric techniques (Chapter 10). Note that spirometric tests require the cooperation of the patient; so does lung acoustic impedance measurement. Acoustic transfer function measurement does not.

13.5 SUMMARY

In this chapter, we have seen how the transmission of audio-frequency acoustic energy (either as sinusoidal or random pressure waves) through the chest and lungs can be used as an inexpensive NI diagnostic tool to detect OLD and fluid in the lungs and pleural space. Such systems are, at present, experimental; as yet they have no clinical application.

Measurement of the acoustic impedance (or admittance) of the ear canal plus tympanic membrane, however, is a widely used, clinical test in audiology. The absence of a normal tympanic reflex to sudden loud sounds is used as a measure of deafness in infants.

14 NI Tests Using Ultrasound (Excluding Imaging)

14.1 INTRODUCTION

The use of ultrasound (sound with frequencies ranging roughly from 30 kHz to more than 30 MHz) in medical diagnosis is best associated with its ability to image internal structures of the body. However, ultrasound, by virtue of its short wavelengths in the body, is also well suited to nonimaging "A-mode" applications where the phase and frequency of the reflected sound is used to measure the distance to and velocity of the reflector or reflecting objects.

In discussing sound waves, recall that the sound wavelength is given by the simple relation $\lambda = v/f$, where v is the sound velocity in the medium and f is its frequency. Also, in dealing with sinusoidal functions, the sine argument is phase in radians, and frequency in general is the time-derivative of phase. That is, if the sound pressure at a point is given by $P_o \sin(2\pi f\, t + \varphi)$, then the phase argument is $(2\pi f\, t + \varphi)$ radians and the frequency is $2\pi f$ r/s.

In this chapter, we first examine the Doppler effect when the source and receiver transducers are collinear and stationary with respect to the moving reflector(s), then consider closed-loop ultrasonic ranging systems that operate under constant phase conditions with a moving reflector. One such experimental system devised by the author used air-coupled ultrasound to measure the ocular pulse (the minute, ± 10 μm expansion of the cornea in response to blood flowing into the eyeball). The no-touch ocular pulse measurement (NOTOPM) system used a voltage-to-frequency oscillator (VCO) to adjust the transmitted frequency so that the phase difference of the transmitted and received waves remains constant. It is shown in Section 14.4.2 that the sensitivity of the NOTOPM system $(v_o/\Delta x)$ is proportional to $1/x_o^2$. The author showed that this nonlinear sensitivity is avoided if a voltage-to-period converter (VPC) oscillator is used instead of a VFC. Use of the VPC permits simultaneous measurement of x and dx/dt in applications such as the NOTOPM system.

Section 14.6 describes an experimental system that may have application in the noninvasive measurement of blood glucose concentration in a tissue such as an earlobe. This system is based on the closed-loop constant-phase principle used in the NOTOPM system, except that the ultrasound is transmitted rather than reflected. Small changes in the velocity of sound caused by changes in tissue density, which, in turn, can be due to changes in glucose concentration in the tissue, will alter the phase lag of the received signal. Other factors, such as the interstitial fluid water concentration, can act as a confounder in this system. The system was tested *in vitro*

301

successfully, but there is a big jump from a test chamber to a living tissue. Further research needs to done.

14.2 THE DOPPLER EFFECT

The Doppler effect can be observed with both electromagnetic and sound waves. We are all familiar with the Doppler effect on sound. A car moving toward us blows its horn. As it passes, there is a perceptible downward shift in the pitch of the horn. In 1842, Johann Christian Doppler delivered a paper entitled, "On the Colored Light of Double Stars and Some Other Heavenly Bodies" before the Royal Bohemian Society of Learning. Doppler was professor of elementary mathematics and practical geometry at the Prague State Technical Academy. He apparently got little recognition for his work, and died of consumption in 1854 at the age of 49. In 1844, a contemporary of Doppler, Buys Ballot, contested Doppler's theory as an explanation for the color shift of binary stars rotating about an axis perpendicular to a line from the observer to the stars. Ballot actually did an experiment using sound waves where a trumpet player sounded a constant note while riding on a flatcar of a train moving at constant velocity. A musician with perfect pitch, standing at trackside, perceived the trumpet note to be a half-tone sharp as the train approached, and a half-tone flat as it receded. In spite of this direct evidence of velocity-related frequency shift, Ballot continued to object to Doppler's theory. Ballot's erroneous publications apparently served to discredit Doppler for a number of years. So much for peer review.

To derive the Doppler effect for sound waves, we will assume a moving reflecting target and a stationary source/observer, as shown in Figure 14.1. Assume that sinusoidal sound waves leaving the stationary transmitter (TRX) propagate at velocity, c, over a distance, d, to the target, T. The target is moving at velocity, $\mathbf{v}$, at an angle θ with the source. Velocity $\mathbf{v}$ can thus be resolved into a component parallel to the line connecting TRX and the reflecting target, T, and a component perpendicular to the TRX-T line. These components are $|\mathbf{v}|\cos(\theta)$ and $|\mathbf{v}|\sin(\theta)$, respectively. The reflected wave from T propagates back to the stationary receiving transducer, RCX, along path d. The receiving sensor output waveform can be written as:

$$V_r = B \sin[\omega_r t + \psi] \qquad\qquad 14.1$$

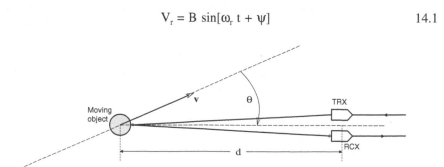

FIGURE 14.1 Basic Doppler geometry for moving reflector with stationary collinear transmitter and receiver.

The received radian frequency is ω_r, the transmitted radian frequency is ω_o, and ψ represents the phase lag between the transmitted signal and the received signal. In general, the phase lag, ψ, is given by:

$$\psi = 2\pi\,(2d/\lambda) = 2\pi\,[2d/(c/f_o)] = \omega_o\,(2d/c) \text{ radians} \qquad 14.2$$

However, the distance 2d is changing because of the target velocity component along the line from the transducers to the target. Thus the frequency of the received signal, ω_r, is the time derivative of its phase:

$$\omega_r = d\big[\omega_o t + \omega_o(2d/c)\big]\big/dt = \omega_o\big[1 + \big(2\,\dot{d}/c\big)\big] = \omega_o\big[1 + (2/c)|v|\cos(\theta)\big] \quad r/s \qquad 14.3$$

The Doppler shift frequency, ω_D, is defined by Equation 14.4. It contains the velocity information:

$$\omega_D = (\omega_o\,2/c)\,|\,\mathbf{v}\,|\cos(\theta) \text{ r/s} \qquad 14.4$$

Note that $\omega_r > \omega_o$, because, in this example, the target is approaching the source/sensor. The sign of ω_D will be negative for a target moving away from the transducers.

As you will see in Section 14.3, the Doppler effect using ultrasound has many important noninvasive diagnostic applications. The Doppler effect is used to measure blood velocity in veins, arteries and capillaries. When the diameter of the vessel's lumen is known, true blood flow can be estimated from Doppler measurements. Doppler ultrasound can also detect fetal heartbeats and those of unconscious persons. When the ensonifying beam is perpendicular to the blood vessel and $\mathbf{v}$, the radial motion of an aneurism, can be sensed by the Doppler technique. Doppler ultrasound can also measure heart valve motion.

14.3 DOPPLER ULTRASOUND FOR BLOOD AND TISSUE VELOCITY MEASUREMENTS

14.3.1 ANGLE-DEPENDENT CW BLOOD VELOCITY MAGNITUDE MEASUREMENT

Doppler velocity measurements of blood suffer from two major problems: one is the angle dependence seen in the equations derived in Section 14.2. The other is noisiness. Practical limitations on noninvasive Doppler measurement geometry restrict $25° \le \theta \le 45°$ with reference to the axis of the blood vessel. Often the angle is not known precisely because of natural anatomical variation, and hand wobble can cause low-frequency noise if the probe is hand-held.

The noise associated with Doppler measurements of blood velocity comes from two sources. First, assuming laminar flow, the blood velocity in larger arteries and veins follows an approximately parabolic velocity profile as a function of radial distance from the center of the vessel; the peak velocity is in the center of the vessel, it is zero at the edges. Because the input ultrasound beam has finite width, it simultaneously interacts with a wide range of velocities in the vessel. The ultrasound reflects off red blood cells (RBCs) being carried along in the blood. The RBCs are biconcave discs in shape; they are about 7.5 µm in diameter, about 1.9 µm thick at their edges, and are about 1 µm thick at their centers. Typical RBC density is about 5.2×10^6 ($\pm$ 3×10^5) cells per cubic mm of plasma for men. Normally, from 40 to 45% of the blood volume is RBCs; this percentage is called the *hematocrit* (Guyton, 1991).

The RBCs spin and turn as they flow along in the larger vessels, providing nonstationary targets with varying cross-sections for the input ultrasound waves. Thus, instead of a sharp single Doppler return frequency, we see a noisy bell-shaped spectrum of return frequencies, S(f), with its peak at the frequency of the Doppler shift of the maximum RBC velocity in the center of the blood vessel. Any calculation of volume flow necessarily must use the peak velocity, the lumen diameter, and the fact that the velocity profile is approximately parabolic.

A simple CW Doppler ultrasound system, such as a Parks Model 811-BTS, typically has an analog (audio) voltage output whose amplitude is proportional to the power in the reflected beam, and whose frequency is proportional to the Doppler frequency shift magnitude, ω_D. Figure 14.2 illustrates the organization of a basic CW Doppler ultrasound blood velocity system. A sinusoidal oscillator coupled to a power amplifier drives the transmitting piezoelectric transducer (TRX) at its mechanical resonant frequency. At resonance, the transducer's power output is maximum, and it appears as a nearly real impedance load in the order of hundeds of ohms to the power amplifier (POA). The transmitting transducer may have a concave plastic ultrasound "lens" that acts to concentrate the transmitted beam at the expected distance where blood vessels are found below the skin. The TRX is placed against the skin with a thin layer of acoustic impedance-matching ultrasound gel between it and the skin. The receiving transducer (RCX) also has the same resonant frequency as TRX, and is often placed in the same probe housing as TRX. TRX and RCX must be acoustically isolated, so that RCX responds only to the reflected Doppler-shifted ultrasound. The Doppler-shifted signal from RCX is amplified, and then mixed or detected by effectively multiplying it by the transmitted signal. One easy way to do this is not to isolate TRX and RCX perfectly, so that the output of RCX contains the sum of the transmitted signal and the Doppler-shifted return signal. Thus:

$$V_r(t) = A \sin(\omega_o t) + B \sin\{\omega_o [1 + (2/c) |\mathbf{v}| \cos(\theta)]t + \psi\} \qquad 14.5$$

Now V_r is conditioned by a square-law transfer nonlinearity, such as a JFET mixer. Squaring V_r we get:

$$V_r^2(t) = \left[A^2 \sin^2(\omega_o t) + 2AB \sin(\omega_o t)\sin\{\omega_o [1 + (2/c)|\mathbf{v}|\cos(\theta)]t + \psi\} \right.$$
$$\left. + B^2 \sin^2\{\omega_o [1 + (2/c)|\mathbf{v}|\cos(\theta)]t + \psi\} \right] \qquad 14.6$$

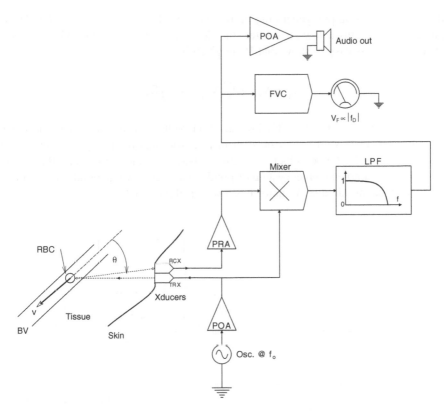

FIGURE 14.2 Block diagram of a typical CW Doppler blood velocity measurement system. *Key*: RBC = reflecting moving red blood cell; FVC = frequency-to-voltage converter; LPF = low-pass filter; PRA = RF preamplifier; POA = power amplifier; Osc. = sinusoidal RF oscillator at frequency f_o.

Now, by trig identity, the two $\sin^2(*)$ terms give dc + double frequency cosine terms. The middle term above, by the $\sin X\ \sin Y = \frac{1}{2}\ [\cos(X - Y) - \cos(X + Y)]$ trig identity, yields the following cosine terms: $\cos[-\omega_o\ (2/c)\,|\mathbf{v}|\cos(\theta)\ t - \psi]$, and $\cos\{2\omega_o\ [1 + (1/c)\,|\mathbf{v}|\cos(\theta)]t + \psi\}$. By passing $V_r^2(t)$ through an audio-frequency bandpass filter, the frequency of the Doppler shift is actually heard as an audio tone, $V_a(t) = kAB\ \cos[\omega_o\ (2/c)\,|\mathbf{v}|\cos(\theta)\ t]$. (We do not hear minus signs, constant phase shifts or dc terms, and terms of frequency ω_o and $2\omega_o$ are not audible.) Thus, the amplitude and frequency of the audio output of the simple CW Doppler ultrasound blood velocity meter is actually a superposition of all the ensonified, low-amplitude, velocity components from the population of RBCs moving at various velocities in the blood vessel under study.

To obtain a dc voltage output proportional to the blood velocity magnitude suitable for a strip-chart recorder, the output of the audio bandpass filter, $V_a(t)$, is further amplified and put through a comparator configured as a zero-crossing detector. The TTL logic output of the comparator is HI when $V_a(t) > 0$, and is LOW when $V_a(t) < 0$. A one-shot multivibrator is set to trigger on the LO $\rightarrow$ HI transitions at the comparator's output, generating narrow positive TTL pulses of width δT. These pulses are put into a low-pass filter, the dc output of which approximates their average, V_F. It is easy to show that V_F is given by:

$$V_F = V_{LO} + \overline{f_D}\left(V_{HI} - V_{LO}\right)\delta T \qquad 14.7$$

Where V_{LO} and V_{HI} are the TTL low and high voltage levels, and $\overline{f_D}$ is the mean Doppler frequency shift ($\overline{f_D} = \omega_D/2\pi$) in Hz. Note that the low-pass filter output will be positive for blood velocity toward or away from the transducers; the analog output of this simple Doppler system responds to the velocity magnitude. This simple frequency magnitude discriminator is shown in Figure 14.3.

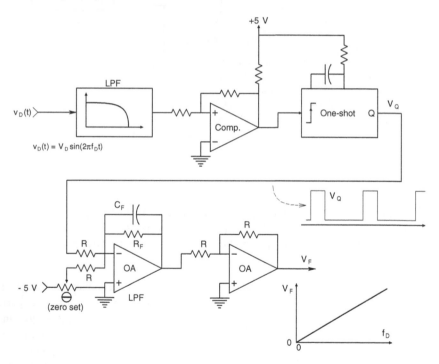

FIGURE 14.3 A VFC that converts an audio-frequency Doppler signal to a voltage proportional to f_o by duty-cycle averaging.

Webster (1992) gives an expression for the average zero crossing rate, r_z, of the comparator. It is not a simple function of the Doppler frequency shift, f_D, but, instead, is given by the relation:

$$r_z = \left[\frac{\int\left(f_r - f_o\right)^2 S(f)\,df}{\int S(f)\,df}\right]^{\frac{1}{2}}$$

Where: $(f_r - f_o) = f_D$, the Doppler frequency shift, S(f) is the power density spectrum of $V_r(t)$, in ms volts/Hz, the denominator is P_r, the total ms volts in the return signal, and the numerator can be considered to be the second moment of the Doppler frequency. Note that S(f) is, in fact, non-stationary because of the pulsatile nature of blood flow. S(f) might be better described by a S(f, t), i.e., by joint time-frequency analysis, as described in Section 3.2.3.

The simple non-directional CW Doppler ultrasound system described above provides more qualitative than quantitative information for NI diagnosis. It can provide left/right comparisons of carotid sinus blood velocity and turbulence. A noticeable L/R difference may indicate a unilateral carotid occlusion from cerebrovascular disease.

More sophisticated Doppler systems exist that: 1) Provide an analog output with the sign of the blood velocity (i.e., they are directional), and 2) are angle independent. These systems are described in the following sections.

14.3.2 A Directional CW Doppler System

The organization of a CW directional Doppler system is shown in block diagram form in Figure 14.4. This system generates a time-varying output voltage whose magnitude is proportional to f_D, and whose sign is + or −, depending whether blood velocity is toward or away from the probe, respectively. To see how this system functions, we will examine its signals and their functions. Assume the oscillator puts out a voltage, $A \cos(\omega_o t)$. The output of the quadrature phase shifter is $A \sin(\omega_o t)$. The received Doppler-shifted return signal is:

$$V_r(t) = B \sin\{\omega_o[1 + (2/c)v \cos(\theta)] t + \Psi\}. \qquad 14.9$$

$V_r(t)$ is added to $A \cos(\omega_o t)$ and $A \sin(\omega_o t)$ to form the analog sums X and Y, respectively. X and Y are squared by high-frequency analog multipliers. Their respective outputs are:

$$W = K_m\{ A^2 \cos^2(\omega_o t) + 2AB \cos(\omega_o t) \sin\{\omega_o[1 + (2/c)v \cos(\theta)] t + \Psi\}$$

$$+ B^2 \sin^2\{\omega_o[1 + (2/c)v \cos(\theta)] t + \Psi\}\} \qquad 14.10$$

$$Z = K_m \{A^2 \sin^2(\omega_o t) + 2AB \sin(\omega_o t) \sin\{\omega_o[1 + (2/c)v \cos(\theta)] t + \Psi\}$$

$$+ B^2 \sin^2\{\omega_o[1 + (2/c)v \cos(\theta)] t + \Psi\}\} \qquad 14.11$$

W and Z are put through audio bandpass filters. The $\sin^2(*)$ and $\cos^2(*)$ terms by trig identity become dc $\pm \cos(2\omega_o t)$ terms, neither of which appear at the audio BPF outputs. The W middle term can be written by trig identity as:

$$2AB \cos(\omega_o t) \sin\{\omega_o(1 + (2/c)v \cos(\theta)) t + \Psi\} \qquad 14.12$$

$$= AB\{ \sin(2\omega_o t + \omega_o (2/c)v \cos(\theta) t + \Psi) + \sin(\omega_o (2/c)v \cos(\theta) t + \Psi)\}$$

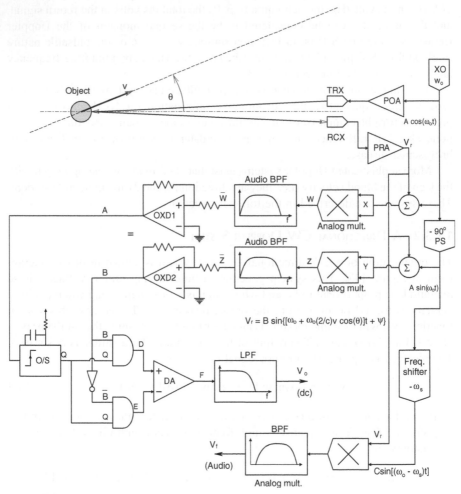

FIGURE 14.4 Block diagram of a CW directional Doppler system. Quadrature detection allows V_o to have the sign of **v**. The audio output has a center frequency and is shifted up or down in frequency depending on whether the object is approaching or receding, respectively.

The $2\omega_o t$ term is filtered out, and the analog signal at the output of the W BPF is:

$$\overline{W} = K_f K_m 2AB\sin\left[\omega_o(2/c)v\cos(\theta)t + \psi\right] \qquad 14.13$$

The audible Doppler frequency is $\omega_D = \omega_o\,(2/c)v\cos(\theta)$ r/s. Similarly, the analog signal at the output of the Z BPF is:

$$\overline{Z} = K_f K_m 2AB\cos\left[\omega_o(2/c)v\cos(\theta)t + \psi\right] \qquad 14.14$$

$\overline{W}$ and $\overline{Z}$ are next put through analog comparators configured as zero-crossing detectors, (0XDs) with some hysterisis to give them noise immunity (the hysterisis is the result of the positive feedback around the comparator). Refer to the two timing diagrams, Figures 14.5 and 14.6 to see how the Doppler signal is demodulated to give an analog V_o whose magnitude is proportional to ω_D, and whose sign follows **v**. When the reflecting objects are moving toward the probe, the gating (Q) pulse from the one-shot is ANDed with the B output from the cosine OXD, producing a pulse of the same width at the D AND gate output. E remains low, so a pulse appears at F at the output of the differential amplifier with amplitude $K_{DA}(V_{HI} - V_{LO})$. The F pulses are periodic at f_D, so the average output voltage, V_o, is:

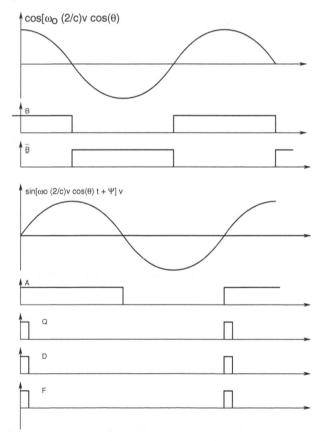

FIGURE 14.5 Waveforms in the detector of the directional Doppler system of Figure 14.4 when the object is approaching the transducers.

$$V_o = f_D \, K_{DA}(V_{HI} - V_{LO}) \qquad 14.15$$

When the objects are moving away from the probe, the sign of the sin(*) term is inverted, and the gating pulse produced by the one-shot ANDS with the HI B input

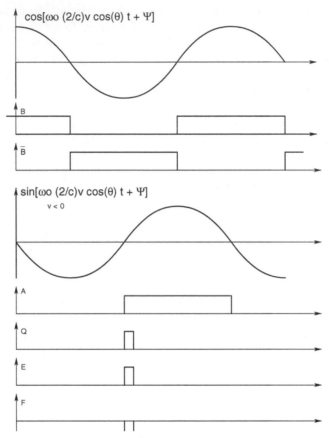

FIGURE 14.6 Waveforms in the detector of the directional Doppler system of Figure 14.4 when the object is receding from the transducers.

to the lower AND gate, producing a pulse at E while D remains low. Now, the peak pulse amplitude at F is $-K_{DA}(V_{HI} - V_{LO})$, and the average output of the low-pass filter is negative:

$$V_o = -\overline{f_D} K_{DA}\left(V_{HI} - V_{LO}\right) \qquad 14.16$$

The phase shift, Ψ, is common to both sine and cosine channels, $\overline{W}$ and $\overline{Z}$, respectively, so its effect cancels out.

It is also possible to obtain an audio frequency output from the directional Doppler system that is also responsive to the sign of the object velocity. In this simple system, the return signal, $V_r(t)$, is mixed with a synthesized constant frequency signal, V_2, that is $\omega_s = 2\pi 10^3$ r/s below the transmitted signal frequency, ω_o. That is, $V_r(t)$ is mixed with $V_2 = C \sin((\omega_o - \omega_s)t)$. Thus:

$$V_r V_2 = K_m BC \sin\{\omega_o[1 + (2/c)v \cos(\theta)] t + \Psi\} \sin((\omega_o - \omega_s)t) \qquad 14.17$$

The mixer output is passed through an audio band-pass filter which blocks all dc and high-frequency terms. Thus the $\sin(\alpha) \sin(\beta)$ term produces an audio-frequency output given by the $\cos(\alpha - \beta)$ term in the trig identity.

$$V_f = K_F K_m (BC/2)\cos\{[\omega_s + \omega_o(2/c)v \cos(\theta)] t + \Psi\} \qquad 14.18$$

If the object is stationary, V_f has frequency f_s; if the object is approaching the probe, V_f's frequency rises by f_D: if the object is receding, the frequency of V_f is lowered by f_D, just like the trumpet sound on the moving train.

14.3.3 Angle-Independent, CW Doppler Velocimetry

A serious problem in obtaining quantitative Doppler velocity measurements is the often imprecise knowledge of the probe angle, θ. Obviously, v is proportional to $f_D/\cos(\theta)$, and an error in θ will give an error in v. In 1985, Fox derived a closed-form solution to the two-dimensional Doppler situation that utilizes the outputs of two independent transmit–receive probes. The probes transmit at two separate frequencies, f_1 and f_2. They are aligned so that their focused beams cross in the volume whose velocity is being measured.

Fox's solution yields the velocity magnitude, $|v| = \sqrt{v_x^2 + v_y^2}$, and the angle θ_1 between the velocity vector v and a line from number 1 probe (see Figure 14.7). Note that the probes lie in the XY plane with the velocity vector. The probes are separated by an angle ψ, and their beams converge on the moving reflecting object. The Doppler frequency shift returned to each probe is given by:

$$f_{D1} = f_{o1} (2/c)|v| \cos(\theta_1) \qquad 14.19A$$

$$f_{D2} = f_{o2} (2/c)|v| \cos(\theta_2) = f_{o2} (2/c)|v| \cos(\theta_1 - \psi) \qquad 14.19B$$

Now, we can solve Equation 14.19 for θ_1:

$$|v| = \frac{f_{D1}c}{f_{o1} 2\cos(\theta_1)} = \frac{f_{D2}c}{f_{o2} 2\cos(\theta_1 - \psi)} \qquad 14.20$$

After some algebra and the trig. identity for $\cos(x - y)$, we find:

$$\frac{f_{D1}}{f_{o1}} = \frac{f_{D2}}{f_{o2}[\cos(\psi) + \tan(\theta_1)\sin(\psi)]} \qquad 14.21$$

Fox defines R as:

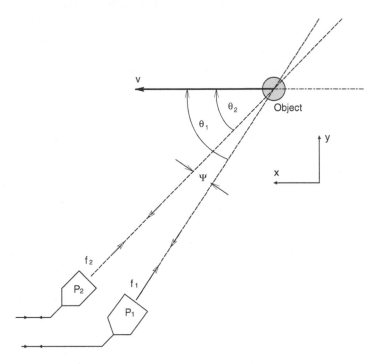

FIGURE 14.7 Geometry relevant to Fox's angle-independent CW Doppler. All vectors are in the plane of the paper.

$$R \equiv \frac{f_{D2}f_{o1}}{f_{D1}f_{o2}} = \frac{1}{\left[\cos(\psi) + \tan(\theta_1)\sin(\psi)\right]}$$ 14.22

From which we find the unknown incidence angle:

$$\theta_1 = \tan^{-1}\left[\frac{R - \cos(\psi)}{\sin(\psi)}\right]$$ 14.23

The arctangent relation for θ_1 suggests a right triangle with angle θ_1; the adjacent side is length $\sin(\psi)$, the opposite side is $(R - \cos(\psi))$, and the hypotenuse is $\sqrt{\sin^2(\psi) + [R - \cos(\psi)]^2} = \sqrt{1 + R^2 - 2R\cos(\psi)}$. Returning to Equation 14.19A, and using the trig definition for $\cos(\theta_1)$, we find:

$$|\mathbf{v}| = \frac{f_{D1}c}{f_{o1}2\cos(\theta_1)} = \frac{f_{D1}c\sqrt{1 + R^2 - 2R\cos(\psi)}}{\sin(\psi)}$$ 14.24

To calculate $|\mathbf{v}|$ and θ_1, one must measure f_{D1} and f_{D2}, knowing f_1, f_2 and ψ. The accuracy of the method is limited by the accuracy with which one f_{D1} and f_{D2} can be determined. Because of the parabolic (laminar) flow profile in blood vessels, the finite size of the ensonified volume (typically 3 mm^3 for a 2.25 MHz carrier, (Fox, 1978)), and the random scattering nature of moving red blood cells, there typically is a bell-shaped distribution of f_Ds, rather than a single sharp peak. The mode of the distribution is generally taken as the desired f_D. The Fox two-probe method of determining the velocity vector in two dimensions is best implemented with a computer system that algorithmically processes the Fourier-transformed Doppler return signals to determine their modes to estimate f_{D1} and f_{D2}, and then calculates $|\mathbf{v}|$ and θ_1 using the relations above and the known parameters Ψ, f_1, and f_2.

Fox and Gardiner (1988) extended the two-dimensional closed-form solution for $|\mathbf{v}|$ to three dimensions. Their equations are too long to include here, but they have the same general form as the simpler two-dimensional case described above. Their results showed that the calculated $|\mathbf{v}|$ remained within 5.6% of the theoretical value for Doppler angles up to 50°. Also, their angle estimate agreed with the theoretical values with a correlation coefficient, r = 0.99937. The two- and three-dimensional Doppler flow velocimetry technique developed by Fox and colleagues is, of course, not restricted to the ultrasonic measurement of blood velocity. Their technique can be extended to the other Doppler modalities (lasers and microwaves), when a two- or three-dimensional estimate of object velocity is required.

14.3.4 PULSED DOPPLER SYSTEMS

A pulsed Doppler ultrasound system emits periodic sinusoidal pulses of ultrasonic energy. The pulses are characterized by their *repetition rate*, f_r, (or period, T_r), their *oscillation frequency,* f_o, and their *pulse envelope*, e(t), which effectively defines the pulse duration and amplitude. A significant advantage of pulsed Doppler ultrasound is that it allows relatively small sample volumes (voxels) to be ensonified, giving the ability to describe blood and tissue velocity in detail around structures such as heart valves, aneurisms, atherosclerotic occlusions in major vessels, kidney vessels, and umbilical cord vessels, etc. The output displays on modern pulsed Doppler systems can generally show velocity vs. time plots for a targeted voxel, or be shown as a 2-D image slice of tissues (B-mode display) showing structures as well as velocities in color.

When measuring blood velocity by pulsed Doppler, the return echoes scattered from the moving RBCs are greatly attenuated compared with the echoes from solid tissues of different densities such as bone, muscle and blood vessel walls. The reflections from blood can be 40 dB less than that from other tissues (Routh, 1996). In measuring blood velocity in deep vessels, the pulsed Doppler system (PDS) must wait for the Doppler-shifted echo to return before transmitting the next pulse. If the pulse has a round-trip distance of 2L meters to a fixed reflector, then it will take T_t = 2L/c = 2 × 0.1/1540 = 1.2987 × 10^{-4} section to travel 10 cm. Thus for no pulse overlap, the maximum rate pulses can be transmitted is f_r = 1/T_t = 7.7 kHz at this distance. Shorter distances permit faster pulse repetition rates (PRRs). In summary:

$$\text{PRR}_{max} = f_r = c/\, 2L \text{ pps} \qquad\qquad 14.25$$

A major engineering trade-off exists in a PDS between the ability to define a voxel in the target, and to simultaneously measure the target velocity. This trade-off is very like the Heisenberg uncertainty principle in quantum physics. The shorter pulse required to define a smaller voxel has a larger transmitted bandwidth and poorer velocity resolution. Another way of stating the trade-off between range and target velocity given by Signal Processing, S.A. (1999), is:

$$L_{max}\, v_{max} = c^2/[8f_r \cos(\theta)] \text{ m}^2/\text{sec} \qquad\qquad 14.26$$

To examine the PDS in the frequency domain, we first consider one pulse alone. In its simplest form, the pulse, $f(t)$, is equal to the time-domain product of a cosine wave at the resonant frequency of the transducer, $\omega_o = 2\pi f_o$ radians/sec, and an envelope or gating function, $g(t)$. That is, $f(t) = g(t) \cos(\omega_o t)$. The simplest envelope function is an (even) rectangular pulse: $g(t) = P_r(T_r/2)$. $P_r(T_r/2) = 1$ for $|t| < T_r/2$, and 0 for $|t| \geq T_r/2$. However, the acoustic output of a transducer initially at rest, given a narrow dc excitation pulse, rises gradually to a peak amplitude and then dies off to zero. Two simple envelope function models can be used to describe the output tone burst. One is the Gaussian model; $g_g(t) = \exp[-\frac{1}{2}(t/\tau)^2]$, $-\infty \leq t \leq \infty$. Another is the cosine on a pedestal function; $g_c(t) = \frac{1}{2}[1 + \cos(\omega_c t)] P_r(\pi/\omega_c)$. This function is zero for $|t| > \pi/\omega_c$ and has unit value for $t = 0$. Note that $\omega_c = 2\pi/T_c$, so $t = \pi/\omega_c$ $= T_c/2$. Thus, the $g_c(t)$ function makes a tone burst T_c seconds in duration. Typically, $T_c = 8T_o$, where T_o is the period of the transducer's natural frequency (i.e., $T_o = 2\pi/\omega_o$). The Gaussian envelope function, while not finite in length, is mathematically more expedient to use as a model.

Let us examine a single PDS pulse in the frequency domain. We will use the Fourier transform pairs:

$$\cos(\omega_o t) \longleftrightarrow \pi[\delta(\omega - \omega_o) + \delta(\omega + \omega_o)] \qquad\qquad 14.27A$$

$$\exp\left[-\tfrac{1}{2}(t/\tau)^2\right] \longleftrightarrow \tau\sqrt{2\pi}\, \exp\left[-\tfrac{1}{2}(\tau\,\omega)^2\right] \qquad\qquad 14.27B$$

The Gaussian-gated pulse in the time domain is represented by the product:

$$g_o(t) = g_g(t) \cos(\omega_o t) \qquad\qquad 14.28$$

Its Fourier transform is given by *complex convolution*:

$$G_0(\omega) = \frac{1}{2\pi} \int_{-\infty}^{\infty} G_g(\omega - u)\, \pi\left[\delta(u - \omega_0) + \delta(u + \omega_0)\right] du$$

$\downarrow$ 14.29

$$G_0(\omega) = \frac{\pi\tau}{\sqrt{2\pi}}\left\{\exp\left[-\tfrac{1}{2}\tau^2(\omega - \omega_0)^2\right] + \exp\left[-\tfrac{1}{2}\tau^2(\omega - \omega_0)^2\right]\right\}$$

Thus, the Fourier spectrum of a single gated pulse has peaks at $\omega = \pm\,\omega_0$, and at $\omega = 0$, has the value of:

$$G_0(0) = \tau\sqrt{2\pi}\,\exp\left[-\tfrac{1}{2}\tau^2\omega_0^2\right]$$ 14.30

Note that the parameter τ is chosen so that a few f_0 cycles are included in the pulse envelope before its amplitude becomes negligible.

Next, we consider an infinite train of pulses, each pulse of the form of Equation 14.28. These pulses have a repetition rate governed by $f_r = c/2L$, where c is ca. 1540 m/sec, and L is the distance in the tissues (in meters) from the source transducer to the target vessel. In general, $f_r \ll f_0$. Let us represent the infinite pulse train in the time domain by

$$g*(t) = \sum_{n=-\infty}^{\infty} g_0\left(t - nT_r\right)$$ 14.31

Because g*(t) is periodic and meets certain other criteria, it can be represented by a complex Fourier series:

$$g*(t) = \sum_{n=-\infty}^{\infty} C_n\, \exp\left[+jn\omega_r t\right]$$ 14.32

The complex Fourier coefficient, C_n, is given by (Papoulis, 1977):

$$C_n = \int_{-T_r/2}^{T_r/2} g*(t)\exp\left[-jn\omega_r t\right] dt = \left(1/T_r\right)G_0\left(n\omega_r\right)$$ 14.33

Thus g*(t) can be written:

$$g*(t) = \left(1/T_r\right)\sum_{n=-\infty}^{\infty} G_0\left(n\omega_r\right)\exp\left[+jn\omega_r t\right]$$ 14.34

Which Fourier transforms to:

$$G*(\omega) = (2\pi/T_r) \sum_{n=-\infty}^{\infty} G_o(n\omega_r)\delta(\omega - n\omega_r)$$

$$= (2\pi/T_r) \sum_{n=-\infty}^{\infty} \frac{\pi\tau}{\sqrt{2\pi}} \left\{ \exp\left[-\tfrac{1}{2}\tau^2 (n\omega_r - \omega_o)^2 \right] \right. \qquad 14.35$$

$$\left. + \exp\left[-\tfrac{1}{2}\tau^2 (n\omega_r + \omega_o)^2 \right] \right\} \delta(\omega - n\omega_r)$$

Thus, the spectrum of the pulse train, $g*(t)$, is a *line spectrum* with lines spaced $\Delta\omega$ = $n2\pi/T_r$ radians/sec apart. The exponential terms have maximum amplitude (1) for $|n| = \omega_o/\omega_r$ (nearest integer).

The Doppler return spectrum from a moving object is also a line spectrum. The return signal frequencies, f_s, for an approaching reflecting object is at frequencies:

$$f_s(n) = nf_r [1 + (2v/c)\cos(\theta)]\ Hz \qquad 14.36$$

Thus, the actual Doppler shift is given by:

$$f_d = (nf_r 2v/c)\cos(\theta)\ Hz \qquad 14.37$$

Note that f_d is not a function of f_o. The Doppler-shifted return signal's line spectrum is thus:

$$G_{ret}(\omega) = \beta(2\pi/T_r) \sum_{n=-\infty}^{\infty} \frac{\pi\tau}{\sqrt{2\pi}} \left\{ \exp\left[-\tfrac{1}{2}\tau^2 (n\omega_r\{1 + (2v/c)\cos(\theta)\} - \omega_o)^2 \right] \right.$$

$$\left. + \exp\left[-\tfrac{1}{2}\tau^2 (n\omega_r\{1 + (2v/c)\cos(\theta)\} + \omega_o)^2 \right] \right\} \qquad 14.38$$

$$\delta\left[\omega - n\omega_r\{1 + (2v/c)\cos(\theta)\} \right]$$

Note that β is the attenuation of the Doppler signal. The entire return line spectrum is thus seen to be distributed approximately symmetrically around ω_o, the transducer's natural frequency.

To gain a heuristic appreciation of how a PDS works in the time domain, refer to Figure 14.8, where $\cos(\theta) = 1$. Pulses are emitted at a fixed rate, f_r, which is set at $\leq c/2L$ to prevent aliasing. L is the mean distance to the moving reflecting target. The returning pulses are amplified and filtered. Each returning pulse is sampled at the same time relative to its emission time; i.e., the sampling rate is f_r. If the target is stationary, each sampled return pulse is sampled at the same time and the sampler output is constant (zero Doppler frequency). In the figure, the target is moving toward the transducer at velocity **v**. Thus, each successive return pulse is advanced in phase, creating a periodic sampled signal, v_s (t). In practice, v_s is noisy and must be averaged over many pulse periods, and then high-pass filtered by a "wall" filter to remove excessive low-frequency "clutter" noise. The averaged filtered v_s can be Fourier transformed to form a root power density spectrum, $\sqrt{P_{Vs}(\omega)}$ rms Volts/$\sqrt{Hz}$. The frequency of v_s is the Doppler shift frequency, which carries the velocity magnitude information. By also sampling the return pulse at a time shift of $1/4f_o$ from the main channel, the quadrature signal obtained can be used to give directional information, i.e., is the target receding or approaching? The electronic analog and digital systems that do this in a PDS are complex. The interested reader can consult the June, 1986 *Hewlett-Packard Journal* for an excellent system-level description of a modern PDS.

Modern PDSs can display their data in a time-frequency format in which the Doppler frequency (proportional to velocity) is coded by amplitude. PDSs are also used in an imaging or "B" mode; more will be said of this in Chapter 16 on imaging. The signal-to-noise ratio in PDSs depends in part on the transmitted ultrasonic power.

A fundamental limit to transmitted power is tissue heating; ultrasonic energy absorbed by tissues causes heating due to viscous (lossy) vibration. Only a small portion of the incident ultrasound energy is reflected back at interfaces between structures having different acoustic impedances in tissues. If not dissipated, the heating can cause pain, and excessive heating can denature proteins and destroy cell structures, "cooking" the ensonified tissues. Extreme ultrasound energy density levels can also cause *cavitation* (the formation of gas bubbles), which can rupture cells and otherwise physically destroy tissues. Naturally, ultrasound dosage is rigorously controlled by the FDA and other regulatory agencies, and the dosage from an approved diagnostic PDS does no harm in the applications for which it is designed.

14.3.5 DISCUSSION

In this section, we have described how the Doppler effect used with CW and pulsed ultrasound can measure blood velocity, as well as the velocity of moving tissues in the body such as aneurisms, fetal heartbeat, etc. Simple instruments that provide output signals proportional to average blood velocity are not blood flowmeters. To obtain flow, we must multiply blood vessel lumen area by the average blood velocity. Lumen area can be found by ultrasound imaging or another imaging modality.

The simple CW ultrasound velocimeter is valuable in screening for obstructive artery disease. When an atherosclerotic plaque forms, partially occluding a blood vessel, Bernoulli's principle dictates that the blood velocity through the restricted area will increase, often causing turbulence. This increase in velocity and the resulting turbulence are easy to spot with a simple Doppler ultrasound system. If the lesion is unilateral, a left-right comparison of velocity at the same anatomical location makes diagnosis easier. The gold standard for verification of arterial obstruction is X-ray angiography.

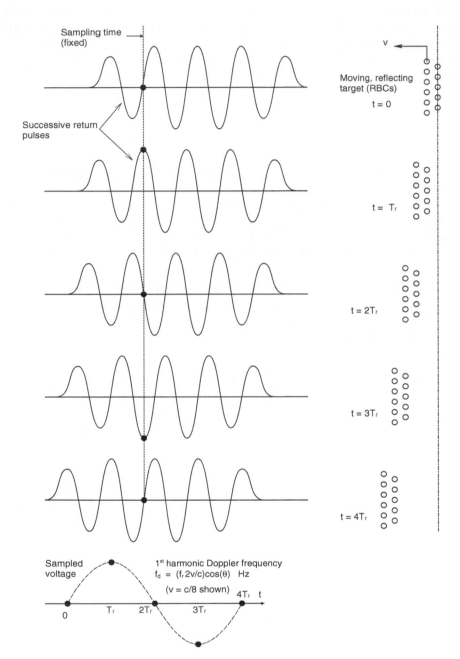

FIGURE 14.8 Description of how pulsed Doppler velocimetry works. The reflecting objects are approaching the transducer. The Doppler frequency voltage is found by sampling the return pulse at a fixed time relative to the transmission time. The samples are held and used to reconstruct the f_D waveform. T_r is the interval between transmitted pulses.

14.4 THE NO-TOUCH OCULAR PULSE MEASUREMENT (NOTOPM) SYSTEM

14.4.1 INTRODUCTION

The ocular pulse (OP) is the minute periodic radial displacement of the corneal surface caused by arterial pressure pulsations in the intraocular circulation acting on the compliance of the cornea. Features of the OP waveform have been shown by several workers to be diagnostic indicators of: 1) Cerebrovascular disease (particularly arteriosclerosis in one or both carotid arteries); 2) Abnormally high intraocular pressure (IOP), aka glaucoma; 3) Autonomic changes in the cerebral circulatory system in response to changes in blood CO_2 and O_2 levels (Northrop and Decker, 1978).

The arterial blood supply for the human eye comes from the *ophthalmic artery* (OA), which branches off the *internal carotid artery* (ICA) below the optic nerve. In addition to the eyes, the opthalmic artery serves to supply other tissues with blood; notably the extraocular muscles, the sinuses, nasal tissues, etc. Here, we will consider only the ophthalmic artery's role in supplying the internal tissues of the eyeball. The central retinal artery (CRA) branches from the OA and enters the optic nerve and runs inside it. The CRA enters the rear of the eyeball along with the optic nerve fibers. Inside the rear of the eye, the CRA makes numerous fine branches; it also supplies the arterial circle of Zinn surrounding the optic disc ("blind spot") of the retina. Two *posterior ciliary arteries* (PCAs) also branch off the OA and divide into some 10 to 20 branches that run forward surrounding the optic nerve and pierce the choroid coat of the rear of the eyeball on the medial and lateral sides of the optic nerve. The branches from the *short ciliary artery* enter the sclera on the medial (nasal) side of the optic nerve, while the *long ciliary artery's branches* enter the lateral side of the eyeball and run forward between the sclera and the choroid to supply the ciliary body. They also anastomose with branches from the *anterior ciliary arteries* (ACAs) to form the *circulus arteriosis iridus major* that supplies the iris. The ACAs arise as branches off the muscle branches of the OA. Although the arterial anatomy of the eyeball is complex, the reader should appreciate that it is all derived from the internal carotid artery (Kronfeld, 1943). Hence, any factor reducing pressure in the ICA will reduce arterial blood flow into the eyeball.

If we take the mean arterial blood pressure (MAP) in the brachial artery to be 100 mmHg, then it can be estimated by *ophthalmodynamometry* that the MAP in the CRA and the PCAs is about 65 to 70 mmHg (Adler, 1933). The static intraocular pressure (IOP) of a normal eyeball is about 16 mmHg (Guyton, 1991). This pressure is due to the constant rate of production of aqueous humor (AH) by the cells of the ciliary process, and the resistance to the outflow of the AH through the trabecular network, the canal of Schlemm and the episcleral veins (Northrop, 2000). If the outflow resistance rises, the IOP will rise; a condition known as *glaucoma*. Elevated IOP presses on the arteries within the eyeball that supply the intraocular tissues, restricting the inflow of arterial blood. Prolonged restriction of arterial inflow leads to tissue anoxia, which can permanently damage sensitive retinal neurons, leading to visual defects and even blindness.

Under normal IOP, the pulsation of internal arteries creates a periodic pressure variation that is added to the IOP. This pressure variation causes the elastic cornea to stretch and contract radially in a Hookean manner. It is this displacement of the cornea that can be measured noninvasively as the ocular pulse. Because the OP depends on the internal arterial pressure transients, the OP is, in effect, a plethysmograph for the ocular circulation. Any factor that alters the pressure as a function of time in the CRA and the ciliary arteries will alter the OP. Such factors can include obstructions in the ICA (or OA), elevated IOP, or changes in the hydraulic loading of the ICA beyond where the OA branches off. These latter changes involve arterial perfusion of the brain, which is under tight autonomic control by the CNS. Of course, cardiac output will also affect the OP; the heart stroke volume and rate being under autonomic nervous control.

Hørven and Nornes (1971), Hørven (1973), and Hørven and Gjønnaess (1974) were among the first researchers to measure the OP and relate it to known circulatory problems and other medical conditions. Hørven and colleagues used an electronic Schiøtz indentation tonometer with a 5.5-gram loading weight. The patient lay supine, with the tonometer applied vertically to the cornea. The tonometer output was 1 mV per μm of corneal displacement. Thus, the static IOP could be measured along with the OP waveform. Sterile technique was observed and the surface of the cornea was anesthetized. The OP waveforms recorded by Hørven and Nornes on strip charts were all very smooth; they contained no high-frequency transients or oscillations. They were not quite sinusoidal in form, apparently containing few harmonics beyond the fundamental frequency (heart rate). Hørven and Nornes examined the OP from six classes of patients — normal patients, and patients having glaucoma, choroidal melanoma, carotid obstruction, giant cell arteritis or carotid carvernous sinus fistula. They recorded IOP, pulse rate, peak-to-peak OP amplitude, and the relative crest time (the time to an OP peak from the previous OP minimum divided by the period of that OP cycle). (Note that the RCT is concerned with the OP wave shape. Another significant OP parameter is the *peak phase delay* (PPD), measured as the time from the ECG R peak to the next OP peak, divided by the period of that cardiac cycle, times 360°. The PPD was not measured by Hørven, et al.)

In normal subjects, Hørven and Nornes found an average IOP of 16.6 mm Hg, and an average peak-to-peak OP amplitude of 30.75 μm ($\sigma = 10.35\mu m$); the relative crest time (RCT) was 41.5% ($\sigma = 2.34\%$). A notable diagnostic parameter was a significant increase in the RCT. Only in the case of melanoma was there no significant change in the RCT. The mean RCT increased significantly to 43.6%, 45.4% and 48.6% for glaucoma, carotid obstruction (degree not noted), and giant cell arteritis, respectively. RCT significantly decreased to 34.8% for carotid cavernous sinus fistula. Of particular note was that the mean amplitude of the OP increased to 34.4 μm in eyes with glaucoma having a mean IOP of 37.7 mm Hg. One might have thought that doubling the normal IOP would reduce the OP amplitude and increase the RCT more than it did. (The slight rise in OP amplitude in glaucoma may have its origin in the nonlinear elastic properties of the arteries in the eyeball; a phenomenon similar to that which gives rise to Korotkoff sounds when measuring brachial blood pressure by sphygmomanometer.)

Another simple contact system for OP measurement was developed by LaCourse and Sekel (1986). A soft EVM rubber cup, used to remove contact lenses, made contact with the cornea. The cup was attached to a piezoelectric bender transducer with a short post. An initial cup displacement of 30 μm produced 260 mV across the crystal and required 2g force. LaCourse and Sekel examined the OP on New Zealand white rabbits under conditions of normal carotid flow and under condition of ipsilateral carotid flow occlusion by an inflatable hydraulic cuff around the artery. Not surprisingly, a marked attenuation of the OP and change in its wave shape were observed when carotid occlusion was applied.

Note that a piezoelectric transducer is a bandpass system. That is, it is characterized by a transfer function (relating output voltage to applied displacement) having a *zero at the origin,* a *low-frequency pole* whose value depends on the transducer's electrical loading, and one or more *high-frequency poles* (Northrop, 1997). Only by connecting a piezoelectric transducer to a *charge amplifier* can one accurately specify the low-frequency pole value. LaCourse and Sekel connected their transducer to an isolation amplifier, thus, the low-frequency pole of their system depended on this amplifier's input resistance as well as the capacitive load presented to the transducer by amplifier's input capacitance, and the wires connecting the transducer to the amplifier. It is not clear from their paper what the value of their measurement system's low-frequency pole was, with or without the isolation amplifier. However, there was no evidence of low-frequency OP waveform differentiation in their figures, so the low-frequency pole was probably lower than 1 Hz. It should be noted that Hørven's electronic Schiøtz tonometer output was dc coupled, hence the OP waveforms he showed in his papers were probably characterized by the frequency response of his strip-chart recorder, typically flat from dc to 50 Hz. No low-frequency waveform differentiation was possible in his data.

To eliminate the need for physical contact with the cornea to measure the OP and the consequent need for sterile technique and corneal anesthetization, this author and Shrikant Nilakhe developed an ultrasonic no-touch means of measuring the corneal displacement. The design and performance of their no-touch ocular pulse measurement (NOTOPM) system is described in the next section.

14.4.2 A Closed-Loop Constant Phase No-Touch Means of Measurement of Ocular Pulse

The NOTOPM system of Northrop and Nilakhe (1977) used continuous-wave air-coupled ultrasound reflected off the corneal surface to noninvasively measure the OP. The no-touch method obviates the need for sterile technique and corneal anesthesia. This system is shown schematically in Figure 14.9. A pair of $^1/_4$-in.-diameter LTZ-2 air-backed transducers were used as independent CW ultrasound transmitter and receiver. The transducers were used at frequencies well below their 3 MHz resonant frequency, typically in the range of 850 to 900 kHz. The system behaved as a constant-phase type 1 servo loop (not a phase-locked loop). Heuristically, the system measures the total airpath distance (transmitter to cornea, cornea to receiver) by adjusting the transmitted frequency so that the same number of ultrasound wavelengths remain in the airpath, regardless of its length. If the cornea expands,

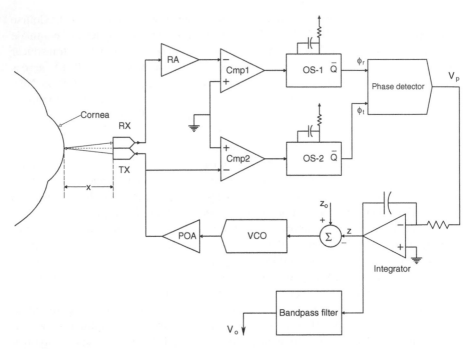

FIGURE 14.9 Block diagram of the no-touch ocular pulse measurement system of Northrop and Nilakhe (1977). *Key*: RA = receiver RF amplifier; POA = power amplifier; VCO = voltage-controlled oscillator; OS-1 = oneshot multivibrator; Cmp1 = amplitude comparator; TX = transmitting transducer; RX = receiving transducer.

the airpath distance is shortened, and the VCO frequency rises; if the cornea contracts, the VCO frequency is lowered to maintain the same number of cycles (phase) in the airpath. Changes in the VCO input voltage are shown to be proportional to the airpath's Δx.

To understand quantitatively how the NOTOPM system works, we first consider it to be in the open-loop steady state (SS), with no motion of the cornea. The transducers are each a distance x_o from the cornea, so that the airpath length is $2x_o$. If the VCO output frequency is f_o, then it is easy to see that the total SS phase lag between the received ultrasound and the transmitted ultrasound is:

$$\phi_m = 2\pi \, (2x_o/c)f_o \text{ radians} \qquad\qquad 14.38$$

Where c is the velocity of sound in air, nominally 344.0 m/s at 20°C and 40% relative humidity. There can be many wavelengths of ultrasound in the SS airpath at any instant, so the SS ϕ_m can be $\gg$ 360°. For example, if the transducer distance is $x_o = 1.5 \times 10^{-2}$ m, and the VCO center frequency is 850,000 Hz, there will be $2x_o$ f/c = 74.128 cycles or wavelengths of ultrasound in the total airpath.

Changes in airpath length are detected by a digital phase detector. Typical digital phase detectors have a limited range of operation. For example, the simple R-S flip-flop phase detector (PD) used in the NOTOPM system gives zero output for a 180° phase difference between its input pulses, and has a linear range of 0 to 360°. If the input phase difference exceeds 360°, its output characteristic is again linear for 360° < ϕ_e < 720°, etc. That is, it has a sawtooth periodic output characteristic, as shown in Figure 14.10. Note that the R-S flip-flop PD has output zeros for input phase differences equal to:

$$\phi_e = 2\pi(k + {}^1/_2) \text{ radians,} \qquad 14.39$$

where k is the nearest integer value of $(2x_0 f/c)$. When the system is initially turned on, the transmitted frequency is $\omega_o = K_v V_r$ r/s. A dc voltage V_r is initially applied to the VCO until the return signal is sensed and pulses ϕ_r are available at the phase detector input. At this time, a PD output voltage, V_p, is presented to the system integrator's input. The integrator's output, V_i, is subtracted from the reference voltage, V_r, changing the input to the VCO from V_r so that its output frequency changes to $\omega = (\omega_o + \Delta\omega) = K_v (V_r - V_i)$. In the steady state, the servo loop forces the integrator *input*, V_p, to be zero. This means that $\phi_e = \phi_m = 2\pi(k + {}^1/_2) = 2\pi(2x_o f/c)$ = $(2x_o/c) K_v (V_r - V_i)$ radians.

Assume SS closed-loop operation: the instantaneous output frequency of the VCO is $\omega_T(t)$. At the cornea, this instantaneous frequency is $\omega_T (t - \tau)$, where the delay τ is just x_o/c section. If the cornea is moving with velocity $\dot{x}$, the reflected ultrasound is given a *Doppler frequency* shift, so that at the cornea, the instantaneous reflected frequency is given by:

$$\omega_{rc} = \omega_T(t - \tau)\left[1 + 2\dot{x}(t - \tau)/c\right] \quad \text{r/s} \qquad 14.40$$

At the receiving transducer, we have:

$$\omega_r = \omega_T(t - 2\tau)\left[1 + 2\dot{x}(t - \tau)/c\right] \quad \text{r/s} \qquad 14.41$$

And the total phase lag between the VCO output and the received signal is:

$$\phi_r = 2\pi\int\omega_r dt = 2\pi\int\omega_T(t - 2\tau)\left[1 + 2\dot{x}(t - \tau)/c\right] dt \quad \text{radians} \qquad 14.42$$

An expression for the total phase error, ϕ_e, must include the periodic finite range characteristics of the phase detector used. Thus, we can write:

$$\phi_e = -2\pi\int\omega_T(t - 2\tau)\left[1 + 2\dot{x}(t - \tau)/c\right] dt - 2\pi(k + \tfrac{1}{2})$$
$$+ 2\pi\int\omega_T(t) dt \quad \text{degrees} \qquad 14.43$$

Equation 14.43 can be rearranged to yield:

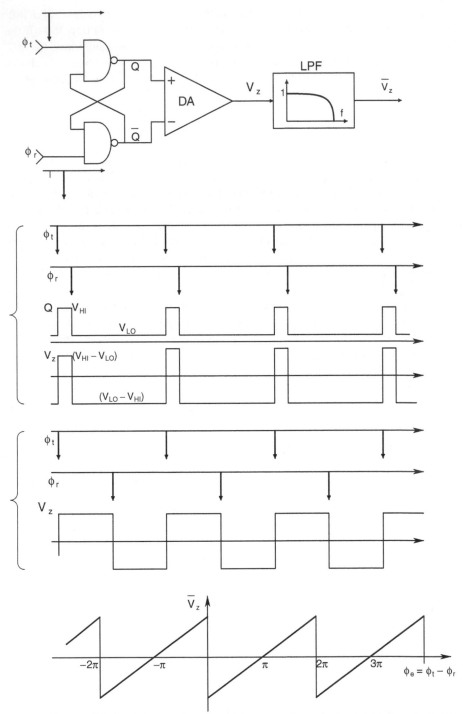

FIGURE 14.10 RS flip-flop phase detector, relevant waveforms, and output voltage vs. input phase difference characteristic.

$$\phi_e = -2\pi \int \left[\omega_T(t - 2\tau) - \omega_T(t) \right] dt - 2\pi(k + \tfrac{1}{2})$$
$$+ 2\pi(2/c) \int \omega_T(t - 2\tau) \dot{x}(t - \tau) dt$$

14.44

In normal closed-loop small-signal operation, k remains constant, because the peak displacement of the OP is $<< x_o$. The phase detector output, V_p, is integrated to form V_i. Thus

$$V_i = -K_i \int (-K_p)\phi_e \, dt$$

14.45

From Equation 14.45 we obtain:

$$\phi_e = \dot{V}_i / \left(K_p K_i \right) \quad \text{radians}$$

14.46

Also, the VCO output instantaneous frequency is given by:

$$\omega_T(t) = K_v (V_r - V_i) \quad \text{r/s}$$

14.47

Substituting Equations 14.46 and 14.47 into 14.44 we obtain:

$$\dot{V}_i = -K \int \left[V_i(t) - V_i(1 - 2\tau) \right] dt - 2\pi K/K_v (k + \tfrac{1}{2}) + K(2/c)V_r x(t - \tau)$$
$$- K(2/c) \int V_i(t - 2\tau) x(t - \tau) \, dt$$

14.48

In which $K \equiv K_p K_i K_v$. Under SS conditions, by definition, $\dot{x} = \dot{V}_i = 0$, $x = x_o$, and $\overline{V}_i = V_i$. Hence Equation 14.48 can be written as

$$0 = -K \overline{V}_i \left(2 x_o / c \right) - \left(K 2\pi / K_v \right)(k + \tfrac{1}{2}) + K(2/c)V_r x_o$$

14.49

From which we find that

$$\overline{V}_i = V_r - \frac{2\pi(k + \tfrac{1}{2})c}{2 x_o K_v}$$

14.50

Thus, we have shown that, in the SS, the average value of the integrator output, V_i, is a nonlinear function of the average distance to the cornea, x_o. The corneal Δx from the OP, however, represents a small fraction of x_o, roughly ± 15 μm out of $x_o = 15,000$ μm. Thus, the ΔV_i from the OP can be represented by:

$$\Delta V_i = \frac{\partial V_i}{\partial x} \Delta x = \frac{2\pi(k + \tfrac{1}{2})c}{2 x_o^2 K_v} \Delta x$$

14.51

Thus, in this system, the dc small-signal sensitivity is proportional to x_o^{-2}. This is a drawback to calibration, because x_o must be precisely known. Northrop and Nilakhe (1977) showed that loop dynamics also impose a high-frequency real pole at $\omega_x = 2\pi f_x$ on the $\Delta V_i/\Delta x$ transfer function. That is:

$$\frac{\Delta V_i}{\Delta x}(j\omega) = \frac{\dfrac{2\pi(k + \frac{1}{2})c}{2\,x_o^2 K_v}}{j\omega/(\omega_b) + 1} \qquad 14.52$$

They also showed that $\omega_b = K_p\,K_i\,K_v\,2x_o/c$ r/s, and the SS value of k is given by the integer value

$$k = INT\,[2x_o K_v V_r/(2\pi c)] \qquad 14.53$$

The steady-state lock frequency is

$$\omega_{TL} = \frac{2\pi(k + \frac{1}{2})c}{2\,x_o}\ r/s \qquad 14.54$$

Let us evaluate numerically some of the NOTOPM system's key parameters: Take c = 344 m/sec, x_o = 15 mm = 1.5×10^{-2} m, K_p = 3.1831 V/radian, K_i = sec^{-1}, K_v = 1.06814×10^6 r/sec/V, k = 74. From Equation 12, the small-signal sensitivity is $S_{Vi}(\Delta x) = 2\pi\,(k + \frac{1}{2})\,c/(2\,x_o^2\,K_v)$ V/m = 3.35×10^2 V/m, or 0.335 mV/μm. The closed-loop system's break frequency is at $f_b = \omega_b/2\pi = K_p\,K_i\,K_v\,2x_o/2\pi c$ Hz. Numerically, f_b = 47.2 Hz for the parameters given. The SS lock frequency is f_{TL} = c (k + $\frac{1}{2}$)/(x_o 2) = 850.827 kHz.

Northrop and Nilakhe (1977) investigated the effectiveness of their ultrasonic NOTOPM system on rabbits and normal human subjects. Adult New Zealand white rabbits were immobilized by IM injection of a mixture of Acepromazine maleate 1.5 mg/kg and Ketamine HCl 15 mg/kg. The animals were immobile in about 6 minutes, and stayed that way for about 45 minutes, unless more drug was given. Recovery was complete in about 2 hours after the last injection. Immobilized rabbits were laid on their sides and their heads were sandbagged. The downward eye was taped shut to prevent drying (the blinking reflex was inhibited by the drugs).

The upper eye was held open with tape on the eyelids, and artificial tears were used to prevent corneal drying. The ultrasound transducers were positioned at x_o = 15 mm from the cornea, and ECG electrodes were attached to shaved spots on the forelimbs.

Examples of rabbit OP waveforms are shown in Figures 14.11 and 14.12. The peak outward corneal deflection occurs at approximately a 175° phase lag following the ECG R spike. Corneal expansion generally proceeds without inflection, i.e., the OP's first derivative does not go to zero once expansion starts until the peak is reached; similarly, the contraction phase has no inflection until minimum corneal radius is reached. Peak-to-peak OP was about 13 μm. The effects of (external,

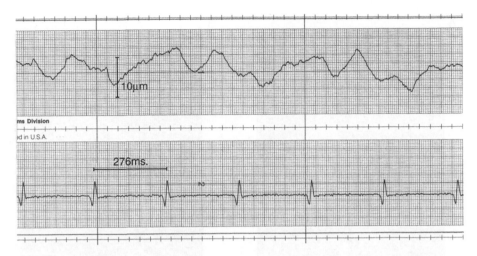

FIGURE 14.11 Strip chart recording of ocular pulse recorded from an anesthetized New Zealand white rabbit along with its ECG QRS complex. Note the noise on the OP waveform.

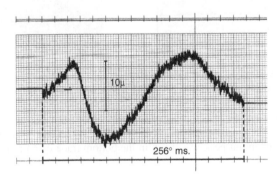

FIGURE 14.12 Rabbit OP averaged over 128 cardiac cycles.

bilateral) carotid compression on rabbit OP were shown to be a reduction in its amplitude. In addition, CNS autonomic changes in cerebral circulation induced by breathing different gas mixtures (pure O_2, air, and air + 5% CO_2) produced OP amplitude changes. In some cases, there was as much as a 50% reduction in OP amplitude when breathing pure O_2. On the other hand, air with 5% CO_2 caused the OP amplitude to increase, sometimes as much as 75% above the air value. The wave-shape of the OP remained substantially invariant, however, regardless of the gas breathed. Rabbit heart rate also changed less than ± 10% with different gases (Northrop and Decker, 1978).

The protocol for measuring human OP used the same transducers and 1.5 cm x_o distance used with the rabbits. x_o was set by a calibrated pulse echo delay. No drugs were used. Monocular OP was measured; the subject rested their forehead on an optometrist's headrest. Instead of a chin rest, extra head stability was achieved

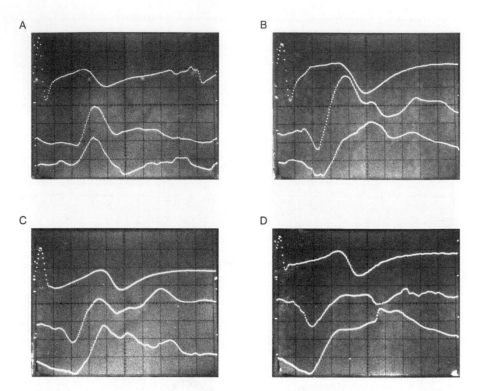

FIGURE 14 13 Averaged normal human bilateral OP wave-forms with ECG. In all wave-forms, top trace = ECG, middle trace = left eye OP, bottom trace = right eye OP. 64 averages done triggered with QRS spike. Upward deflection of OP is expanding cornea. A) Male age 31, normal vision. B) Male age 23, normal vision. C) Male age 24, farsighted. D) Male age 24, normal vision. Note that no subject's eyes had identical OP waveforms. Vertical scale in all figures: height of initial peak waveform in the bottom trace of A) is 12 μm.

by using a bite bar. In later measurements, we adapted a pair of optometrist's trial frames worn by the subject to carry transducers for the left and right eyes, permitting simultaneous binocular OP recordings.

One salient feature of all OP recordings done on human subjects was their noisiness. The sources of noise were found to be eyelash tremor, micronystagmus of the eyeball, air currents, weak return signal due to misalignment of the transducers, electronic noise from the phase tracking loop's amplifiers, etc. Some of the noise could be minimized by instructing the subjects to open their eyes wide and fixate on an LED fixation spot on the centerline of the transducers. Bandpass filtering was also used to restrict the noise to the OP bandwidth. It was generally necessary to average 32 OP waveforms synchronized by the ECG R spike to reduce the noise to an acceptable level. Figure 14.13 illustrates some of the variability in normal averaged human OP waveforms.

Northrop and Nilakhe's (1977) research on normal human OP, and Northrop and Decker's (1978) study of the effect of respiratory gases on the OP led to some surprising observations and conclusions about using the OP as a noninvasive diagnostic screening tool for the detection of cerebrovascular disease. First, human OP was found to have a more complex shape than that of rabbits; there were generally more inflections, and often two positive peaks in a cardiac cycle. There were also differences between individuals, and often left/right OP differences in the same individual. As a further complication, we discovered that, when subjects held their breath in the process of concentrating on holding their eyes wide open and fixating their gaze, their OP waveforms increased in amplitude. This increase was probably due to an increase in blood pCO_2, and a compensatory increase in flow in the internal carotid artery to the brain.

While their OP was being measured, human subjects were asked to breathe either USP oxygen, air, or air + 5% CO_2. There was a consistent and significant OP amplitude decrease with O_2 with reference to air, and a consistent and significant OP amplitude increase when breathing air with 5% CO_2. Clearly, there was an autonomic compensation for both high O_2 and high CO_2 partial pressures. The stroke/volume of the heart and the hydraulic admittance of the internal carotid artery may have been increased by the high pCO_2, and decreased by pure O_2.

14.4.3 DISCUSSION

Besides the labile nature of the human NOTOP waveform and its relative noisiness, another drawback to the NOTOPM system is that it requires patient cooperation (and some practice) in keeping the eyes open wide and fixated over the 30-second or so interval required to average 32 pulse cycles. The NOTOPM system is not suitable for use on persons who cannot or will not cooperate in this manner. These problems mean that it cannot be used as an absolute indicator of reduced carotid blood flow. It must be used under controlled conditions, generally on the same individual. The NI contact methods of OP measurement used by Hørven and Nornes (1971), and by LaCourse and Sekel (1986) are far less noisy than the NOTOPM system. They do require sterile technique and corneal anesthesia, however.

It is clear that more work needs to be done in establishing the OP diagnostic parameters for cerebrovascular diseases that are transferable among individuals. No one appears to have examined the OP in the frequency domain, either as an impulse response (to the ECG R wave) or to display the OP's Fourier series harmonics under various conditions.

14.5. THE CONSTANT-PHASE CLOSED-LOOP TYPE-1 RANGING SYSTEM (CPRS)

14.5.1 INTRODUCTION

Several years ago, this author described a means of linearizing CW constant-phase, closed-loop ultrasonic distance measuring systems such as the NOTOPM system described in Section 14.4 above. This innovation was also extended to laser and microwave distance measurement systems (Northrop, 1997; Nelson, 1999). At the heart of the CPRS is the use of a *voltage-to-period converter* (VPC) instead of a voltage-to-frequency converter (VFC). The VPC is a voltage-controlled oscillator in which the period of the output waveform is directly proportional to the input (control) voltage, that is,

$$T = 1/f = b + K_p V_c \text{ seconds} \qquad 14.55$$

(In a VFC, $f = 1/T = a + K_v V_c$ Hz.) Thus the output frequency of a VPC is given by:

$$\omega_o = 2\pi[b + K_p V_c] \quad \text{r/s} \qquad 14.56$$

For small changes in V_c, we can write:

$$\Delta\omega = \left(\frac{\partial\omega_o}{\partial V_c}\right)\Delta V_c = \frac{-2\pi}{\left(b + K_p V_{co}\right)^2}\Delta V_c \qquad 14.57$$

If the closed-loop CPRS system is made a type 2 system by the inclusion of an integrator in the feedback path, then it is easy to show that the input to the integrator is proportional to target (reflecting object) velocity, and the integrator output is linearly proportional to target range ($2x_o$). Unlike the NOTOPM system described above, there is no distance dependence in the velocity and range sensitivity expressions; they remain constant over the system's operating range. Examples of an analog and a digital VPC are shown in Figures 14.14 and 14.15. Note that the AVPC uses a standard VFC but takes the reciprocal of the input analog control voltage. As in the case of VFCs, there are practical limits to the range of the output frequency in VPCs.

We now examine how use of a VPC linearizes the distance and velocity sensitivities of the NOTOPM system.

14.5.2 Analysis of a Linear NOTOPM System Using a VPC

Figure 14.16 shows the organization of a NOTOPM system using a VPC. Its system block diagram is shown in Figure 14.17. In addition to the VPC, this system uses a compensating zero in its integrator to ensure closed-loop stability. The transfer function of this integrator is:

$$\frac{V_o}{V_p} = \frac{-K_i(\tau s + 1)}{s} \qquad 14.58$$

From Equation 14.58, we can write the ODE:

$$\dot{V}_o = -K_i\left(\tau\dot{V}_p + V_p\right) \qquad 14.59$$

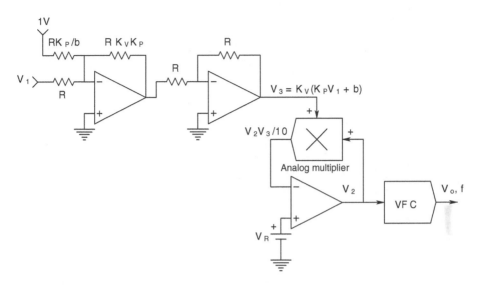

FIGURE 14.14 An analog voltage-to-period converter. A conventional voltage-to-frequency converter (VFC) is driven by a voltage V_2. It is easy to show that $V_2 = 10V_R/V_3$, $(V_3 > 0)$. V_R is made 0.1 V so $V_2 = 1/V_3$. Now, as shown in the figure, $V_3 = K_V (K_P V_1 + b)$. The VCO generates $f_o = K_V V_2$ Hz $= K_V/K_V (K_P V_1 + b)$, hence the output period is $T_o = 1/f_o = K_P V_1 + b$, which is the desired characteristic of a VPC given input V_1.

The phase error is given by the expression:

$$\phi_e = -\int \omega_T(t - 2\tau)\left[1 - 2\,\dot{x}(t - \tau)/c\right]dt - 2\pi(N + \tfrac{1}{2}) + \int \omega_T(t)\,dt \qquad 14.60$$

Rearranging terms in the integral equation above, we have:

$$\phi_e = -\int\left[\omega_T(t - 2\tau) - \omega_T(t)\right]dt - 2\pi(N + \tfrac{1}{2}) + (2/c)\int \omega_T(t - 2\tau) \qquad 14.61$$

From the VPC:

$$\omega_T(t - 2\tau) = \frac{2\pi}{b + K_p\left[V_r + V_o(t - 2\tau)\right]} \qquad 14.62$$

We now note that $V_p = -K_d\,\phi_e$ can be substituted into Equation 14.59, giving

$$\dot{V}_o = K_i\left[\tau\left(-K_d\phi_e\right) - \left(K_d\phi_e\right)\right] \qquad 14.63$$

Which is solved for ϕ_e:

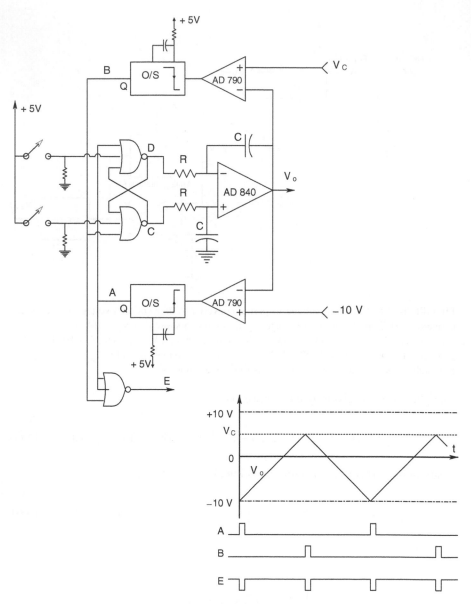

FIGURE 14.15 A digital VPC. The AD840 high-speed op amp integrates the complementary TTL output, D and C, of the RS flip-flop. Assume initially D is HI and C is LO. V_o ramps negative. When V_o reaches −10 V, the lower AD 790 comparator threshold, this comparator goes HI, producing a narrow positive TTL pulse at A that resets the flip-flop so D is LO and C HI. The integrator now ramps positive until V_o reaches V_C. Now, the upper AD 790 comparator output goes LO, triggering a narrow positive pulse at the upper one-shot's output, B. This B pulse again resets the FF so D is HI and C LO, and V_o again ramps negative. You can see intuitively that the lower the V_C, the higher will be f_o and the smaller the period. It can be shown that the pulses at E have a period given by: $T = K_P V_C + b$, as in Equation14.55.

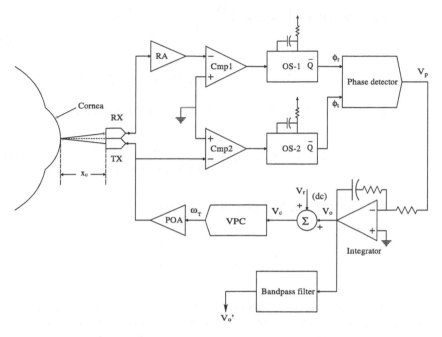

FIGURE 14.16 Block diagram of a no-touch ocular pulse measuring system using a VPC instead of a VFC.

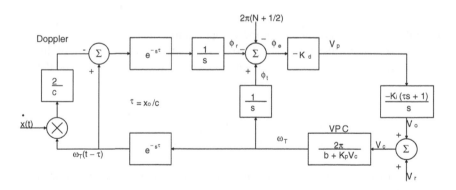

FIGURE 14.17 Systems block diagram of the NOTOP system of Figure 14.16.

$$\phi_e = -\left[\tau\,\dot{\phi}_e + \dot{V}_o\big/\left(K_i K_d\right)\right] \qquad 14.64$$

Thus, we can write:

$$-\left[\tau\dot\phi_e+\dot V_o/(K_iK_d)\right]=-2\pi K_p\int\frac{\left[V_o(t)-V_o(t-2\tau)\right]}{\left[b^2+\ldots\right]}dt-2\pi(N+\tfrac12)$$

$$+(4\pi/c)\int\frac{\dot x(t-\tau)}{b+K_p\left[V_r+V_o(t-2\tau)\right]}dt$$

14.65

In the steady state: $\dot V_o = \dot\phi_e = 0$, $V_o = \bar V_o$, $x = \bar x = x_o$. Thus, Equation 14.65 becomes:

$$0=0-2\pi(N+\tfrac12)+\frac{4\pi\,\bar x}{c\left[b+K_p\left(V_r+V_o\right)\right]}$$

14.66

Let $V_r\equiv-b/K_p$. Rearranging Equation 14.66, we find

$$V_o = x_o\left[\frac{2}{K_p c(N+\tfrac12)}\right]$$

14.67

The small-signal range sensitivity is obviously $[2/(K_p\,c(N+\tfrac12)]$ at frequencies $\ll$ the closed-loop system's ω_n. From algebraic manipulation of the equations above, it also can be shown that the system's response to *target velocity* is:

$$\frac{V_p}{\dot X}(s)=\frac{\dfrac{-2}{K_iK_p c(N+\tfrac12)}}{\tau s+1}$$

14.68

The pole at $s = -1/\tau$ is inherent in the compensation filter.

We now examine the dynamics of the closed-loop system. Figure 14.18 illustrates the negative feedback loop that determines the closed-loop system's ω_n and damping. The loop gain is:

$$A_L(s)=\frac{-(\tau s+1)}{s^2}\,\frac{K_d K_i 2\pi c^2(N+\tfrac12)^2}{4\,x_o^2}$$

14.69

The closed-loop system's transfer function's denominator is the numerator of $F(s)$ $= 1 - A_L(s)$. Thus:

$$DEN =s_+^2 s2\xi\omega_n+\omega_n^2=s^2+s\tau\frac{K_d K_i 2\pi c^2(N+\tfrac12)^2}{4\,x_o^2}+\frac{K_d K_i 2\pi c^2(N+\tfrac12)^2}{4\,x_o^2}$$

14.70

The right-hand term in Equation 14.70 is ω_n^2. The damping factor can be shown to be equal to

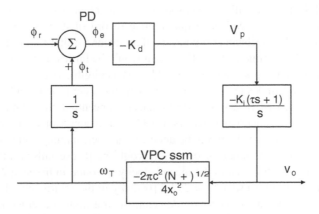

FIGURE 14.18 Linearized systems block diagram of the system of Figure 14.16. From the single-loop system we can deduce the linearized closed-loop system's poles.

$$\xi = \tau \sqrt{2\pi K_d K_i} \; \frac{c(N + \frac{1}{2})}{2 x_o}$$ 14.71

It is now useful to define and to calculate some of the system parameters. The mean distance to the moving object is taken as $x_o = 1.5 \times 10^{-2}$ m = 15 mm, the speed of sound in air is c = 344 m/s, and the closed-loop center frequency of the system is to be $f_o = 850$ kHz. Thus, in the air path under steady-state (SS) conditions, there are $(2x_o/\lambda_o) = (2x_o f_o/c) = 74.128$ cycles. Hence, we take N = 74. Take $K_i = 0.01$ and $K_d = 0.1$ V/radian. The VPC was designed so that with b = 0, $V_c = 5$ V will produce $f_o = 850$ kHz. That is, $8.5 \times 10^5 = 1/(K_p 5V)$, so $K_p = 2.353 \times 10^{-7}$ sec/volt. Hence the range sensitivity is $2/[c \, K_p \, (N + \frac{1}{2})] = 3.317 \times 10^2$ V/m or 3.317×10^{-1} mV/μm. The velocity sensitivity is $-2/[K_i \, K_p \, c(N + \frac{1}{2})] = -3.317 \times 10^4$ V/m/s. The undamped natural frequency, ω_n, of the system is 6.77×10^4 r/s, or $f_n = 1.078 \times 10^4$ Hz. In order for the damping factor to be 1 (critically damped), the compensation zero's time constant must be $\tau = 1.478 \times 10^{-5}$ seconds (15.8 μs). These parameter values are entirely reasonable for the NOTPM system.

14.5.3 OTHER APPLICATIONS OF THE CPRS SYSTEM ARCHITECTURE USING ULTRASOUND

In the sections above, we have considered the use of air-coupled ultrasound to noninvasively measure the periodic corneal displacements caused by the ocular arterial blood supply. This ocular pulse was shown to have some diagnostic value in screening for severe cerebrovascular disease. In this section, we will examine the possible use of a CPRS ultrasound system to detect aneurisms of the aorta and common carotid arteries. Because the CPRS system architecture provides simultaneous outputs proportional to both target velocity and position that are range-independent, it has the potential to provide useful data on aneurism size and type, without the risk of dye-injection angiography. Its use would be similar to conventional directional Doppler ultrasound except the CPRS method will give an exact displacement measurement of the aneurism surface as it pulsates, as well as a quantitative record of its velocity. It will allow quantification of the mechanical properties of an aneurism that might have been first seen on a static X-ray image. A CPRS system would be far less expensive than a real-time ultrasound imaging system, and would carry negligible risk.

The CPRS system design for an aneurism-sensing system can use a CW ultrasound frequency of about 1 MHz, and an acoustic lens to concentrate the sound energy at the expected depth of the aneurism (Macovski, 1983). Sufficient acoustic energy would be reflected from the interface between the aneurism and surrounding soft tissue to enable phase-lock. An alternate mode of operation would be to use pulsed ultrasound. For example, taking c = 1540 m/s as the mean velocity of sound in tissue, a 2 cm distance to the aneurism would cause a δT = 25.97 μs delay in the return echo. For this δT to represent a 45° phase lag at the phase detector, the transmitted average pulse rate, f_o, would have to be 4.81 kHz. The CPRS system keeps this 45° phase lag constant as the target distance x varies around x_o by adjusting the pulse rate with the VPC. If the aneurism is aortic, say at x_o = 10 cm, then the average pulse rep rate would be 962.5 pps for a 45° phase shift. Even at this slower f_o, the system bandwidth would be high enough to characterize an aneurism moving with a period of about 1 second.

Besides aneurisms, the pulsed ultrasonic CPRS system could be used to measure distance to, and motion of, such organs as the heart, the uterus, and the bladder. The CPRS system is not intended to replace conventional real-time tomographic systems, which can image the heart in 3-D. However, it could find application in emergency medicine to see quickly whether a patient's heart is beating, or a uterus is contracting in an unconscious patient.

14.5.4 DISCUSSION

The CPRS makes use of the voltage-to-period oscillator rather than the conventional VFC/VCO. By doing so, its simultaneous range and velocity output gains are independent of range, i.e., are properly constants, unlike the same system using a VFC/VCO. Nelson (1999) successfully designed, built and tested a pulsed laser range finder using the CPRS architecture. The CPRS system architecture can easily be adapted to CW or pulsed ultrasound, It does not appear that CPRS is suitable to measure blood velocity; it requires a coherent, relatively noise-free return signal for closed-loop constant-phase operation.

14.6 MEASUREMENT OF TISSUE GLUCOSE CONCENTRATION BY CLOSED-LOOP CONSTANT-PHASE CW ULTRASOUND (A PROTOTYPE SYSTEM)

14.6.1 INTRODUCTION

The design of an instrument to make rapid accurate *noninvasive* measurements of blood glucose in diabetic patients has been an elusive technical objective for biomedical engineers for over 20 years. One physical means proposed by the author would make use of the fact that excess dissolved glucose solute in extracellular body fluids slightly raises the density of those fluids, hence slightly reducing the speed of sound, c, in tissues containing those fluids. If it were possible to accurately and consistently measure the speed of sound or a quantity dependent on it, such as phase, one could estimate the glucose concentration, *providing no other confounding physiological factor alters tissue density,* hence c.

The system described below is a prototypical constant-phase self-nulling type 1 control loop that maintains a constant phase lag in the transmitted CW ultrasound wave path by automatically adjusting the frequency of a voltage-controlled oscillator (VCO). The system's block diagram is shown in Figure 14.19. The small changes in tissue density due to changes in blood glucose concentration produce changes in the velocity of sound in the tissue, leading to small changes in the VCO input voltage, hence its frequency. Theoretically, the system is linear in that Δf and ΔV_o are linearly proportional to ΔG, the change in glucose concentration.

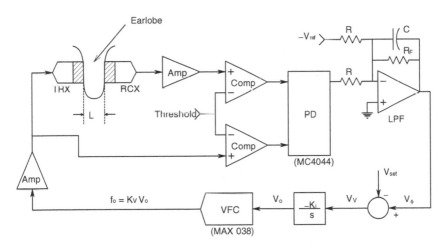

FIGURE 14.19 Block diagram of a proposed system to estimate blood glucose concentration by nulling the difference between the transmitted and received ultrasound phase through the earlobe. It is shown that the fractional change in VCO frequency required to null the system's phase detector output is proportional to the change in the glucose concentration in the earlobe.

14.6.2 An Approximate Model of How c Varies with Density, ρ

For a homogeneous liquid medium, such as sea water at 12.5° C, the speed of sound is given by: $c = \sqrt{(B/\rho)} = \sqrt{(3.31 \times 10^9 N/m^2 / 1025 kg/m^3)} = 1501.2$ m/s. B is the liquid's bulk modulus, ρ is its density. We assume that soft vascular tissue such as an ear lobe or the web between the thumb and forefinger can be treated in the same manner as sea water as far as sound velocity is concerned. (Obviously, soft tissues contain inhomogeneities including skin, fat, muscle, cartilage, blood vessels etc., that complicate the picture.) The vascular tissue is assumed to be uniformly perfused with glucose at a concentration equal to the plasma glucose concentration, [pG]. Normally, the tissue density includes the normal [pG] = 1 g/l = 1 kg/m³. A frequent condition in untreated or poorly treated diabetes is an elevated [pG], which can rise to 4 or 5 g/l above the normal level. A concentration rise above the normal glucose concentration of 1 g/l is defined as ΔG. Thus, we can write:

$$c(\Delta G) \cong \sqrt{B/\rho_o + \Delta G} = \sqrt{B/[\rho_o(1 + \Delta G/\rho_o)]} \cong c_o/(1 + \Delta G/2\rho_o)$$

$$\cong c_o(1 - \Delta G/2\rho_o)$$

14.72

Here we have assumed that $1 >> \Delta G/\rho_o$, $\sqrt{(1 + \varepsilon)} \cong (1 + \varepsilon/2)$, and $1/(1 + \varepsilon/2) \cong 1 - \varepsilon/2$.

Thus, a small increase in the density of the sound-conducting medium from elevated plasma glucose concentration results in a small decrease in the speed of sound in the medium.

14.6.3 PHASE LAG BETWEEN THE TRANSMITTED AND RECEIVED CW ULTRASOUND WAVES

It is easy to show that the received wave's phase lags the transmitted wave's phase by φ_r.

$$\varphi_r = 360° L f_o/c(\Delta G) \cong \frac{360° L f_o(1 + \Delta G/2\rho_o)}{c_o} \text{ degrees}$$

14.73

Where L = sound transmission path length in tissue in m., f_o = VCO output frequency in Hz.

14.6.4 SYSTEMS BLOCK DIAGRAM FOR THE CONSTANT-PHASE GLUCOSE SENSOR SYSTEM

Figure 14.20 illustrates the closed-loop system that adjusts the VCO output frequency so that the steady-state phase difference remains fixed, regardless of the small changes in the speed of sound in the transmission medium (vascular tissue). The sound transmission path length, L, is assumed to be constant. Because the system is a type 1 control system, there will be zero steady-state error in φ_r. Thus, in the SS, $V_V = 0$, hence $V_{set} = V_\varphi$, and we can write:

$$V_{set} = \frac{K_\varphi 360 L K_V V_o}{c_o}[1 + \Delta G/(2\rho_o)]$$

14.74

From this equation we find that:

$$V_{oss} = \frac{V_{set} c_o}{K_\varphi 360 L K_V}[1 - \Delta G/(2\rho_o)]$$

14.75

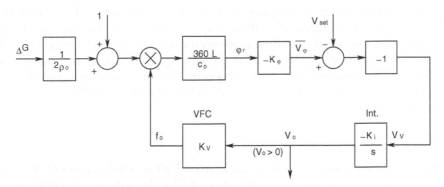

FIGURE 14.20 Block diagram of the system of Figure 14.19. Note that the system is nonlinear because of the multiplier in the loop.

Also, the VCO output frequency is:

$$f_o = \frac{c_o V_{set}}{K_\varphi 360 L}\left[1 - \Delta G/(2\rho_o)\right]$$ 14.76

The change in frequency due to an incremental increase in glucose concentration is simply:

$$\Delta f = \frac{-c_o V_{set}}{2 K_\varphi 360 L \rho_o}\Delta G$$ 14.77

Also in the SS, it is obvious that $\varphi_r = V_{set}/K_\varphi$.

The dynamics of the system can be estimated from consideration of the system's loop gain, $A_L(s)$. Input ΔG and dc quantities are $\to 0$.

$$A_L(s) = -\frac{360 L\, K_\varphi K_i K_V}{s c_o}$$ 14.78

The denominator of the linearized closed-loop transfer function is the so-called return difference, $F(s) \equiv 1 - A_L(s)$. The zeros of the return difference are the poles of the closed-loop system transfer function. In this case, the closed-loop system has one real pole.

$$F(s) = 1 + \frac{360 L\, K_\varphi K_i K_V}{s c_o} = \left[s + \frac{360 L\, K_\varphi K_i K_V}{c_o}\right]\Big/ s$$ 14.79

Thus, we see that the closed-loop system's real pole has a break frequency ω_b:

$$\omega_b = \frac{360 L\, K_\varphi K_i K_V}{c_o} \quad \text{radians/sec.}$$ 14.80

Substituting system design parameters: $K_i = 1$, $c_o = 1501$ m/sec, $K_V = 10^5$ Hz/V, $V_{set} = 6$ V, $K_\varphi = 0.2$ V/degree, L = 0.0035 m, $c_o = 1501$ m/s, we find $\omega_b = 16.79$ r/s, $f_b = 2.67$ Hz. This small bandwidth describes the speed with which the system will come to SS lock with $\varphi_r = 30°$. The low closed-loop bandwidth is beneficial in that it limits output noise arising within the system. The same parameters yield $V_{oSS} = 0.35738$ V, $f_o = 35.738$ kHz, and $\Delta f = -17.433 \Delta G$ Hz. ΔG is in g/liter or kg/m^3 of glucose.

14.6.5 Discussion

Even though tissue density changes due to $\Delta G = 1$ g/l are on the order of 0.1%, the absolute frequency changes are of the order of 17.4 Hz, and are easily detectable. If the VCO output frequency is mixed with a fixed frequency f_r, and the lower sideband extracted by a LPF, the resultant mixed frequency will be:

$$f_m = f_r - [f_o - \Delta f] = 35.838 \times 10^3 - [35.738 \times 10^3 - (-17.433 \Delta G)]$$

$$= 100 - 17.4 \Delta G \text{ Hz} \qquad\qquad 14.81$$

Thus, the percentage change of $\Delta f/f_o{}'$ can be made much larger after mixing. Note that f_r must be a very stable frequency source.

The path length L can be held constant by mechanical means. The tissue temperature is relatively constant if the patient is indoors at room temperature. One possible confounding factor that must be explored in the future development of this instrument is how much the effective tissue density changes with normal water intake (drinking) in normal and diabetic subjects.

It is anticipated that, because of anatomical differences between individuals, the ultrasonic glucose estimator will have to be calibrated for every patient by direct blood glucose measurement.

Figure 14.21 illustrates the circuit of a prototype ultrasonic, glucose sensor built by the author. It was tested on a 1 cm *in vitro* chamber containing glucose in normal saline rather than an earlobe, however. Linear regression fits of output voltage to chamber glucose concentration were not as tight as might have been expected, probably because of standing waves in the test chamber. Typical fit correlation values ranged from 0.987 to 0.993.

14.7   Summary

We have seen in this chapter that there are many important nonimaging uses for ultrasound in noninvasive medical diagnosis. The Doppler blood velocimeter is an accepted clinical instrument. In its simplest form, it has about 3-bit resolution because of noise and uncertainty of the incidence angle, θ. The uncertainty comes from estimation of the external probe angle as well as a poor knowledge of the internal path of the ensonified vessel.

I have also included descriptions of three prototype instruments using ultrasound. All three instruments use a closed-loop architecture in which the period of an

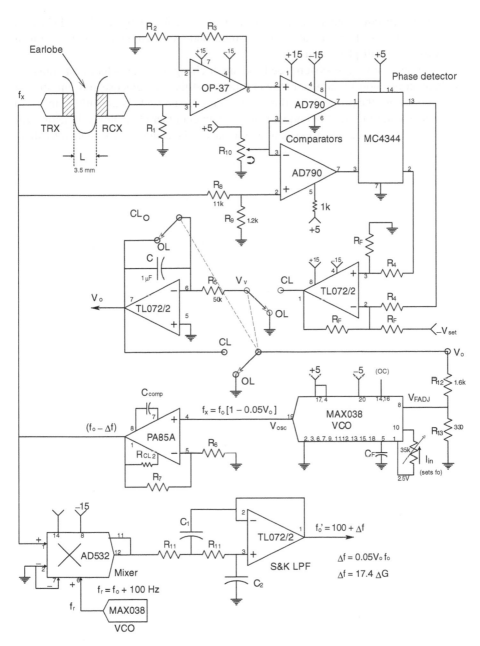

FIGURE 14.21 Schematic diagram of an ultrasonic tissue glucose sensor built by the author and tested *in vitro*. Operating frequency range was around 35.7 kHz.

oscillator is adjusted to maintain a constant phase difference between the transmitted and reflected ultrasound waves. The no-touch ocular pulse measurement (NOTOPM) system was used to experimentally study the minute pulsations of the cornea of the eye (the ocular pulse) in response to blood flow into the eye. The CPRS system used a systems improvement in which the VCO was replaced by a VPC/VFO. This replacement was shown to allow range-independent measurement of the corneal velocity and its displacement.

The third prototype system used the small changes in the velocity of sound in a chamber of known width and temperature to estimate its glucose concentration. I propose testing the principle of this system on a tissue such as an earlobe to try to estimate blood glucose. Not known is to what extent other physiological factors will change c in the tissue. Such a system would have to be calibrated for each individual.

15 Noninvasive Applications of Photon Radiation (Excluding Imaging)

15.1 INTRODUCTION

Photon radiation is also electromagnetic radiation (EMR), a wave phenomenon traditionally described by Maxwell's equations. At very low power levels and at high frequencies, the quantum photon description of EMR is used. For example, we count "single photons" at ultra-low light levels with photomultiplier tubes, not single waves, yet most optical phenomena such as reflection, refraction, interference, polarization and imaging make use of the mathematics of waves and EMR.

Wavelength bands used in nonimaging, diagnostic applications range from X-ray and gamma radiation (0.2 pm to 50 nm), ultraviolet (50 to 400 nm), visible (400 to 700 nm), and infrared (0.7 to 1000 μm). Little diagnostic use is made of radio-frequency EMR, including microwaves. The energy in a photon is given by the simple relation $E = h\nu$, where E is the energy (joules, or electron volts), h is Planck's constant ($6.624 \times 10{-}34$ joule sec.), and ν is the frequency of the EMR in Hz. Note also that $\nu\lambda = c$, where λ is the EMR wavelength (meters) and c is the speed of light in the medium in which the photons are traveling ($c = 3 \times 10^8$ m/s *in vacuo*). Often, X- and gamma "rays" are described by the energy of their photons in electron Volts (eV). (1 eV = 1.603×10^{-19} joules.) For example, an X-ray with a wavelength of 50 pm has a frequency of $\nu = 3 \times 10^8/5 \times 10^{-11} = 6 \times 10^{18}$ Hz. A 50 pm photon thus has an energy of $E = h\nu = 3.974 \times 10^{-15}$ joules, or $3.974 \times 10^{-15}/1.603 \times 10^{-19} = 24.8$ keV. In general, the wavelength in pm of an X- or gamma ray is related to its eV energy by:

$$\lambda = \frac{1.2397 \times 10^{-6}}{W(\text{in eV})} \quad \text{pm} \qquad\qquad 15.1$$

When directed at the body, the EMR used for medical diagnosis interacts with the biomolecules of the body in several interesting ways. Incident photon energy is reflected or backscattered, absorbed, or transmitted through the tissues to emerge. The energy spectrum of emergent and back-scattered radiation can show peaks and valleys at wavelengths where certain biomolecules have absorbed more energy than at others. This selective absorption is the basis for several interesting kinds of

343

absorption spectroscopy; it is due to "tuned" energy absorption by different classes of interatomic bonds. Energy absorption at selected frequencies by interatomic bonds is also the basis for *Raman spectroscopy*, where scattered light from an incident monochromatic beam exhibits spectral peaks and valleys. Incident photons with sufficient energy (e.g., blue light) can also produce *fluorescence* in biological molecules. Fluorescence is where an incident photon strikes a particular molecule where it is absorbed and causes secondary photon(s) having longer wavelength(s) (lower energy) to immediately be generated. The spectrum of the emitted fluorescent light is unique for each species of fluorescing molecule, and thus, can be used for detection and measurement of an analyte's concentration.

Very-high-energy photons, e.g., from UV light, X- and gamma rays, can actually break molecular bonds and destroy critical biomolecules such as DNA and RNA, causing genetic damage, mutations, cancer and leukemia. These high-energy photons are called *ionizing radiations*, and as you might expect, their use in diagnosis is not without statistical risk to the patient for diseases such as cancer and leukemia. The reason they are classified as ionizing radiation is that when these photons interact with certain molecules or atoms, they can cause the net loss or gain of one or more electrons, creating an ion. Generally, UV has little penetration and affects surface molecules. Long-term UV exposure is associated with skin cancers (melanomas), corneal damage and cataracts. High-energy X- and gamma rays penetrate the entire body, and can cause radiation damage to biomolecules anywhere in the body. Particularly sensitive are tissues in which cell division is continuously underway to replace cells lost by natural turnover *(apoptosis)*. These cells include *blood stem cells* in bone marrow, *intestinal epithelial cells*, and skin cells. A 1 meV gamma ray has ca. 2×10^6 times the energy of visible light, and can generate tens of thousands of ions as it passes through the body. It also can break DNA and RNA strands, which, if not repaired by natural enzymes, can lead to cell mutation or premature cell death. The reader interested in probing the effects of ionizing radiation in greater depth can begin by visiting the U.S. Government DOE ACHRE web site, which contains an excellent primer on the basics of radiation science.

The following sections of this chapter treat the use of photon radiation in:

- Bone density analysis by X-rays (15.2)
- Tissue fluorescence to detect cancers (15.3)
- Interferometry to measure nanometer displacements of body surfaces (15.4)
- Laser Doppler velocimetry to measure capillary blood flow (15.5)
- Transcutaneous IR spectroscopy to measure blood analytes (15.6)
- Gilham polarimetry to measure glucose on the aqueous humor of the eyes (15.7)
- Pulse oximetry to measure the percent of oxyhemoglobin in capillary blood (15.8)
- Applications of Raman spectroscopy in NI medical diagnosis (15.9)

15.2 BONE DENSITOMETRY

15.2.1 INTRODUCTION

The disease of *osteoporosis* is a slow, progressive loss of bone calcium (and bone strength) that affects an estimated 250 million women worldwide and more than 25 million people in the United States alone, where it leads to c.1.5 million fractures each year, having an estimated treatment cost, including physical therapy, of $18 billion. Most of the persons at risk for osteoporosis are postmenopausal women who are not on estrogen therapy. In osteoporosis, there is a decrease in the activity of *osteoblasts* (cells that build the bone matrix) and in the rate of production of bone growth factors. Also, estrogen deficiency causes a rise in the concentrations of the following cytokines: interleukin-1, tumor necrosis factor-α, granulocyte-macrophage colony-stimulating factor, and interleukin-6. These cytokines enhance bone resorption through the stimulation of *osteoclasts*, cells that break down bone and bone matrix. Many external factors increase the rate of osteoporosis in both men and women. These include malnutrition, prolonged physical inactivity, a prolonged zero-gravity environment (space travel), lack of dietary calcium, lack of exposure to sunlight (to generate endogenous vitamin D), excessive dietary protein consumption, smoking, alcoholism, excessive caffeine consumption and taking corticosteroids (see: http://medlib.med.utah.edu).

The natural decline in bone density and consequent decrease in bone strength following menopause can eventually lead to debilitating and sometimes fatal bone fractures. Falls can lead to broken wrists, fractures to the head of the femur, the pelvis, the spine, and other bones. The rate of osteoporosis in postmenopausal women can be slowed by avoiding some of the aggravating factors listed above. A good diet, moderate exercise, and moderation in caffeine and alcohol consumption are indicated.

To assess the degree of osteoporosis in a patient, there are several invasive tests (bone biopsy, certain chemicals in blood) that we will not consider here, and some fairly definitive noninvasive tests. Bone density can be measured by quantitative CAT scan techniques, and, less expensively, by dual-energy X-ray absorption (DEXA) scans of bones (described in the following section), and tests of urine of a fasting patient for excess Ca^{++}, hydroxyproline-containing peptides and pyridinium peptide (from the breakdown of bone matrix) (visit the online Merk Manual: www.merk.com/pubs/mmanual/sections.htm). The purpose of these NI tests is to assess the a person's degree of risk for broken bones and other orthopedic complications of osteoporosis.

15.2.2 DUAL-ENERGY X-RAY ABSORPTION METHOD

The dual-energy X-ray absorption (DEXA) method is an inexpensive and accurate means of measuring bone mineral density, primarily from the calcium content in bone salts (Bonnick, 1998). DEXA is typically used on the heel, wrist or forearm, proximal femur, or lumbar spine. A typical DEXA system is shown schematically in Figure 15.1.

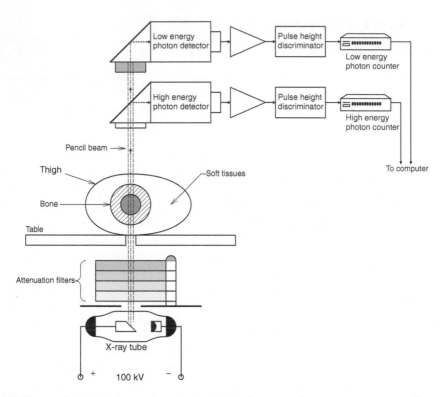

FIGURE 15.1 A typical DEXA system. Note that it has two X-ray photon counters for the two energy levels used.

X-rays are characterized by their photon energy, hv, in thousands of electron volts (keV) (or, alternately, by their wavelengths, λ, in picometers), and their intensity in Watts/m^2. X-rays can be formed into fairly collimated pencil beams or floodlight-like fan beams. Both types are used in various DEXA systems. The operation of a DEXA system is reminiscent of spectrophotometry at two wavelengths (see Section 15.8 on pulse oximetry). To obtain a heuristic appreciation of how a DEXA system works, consider X-ray transmission through a homogeneous dense material (e.g., bone) of thickness L. Some of the X-rays entering the material are absorbed and do not exit. Most of these absorbed X-rays are ultimately converted to heat, and some cause chemical bonds to rupture, creating ions and free radicals that can lead to genetic damage, even cancer. The X-rays that emerge are "counted" by an X-ray sensor. Some X-ray sensors are of the ionozation type (acting like Geiger counters), producing a current pulse for every X-ray photon that creates an ion pair. Another type of X-ray sensor uses a scintillation crystal that emits secondary visible photons when struck by an X-ray photon; the visible photons are, in turn, sensed by a photomultiplyer tube. The law that governs X-ray absorption (or transmission) in bone is very like Beer's law in spectrophotometry.

$$\frac{I_{out}}{I_{in}} = \exp\left[-\mu_\lambda \rho L\right] \qquad 15.2$$

Where I_{out} is the intensity of the transmitted X-rays, I_{in} is the intensity of the input X-rays, μ_λ is the wavelength-dependent *mass attenuation coefficient* (aka X-ray cross-section) in cm²/g, ρ is the volume density of the absorbing medium in g/cm³, and L is the length of the path the X-rays travel in the medium. μ_λ is a function of the absorbing element (in the case of bone it is significantly calcium) as well as the X-ray's wavelength, λ. Note that X-ray photon energy is hν, and ν = c/λ. "Soft" X-rays have energies in the range of 1 to 20 keV. Intermediate energies range from 20 keV to 0.1 MeV. Hard X-ray energies are above 0.1 MeV. Figure 15.2 illustrates the relative intensity/hν vs. X-ray photon energy hν in keV for various conditions in a DEXA X-ray system. The top curve is the intensity spectrum of X-ray photons leaving the X-ray tube. The second curve is the intensity spectrum of attenuated photons entering the tissue and bone, and the bottom curve is the intensity spectrum of photons exiting the bone. In this example, the X-ray tube's tungsten anode is bombarded with 100 keV electrons. Note the presence of line spectra added to the smooth *bremsstrahlung* spectra. Tungsten has line spectra at 57.9, 59.3, 67.4, and 69.3 keV photon energies. The total energy in these spikes amounts to c. 10% of the total emitted energy. The spikes are generated by the bombarding electrons in the X-ray tube interacting with K-shell electrons in the tungsten atoms (Jacobsen and Webster, 1977). The two triangular graphs on the spectrum plots represent the spectral sensitivities of low- and high-energy X-ray detectors that respond to the photon intensities in the exiting X-ray beam.

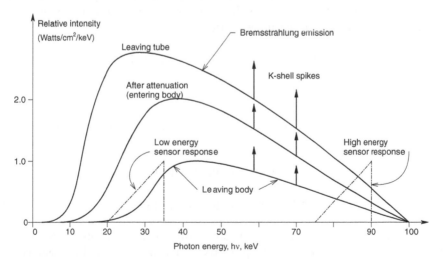

FIGURE 15.2 X-ray energy spectra in a DEXA system.

The general X-ray absorption equation (Equation 15.2) can be modified to find the effective density of calcium in a bone of thickness L. One approach to this problem is to consider the incident X-ray spectrum to be absorbed by calcium in the bone and "other tissue" including soft tissue surrounding the bone, and the collagen in the bone matrix. Because the X-ray photon detectors select low- and high-energy photons and two absorbers have been defined (Ca and "other"), there are four mass attenuation coefficients (MACs) associated with the DEXA system:

1. μ_{Hc}: the mean MAC for Ca at high hv
2. μ_{Lc}: the mean MAC for Ca at low hv
3. μ_{Ho}: the mean MAC for other tissue at high hv
4. μ_{Lo}: the mean MAC for other tissue at low hv.

For example, the MAC for Ca at hv = 30 keV is 3.97 cm^2/g; the MAC for Ca at hv = 62 keV is 0.63 cm^2/g, a ratio of 6.3:1 All four MACs are assumed to be known from prior measurements. Thus, the detected X-ray intensities can be written:

$$I_L = I_{inL} \exp[- \mu_{Lc}\, \rho_c\, L]\, \exp[- \mu_{Lo}\, \rho_o\, L] \qquad\qquad 15.3A$$

$$I_H = I_{inH} \exp[- \mu_{Hc}\, \rho_c\, L]\, \exp[- \mu_{Ho}\, \rho_o\, L] \qquad\qquad 15.3B$$

where: I_{inL} is the total input intensity of X-rays to the tissue defined by the low-energy detector's acceptance spectrum, I_{inH} is the total input intensity of X-rays to the tissue defined by the high-energy detector's acceptance spectrum. I_L is the transmitted intensity of the low-energy X-rays, I_H is the transmitted intensity of the high-energy X-rays, L is the path length through the sample, ρ_c is the unknown density of Ca in the bone, and ρ_o is the mean mass density of other tissues in the sample. The equations above can be rewritten:

$$I_L = I_{inL} \{\exp[- \mu_{Lc}\, \rho_c\, L - \mu_{Lo}\, \rho_o\, L] \qquad\qquad 15.4A$$

$$I_H = I_{inH} \exp[- \mu_{Hc}\, \rho_c\, L - \mu_{Ho}\, \rho_o\, L] \qquad\qquad 15.4B$$

When we take the natural logarithm of both sides of each equation above, we have the simultaneous equations:

$$\ln(I_{inL}/I_L) = + \rho_c\, \mu_{Lc}\, L + \rho_o\, \mu_{Lo}\, L \qquad\qquad 15.5A$$

$$\ln(I_{inH}/I_H) = + \rho_c\, \mu_{Hc}\, L + \rho_o\, \mu_{Ho}\, L \qquad\qquad 15.5B$$

These equations are solved for the calcium density, ρ_c, g/cm^3 by the DEXA system computer, which has values for the μ matrix, L, I_{inL} and I_{inH} stored in memory.

$$\rho_c = \frac{\mu_{Ho}\, \ln(I_{inL}/I_L) - \mu_{Lo}\, \ln(I_{inH}/I_H)}{L[\mu_{Lc}\mu_{Ho} - \mu_{Hc}\mu_{Lo}]} \qquad\qquad 15.6$$

Once measured on a patient, ρ_c and ρ_o are compared with the database value for the same bone in a healthy 30-year-old person (peak calcium density). A measured bone density (ρ_c) of less than one standard deviation from the peak bone mass mean is considered to be a normal or safe bone mass loss in aging. The condition of *osteopenia* is considered to exist when the measured ρ_c is between -1 and -2.5 SD down from the peak mean. When ρ_c is < -2.5 SD from the peak mean bone mass, the patient is considered to have severe osteoporosis and to be at risk for stress fractures, falls, etc. These classifications with respect to peak bone mass are called a T-score. Another type of scoring (the Z-score) for bone mass loss compares the measured ρ_c with that for age- and sex-matched controls. The Z-score can be misleading, however, because of its relative nature.

If a CT scanner is used to measure bone density, it must be calibrated with a standard of reference to give quantitative output. Such physical bone density standards are made by CIRS (Computerized Imaging Reference Systems, Inc.) of Norfolk, VA. Physical standards are also used to field-calibrate DEXA systems.

15.2.3 DISCUSSION

Modern pencil-beam DEXA systems, such as those made by Norland Medical Systems, Inc., minimize patient exposure to X-rays. A typical DEXA system uses a 100 kV Xray source, which is attenuated by a bank of eight samarium metal filters, giving 256 possible intensity levels. Hence, the system can be adjusted to minimize patient exposure and, at the same time, to optimize the dynamic range of the low- and high-energy X-ray photon counting sensors over a range of tissue thickness from 12 to 22 cm. Norland also calibrates its DEXA machines with a 77-step double step wedge (phantom) calibrator.

The DEXA method is definitely the "gold standard" of bone densitometry. It is an accurate noninvasive procedure that can be done in a doctor's office or clinic at low patient cost (use of a quantitative CT scanned for the same purpose costs about 10 times the DEXA procedure's cost).

15.3 NONINVASIVE DIAGNOSIS BY TISSUE FLUORESCENCE

15.3.1 INTRODUCTION

Fluorescence occurs when a molecule absorbs one or more high-energy photons (generally from blue or UV light, depending on the molecule), and immediately re-radiates a low-energy photon, generally in the visible range of wavelengths. Many naturally occurring molecules in cells exhibit fluorescence, and specially engineered fluorescing *fluorophore molecules* can be attached to probe molecules that have affinities for various natural cellular components. Thus, fluorophore tags can be used to identify specific cellular components (surface proteins and receptors). Fluorophore taggants are now generally used in *in vitro* studies, but will become common for *in vivo* applications as their safety is established. One reason for the intense interest in fluorescence in NI medical diagnosis is the incredible analytical sensitivity of the method. Conventional spectrophotometric absorbance methods can reliably detect a molecular species at concentrations of tenths of a μmole/liter; fluorescent techniques can accurately measure concentrations one million times smaller — in the range of picomoles/liter. As techniques improve, quantities less than an attomole ($< 10^{-18}$ mole) may be detected (cf. PTIwebsite (1999): www.pti-nj.com/fluorescence _2.html).

The short-wavelength light required to excite fluorescence is rapidly attenuated in the skin and other tissues, so noninvasive *in vivo* studies of cell fluorescence are limited to the first few mm of tissue depth. Two major sources of excitation light exist: (1) lasers, including the 337 nm nitrogen laser, the argon ion laser with 7 emission lines between 457 and 529 nm, and various solid-state diode lasers; and (2) Xenon tubes coupled to grating monochromators. The latter source is commonly used in research spectrofluorometers, and can produce wavelengths from 200 to 700 nm. Quartz lenses and optical fibers are used for wavelengths < 400 nm. UV light is classified as UVA (320 –400 nm), UVB (280 – 320 nm) and UVC (100 – 280 nm).

15.3.2 PROPERTIES OF FLUORESCENT MOLECULES

Fluorescent molecules used in diagnosis include intrinsically fluorescent substances, as well as the fluorophore tags mentioned above. Table 15.3.2.1 lists some of the major intrinsic fluorescent molecules, their optimum excitation wavelength, their peak emission wavelength, and where they are found. It should be stressed that all fluorescent molecules have a broad excitation action spectrum, sometimes with two peaks. Their emission spectra are also broad and can have more than one peak; often the long wavelength tail of the excitation spectrum overlaps the short wavelength tail of the emission spectrum. Also, conditions of pH, ionic environment, and the proximity (< 6 nm) of other non-fluorescing molecules can shift or attenuate the excitation and emission spectra. The intensity of the induced fluorescent irradiance is thousands of times lower than the irradiance of the excitation source. In cancerous lung tissue, the ratio of blue laser light irradiance to fluorescent emission irradiance is about $64 \times 10^6 : 1$ (Turner Designs, 1998).

Table 15.3.2 lists common fluorophore molecules used for marking specific cellular molecules and structures. The marking can be due to one of the following mechanisms:

- The fluorophore is bound to another molecule (e.g., an antibody) that has a high selective affinity to a molecular species within (or without) a cell.
- The fluorophore can be bound to the active site of an antigen, and thus be used to detect specific circulating antibodies.
- The fluorophore may fluoresce when in the presence of a high ionic concentration of calcium, or some other molecule or ion that activates it.

Note that each fluorophore molecule has a finite working lifetime. Typically, < 10^5 photons can be emitted before the molecule is damaged and undergoes a structural change that makes it non-fluorescent. Thus, fluorophore-tagged cells cannot be illuminated by CW UV excitation without gradual loss of fluorescence or "bleaching." Often, nanosecond-length pulses having a very low duty cycle are used. The

TABLE 15.3.1
Naturally Occurring Biomolecules that Fluoresce

Molecule	Excitation Peak, nm	Emission Peak, nm	Comment
Tryptophan	285 (290)	340 (330)	amino acid emits; in UV
Tyrosine	274	303	"
Phenylalanine	257	282	"
GFP	490	509	Green fluorescent protein from jellyfish
NADH	350	450	Nicotinamide adenine dinucleotide Found in mitochondria
FAD	450	525	Flavin adenine dinucleotide. Concentated in mitochondria, also found in cytoplasm
Flavins	445–470	500–700	"
Protoporphyrin IX	375–440	520, 635 and 704 (3 peaks; 635 largest)	In erythroid cells, and Ca cells treated with 5-ALA

TABLE 15.3.2
Partial List of Synthetic Fluorophore Molecules

Fluorophore	Excitation peak, nm	Emission peak, nm	Specificity
Bisbenzimide Hoechst 33342	UV	390–440	Binds to DNA
Rhodamine 123	545, (485)	red, (green)	Binds to mitochondria
Wheat germ agglutinin + fluorescein isothiocyanate	488 (Ar laser)	520	Plasma membrane and endosomes, but not mitochondria
Texas Red coupled to streptavidine	595 (dye laser)	620	Binds to biotin
FURA-2	340	515	Fluorescence depends on [Ca^{++}]. Chelates Ca^{++}
Alexa	?	603 or 617	These fluorophores attach to taggants
Phenol red	?	575	"
Resorufin	?	587	"
Red phycoerythrin (R-PE)	488 (Ar laser)	576	"
Allophycocyanin (APC)	595 (dye laser)	660	"
Cy-3 (cyanine dye)	?	565	"
Cy-5	488 (Ar laser)	667	"
Cy-Chrome tandan Conj. of R-PE and cyanine	?	670	"
Cascade blue	406 krypton	430	"
EDANS aminonaphthalene-1-sulfonic acid	336	490	"

use of excitation pulses allows the dynamics of the fluorescence to be studied at a given wavelength, including the latency, the time to peak, the emitted pulse shape, and the decay time. *Phase fluorometry* looks specifically at the dynamics of pulse-excited fluorescence.

15.3.3 FLUORESCENCE IN NI CANCER DIAGNOSIS

A recent important trend in medical diagnosis is the use of fluorescent molecules to screen for superficial cancers, i.e., cancers that lie on or near the skin surface, or on or near the surface of the tissues that are accessible to endoscopes, such as the lungs, bladder and cervix. At the present time, cancer diagnosis by fluorescence is generally done as an imaging process. The examining physician illuminates the tissue being evaluated with monochromatic light ranging from 330 nm wavelength (UVA) to green light, depending on the optimum excitation range of the fluorescing molecules. UV light with wavelengths shorter than 330 nm is known to damage cellular DNA by inducing thymine dimers (Heintzelman et al. 2000), and so is avoided when examining tissues *in vivo*.

Xillix, a Canadian medical imaging company, has developed a fiber optic system used to detect lung cancer. Called LIFE-Lung Fluorescence Endoscopy System™, it is used as an adjunct to white-light endoscopy. A HeCd laser produces deep blue light at 442 nm with an irradiance of c. 64 mW/mm^2 that is shone on lung tissues from a bronchoscope probe inserted into the bronchi. Both normal and precancerous lung tissues emit similar quantities of red light, but normal cells also emit about eight times the intensity of green light. The fluorescence is picked up by more than 10^4 optical fibers in a coherent (imaging) bundle. The emitted light is split into green and red color bands by a dichroic mirror and further refined in bandwidth by interference filters. The intensity of the faint red and green spectral images is then amplified by two image intensifiers up to $\times$ 10^4. The images are captured on two 512 $\times$ 512-pixel CCD cameras and encoded as digital video signals. To compensate for the 1/r^4 law of *in vivo* fluorescence attenuation with distance, the red emission, which is the same for both healthy and cancerous cells, is used to normalize the green channel signals. Lung tissues fluorescing proportionally less green light than red then can be marked as suspect regardless of their distance from the endoscope tip. The Xillix system is approved to be used with the Olympus-type BF20D bronchoscope.

Xillix claims that, following a large multi-center clinical study of their LIFE system vs. white-light endoscopy done on suspected lung cancer patients, detection improved from 37% to 75% on a per-patient basis, and on a per-lesion basis, detection improved from 25% to 67%.

In summary, the Xillix LIFE-Lung system is a mildly invasive diagnostic system that uses computer-enhanced spectral imaging of lung tissues to detect precancerous cells by fluorescence. The blue light used does not damage tissues like UVA and B wavelengths. No special systemic drugs are required for the Xillix diagnostic system; it works with endogenous fluorescent molecules.

The cytochrome proteins found in the mitochondrial oxidative phosphorylation process are *heme proteins*, i.e., they contain one or two heme residues in one polypeptide chain. *Cytochrome c* contains a modified iron protoporphyrin called

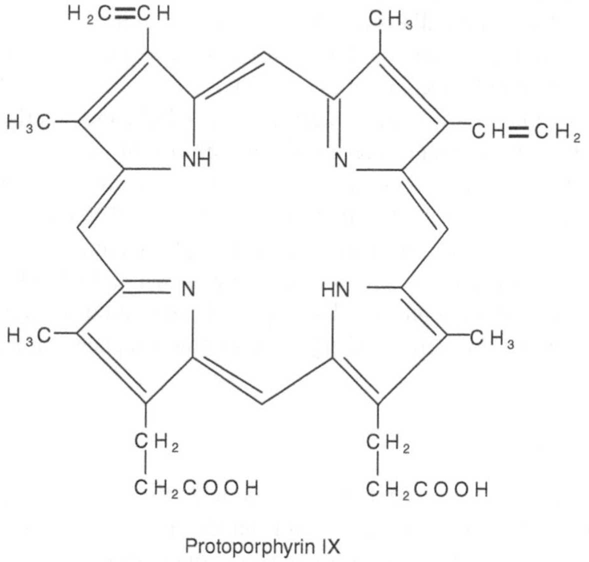

Protoporphyrin IX

FIGURE 15.3 The fluorescing protoporphyrin IX molecule.

heme c. All three forms of heme found in cytochromes are derived biochemically from *iron protoporphyrin IX* (PpIX), also called *heme b.* The 2-D molecular schematic of PpIX is shown in Figure 15.3. PpIX has emission peaks at 520, 635 and 704 nm.

The red (635 nm) major fluorescent emission peak from PpIX has been investigated as a marker for oral carcinoma. In one study, 410 nm excitation elicited PpIX-like fluorescence spectra from 85% of oral carcinomas irradiated. Analysis of the emissions was by spectrofluorometer (Inaguma and Hashimoto, 2000). In another study, topical application of 5-aminolevulinic acid (5-ALA) was found to enhance the PpIX fluorescent emission from neoplastic tissue in the oral cavity. There was a maximum fluorescent contrast of 10:1 between cancers and normal tissues at about 1 to 2 hours after the 5-ALA treatment, allowing a demarcation of tumors visible even to the naked eye (Leunig et al., 1996). In a similar study, 5-ALA (a 0.4% solution) used as a topical rinse was used to enhance PpIX red fluorescence of oral leukoplakias (squamous cell carcinomas). The identified lesions were treated with *retinyl palmitate* (vitamin A) which caused complete remissions in 15 out of 20 cases. The cured cancers lost their PpIX fluorescence (Leunig et al., 2000). In another study of basal cell (skin) carcinoma, varied doses of orally administered 5-ALA were given to determine optimum fluorescence response of PpIX in the cancers vs. side effects. *In vivo* spectrofluorometry was used (Tope et al., 1998).

NADH stands for (reduced) nicotinamide adenine dinucleotide. NADH plays an important biochemical role in Complex 1 of the mitochondrial oxidative phosphorylation process. As we have seen above, NADH has an intrinsic blue fluorescence emission with a peak at 450 nm, which can be excited by 337 nm UV pulses from a nitrogen laser. NADH fluorescence of bladder cancer cells was observed using a quartz fiber to deliver the short laser pulses and another fiber to collect the fluorescence radiation. The optical fibers and a conventional white-light FO cystoscope are inserted up the urethra, a process that is arguably as about as invasive as a semi-invasive procedure can be (König et al., 1994).

In an *in vitro* fluorescence study, cervical epithelial cancer cells were shown to have high levels of tryptophan, offering the possibility of their being discriminated from inflammatory immune system cells (leucocytes) and normal cervical cells (Heintzelman et al., 2000). Unfortunately, the wavelength required to excite tryptophan fluorescence is 290 nm, which can cause DNA damage in normal cells *in vivo*. Clearly, what is needed is a fluorescent taggant with a high affinity to a surface protein unique to cervical cancer cells, and with an excitation wavelength longer than 330 nm. Direct excitation of tryptophan fluorescence appears to carry an unacceptable risk.

15.3.4 Discussion

The use of noninvasive fluorescent imaging methods to detect surface cancers on the skin, oral mucosa, lung tissues, cervix and bladder is an area of medical diagnosis being rapidly developed. Because most intrinsic fluorescent biomolecules generally require potentially tissue-damaging short wavelengths for excitation, the use of fluorophore taggants excitable at wavelengths longer than 330 nm is expected to grow.

The most satisfactory approach for fluorescent diagnosis appears to be digitally enhanced endoscopic imaging using appropriate interference filters to contrast the cancerous cells with the normal surround. A more complex approach is to use quantitative spectrofluorometry to map the lesion, and to use pulsed excitation so the dynamics of the fluorescence can be studied. The behavior of fluorescent molecules changes with their chemical environment, a fact that offers another tool to differentiate what molecules are fluorescing, and how much of each is there.

15.4 OPTICAL INTERFEROMETRIC MEASUREMENT OF NANOMETER DISPLACEMENTS OF BIOLOGICAL SURFACES

15.4.1 Introduction

Several areas of noninvasive diagnosis exist in which information is gained by the no-touch optical interferometric measurement of extremely small (e.g., on the order of nanometers) mechanical displacements of external surfaces. One such displacement is the extremely small vibration of the eardrum in response to incident sound pressure. Such measurement can be useful in the study of the mechanics of hearing, including the tympanal reflex in response to sudden loud sounds. Another physical displacement is the movement of a tooth *in situ* in response to a lateral force. Such measurement of the mechanical compliance of teeth can be useful in orthodontic research and in the study of dental health. Still another application of optical interferometry lies in the measurement of very small displacements of the skin caused by blood flow in capillary beds. Microplethysmography of the skin surface can have application in studies of the control of peripheral circulation, and in assessing microcirculation following vascular surgery. Quantitative measurement (amplitude and frequencies) of skin displacement caused by fine tremors in underlying muscles can have application in studies of neurological disorders such as Parkinson's disease.

There are many types of optical interferometers that can be used to make the measurements described above; most use one coherent light source (i.e., a laser) and split the coherent beam into two optical paths, R and M, then combine the beams so that there is a linear summation of the output beam E vectors ($\mathbf{E_M}$ and $\mathbf{E_R}$) at a common output plane or photo-sensor. At the output plane, there is alternate constructive and destructive interference. There are bright rings or lines where there is constructive addition; dark rings or lines appear where there is destructive interference. To measure a physical quantity such as surface displacement, it must change the phase between $\mathbf{E_M}$ and $\mathbf{E_R}$ by changing the M beam's path length. As you will see, a convenient way of doing this is to stick a mirror on the moving surface and use the phase change in the reflected light in the M path. (Other physical quantities can be measured by interferometry when they cause a phase change between the M and R beams.) For an elementary discussion of the use of interferometry in length or displacement measurement, see Chapter 4 and others in the text by Sirohi and Kothiyal (1991). A detailed mathematical analysis of several major types of interferometer can be found in Chapter 9 in *Optics* by Hecht (1987).

Direct measurement of an object's displacement with an interferometer is limited to motions of less than $\pm \lambda/4$. Greater motion will result in a periodic output of the interferometer, and some means must be used to count interference "fringes" during the motion of the object to keep track of the total object displacement.

Before describing specific types of interferometers, let us examine a general heuristic treatment of optical interference. For interference to occur, the electromagnetic light wave must be temporally and spatially *coherent*. That is, the frequency and phase of the E vectors of the interfering waves must remain constant in time and space for interference to occur. A stable monochromatic source such as a laser is ideal for interferometry. The optical intensity changes associated with interference occur as the result of the superposition of the E vectors at a point on the detector. The intensity at the detector is proportional to the net E vector squared. That is:

$$I_d \propto (e_r + e_m)^2 \text{ Watts/m}^2 \qquad\qquad 15.7$$

Where

$$e_r = e_r(t) = E_{Ro} \cos[(2\pi c/\lambda)t)] \qquad\qquad 15.8$$

$$e_m = e_m(t) = E_{Mo} \cos[(2\pi c/\lambda)t + 2\phi_m + (2d/\lambda)2\pi] \qquad\qquad 15.9$$

e_m and e_r are the time-varying E vectors of EM plane waves at a point at the detector surface. The fixed phase of e_r is taken as zero; the phase of the measurement wave, e_m, has a fixed component, $2\phi_m$, due to the out and back propagation delay, and a variable component, $(4\pi d/\lambda)$ radians, due to the small, relative displacement of the reflecting surface, d. Note that the frequency of both waves is $v = c/\lambda$ Hz. Substituting Equations 15.8 and 15.9 into Equation 15.7, we find:

$$1_d = \left(E_{Ro}^2/2\right)\left[1 + \cos(4\pi vt)\right] + \left(E_{Mo}^2/2\right)\left[1 + \cos\left(4\pi vt + 4\phi_m + (4d/\lambda)2\pi\right)\right]$$

$$+ E_{Ro}E_{Mo}\left\{\cos\left[4\pi vt + 2\phi_m + (2d/\lambda)2\pi\right] + \cos\left[2\phi_m + (2d/\lambda)2\pi\right]\right\} \qquad 15.10$$

Watts/cm^2

Of course the photodetector does not respond to terms at frequency $2v$ Hz. Thus the detector output is given by:

$$V_o = -K_d\overline{1_d} = -K_d\left\{\left(E_{Ro}^2/2\right) + \left(E_{Mo}^2/2\right) + E_{Ro}E_{Mo}\cos\left[2\phi_m + (2d/\lambda)2\pi\right]\right\} \qquad 15.11$$

Volts.

We use the trig identity, $\cos(A + B) \equiv [\cos(A)\cos(B) - \sin(A)\sin(B)]$. If d is slowly varying (i.e., is a dc quantity), we can make $2\phi_m = q\pi/2$, (q 1, 5, 9, 13, ...) so that $\cos(2\phi_m) = 0$, and $\sin(2\phi_m) = +1$. Thus the detector output is given by:

$$V_o = -K_d\left\{\left(E_{Ro}^2/2\right) + \left(E_{Mo}^2/2\right) - E_{Ro}E_{Mo}\sin\left[(2d/\lambda)2\pi\right]\right\} \qquad 15.12$$

If d is moving at an audio frequency so that $d = d_o\sin(\omega_m t)$, the dc terms are filtered out by high-pass filtering, and again, $2\phi_m$ is made equal to $q\pi/2$, q = 1, 5, 9, 13, ..., so

$$v_o(t) = K_d E_{Ro} E_{Mo} \sin[(4\pi/\lambda)d_o \sin(\omega_m t)] \qquad 15.13$$

To keep the system in its linear output range, the argument of the sin[.] term must not exceed $\pm \lambda/4$. That is, d_o must be $< \lambda/4$. If $d_o > \lambda/4$, periodicity in the output vs. d_o is observed, and unless one counts output maxima and minima, there will be ambiguity in the true value of d_o.

Equation 15.13 can be expanded by the Bessel-Jacoby identity (Stark, Tuteur and Anderson, 1988).

$$v_o(t) = K_d E_{Ro} E_{Mo} \sum_{n=-\infty}^{\infty} J_n(\xi)\sin(n\omega_m t) \qquad 15.14$$

Where, obviously, $\xi \equiv (4\pi/\lambda)d_o$, and $J_n(\xi)$ is a *Bessel function of the first kind*. It can be shown that $J_n(\xi)$ can be approximated by the series (Stark, Tuteur and Anderson, 1988):

$$J_n(\xi) = \sum_{k=0}^{\infty} \frac{(\xi/2)^{(n+2k)}(-1)^k}{(n+k)!k!} \qquad 15.15$$

If $\xi \ll 1$, Equation 15.15 can be approximated by:

$$J_n(\xi) \cong (\xi/2)^n/n! \quad n > 0, \text{ integer} \qquad 15.16$$

and in general (Dwight 807.4, 1969),

$$J_{-n}(\xi) \equiv (-1)^{|n|} J_n(\xi) \qquad 15.17$$

Thus the first few terms of Equation 15.14 can be written, assuming $\xi \ll 1$:

$$v_o(t) \cong \overset{n=0}{0} + K_d E_{Ro} \overset{n=\pm 1}{E_{Mo}}$$

$$\left\{ \xi \sin(\omega_m t) + \overset{n=\pm 2}{0} + (\xi^3/24) \overset{n=\pm 3}{\sin}(3\omega_m t) + \overset{n=\pm 4}{0} + (\xi^5/1920) \overset{n=\pm 5}{\sin}(5\omega_m t) + \overset{n=\pm 6}{0} + ... \right\}$$

$$15.18$$

Because even high-order harmonic terms are zero, and $\xi \ll 1$, the fundamental frequency term dominates the series of Equation 15.14. d_o, the quantity under measurement can be found by phase-sensitive rectification of $v_o(t)$ using a ω_m-frequency reference signal, followed by low-pass filtering. If the low-pass filter has gain K_F, then its dc output, V_o', will be:

$$V_o' = K_F\, K_d\, E_{Ro}\, E_{Mo}\, (4\pi/\lambda)d_o \quad \text{dc volts} \qquad 15.19$$

We next examine some examples of optical interferometers that have been used in biomedical applications. The first is the fiber optic Fizeau interferometer developed by Drake and Leiner (1984).

15.4.2 Measurement of Tympanal Membrane Displacement by Fizeau Interferometer

This prototype instrument, shown in Figure 15.4, was used to sense the minute displacement of the tympanal membrane of a common cricket subjected to external audible sound. Drake and Leiner used a 15 mW HeNe (633 nm) laser as their source. The half-wave plate was rotated to minimize the observed intensity, indicating that all of the linearly polarized light from the laser was going into the 10×0.255 NA microscope objective used to direct all of the incident light into the proximal end of the polarization-preserving, glass optical fiber (PPOF). The PPOF was of two-step design; it had a 5 μm core diameter and a 125 μm cladding diameter. By experimentally adjusting the PPOF loop diameter D, and twisting it some small angle, θ, around the axis from the objective to the object, the PPOF loop could be made to act as a quarter-wave plate. Thus, the light returning to the proximal end of the PPOF was rotated 90° with respect to the entering light. Drake and Leiner stated:

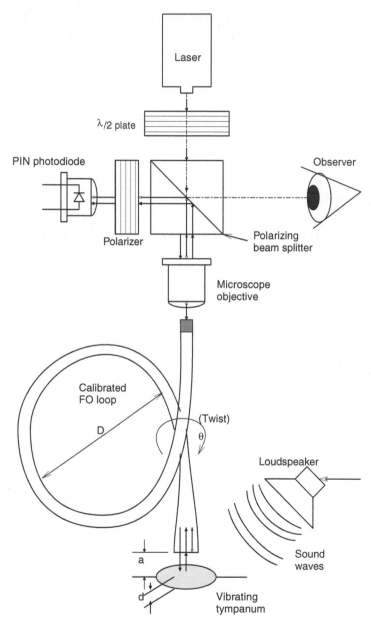

FIGURE 15.4 Schematic of the fiber optic Fizeau interferometer used by Drake and Leiner to measure very small deflections of a tympanal membrane. The linear range measured was 0.01 to 30 nm.

"All of the interfering light is then reflected toward the detector by the polarizing beamsplitter, while light reflected from the back side of the beamsplitter, from the elements of the microscope objective, and from the proximal end of the fiber, all pass straight back through the polarizing beam splitter and does not contribute unwanted radiation at the detector."

Because the Fizeau interferometer gives an output signal proportional to *relative object displacement,* Drake and Leiner mounted their object (cricket tympanum) on a piezoelectric crystal that could be displaced toward or away from the PPOF's distal end by $> \pm \lambda/2$ by applying a 10 Hz, triangular, voltage waveform and observing the magnitude of the ac signal output at the acoustic stimulus frequency, f_m. The ac output was maximum when the distance, a, was some multiple of $\lambda/4$. This particular dc voltage was applied to the crystal for subsequent tests of tympanal membrane response, d. Calibration of the Fizeau interferometer was accomplished by applying a 1 kHz triangular wave around the dc bias voltage to the piezocrystal. The triangle wave amplitude was adjusted until the output peaks just began to fold over as seen on an oscilloscope display. The target was then known to be undergoing a $\pm \lambda/4$ displacement. Thus, an output calibration factor was determined in volts/nm displacement. ($\lambda/4 = 158.2$ nm.)

Drake and Leiner displayed their output signal on an oscilloscope and on a spectrum analyzer. The typical ratio of fundamental frequency to second harmonic amplitude was 0.16. They found that their instrument could resolve 0.01 nm $< d_o <$ 30 nm linearly . This is an amazing sensitivity, considering that a lock-in amplifier was not used. They commented that the working distance, a, from the distal end of the fiber to the moving object can be increased to over a few mm by adding a Selfoc® lens to the tip of the PPOF cable.

Drake and Leiner mention that future applications of their Fizeau interferometer can include studies of human eardrum displacement, measurement of the ocular pulse (a typical human ocular pulse is ± 8 µm, beyond the described range of their instrument), basilar membrane deflection in the cochlea (presumably done *in vitro*), measurement of nerve axon displacement during an action potential, and dental strain measurements.

15.4.3 Measurement of Skin Vibration by Optical Interferometry

The Michelson interferometer has been used to measure skin surface microvibrations (Hong and Fox, 1993; Hong, 1994). A true Michelson interferometer is illustrated in Figure 15.5 (Hecht, 1987). Note that it uses a compensating plate in optical path L_1 so that each beam travels the same distance through glass. The compensating plate is identical to the half-silvered mirror beam splitter, except that it does not have silvering. Use of the compensation plate corrects for refractive index dispersion with λ, and lets the Michelson interferometer be used with broadband (semi-coherent) light sources. If a monochromatic laser source is used, the compensation plate is not necessary. A Michelson interferometer without the compensation plate is often called a *Twyman-Green interferometer* (Sirohi and Kothiyal, 1991). As shown above with the Fizeau interferometer, the optical intensity at the photodetector is proportional to the square of the sum of the two E vectors impinging on the detector. Let us take point **O** on the half-silvered mirror as the phase origin. Neglecting the half-silvered mirror thickness, we can write for the Twyman-Green/Michelson interferometer:

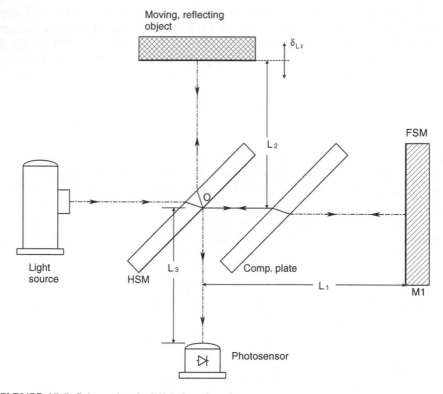

FIGURE 15.5 Schematic of a Michelson interferometer.

$$e_r(t) = E_{Ro} \sin[2\pi v t + 2\pi(2L_1 + L_3)/\lambda] \qquad\qquad 15.20$$

$$e_m(t) = \eta E_{Ro} \sin[2\pi v t + 2\pi(2L_2 + L_3)/\lambda] \qquad\qquad 15.21$$

Where the lightwave frequency $v = c/\lambda$ Hz, the distances are defined in Figure 15.5, and $\eta < 1$ represents the fraction of incident light reflected back to the detector. The intensity at the detector is proportional to $[e_r(t) + e_m(t)]^2$. That is,

$$1_d \propto \left(E_{Ro}^2/2\right)\left\{1 - \cos\left[4\pi\left(vt + 2L_1 + L_3\right)/\lambda\right]\right\}$$

$$+ \eta^2\left(E_{Ro}^2/2\right)\left\{1 - \cos\left[4\pi\left(vt + 2L_2 + L_3\right)/\lambda\right]\right\} \qquad\qquad 15.22$$

$$+ 2E_{Ro}\eta E_{Eo} \sin\left[2\pi vt + 2\pi\left(2L_1 + L_3\right)/\lambda\right]\sin\left[2\pi vt + 2\pi\left(2L_2 + L_3\right)/\lambda\right]$$

Because the detector does not respond to the double light frequency terms, Equation 15.22 reduces to:

$$l_d \propto \left(E_{Ro}^2/2\right)\left(1+\eta^2\right) + \eta E_{Ro}^2\left\{\cos\left[4\pi\left(L_1 + L_2\right)/\lambda\right]\right.$$
$$\left. - \cos\left[4\pi vt + 4\pi\left(L_1 + L_2 + L_3\right)/\lambda\right]\right\}$$

15.23

Again, the double light-frequency term drops out, and we have:

$$l_d \propto \left(E_{Ro}^2/2\right)\left(1+\eta^2\right) + \eta E_{Ro}^2 \cos\left[4\pi\left(L_1 - L_2\right)/\lambda\right]$$

15.24

Using the cos(A − B) = [cos(A)cos(B) + sin(A)sin(B)] identity, we can write:

$$l_d \propto \left(E_{Ro}^2/2\right)\left(1+\eta^2\right) + \eta E_{Ro}^2\left\{\cos\left(4\pi L_1/\lambda\right)\cos\left(4\pi L_2/\lambda\right)\right.$$
$$\left. + \sin\left(4\pi L_1/\lambda\right)\sin\left(4\pi L_2/\lambda\right)\right\}$$

15.25

Now we adjust L_1 so that $\cos(4\pi L_1/\lambda) \to 0$ and $\sin(4\pi L_1/\lambda) = 1$. We can now consider a small sinusoidal skin vibration at frequency f_s and peak amplitude, $\delta_{L2o} < \lambda/4$:

$$L_2(t) = L_{2o} + \delta_{L2o}\sin(2\pi f_s t)$$

15.26

Thus:

$$l_d \propto \left(E_{Ro}^2/2\right)\left(1+\eta^2\right) + \eta E_{Ro}^2 \sin\left\{\left(4\pi/\lambda\right)\left[L_{2o} + \delta_{L2o}\sin\left(2\pi f_s t\right)\right]\right\}$$

15.27

Using the sin(A + B) = [sin(A)cos(B) + cos(A)sin(B)] trig identity, we can finally write:

$$l_d \propto \left(E_{Ro}^2/2\right) + \eta^2\left(E_{Ro}^2/2\right) + \eta E_{Ro}^2\left\{\sin\left(4\pi L_{2o}/\lambda\right)\cos\left[\left(4\pi\delta_{L2o}/\lambda\right)\sin\left(2\pi f_s t\right)\right]\right.$$
$$\left. + \cos\left(4\pi L_{2o}/\lambda\right)\sin\left[\left(4\pi\delta_{L2o}/\lambda\right)\sin\left(2\pi f_s t\right)\right]\right\}$$

15.28

The $\cos(\xi \sin(2\pi f_s t))$ and $\sin(\xi \sin(2\pi f_s t))$ terms can be represented as Bessel functions (Stark, Tuteur and Anderson, 1988), thus:

$$\cos\left[\xi\sin\left(2\pi f_s t\right)\right] = \sum_{n=-\infty}^{\infty} J_n(\xi)\cos\left(n2\pi f_s t\right)$$

15.29

$$\sin\left[\xi\sin\left(2\pi f_s t\right)\right] = \sum_{n=-\infty}^{\infty} J_n(\xi)\sin\left(n2\pi f_s t\right)$$

15.30

Where $\xi \equiv (4\pi\delta_{L2o}/\lambda)$. Thus, the electric output of the detector contains dc terms, a fundamental frequency term (at f_s), and harmonics (at nf_s, $n \geq 2$). The dc terms can be eliminated by a high-pass filter, but there is no way to eliminate the harmonics; however, they will be small for small ξ. Thus, the output of the Michelson interferometer is nonlinear, even with a reflecting object's small motion.

If the object motion is fast enough, there will also be a significant *Doppler frequency shift* associated with the lightwave frequency of $e_m(t)$. This shift can be expressed as a change in frequency of the e_m E vector:

$$e_m(t) = \eta E_{Ro} \sin[2\pi v_m/c)t + (2\pi v/c)(2L_2 + L_3)] \qquad 15.31$$

and

$$e_r(t) = E_{Ro} \sin[2\pi vt + (2\pi v/c)(2L_1 + L_3)] \qquad 15.32$$

Where $v_m \equiv v + \Delta v$. The Doppler shift is $\Delta v \equiv v(2\dot{L}_2/c)$ Hz. Now, ignoring light-frequency terms, the intensity is of the form:

$$1_d \propto \left(E_{Ro}^2/2\right)\left(1+\eta^2\right) + 2\eta E_{Ro}^2 \cos(A)\cos(B) \qquad 15.33$$

Where $A \equiv [2\pi vt + (2\pi v/c)(2L_1 + L_3)]$, and $B \equiv [2\pi v(1 + 2\dot{L}_2/c)t + (2\pi v/c)(2L_2 + L_3)]$. Using the identity $\cos (A) \cos(B) \equiv (^1/_2) (\cos(A - B) + \cos(A + B))$, we have:

$$1_d \propto \left(E_{Ro}^2/2\right)\left(1+\eta^2\right) + \eta E_{Ro}^2\left\{\cos\left[\left(2\pi v2\dot{L}_2/c\right)t + (4\pi v/c)(L_2 - L_1)\right] + \right.$$
$$\left. + \cos\left[4\pi vt + \left(2\pi v2\dot{L}_2/c\right)t + (4\pi v/c)(L_1 + L_2 + L_3)\right]\right\} \qquad 15.34$$

The second term in the $\{_*\}$ is dropped because it is twice lightwave frequency. The first term is at the Doppler shift frequency, Δv Hz, which is generally in the audio range and resolvable by the photosensor. We can now use the trig. identity, $\cos(C + D) \equiv (\cos(C)\cos(D) - \sin(C)\sin(D))$, to find:

$$1_d \propto \left(E_{Ro}^2/2\right)\left(1+\eta^2\right) + \eta E_{Ro}^2\left\{\cos\left[\left(2\pi v2\dot{L}_2/c\right)t\right]\cos+\left[(4\pi v/c)(L_2 - L_1)\right]\right.$$
$$\left. - \sin\left[\left(2\pi v2\dot{L}_2/c\right)t\right]\sin\left[(4\pi v/c)(L_2 - L_1)\right]\right\} \qquad 15.35$$

If the skin motion is sinusoidal so that

$$L_2 = L_{2o} + \delta_2 \sin(\omega_s t) \qquad 15.36$$

Then

$$\dot{L}_2 = \omega_s\delta_2 \cos(\omega_s t) \qquad 15.37$$

We set $L_1 = L_{2o}$, and after some mild algebra, we get the messy result:

$$1_d \propto \left(E_{Ro}^2/2\right)\left(1+\eta^2\right) + \eta E_{Ro}^2 \left\{\cos\left[\left(4\pi\delta_2/\lambda\right)\left(\omega_s \cos(\omega_s t)\right)t\right]\right.$$

$$\cos\left[\left(4\pi\delta_2/\overset{\xi}{\lambda}\right)\sin(\omega_s t)\right]$$

15.38

$$\left.-\sin\left[\left(4\pi\delta_2/\lambda\right)\left(\omega_s \cos(\omega_s t)\right)t\right]\sin\left[\left(4\pi\overset{\xi}{\delta}_2/\lambda\right)\sin(\omega_s t)\right]\right\}$$

The $\cos(\xi\sin(\omega_s t))$ and $\sin(\xi\sin(\omega_s t))$ terms in Equation 15.38 give rise to the motion-frequency Bessel function series of Equations 15.29 and 15.30. It is not known what sort of temporal modulation of the Bessel series the Doppler $\cos(\xi\omega_s t \cos(\omega_s t))$ and $\sin(\xi\omega_s t \cos(\omega_s t))$ terms will provide. For example, let us calculate the maximum Doppler shift for a peak sinusoidal skin deflection of 120 nm at 1 Hz, using a HeNe laser with $\lambda = 633$ nm. From above, $\Delta v_{max} = 2_{max}/\lambda$ Hz. So:

$$\Delta v_{max} = [2 \times 2\pi(1) \times 1.2 \times 10^{-7}/(633 \times 10^{-9})] = 2.38 \text{ Hz} \qquad 15.39$$

Thus, the peak Doppler shift is about three times the 1 Hz displacement frequency.

Hong and Fox (1993) reported on an "optical stethoscope" that used a 670 nm laser diode as a coherent light source with a Michelson (actually, a Twyman-Green) interferometer to sense skin vibrations. Their interferometer was housed in a metal box about 5 in. × 3.5 in. × 3.5 in.; its accoupled photodiode output was observed in real time on a digital oscilloscope with FFT spectrum analysis capability. A more refined version of this instrument was described by Hong (1994), in which he used a HeNe laser source and a fiber optic cable to impinge the light on the skin. In most of the phantoms and human subjects studied by Hong, object displacements were periodic at the heart rate, but displacements were in hundreds of μm rather than hundreds of nm. Thus, the Twyman-Green interferometer was well out of its ± λ/4 linear range, and the apparatus served only as a mixer to extract the light-wave Doppler shift frequency in the measurement beam. The Doppler frequency shifts extracted followed the shape of the *magnitude* of the time derivative of the pressure waveform in the phantom studies, as evidenced by the output of a frequency-to-voltage converter (VFC). (Apparently, the "skin" surface displacement of the phantom was proportional to the vessel pressure.) In human studies, Hong cites the peak displacement of the skin over the common carotid artery to be 510 μm over 86 ms. This is a velocity of 5.93×10^{-3} m/s, and the peak Doppler light-wave frequency is $\Delta v = 2 \times 5.93 \times 10^{-3}/633 \times 10^{-9} = 18.74$ kHz. Obviously, this output frequency will vary over the cardiac cycle. Because there is no way to sense the sign of Δv, the VFC V_o was determined by:

$$V_o \propto \Delta v \propto |\dot{L}_2| \propto |\dot{p}| \qquad 15.40$$

Thus, in summary, Hong's interferometer was apparently used as a Doppler mixer, not an nm distance measuring system.

15.4.4 Discussion

Interferometers are generally suited for precise displacement measurements of body surfaces when the range of deflection is < $\lambda/4$. When the surface is moving at a high frequency, the interferometer output contains many harmonics due to the $\cos(\xi\sin(\omega_s t))$ terms, and light-wave Doppler shift terms. They are better suited to measuring small, slow displacements, such as tooth drift in orthodontic research.

15.5 LASER DOPPLER VELOCIMETRY

15.5.1 Principles of Laser Doppler Velocimetry

Laser Doppler velocimetry (LDV) provides a "no-touch" means of measuring the linear velocity of fluids, including air, water, hydraulic fluid, and, for our purposes, blood. The Doppler effect is observed as a frequency shift in coherent monochromatic light waves reflected or scattered from particles moving in the fluid whose velocity is to be measured. As in the case of Doppler ultrasound used to measure blood velocity, the reflecting particles are the erythrocytes (RBCs) in the blood. However, unlike Doppler ultrasound, the return wave path is seldom colinear with the path from the laser source to the reflecting particle, P.

To understand how LDV works, let P move with a velocity **V**, which is to be measured. Refer to Figure 15.6, in which all vectors lie in the x-y plane. Define a *unit vector*, **i**, directed from the source S to P. Assume that $|\mathbf{V}|/c \ll 1$, so that relativistic effects are negligible. When **V** = 0, the number of wave fronts striking the object per unit time is

$$f_s = c/\lambda_s. \qquad 15.41$$

Where c is the velocity of light in the medium in which V is being measured, and λ_s is the wavelength of the source laser (f_s for a HeNe laser in plasma striking an RBC is (3 × 10^8/1.336)/632.8 × 10^{-9} = 3.5348 × 10^{14} Hz. n_p = 1.336 is taken as the refractive index of plasma). It is easy to show that the number of wavefronts hitting a moving RBC is:

$$f_p = ((c/n_p) - \mathbf{V}\cdot\mathbf{i})/\lambda_s \qquad 15.42$$

The *vector dot product* gives the RBC velocity component parallel to the *unit vector*, **i**. **i** points in a line from the source to the moving RBC. Thus, the wavelength apparent to the RBC is:

$$\lambda_p = c'/f_p = (\lambda_s c')/(c' - \mathbf{V}\cdot\mathbf{i}) = (\lambda_s c')/(c' - V\cos(\mu)) \qquad 15.43$$

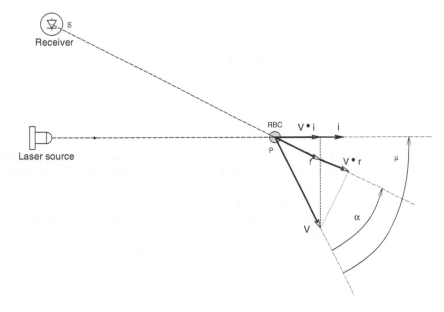

FIGURE 15.6 Vectors required to explain laser Doppler velocimetry (LDV). All vectors lie in the x-y plane (plane of the paper).

Where $c' = c/n_p =$ the velocity of light in the medium (plasma) in which the RBC is moving. Now the *unit vector,* **r**, points from the instantaneous position of the moving RBC, P, to the stationary receiver, R. An observer at R sees a scattered wavelength, λ_r, emanating from P. This is:

$$\lambda_r = (c' - \mathbf{V\cdot r})/f_p = [c' - V\cos(\alpha)]/f_p \qquad 15.44$$

The dot product, **V·r**, gives the velocity component of the RBC in the **r** direction. Thus, the frequency of the received, scattered, Doppler-shifted radiation is:

$$f_r = c'/\lambda_r \qquad 15.45$$

Substituting from Equations 15.44 and 14.45, we find:

$$f_r = c'(c' - \mathbf{V\cdot i})/[\lambda_s(c' - \mathbf{V\cdot r})] = f_s\frac{(c' - \mathbf{V\cdot i})}{(c' - \mathbf{V\cdot r})} \qquad 15.46$$

Now, if the f_s and f_r signals are mixed, and the difference term is examined, the Doppler shift is:

$$f_D \equiv \left(f_s - f_r\right) = \left(c'/\lambda_s\right) = \left[1 - \frac{\left(c' - \mathbf{V} \cdot \mathbf{i}\right)}{\left(c' - \mathbf{V} \cdot \mathbf{r}\right)}\right] \qquad 15.47$$

Now, because $V \ll c'$, Equation 15.47 reduces to:

$$f_D \equiv \frac{V\left[\cos(\mu) - \cos(\alpha)\right]}{\lambda_s} \quad \text{Hz} \qquad 15.48$$

For example, if $V = 0.1$ m/s, $\lambda_s = 632.8 \times 10^{-9}$ m, $\mu = 50°$, and $\alpha = 30°$, f_D is equal to -35.278 kHz. f_D is negative because the object is receding. There is no simple way to extract the sign of $\mathbf{V}$.

The mixing of the input and return (Doppler-shifted) signals can be thought of as occurring on the photocathode (PC) of the receiver photomultiplier tube (PMT). The transmitted and received light sinusoidal $\mathbf{E}$ vectors add linearly and vectorially at the PMT PC surface. However, the PMT responds to the net intensity of light at its PC surface. The intensity is proportional to the net, instantaneous, $\mathbf{E}$ vector magnitude squared. Thus, the PMT photocurrent can be written as:

$$i_p(t) = K_p \int \left|\mathbf{E}_s(t) + \mathbf{E}_r(t)\right|^2 dt \qquad 15.49$$

Where: $\mathbf{E}_s(t)$ is the electric field vector of non-Doppler-shifted laser source light of frequency c'/λ_s. $\mathbf{E}_r(t)$ is the sum total of Doppler-shifted, backscattered light electric field vectors. Thus, when the resultant $\mathbf{E}$ vector magnitude at the PC surface is squared, it gives terms with frequencies of $2f_s$, $2f_r$, $(f_s + f_r)$, $(f_s - f_r)$, and 0 (dc). Of course, the $f_D = (f_s - f_r)$ term is of interest. (Normally, the PMT responds to the 0 frequency terms, but, in this case, they are filtered out by a band-pass filter to select the distribution of f_D frequencies in $i_p(t)$.

15.5.2 LDV Applied to Retinal Blood Vessels

Figure 15.7 illustrates a simple geometry for sensing RBC velocity in the large blood vessels surrounding the head of the optic nerve (macula) at the rear of the eyeball. Measurement of the flow in these vessels is important in diagnosing glaucoma. The system is responsive to velocity vectors lying in a plane defined by the $\mathbf{i}$ and $\mathbf{r}$ vectors. The Doppler frequency shift from the component of RBC velocity lying in the $\mathbf{i}$-$\mathbf{r}$ plane can be shown to be equal to that derived in the section above. That is:

$$f_D \cong \frac{V\left[\cos(\mu) - \cos(\alpha)\right]}{\lambda_s} \qquad 15.50$$

Note that both angles, μ and α, must be known to obtain accurate velocity estimates. These angles are very difficult to estimate, so simple ocular blood vessel LDV lacks

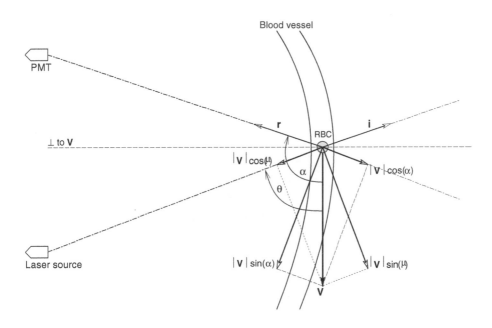

FIGURE 15.7 Vectors required to describe the application of LDV to retinal blood vessels. The vectors **i** and **r** define the plane in which the vectors lie.

accuracy. To overcome the uncertain angle problem, a system was designed by Feke et al. (1987) that uses two PMT receivers with their optical axes separated by a small fixed angle, γ. Figure 15.8 illustrates the vector geometry of their system in three dimensions. The RBC velocity vector **V** is described in a spherical coordinate system by its length, V, angle ϕ with the z-axis (vertical), and angle θ with the x-axis (horizontal). We assume that the input laser beam and the two receiver axes all lie in the x-y (horizontal) plane. The vector component of **V** in the x-y plane is relevant in finding the system output. The magnitude of this projection is $V_{xy} = |\mathbf{V}|\sin(\phi)$. For simplification, Figure 15.9 shows the relevant vectors in the x-y plane. As in the previous developments, the moving RBC at P "sees" an illuminating frequency, f_p:

$$f_p = \frac{c' + \mathbf{V}_{xy} \cdot \mathbf{i}}{\lambda_s} = \frac{c' + V_{xy}\cos(\pi - \mu)}{\lambda_s} = \frac{c' - V_{xy}\cos(\mu)}{\lambda_s} \qquad 15.51$$

A + sign is used in the numerator of Equation 15.51 because the object has a velocity component parallel with the **i** vector adding to the apparent light speed from the source. Thus, the wavelength of the laser light seen by the RBC is given by:

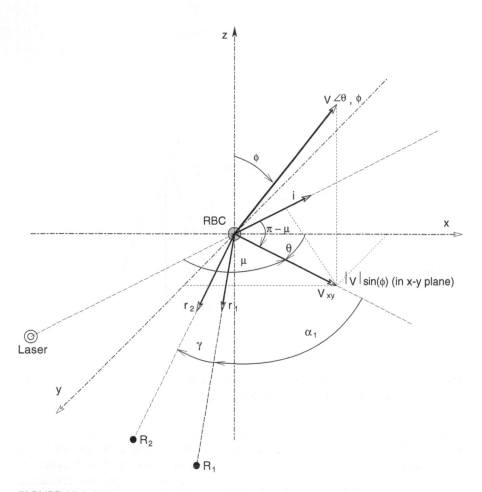

FIGURE 15.8 LDV vectors in 3-D space, following the system of Feke et al. (1987). The projection of the object velocity **V** into the x-y plane is **V**$_{xy}$.

$$\lambda_p = c'/f_p = \frac{c'\lambda_s}{c' - V_{xy}\cos(\mu)} = \frac{\lambda_s}{1 - (V_{xy}/c')\cos(\mu)} = \lambda_s\left[1 + (V_{xy}/c')\cos(\mu)\right] \quad 15.52$$

Note that there is a "red shift" (stretching of the perceived source wavelength) at a receding RBC. Now an observer at R_1 sees a scattered wavelength, λ_{r1}, emanating from the RBC.

$$\lambda_{r1} = \frac{c' + \mathbf{V_{xy}} \cdot \mathbf{r_1}}{f_p} = \frac{c' + V_{xy}\cos(\alpha_1)}{f_p} = \frac{\lambda_s\left[c' - V_{xy}\cos(\alpha_1)\right]}{c' - V_{xy}\cos(\mu)} \qquad 15.53$$

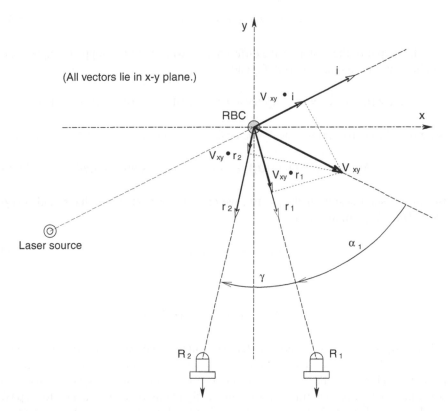

FIGURE 15.9 LDV vectors in the x-y plane. The laser and two detectors lie in the x-y plane.

Now, $f_{r1} = c'/\lambda_{r1}$, so:

$$f_{r1} = (c'/\lambda_s)\frac{1-(V_{xy}/c')\cos(\mu)}{1+(V_{xy}/c')\cos(\alpha_1)} \qquad 15.54$$

The Doppler frequency of the RBC at R_1 is found by mixing f_s and f_{r1} at the R_1 photocathode:

$$f_{D1} = (f_s - f_{r1}) = (c'/\lambda_s)1 - \frac{1-(V_{xy}/c')\cos(\mu}{1+(V_{xy}/c')\cos(\alpha} \qquad 15.55$$

If we assume that $(V_{xy}/c') \ll 1$, then Equation 15.55 reduces to:

$$f_{D1} \cong (V_{xy}/\lambda_s)\,[\cos(\alpha_1) + \cos(\mu)] \qquad 15.56$$

By the same development, we can show that:

$$f_{D2} = (V_{xy}/\lambda_s) \left[\cos(\alpha_1 + \gamma) + \cos(\mu)\right] \qquad 15.57$$

The output of the system is the difference between the two Doppler frequencies, obtained by mixing and filtering f_{D1} and f_{D2}.

$$\Delta f_D = (f_{D1} - f_{D2}) = (V_{xy}/\lambda_s) \left[\cos(\alpha_1) + \cos(\mu) - \cos(\alpha_1 + \gamma) - \cos(\mu)\right] \quad 15.58$$

Note that the $\cos(\mu)$ terms cancel. The $\cos(\alpha_1 + \gamma)$ can be expanded by trig identity:

$$\Delta f_D = (V_{xy}/\lambda_s) \left[\cos(\alpha_1) - \cos(\alpha_1)\cos(\gamma) + \sin(\alpha_1)\sin(\gamma)\right] \qquad 15.59$$

Because system design made $\gamma < 10°$, we can let $\sin(\gamma) \rightarrow \gamma$ in radians, and $\cos(\gamma) \rightarrow 1$. Thus Δf_D simplifies to:

$$\Delta f_D = (V_{xy}/\lambda_s) \, \gamma \sin(\alpha_1) \qquad 15.60$$

or:

$$V_{xy} = \Delta f_D \, \lambda_s/[\gamma \sin(\alpha_1)] \qquad 15.61$$

Where: Δf_D is measured, λ_s and γ are known, and now only α_1 needs to be estimated.

Figure 15.10 shows a very simplified schematic of the optical setup used by Feke et al. (1987). A flat, front-surface contact lens (a Goldmann-type fundus lens) was fitted to the eye to permit precise optical alignment. After attenuation to 18 μW, a collimated HeNe laser beam was directed at the large blood vessels surrounding the head of the optic nerve. The area illuminated was about $3.14 \times 10^4 \, \mu m^2$. The backscattered Doppler-shifted light rays were directed through two apertures to a pair of matched photomultiplier light sensors. The vergence angle on the sensor optics was 11.5°, which translates to an internal γ angle of 8.3° in an eye with normal vision (emmetropic eye). The Doppler frequency signals from the PMTs were processed by voltage-to-frequency converters (e.g., comparators, one shots, and low-pass filters), and their difference was used to estimate the $|V_{xy}|$ of RBCs in retinal veins and arteries using Equation 15.61 above.

Figure 15.11 was redrawn from a Figure 8 in Feke et al., 1987. It shows a plot of Δf_{Dmax} vs. time (one cardiac cycle) for a superior temporal retinal artery in the right eye of a normal subject, without the noise. Peak (systolic) velocity was 2.7 cm/sec; minimum (diastolic) velocity was 1.0 cm/sec. Corresponding Δf_Ds are shown on the vertical axis. Feke et al. calculate the mean blood flow rate in these retinal arteries from the formula:

$$\dot{Q}_s = \overline{V_{xy}} \, S/2 \quad cm^3/sec. \qquad 15.62$$

Where S is the cross-sectional area of the artery in cm^2, estimated from fundoscopy, and $\overline{V_{xy}}$ is the mean blood velocity in the vessel in cm/sec.

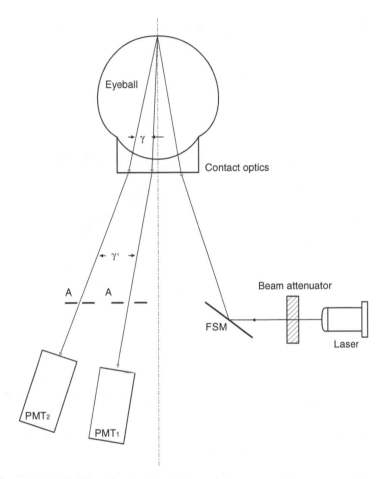

FIGURE 15.10 The Feke LDV system applied to an eye to measure retinal blood flow. A contact lens is required to match the refractive index of the cornea.

A commercial ophthalmic laser Doppler velocimeter, the Oculix 4000®, measuring V_{xy} in a 160 µm diameter spot on retinal vessels, is currently available (Boehm et al., 1999).

15.5.3 LDV Applied to Skin and other Tissues

At the time of this writing, several manufacturers make percutaneous LDV systems for experimental and diagnostic study of the microcirculation in the surface of various tissues. These instruments are generally called laser Doppler blood flowmeters, even though they respond to the velocity of erythrocytes in sub-dermal blood vessels. The noninvasive use of LDV systems includes measuring RBC velocities in blood vessels under the skin, in teeth, and in internal sites still considered to be NI, including the inner surface of the trachea, the colon, nose, rectum, esophagus, etc. Some of the companies that make LDV blood velocity systems are: Moor Co.

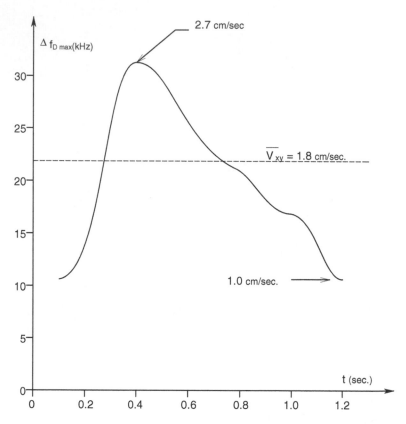

FIGURE 15.11 Representative plot of Δf_{Dmax} vs. time over one cardiac cycle for a retinal artery. (Based on data from Feke et al., 1987.)

(U.K.), Advance Co. (Japan), Kent Scientific Corp. (U.S.), Oxford Optronix Corp., Biopac Systems Corp. (U.S.), etc.

Most of these LDV systems use diode lasers that couple the laser light to the tissue and the Doppler-shifted backscattered light back to the photomultiplier, with optical fibers. Both source and output fibers are terminated in a small probe, not unlike that used in Doppler ultrasound applications. LDV probes have various sizes and shapes, depending on the application. Here, we will focus our attention on dermal circulation. Figure 15.12 illustrates some of the circulatory features of the skin. In the deep layers (4000 μm below the surface), we find horizontal networks of arterioles and venules. Closer to the surface (1000 to 4000 μm) are arteriovenous shunts under autonomic control and vertical branches of arterioles and venules. Just below the epidermis (150 μm) are extensive capillary beds running parallel to the skin's surface. The effective penetration of the input laser light depends on its wavelength, with red HeNe light (633 nm) penetrating between 0.6 and 1.5 mm. The HeNe beam allows the observance of blood Doppler signals from throughout the dermis, while blue argon (458 nm) laser light penetrates c. 250 μm, and so is responsive to the blood velocity in the upper subpapillary capillary plexus beneath the epidermis (Duteil et al., 1985).

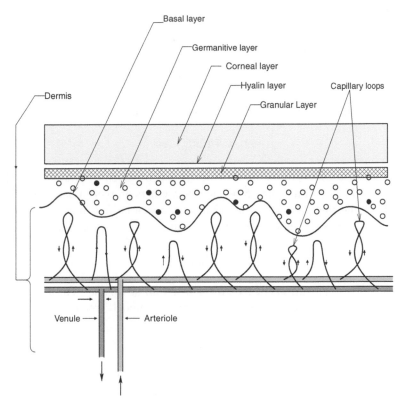

FIGURE 15.12 A highly schematic vertical section through human skin. Not shown are the hairs, sweat glands and ducts, and sensory nerves. Note that blood flow in larger vessels is parallel to the skin surface, while the smaller capillary loops carry vertical flow.

The laser illumination of many sub-epidermal capillaries, the paths of which are generally horizontal but nevertheless torturous, means that the RBCs in them are moving with a broad spectrum of angles {μ} and speeds with respect to the **i** vectors of the divergent rays from the optical input fiber. There is also a broad spectrum of **r** vectors that can pass into the acceptance cone of the pickup optical fiber. Thus, there is a broad low-frequency spectrum of Doppler frequencies generated by the skin's microcirculation.

Because the PMT photocurrent, $i_p(t)$, is a random signal derived from the random distribution of **i** and **r** vectors with respect to many RBCs moving in many different directions, it can be characterized by its two-sided *autocorrelation function*, $R_{ii}(\tau)$, and its *power density spectrum*, $\Phi_{ii}(f)$. ($\Phi_{ii}(f)$ is simply the Fourier transform of $R_{ii}(\tau)$; it shows how the power in the frequency spectrum of Doppler signals is distributed.) Duteil et al. (1985) describe and discuss mathematical models that describe the observed $\Phi_{ii}(f)$s seen in percutaneous LDV. They chose an exponential form to fit the measured autocorrelation functions:

$$R_{ii}(\tau) = \sigma_i^2 \, \exp(-|\tau|/\tau_D) \qquad\qquad 15.63$$

The two-sided power density spectrum thus has the Lorentzian form:

$$\Phi_{ii}(\omega) = \frac{2\sigma_i^2(1/\tau_D)}{\omega^2 + 1/\tau_D^2}$$

15.64

Where $(1/\tau_D)$ is the half-power frequency in r/sec, and:

$$\tau_D = 1/(2\pi f_D) \text{ sec}$$

15.65

Many of the LDV skin blood flow power spectra given by Duteil et al. (1985) do appear to be fit by Equation 15.64, however, others drop off more sharply at low frequencies and might be better modeled by exponential functions or simple rectangular hyperbolas (Hill functions) of the form:

$$\Phi_{ii}(f) = \Phi_{max} \, \varepsilon/(\varepsilon + f)$$

15.66

In addition to parameters of the power spectrum of Doppler return signals such as the half-power frequency, and the peak power (modal) frequency, a parameter known as the "flux" is also used:

$$\text{flux} = k_1 \int_{f_L}^{f_H} \frac{f\Phi_{ii}(f)}{I^n} df = k_2(\text{Ave. speed of RBCs})$$

15.67

$$\times (\text{Number concentration of RBCs})$$

The integral computes the normalized first moment of the PDS over bandwidth, $\{f_H - f_L\}$. I is the mean light intensity on the PMT, and n is an exponent, generally 2. If, instead of illuminating a small fixed subcutaneous voxel with a fiber optic probe, a laser beam in air is scanned over an area of skin with moving mirrors, a two-dimensional LDV plot of the subcutaneous blood flow can be constructed. The Doppler-shifted backscattered light propagates back through the same mirror assembly that scans the laser, through telescope lenses to the detector PMT. This type of LD imaging (LDI) system can be used on a whole torso, or on smaller skin surfaces such as a breast or a face. Here, left/right differences in velocity signature or local changes may signal asymetrical cerebrovascular disease or a tumor. LDI applications on the skin surface also include assessment of wound and burn healing, studies of angiogenesis in plastic surgery, and success in reattaching accidentally amputated limbs and appendages. Although accurate measurement of subcutanous blood flow is impossible with LDV and LDI, these techniques do allow precise comparisons between normal and abnormal skin circulation on a given individual, and allow quantitative measurement of how vasoactive drugs affect skin perfusion.

15.5.4 DISCUSSION

Laser Doppler velocimetry has the advantage over ultrasound velocimetry because it can measure blood velocity in extremely small vessels, such as capillaries in the skin and in mucous membranes, and also in larger vessels in the retina. The laser beam can be focused down to illuminate an area of only a few μm^2. The probe beam will penetrate only a few mm into the skin, so is suited to measure average blood velocity in the subdermal capillaries. Thus, LDV can be used to assess the angiogenesis that accompanies wound, burn, and skin-graft healing. LDV signals from the skin are very noisy, not because of laminar velocity in capillaries, but because the capillaries run in different directions and twist and turn. In an effort to treat LDV output signals quantitatively, autocorrelation and autopower spectrums are sometimes used.

15.6 TRANSCUTANEOUS IR SPECTROSCOPY

15.6.1 INTRODUCTION

Infrared light is electromagnetic radiation whose wavelengths are too long for human eyes to perceive. IR light wavelengths cover from 750 nm to over 1000 μm; the IR spectrum is subdivided somewhat arbitrarily into *near* (750 to 1500 nm), *intermediate* (1500 nm to 7 μm) and *far infrared* (7 to 1000 μm) (Barnes, 1983). (Different references differ slightly on their IR band definitions.)

Many biological molecules absorb IR energy in narrow bands of wavelength due to the transfer of energy from photons to the molecular bonds binding various molecular subgroups together, exciting the vibration and stretching of bonds connecting, for example, hydroxyl, methyl and amino radicals in various modes. Figure 15.13 illustrates the approximate wavelengths at which certain types of chemical bonds absorb photon energy (Young, 1996). These narrow absorption bands provide unique signatures that make *in vitro* IR spectrographic analysis effective, and offer many possibilities for identifying biomolecules *in vivo* through the skin, either by transmitted or backscattered IR light.

Often, IR absorbance or percent transmittance spectra are plotted vs. wavenumber in cm^{-1}. Wavenumber in cm^{-1} is related to wavelength in μm by: $WN = 10^4/\lambda$. When monochromatic light passes through a cuvette containing the analyte in solution, the intensity is attenuated exponentially. That is, by the Beer's law model,

$$I_{out} = I_{in} \, 10^{-\alpha(\lambda)L[C]} \qquad\qquad 15.68$$

If the input intensity is I_{in}, and the output intensity is I_{out}, the % $T \equiv 100(I_{out}/I_{in})$, and the absorbance, A, is defined as:

$$A \equiv \log_{10}(I_{in}/I_{out}) = 2 - \log_{10}(\%T) = \alpha(\lambda)L[C] \qquad\qquad 15.69$$

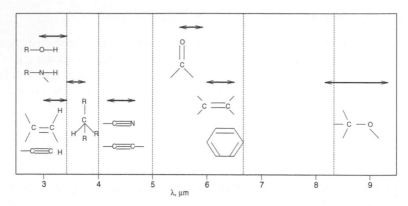

FIGURE 15.13 Wavelength bands where certain molecular groups selectively absorb IR photon energy. Absorption bandwidth depends in part on the presence of other nearby groups and the solvent.

A depends on the wavelength-dependent *molar absorptivity* (*molar extinction coefficient*), $\alpha(\lambda)$, the concentration of the analyte, [C], as well as the optical path length, L. The absorbance is also called the *Optical Density* (OD).

One of the better known uses of NIR light is in the two-wavelength pulse oximeter used to measure the oxygen saturation of hemoglobin in the capillaries. (Pulse oximetry is described in detail in Section 15.8.) A general problem in applying IR spectroscopy to percutaneous measurements is the absorption and attenuation of IR intensity by skin (stratum corneum and other layers), skin pigment, fat cells, and water in extracellular tissues, all of which can overwhelm the absorption by the targeted analyte. Water absorbs IR strongly between 5.5 and 7 µm and also around 2.7 µm, and beyond 25 µm (Barnes, 1983).

A very active area of research at present is the development of a noninvasive transcutaneous IR (TIR), blood glucose sensor. The perfection and FDA approval of such an NI device will revolutionize the management and care of persons with diabetes mellitis and other glucoregulatory dysfunctions. By analyzing the intensity of backscattered IR light at two or more wavelengths, it is theoretically possible to estimate blood glucose concentration from the glucose absorption signature. Such a device would need to have a two-point calibration based on actual blood samples from the individual using it. The IR can come from LEDs, tunable IR diode lasers, from a globar IR source passed through a grating monochromator, or even the blackbody radiation from deep body tissues (at c. 310° K). (Recall that Section 8.2.2 described dispersive spectroscopy and Beer's law.) When non-dispersive IR spectrophotometry is used, an interference-type optical band-pass filter selects the input band from a broadband IR source such as an incandescent filament lamp. For reasons of noise reduction, all radiation sources are chopped to permit synchronous detection (e.g., with a lock-in amplifier). Transduction of the backscattered light can be done with one sensor that covers the IR wavelengths used. This can be an InGaAs photodiode (covers 0.9–2.6 µm), a HgCdTe photodiode (covers 2–11 µm) or a pyroelectric IR sensor (covers 2–25 µm). Pyroelectric sensors have lower temporal signal bandwidths than photodiodes. IR sensors are often thermoelectrically or cryogenically cooled to reduce noise and improve IR photon detection efficiency.

Many medically important molecules theoretically can be measured by transcutaneous IR (TIR) spectroscopy. These include: cholesterol, cocaine, codeine, diacetyl morphine (heroin), ethanol, glucose, morphine, Δ^9-tetrahydrocannabinol, other opioids, etc. Many of these molecules have unique absorption peaks in the range from 6.5 to 14 μm.

Complications arise in TIR measurements because everyone's anatomy is different in terms of skin thickness, pigment, vascularization, fat deposits, etc. To make TIR spectrophotometric measurements, we need body parts with high vascularization, thin skin, low pigment and low fat. For transmission TIR measurements, the earlobes and the webs between the fingers are suitable. For backscattered light, the tissues under the fingernails, the thin skin on the medial surface of the forearms, the tongue, and the lips offer possible sites.

15.6.2 DIRECT MEASUREMENT OF BLOOD GLUCOSE WITH IR SPECTROSOPY

At present, the only practical and inexpensive means to measure blood glucose is the finger-prick blood drop on chemical strip, colorimetric analysis (FPCA) method. Because obtaining a blood sample requires breaking the skin, the FPCA method is mildly invasive, causes discomfort and the risk of possible infection. Couple these "cons" with the fact that Type II , to try to achieve normoglycemia, often have to test their blood four or more times a day to adjust their diet, insulin dose and exercise. Clearly, an accurate glucose-measuring system is needed that is truly noninvasive and can be used as many times as needed without pain or risk. In Section 15.7, we describe one possible NI means of estimating blood glucose using the natural optical rotation of linearly polarized light by glucose molecules in the aqueous humor of the eye. In this section, we consider the use of IR absorption by glucose molecules in tissues under the skin. For reference, Figure 15.14 illustrates an IR percent transmittance spectrogram of pure anhydrous glucose (dextrose). The glucose powder was suspended in nujol. Note the three evenly spaced absorption peaks at c. 11.0, 12.0 and 13.0 μm; also, there are smaller peaks at c. 8.7, 9.0, and 9.6 μm (not shown). In the body, in blood, cells and interstitial fluid, glucose is dissolved in water and surrounded with proteins, lipids, etc., that significantly change the character of its percent transmittance spectrum.

Between the strong IR absorbance regions for water, there are three "windows" that permit *in vivo* NIR absorption spectroscopy to proceed with minimum interference from water absorption:

1. The *combination region*, from 2.0 to 2.5 μm (5000–4000 cm⁻¹)
2. The *first overtone region*, from 1.54 to 1.82 μm (6500–5500 cm⁻¹)
3. The *short wavelength NIR region*, from 0.7 to 1.33 μm (14,286–7500 cm⁻¹)

Glucose also has measurable NIR absorbance peaks at 1.61, 1.69, 1.73, 2.10, 2.27 and 2.32 μm (Burmeister et al., 1998).

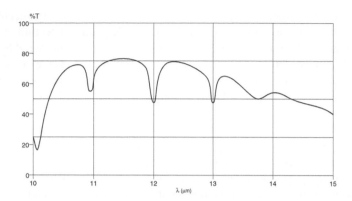

FIGURE 15.14 Percent transmittance of anhydrous glucose in the range from 10 to 15 μm.

One of the first *in vitro* studies of IR spectroscopy of whole blood using an *attenuated total reflection* (ATR) prism was reported by Kaiser (1979). Kaiser first made a percent transmittance spectrogram of distilled water over 2.5 to 20 μm. Then, citrate-buffered blood was scanned with a conventional spectrometer using a 25 μ cell, and again using the ATR prism in direct contact with the blood. Finally, a tunable CO_2 laser IR source was used in a two-beam ATR spectrometer to resolve ethanol from glucose in the 1060 to 1030 cm^{-1} range. Measurement sensitivity for glucose and ethanol was c. 3.5 mg/dl, or 35 ppm. (Normal fasting blood glucose concentration is c. 100 mg.dl.)

Another *in vitro* study that demonstrated that the concentration of glucose in whole blood could be measured accurately by IR absorption was reported by Mendelson et al. (1990). They first made an IR percent transmittance spectrogram of distilled water over a wave-number range of 1900 cm^{-1} to 800 cm^{-1} (5.26 μm to 12.5 μm wavelength) using an ATR prism. An ATR prism (or plate) is an optical surface-effect device used to couple the source IR energy to the sample where absorption occurs. An entering beam of IR energy reflects back and forth between the ATR plate's inner surfaces. Mendelson et al. used a ZnSe, IR-transmitting ATR plate that was 20 mm × 50 mm × 3 mm thick. There were 17 internal reflections of the IR beam before it exited (see Figure 15.15). The refractive index, n_1, of the ZnSe is approximately 2.42 for 9.66 μm light; n_2 of water is 1.33. (n is the ratio of the speed of light *in vacuo* to the speed of light in the medium at a given wavelength.) With water as the absorbing medium, Mendelson et al. calculated that the penetration depth of the light at the interface was only 1.3 μm at λ = 9.6 μm. They passed the sample (water or blood) over both flat surfaces of the ATR plate. When Mendelson et al. used whole human blood as the sample with glucose added to give 10 g/liter (10 × higher than normal blood glucose), definite absorption "wiggles" were seen in the spectrogram between 1000 and 1200 cm^{-1}. By subtracting the percent transmittance spectrum for distilled water, and expanding the wavenumber scale, a very sharp absorption peak was observed (% T went from c. 90 down to 66.5) at 1035 cm^{-1} (9.663 μm). This wavelength was also available from an 8 W, tunable, CO_2 laser. Mendelson et al. built a single-wavelength ATR-based blood glucose measuring system around their CO_2 laser source; they chopped the beam at 193 Hz, and used a pyroelectric IR detector to sense the emergent beam. A reference channel was used to compensate for laser intensity fluctuations. Because the output power of the CO_2 laser was 3 W (c. 10^3 to 10^5 times the power from a standard IR spectrophotometer), and the CO_2 laser has a spectral line width that is between 10^{-3} to 10^{-6} cm^{-1} (vs. 1 to 10 cm^{-1} for a grating monochromator), the *in vitro* measurement of blood glucose with the ATR plate was quite accurate. Mendelson et al. (1990), used pig blood samples doped with glucose between 90 and 270 mg/dl and plotted relative absorption vs. glucose concentration [G] in mg/dl (measured with a YSI Model 23A, "gold standard" electrochemical glucose analyzer). The regression line was RA = 0.64 + 1.37×10^{-3} [G]. The correlation coefficient was r = 0.98, and the standard error of the estimate (SEE) was 0.001. Mendelson and co-workers pointed out that the non-zero intercept (0.64) was due to the other absorbing substances in the blood; whole blood is a biochemically complex substance.

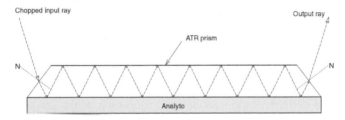

FIGURE 15.15 An ATR prism.

15.6.3 TRANSCUTANEOUS IR MEASUREMENT OF GLUCOSE

To achieve a truly noninvasive means of estimating blood glucose concentration, the measurement must be made through the skin without direct contact with the blood. From the success described above with ATR plates in direct contact with blood, it was suggested by Kaiser (1979) that an ATR plate could be placed over lip tissue to measure glucose absorption in the underlying vascular tissue. Heise et al. (1999) attempted to measure tissue glucose by its absorbance spectrum using an ATR prism pressed against the tissues of the inner lip. IR from 1750 to 750 cm^{-1} (5.71 to 13.3 μm) was used. Heise et al. found that there was no good correlation between the spectral features measured and the subjects' measured blood glucose concentration. This is probably because the evanescent light from the ATR prism scarcely penetrates the stratum corneum into the underlying vascular tissue layers. The ATR method works with direct blood contact because glucose molecules are at the prism's surface(s).

Blank et al. (1999) made a study of diffuse reflectance from tissue in the forearm using NIR light in the range from 1.05 to 2.45 μm. A custom-built scanning NIR spectrophotometer was used with a sampling interval of 1 nm. Indium-gallium-arsenide detectors were used. The authors claimed an SNR of 90 dB at the peak (reflectance intensity). The authors concluded:

"The results reported here lead to a cautious optimism that noninvasive glucose measurement using NIR spectroscopy in the 1050-2450 nm range is possible." ... "Many
factors, including variations in skin surface roughness, variations in measurement
location, skin hydration on the surface and [in] underlying tissue, the effect of tissue
displacement (contact pressure) by the [fiber optic] probe interface, and variations in
skin temperature can contribute to significant changes in the sampling of the tissue
volume elements. Parameters that are internal to the tissue sample may not be control-
lable but their impact on the measurement must be compensated".

The big problems with the glucose measurements of Blank et al. were consis-
tency, repeatability and the maintenance of calibration. In fact, many workers who
have tried the transcutaneous NIR spectrophotometric approach using either transmitted or reflected light conditioned by passing through vascular tissue have encountered these same problems.

Burmeister et al. (1998) claimed that an effective human tissue phantom for the
finger web can be made from a water layer of 5.0 to 6.3 mm, and a fat layer of 1.4
to 4.2 mm thick. The water in such a phantom can contain dissolved glucose, and
the phantom can be "tuned" as a reference for a given subject. Burmeister and co-
workers concluded:

"Successful noninvasive clinical measurements [of glucose] require the ability to collect
reproducible noninvasive spectra from human subjects. Between run variations must
be avoided in the thickness, composition, and temperature of the sampling site. This
demand for spectral reproducibility makes the human-to-spectrometer interface critical.
The temperature of the interface must be controlled to minimize thermal induced
spectral shifts. The compressibility of human tissue further complicates the interface
which must fix the amount and thickness of the tissue being sampled while avoiding
excess pressure which can degrade tissue integrity."

Thus, we see that, to obtain consistent accurate readings, the interface-to-tissue
geometry must be preserved from measurement to measurement, and the optical
path length in the tissue must also be as long as possible and remain constant during
a measurement, and from measurement to measurement. The tissue chosen to measure, and the optical and mechanical details of the spectrophotometer/tissue interface
appear to be critical

The idea of using vascular body tissues in place of a cuvette in a dispersive NIR
spectrophotometer was patented by Dähne and Gross (1987). Their system used the
earlobe. A patent is not a research paper, so the performance of the instrument
described was not evaluated. In 1989, Schlager patented a non-dispersive correlation
NIR spectrophotometer (see Section 8.2.3 of this text) designed to measure tissue
glucose, again in the earlobe. By placing an IR mirror at the back of the earlobe,
glucose absorption resulting from two passes through the lobe was obtained. The
principal advantage of this instrument's architecture is that it does not require an
expensive NIR monochromator. After passing the broadband light from the source
through the tissue, the beam is imaged on a slit, then the slit (as a source) is refocused
on a beamsplitter. Half the beam energy is passed through a *negative correlation
filter* (NCF), i.e., a cuvette, containing a glucose solution that absorbs strongly at

the glucose absorption wavelengths. Light emerging from the NCF is sensed by a lead sulfide IR sensor. The other half beam from the tissue sample is passed through a neutral density filter (NDF), thence to a (matched) lead sulfide sensor. Figure 15.16 illustrates the Schlager system, and shows the necessary chopper. Note that this is a proposed NI glucose sensor architecture that needs clinical evaluation. The tissue phantom devised by Burmeister et al. (1998) may be useful as the NCF in a Schlager-type non-dispersive NIR spectrophotometer.

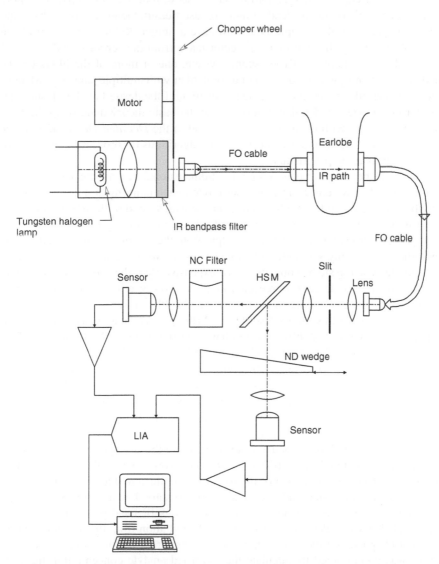

FIGURE 15.16 Schematic of a proposed non-dispersive IR spectrophotometer used to measure glucose concentration in earlobe tissue. (Based on a system patented by Schlager, 1989.)

A relatively new spectrophotometric approach to the measurement of blood glucose uses the *Kromoscopy* system architecture (Sodickson and Block, 1994, 1995). Kromoscopy is simply a non-dispersive technique in which broadband IR is passed through the sample (*in vitro* or *in vivo*). The emergent beam is split into four equal-intensity beams using three half-silvered mirrors, or beamsplitters; each separate beam is then passed through a particular broadband optical band-pass filter, thence to an InGaAs IR photodiode. The transmittance curves of the four filters overlap at their edges. There is nothing sacred about four detection channels; more channels could theoretically lead to more robust measurements. A given absorbing chemical species in the sample is said to have a unique *Kolor vector* (sic) as the result of processing the four-element vector made from the sensor signals.

In other aspects of the Kromoscopic system, one or more of the filters can be made narrow band-pass, band-reject or a comb filter with multiple narrow passbands. Such complex filters can aid in the discrimination of the desired analyte from other interfering analytes. A detailed description of the basic theory underlying the Kromoscopic system, with examples, can be found in the *Detailed Description of the Invention* of Sodickson and Block (1995). The algorithms for processing the detector outputs appear to be proprietary.

It should be noted that a similar multidimensional Kolor-type vector can be generated with a system using NIR laser diodes, each emitting at a different wavelength. (The wavelengths are chosen to coincide with several of the absorption peaks and valleys of the analyte being measured.) After normalizing for the intensity of each laser, the transmitted or reflected output from the sample can be sensed by one photodiode, assuming sequential chopping is used. No filters are required. Such a laser diode based system would be more expensive than the Kromoscopy system with its simple incandescent source and four filters; however, it may be more accurate and robust because of the narrow emission bandwidths of the lasers.

Finally, it is worthwhile to describe the MIR spectroscopic measurement blood glucose using the 310° K blackbody radiation of the body as the IR source. First, the tissue containing the glucose to be measured must itself be at a temperature less than the 310° source, or else no absorption spectrum will be seen. If, at 310°, the sample will radiate only as a blackbody (Klonoff, Braig et al., 1998), Figure 15.17 shows the spectral emission of an ideal blackbody, calculated using Planck's radiation equation, at 25°, 36°, 37° and 38° C. Note that the peaks are at about 10 μm, and W_0 is down to 10% of the peak at c. 4μm.

Braig et al. (1997) described a means to measure the absorption of certain blood analytes in U.S. Patent # 5,615,672, using the body's own 310° K blackbody radiation as a source. The medial surface of the forearm was illustrated as the source/analyte for the system. The system did not use a monochromator, but, as in the Kromoscopy approach, a filter wheel was used containing various IR band-pass filters; a single cryo-cooled HgCdTe detector was used. The IR radiation from the object (forearm) was first chopped and then filtered, before impinging on the detector. A microprocessor was programmed to calculate the estimated analyte concentration from the detector outputs for the various filters. It should be pointed out that this system works only because there is a temperature gradient from the 310° K core of the

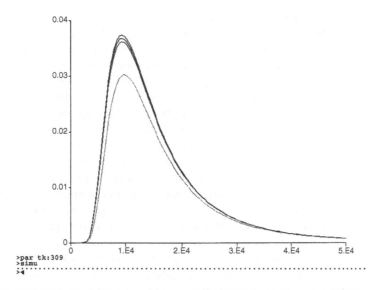

FIGURE 15.17 Theoretical energy spectrum of an ideal blackbody at 25, 36, 37, and 38° C (the top curve is for 38° C). W_λ units are (watts/m^2)/nm. Note linear scales.

forearm, and the skin (298° K). The absorption from the analyte in capillaries immediately underlying the skin would provide the system's signal.

Klonoff et al. (1998) tested the invention of Braig on human subjects. The system, built by Optiscan Biomedical Corp, was reported to estimate blood glucose (verified by the YSI blood glucometer) with an $r^2 = 0.94$ and an overall standard error of 24.7 mg/dl. (The relative glucose absorption around 9.8 μm was examined.) This performance needs improvement before clinical application of the instrument. This type of instrument will always be bothered with sequential non-repeatability and the need for calibration when used on different individuals and on the same individual at different times; the exact site on the skin, the skin temperature, the optical distance, etc., all need to be controlled.

M.J. Block was awarded U.S. patent # 6,002,953, 1999, for Noninvasive IR Transmission Measurement of Analyte in the Tympanic Membrane. In Block's system, the 310° K blackbody IR from the inner ear acts as the radiation source for a cooler eardrum (tympanic membrane).

The tympanic membrane is oval in shape, contains many fine blood vessels, and is about 100 μm thick with an area of c. 40 mm^2. It consists of three anatomical layers:

1. On the outside, a thin skin layer without papillae
2. On the inside, a thin layer of simple, cuboidal ciliated epithelium
3. In the center, a layer of radial fibers of connective tissue, and a layer of circularly ordered connective tissue fibers

It is the connective tissue layers that give the eardrum its stiffness. The tympanum is also supplied with pain-sensing nerve endings. Block cooled the eardrum by exposing it to a heatsink consisting of a thermoelectrically cooled element inserted into the ear canal. Eardrum temperature reduction is by radiation from the eardrum to the chilled element, and by conduction to air molecules in the ear canal. The sensing elements can be a cluster of four miniature MIR-sensing photodiodes covered with appropriate miniature optical band-pass filters, forming a Kromoscopy system. IR radiation from the inner ear passes through the cooler vascular tympanic membrane, where absorption of photon energy occurs at certain wavelengths depending on the concentration of analytes in the blood, including glucose. The emergent radiation from the tympanic membrane can be analyzed by a four-channel Kromoscopy system, as described above, or can be passed to another dispersive or non-dispersive spectrophotometer outside the ear canal by direct focused radiation, or by an MIR-conducting optical fiber. A problem with the use of the tympanic membrane to measure blood glucose is that it is thin, and from Beers' law, the resultant short optical path length produces a poor signal-to-noise ratio. Also, it is a mechanical challenge to chop the output radiation in the ear canal. Because the peak of the natural stable 310° K blackbody radiation is from 7 to 13 µm, the complex absorption peaks of glucose from 7 to 10 µm can be used, as well as its three single peaks at 11, 12 and 13 µm. When working in the MIR, one needs special optics: gold-plated mirrors; IR transmitting lenses such as Ge, Irtran, or plastic Fresnel lenses; special MIR conducting optical fibers; and detectors such as pyroelectric or cryo-cooled HgCdTe sensors. It will be interesting to see if Block's tympanic membrane system, when developed, is accurate and robust enough for use as an NI blood glucose measurement instrument.

15.6.4 DISCUSSION

All of the systems described above are ingenious, and their development to FDA-approved versions faces all of the problems cited. At best, such systems might be adjusted to work with a given individual after a two-point calibration using drawn blood and a gold-standard YSI glucometer. Repeatability will always be a problem because of anatomical differences over a given body region, and changes in instrument placement geometry. At this writing, just one fairly reliable means for personal monitoring of blood glucose exists; the unpopular fingerprick-chemical-strip-colorimetric method.

While this section has focused on the measurement of glucose using transcutaneous IR light, the reader will recall other intrinsic analytes in blood that IR absorption/transmittance/reflection techniques may be able to measure, including cholesterol. Extrinsic drug molecules that show promise for NI transcutaneous IR spectroscopic measurement include ethanol, cocaine, THC, etc. However, because of the problems of individual anatomical differences in skin and underlying tissues (fat, blood vessels), reliable calibration and repeatability remain overwhelming obstacles.

15.7 ESTIMATION OF BLOOD GLUCOSE FROM NI MEASUREMENT OF OPTICAL ROTATION OF THE AQUEOUS HUMOR (A PROTOTYPE SYSTEM)

15.7.1 INTRODUCTION

Over the past two decades and more, a number of researchers have tried to develop effective accurate sensors for blood glucose measurement to aid in the management of diabetes mellitus. Most of these sensors require samples of a body fluid such as blood or interstitial fluid, and are, by nature, invasive. More recently, attention has been given to the development of truly noninvasive blood glucose measurement means. One such approach has attempted to use the wavelength-selective absorption or transmission of NIR light by glucose in vascular tissues.

Another approach, which was followed by the author and his graduate students, was first described by March (1977), March et al., 1982; Rabinovitch et al., 1982. March and Rabinovitch realized that the *aqueous humor* (AH) in the anterior chamber of the eye could be used to estimate blood glucose (BG) concentration. The glucose concentration of AH follows that of the BG with a few minutes' time lag, and at about an 80% level. They proposed to measure the optical rotation (OR) of a beam of linearly polarized light directed through the anterior chamber of the eye. This optical rotation is mostly due to the glucose dissolved in the AH. Hence, measurement of the OR should enable an estimate of the blood glucose concentration to be made. The approach of March and Rabinovitch made use of the fact that aqueous solutions of glucose are *optically active,* i.e., they rotate the vibration axis of the **E** vector of transmitted linearly polarized light by an angle given by the simple relation:

$$\phi = [\alpha]_\lambda^T \, L \, C \qquad\qquad 15.70$$

Here, L is the optical path length through the solution, C is the concentration of the optically active solute (i.e., glucose), T is the Kelvin temperature, λ is the wavelength of the light, and $[\alpha]_\lambda^T$ is the specific rotation constant in degrees/(cm path length times concentration unit); α is both temperature- and wavelength-dependent. In general, the magnitude of $[\alpha]_\lambda^T$ increases as the wavelength gets shorter. $[\alpha]_\lambda^T$ can have either sign (L or D optical rotation), depending on the solute.

If more than one optically active solute is in solution together, the net rotation is given by the relation below, which implies linear superposition of optical activities:

$$\phi = \sum_{k=1}^{N} [\alpha]_{\lambda k}^{T} \, C_k L \qquad\qquad 15.71$$

Finding the concentration of the desired substance under this condition can be as simple as assuming the other optically active constituents are at negligible or constant concentrations, or it may require N measurements of ϕ at N different λs. From the

N simultaneous equations, C_1 ... C_N can be solved for using Cramer's rule, the N measured ϕs, and the N^2 known $[\alpha]_{\lambda k}^{T}$.

The author and certain of his graduate students have developed a prototype NI instrument to measure the optical rotation of glucose in the AH. The small rotation caused by the glucose in the AH was accurately measured in the presence of "confounders," i.e., other optically active substances in the AH, and the birefringence of the cornea in an optical model eye.

Browne (1998) built a proof-of-concept optical model system that has demonstrated the validity of our instrument design. This prototypical noninvasive electro-optical instrument hopefully will lead to the development of an inexpensive approved medical instrument that will allow diabetics to quickly, accurately, and painlessly estimate their blood glucose concentrations. The chemical composition of AH has been well described (de Berardinis et al., 1965). D-glucose is known to be the principal optically active substance in the AH that rotates linearly polarized light (Rabinovitch et al., 1982) Thus, a means of measuring the optical rotation of the AH can be used to estimate blood glucose concentration.

Our prototype system used an improved microdegree ocular polarimeter based on the original design by Gilham (1957). (Gilham's original system is shown in Figure 15.18.) We developed this microdegree polarimeter as part of a Phase I SBIR research project in 1995; it is applied to the noninvasive measurement of the optical rotation caused by D-glucose in the AH. In our configuration of the instrument, a beam of monochromatic linearly polarized light of innocuous intensity is polarization-angle-modulated by a Faraday rotator, then directed through the cornea, the pupil, the AH, and is reflected off the front surface of the lens. The reflected beam emerges from the eye with a greatly reduced intensity, and an additional small optical rotation due to other optically active substances in the AH, and the birefringence of the cornea.

The emergent beam is directed to a polarizer/analyzer, P2, and thence to a photomultiplier light sensor. Details of the operation of the modified closed-loop Gilham-type polarimeter are given below. A schematic of the proposed system is shown in Figure 15.19. Browne (1998) demonstrated theoretically and physically, with a model system, that there is a restricted range of entry angle relative to the gaze vector over which the system will work.

15.7.2 The Open-Loop Gilham Microdegree Polarimeter

The heart of the ocular polarimeter for blood glucose estimation is the modified Gilham polarimeter developed by the author and graduate students Aidan Browne and Todd Nelson. Before describing the operation of the modified closed-loop Gilham polarimeter, it is important to understand how an open-loop Gilham polarimeter works. Figure 15.20 illustrates the open-loop system.

Linearly polarized monochromatic light is derived by passing collimated monochromatic polarized light from a source through a high-quality Glan calcite polarizer, P1. Polarizers P1 and P2 have extinction ratios of $> 5 \times 10^4:1$. P1 and the laser source are aligned so that the linearly polarized electromagnetic **E** vector vibrates

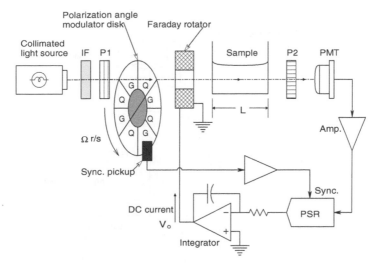

FIGURE 15.18 Schematic of Gilham's original closed-loop microdegree polarimeter. PSR = phase-sensitive rectifier. Square-wave polarization angle modulation was done by the rotating disk that had alternating windows of glass and polarizing quartz.

in the XZ plane at a frequency $\nu = c/\lambda$ Hz as it propagates with velocity c. This linearly polarized light is next passed through a *Faraday rotator* (FR). The FR consists of a dense glass rod with optically polished and antireflection (AR)-coated flat ends. An axially directed magnetic **B** field passes through the axis of the rod. The linearly polarized electromagnetic light waves interact with the material of the rod and the axial B field (**B_z**) to cause a total optical rotation, θ_{mo}, as they exit the rod (Hecht, 1987). The total **E** vector axis rotation is given by the relation:

$$\theta_{mo} = V\, B_z\, L \qquad\qquad 15.72$$

Where V is the rotator material's *Verdet constant,* which is material-, temperature-, and wavelength-dependent. In general, V increases with decreasing wavelength. **B_z** is the mean Z axis component of the magnetic field (parallel to the *Poynting vector*), and L is the length the light travels in the Faraday rod and B field. Practically all transparent liquids (e.g., water) and solids (e.g., glass) exhibit the Faraday magneto-optic effect. That is, they can rotate the axis of the **E** vector of linearly polarized light when subjected to an axial magnetic field.

In the open-loop Gilham polarimeter, the Faraday rotator is used to sinusoidally modulate the axis angle θ_m of the emergent **E** vector. This modulation is accomplished by passing an audiofrequency ac current through a solenoidal coil wound around the Faraday rotator rod. This current causes the axial B field to vary as $B_z(t) = B_{zo}\sin(2\pi f_m t)$. Thus, from Equation 15.72, the polarization angle of the emergent **E** vector varies as:

$$\theta_m(t) = (V\, L\, B_{zo})\sin(2\pi f_m t) = \theta_{mo}\sin(2\pi f_m t) \qquad\qquad 15.73$$

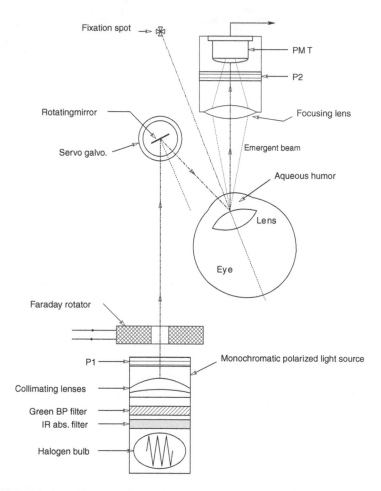

FIGURE 15.19 Optical layout of a proposed ocular polarimeter that can measure the optical rotation of the aqueous humor in the eye which is largely due to glucose. This measurement of glucose in the AH can be used to estimate blood glucose. The sinusoidal polarization angle modulation of the incident beam is done by the Faraday rotator. The moving mirror is to align the beam; it is stationary during a measurement. P1 and P2 are linear polarizers, PMT = photomultiplyer tube.

System parameters are chosen so θ_{mo} typically ranges from 1° to 3°. The modulation frequency, f_m, can range from 20 Hz to 2 kHz, depending on coil design.

After modulating the angle of the **E** vector of the LPL light emerging from the Faraday rotator, the light is passed through an optically active (e.g., glucose) solution, where the **E** vector picks up a fixed clockwise rotation, ϕ_s, from the D-glucose in solution following Equation 15.71. From Figure 15.20 we see that the **E** vector of the polarized light emerging from the sample cuvette swings sinusoidally from $(\phi_s - \theta_{mo})$ to $+ (\phi_s + \theta_{mo})$ in the XY plane. The next critical optical element in the open-loop Gilham polarimeter is the calcite analyzer polarizer, P2.

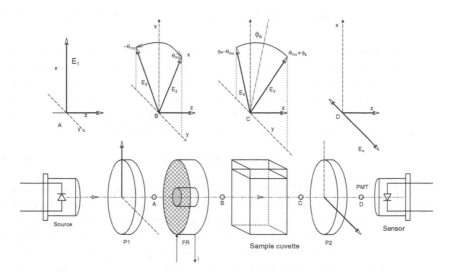

FIGURE 15.20 Schematic of an open-loop Gilham polarimeter. The Faraday rotator sinusoidally modulates the polarization angle of the input beam. Mathematical analysis of this system is in the text.

The pass axis of polarizer P2 is adjusted to be exactly 90° from the input beam **E** vector axis, along the y axis. If we assume P2 is an "ideal" polarizer, then only the y-component of the **E** vector at point C emerges from P2 at D. The peak amplitude of $\mathbf{E}_x$ at D is $\mathbf{E}_4$. By *Malus' law*, the peak E_4 is given by:

$$E_4(t) = E_{4o} \sin[\phi_s + \theta_{mo} \sin(2 \pi f_m t)] \qquad 15.74$$

The irradiance of this beam, i_4, is proportional to $E_4{}^2$ (Hecht, 1987). Thus:

$$i_4(t) = E_{4o}^2 \left(c\varepsilon_o/2\right)\sin^2\left[\phi_s + \theta_{mo} \sin\left(2\pi f_m t\right)\right] \quad \text{Watts}/\text{m}^2 \qquad 15.75$$

Now by trig identity, $\sin^2(x) = (1 - \cos(2x))/2$, so

$$i_4(t)E_{4o}^2 \left(c\varepsilon_o/2\right)\left[1 - \cos\left\{2\phi_s + 2\theta_{mo} \sin\left(2\pi f_m t\right)\right\}\right]\bigg/2 \qquad 15.76$$

The photosensor output is proportional to the irradiance; thus:

$$V_D(t) = K_p i_4(t) = K_p E_{4o}^2 \left(c\varepsilon_o/2\right)\left[1 - \cos\left\{2\phi_s + 2\theta_{mo} \sin\left(2\pi f_m t\right)\right\}\right]\bigg/2 \quad 15.77$$

Since the cos(*) angle argument is small, i.e., $|2(\phi_s + \theta_{mo})| < 3°$, we can use the approximation, $\cos(x) \cong (1 - x^2/2)$ in Equation 15.77. Thus, the photosensor output can be written:

$$V_D(t) = K_p I_{4o}\left[\phi_s^2 + 2\phi_s\theta_{mo}\sin(2\pi f_m t) + \theta_{mo}^2\left\{1 - \cos(4\pi f_m t)\right\}\right] \qquad 15.78$$

Thus, in the photosensor output voltage we see 2 dc (average) terms, a sinusoidal term at the modulation frequency, f_m, whose amplitude is proportional to the unknown ϕ_s, and a double frequency cosine term. The phase-sensitive rectifier (PSR) (or lock-in amplifier) responds only to the fundamental frequency term. The dc photosensor output to the PSR is blocked by a simple RC high-pass filter. After suitable low-pass filtering, the PSR's dc output can be written:

$$V_L = K_L K_P I_{4o} 2\phi_s \theta_{mo} \text{ dc volts} \qquad 15.79$$

V_L is seen to depend not only on the unknown ϕ_s, but also on the beam intensity, I_{4o}, and on the depth of modulation, θ_{mo}. While θ_{mo} can be held constant, I_{4o} can be subject to considerable variation, especially from a non-stabilized laser source. It is this dependence on the constancy of I_{4o} that can be troublesome in open-loop operation. We show below that the type 1 closed-loop operation of the Gilham polarimeter yields robust results, including independence from certain system parameters, including I_{4o}.

15.7.3 DYNAMICS AND SENSITIVITY OF THE CLOSED-LOOP POLARIMETER

In the author's version of the closed-loop Gilham polarimeter, a dc current proportional to the dc error angle, ϕ_E, is fed back to the solenoid coil of the FR to produce a dc component of the magnetic field that causes a counter rotation of the **E** vector axis, ϕ_F, that exactly cancels the rotation, ϕ_s, caused by the sample. Thus, at any instant, the dc error angle is:

$$\phi_E = \phi_s - \phi_F \qquad 15.80$$

Figure 15.21 illustrates our modified closed-loop Gilham system shown measuring the optical rotation of a sample in a 1 cm cuvette. The average (dc) output of the PSR is now proportional to the error angle in optical rotation, ϕ_E. Nulling of the system occurs when $\phi_s = \phi_F$. The effective gain of the PSR is $2K_L K_P I_{4o}\theta_{mo}$. (The intensity I_{4o} is proportional to the source laser's beam intensity.) A first-order low-pass filter with dc gain =1 and time constant, τ_L, follows the PSR to extract its average output voltage, V_L. V_L is then input to a proportional + integral (PI) controller element to make the closed-loop system type 1 with zero steady-state error. The dc output of the PI element drives a voltage-controlled current source (VCCS) that sets the dc nulling current though the Faraday rotator solenoid coil. A high-voltage power op amp is used as the actual FR coil driver, supplying both the dc nulling current and the ac modulation current.

The block diagram of the system is shown in Figure 15.22. If we examine the closed-loop transfer function relating $V_o{}'$ to ϕ_s, we find that it has a quadratic

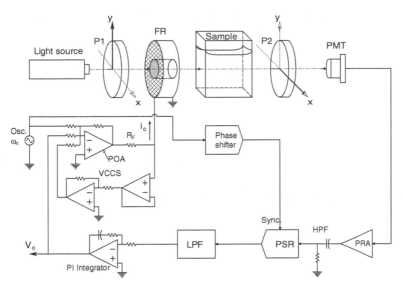

FIGURE 15.21 Schematic of the improved closed-loop Gilham polarimeter developed by the author. The same Faraday rotator is used for polarization angle modulation, and for dc feedback to automatically null the system.

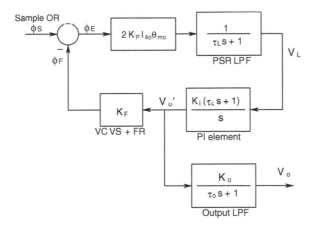

FIGURE 15.22 Block diagram describing the linearized dynamics of the polarimeter of Figure 15.21.

denominator. This transfer function can be used to describe the system turn-on transient, or the transient response of the system to transient changes in ϕ_s. It is:

$$\frac{V_o'}{\phi_s} = \frac{2\,K_p I_{4o}\theta_{mo}G_M K_i \left(\tau_c s + 1\right)/\tau_L}{s^2 + s\left(1 + 2\,K_p I_{40}\theta_{mo}G_M K_i \tau_c K_F\right)/\tau_L + 2\,K_p I_{4o}\theta_{mo}G_M K_i\, K_F/\tau_L} \qquad 15.81$$

From the transfer function above, we see that the closed-loop system has an undamped natural frequency of:

$$\omega_n = \sqrt{2\,K_p I_{4o} \theta_{mo} G_M K_i \, K_F / \tau_L} \quad r/s \qquad 15.82$$

And a damping factor:

$$\zeta = 1/(2\omega_n) + \tau_c/2 \qquad 15.83$$

In the steady state, the system's dc gain is simply:

$$\frac{V_o'}{\phi_s} = \frac{1}{K_F} \qquad 15.84$$

Equation 15.84 is a rather profound result because it tells us that determination of the steady-state ϕ_s does not depend on the laser beam intensity or the peak modulation angle, θ_{mo}, or certain other system constants. To be sure, the beam intensity and θ_{mo}, etc., must have values chosen for practical reasons for satisfactory robust system operation. Thus, only the physical factors affecting K_F affect system accuracy. By using a VCCS to drive the FR coil, the effect of coil resistance changing with temperature is eliminated. However, the Verdet constant of the FR glass rod is a function of temperature; the rod will be heated by the power dissipation of the coil. Unfortunately, there is no easy way to keep the FR glass rod temperature constant. If we measure the rod's Verdet constant's tempco, and put a temperature sensor in intimate contact with the rod, we can then compensate for temperature-caused changes in the Verdet constant. The system's steady-state sensitivity is independent of source intensity fluctuations and modulation depth, θ_{mo}, contributing to its robustness. However, electronic noise arising within the loop can degrade system resolution and accuracy.

A significant source of broad-band noise injected into the loop is from the photosensor and its signal conditioning amplifier. A wise choice of components, PSR filtering time constant, and further low-pass filtering of V_o' will help maximize the system signal-to-noise ratio. The closed-loop system should be designed to have a low ω_n (c. 12 r/s), and a damping factor lying between 0.5 and 0.707.

In bench tests of the self-nulling polarimeter, we found that its resolution was better than 150 microdegrees of optical rotation. The polarimeter was able to measure the optical rotation of aqueous D-glucose solutions in the physiological range of concentrations in a 1 cm cuvette with a LMS linear data fit having an $r^2 = 0.9986$. (The average rotation of a 100 mg/dl dextrose solution in a 1cm path at 633 nm wavelength was 4.53 millidegrees.)

15.7.4 APPLICATION OF THE MODIFIED GILHAM POLARIMETER TO THE MEASUREMENT OF THE OPTICAL ROTATION OF AQUEOUS HUMOR IN A MODEL SYSTEM

Figure 15.23 illustrates the modified Gilham system's components in the horizontal plane, illustrating how a monochromatic beam of linearly polarized light is directed into the eye, reflected off the front surface of the lens, and passed out through the cornea to the analyzer and photomultiplier. The input beam intensity is adjusted to be at an eye-safe level; bright, but not harmful.

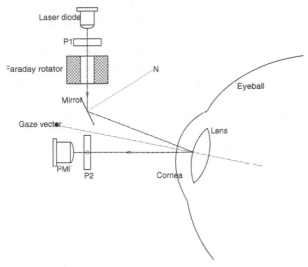

FIGURE 15.23 Simple optical architecture of the polarimeter applied to measuring glucose concentration in the AH.

Browne (1998) mathematically analyzed the optics of polarized light reflection at a dielectric reflecting surface, with particular attention to the AH of the eye and the front surface of the lens.

In discussing the optics of the reflection of linearly polarized light off plane surfaces, we first define the *plane of incidence*, which holds the incoming and reflected rays and the normal vector to the reflecting surface. In general, it is always perpendicular to the plane reflecting surface. For our purposes, we will define it as the XZ plane. A ray always propagates in the direction of its Poynting vector, here defined as the local y axis. In general, the unit vectors are related by the cross-product: $x \times y = z$. A simple planar surface diagram of the boundary and reflection is shown in Figure 15.24.

The reflecting surface is transparent and has an index of refraction, $n_2 = c/v_2$ (c is the velocity of light in free space, and v_2 is the velocity of light in the reflecting medium). Reflection occurs at the interface of aqueous humor with index of refrac-

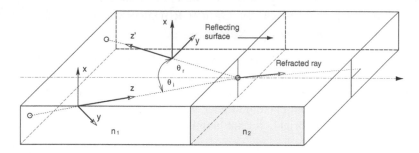

FIGURE 15.24 Relevant vectors describing how TEM linearly polarized light acts at a plane boundary between two transparent media with different refractive indices.

tion, n_1, and the reflecting front surface of the lens having index, n_2 ($n_2 > n_1$). The incident ray's **z** can be normal to the reflecting surface, but, more generally, it is at some angle β to the unit vector, **n**, which is normal to the reflecting surface at the point where the ray strikes it.

The incident **E** vector of the linearly polarized light can have a component in the y direction, which lies in the plane of incidence; this is called the *TM component* of **E**. The **E** component parallel with the x axis (and thus normal to the plane of incidence) is called the *TE component*.

We are interested in what happens to the intensity of the reflected ray at the n_1/n_2 interface, and what happens to its **E** vector when it reaches the corneal boundary. The n_1 medium (aqueous humor) is optically active because it contains glucose, hence the axis of the **E** vector of the incoming ray is rotated by a small clockwise angle, α. What happens to the reflected **E** vector depends on the incidence angle, θ_i, the initial angle of **E**, the optical rotation, α, and n_1 and n_2. In his analysis, Browne (1998) considered three input angle conditions: $\theta_i < \theta_B$, $\theta_i = \theta_B$, and $\theta_i > \theta_B$. θ_B is the Brewster angle (Sears, 1949), defined by

$$\theta_B \equiv \tan^{-1}(n_2/n_1)$$
15.85

When the **E** vector of linearly polarized light (LPL) of the input beam is all in the TM mode (**E** lies in the plane of incidence), there will be zero light intensity reflected when $\theta_i = \theta_B$. Browne assumed an arbitrary polarization angle with respect to the x axis; that is, the polarization angle of the input beam of LPL is ϕ just as it enters the n_1 medium. As it propagates to the n_1/n_2 boundary, the optical activity of the n_1 medium causes **E** to rotate an additional α degrees.

Thus, just before the reflection boundary, the incoming beam has a TM component (in the plane of incidence) of $E_o \sin(\phi + \alpha)$, and the TE component of **E** (in the x-direction) is $E_o \cos(\phi + \alpha)$ as the input wave strikes the n_1/n_2 boundary. In the reflected wave, the TE component of **E** undergoes an 180° phase change for all input angles. The TM component behaves differently depending on θ_i: For $\theta_i < \theta_B$, there is no phase change. For $\theta_i = \theta_B$, the reflected TM component = 0. For $\theta_i > \theta_B$, there is an 180° phase change in the reflected TM component of **E**. The bottom line of

Browne's analysis was that when $\theta_i > \theta_B$, the polarization angle of the ray emerging from the n_1 medium into air was shown to be $\beta = \phi + 2\alpha$. When $\theta_i < \theta_B$, $\beta = \phi$, i.e., there is no sensitivity to optical rotation; the outward rotation cancels the inward rotation. For a real eye, $\theta_B \cong 46.9°$.

Browne concluded:

> "A reflection angle relative to gaze normal [the gaze vector] anywhere in the range of fifty to fifty-five degrees is achievable for all cases. Over this range, the incident beam input angle can be any value in the range of fifty-five to sixty degrees, relative to gaze normal; this range is well within the limits of the Brewster angle on the low end and the maximum angle due to physical limitations on the high end.
>
> These results clearly show that the geometry of the eye is very tolerant of parameter changes in regard to light pathway through the anterior chamber."

Browne also considered the light intensity budget of the eye and the safe exposure energy for the retina. Calculable losses due to reflections occur at every boundary between two media with different refractive indices. At the lens, most of the light is refracted and sent to the retina; only a small fraction is reflected. Assuming 5 mW of 512 nm laser light enters the eye, about 6.1 µW exits the cornea as a result of reflection off the front surface of the lens. This amounts to an attenuation factor of 9.37×10^{-4}. Safety standards for laser light shone into the eye are quite strict (OSHA, 1996; FDA, 1996). The maximum power density that is considered eye safe at 512 nm is 2.5 mW/cm^2 for 0.25 seconds. This is the same as 25 µW/mm^2 over 0.25 seconds. Thus, if the laser beam has a diameter of 2 mm on the retina, its area is 3.14 mm^2, and the maximum beam power cannot exceed 78.5 µW for 0.25 seconds. This power translates to an output beam power from the eye of 95.8 nW for 0.25 seconds. This is adequate power for a photomultiplier tube to sense. If the modulation frequency, f_m, is 2 kHz, the phase-sensitive rectifier has a total of 500 modulation cycles to average to find $V_o' \propto \alpha$. If the SNR is poor, this may not be enough time to average out the noise.

To avoid the government safety restrictions on laser input power to the eye, the polarized light can be derived from a conventional tungsten (quartz-halogen) lamp. The light is filtered to exclude IR, bandpass filtered with an interference filter to define a narrow bandwidth, and then collimated. It is then linearly polarized and sent to the Faraday rotator, and thence to the eye. Optometrists' and ophthalmologists' ophthalmoscopes and slit lamps use high-intensity quartz-halogen lamps, and are considered safe for prolonged use in eye exams. Tungsten lamps are considerably less expensive than stable diode lasers, and are a viable alternative in configuring this type of instrument.

Browne evaluated the modified Gilham ocular polarimeter with an *analog model eye*. This eye was built with a glass meniscus lens "cornea" having a refractive index of 1.439. It was 0.8 mm thick at the center; 11.78 mm in diameter; front radius of curvature, 7.7 mm; rear radius of curvature, 6.8 mm. The inside apex of the meniscus lens was mounted about 3 mm from the outer apex of the inner lens. The plano-convex inner lens was made from SF5 glass; its front radius of curvature was 10.09 mm. Artificial aqueous humor containing various glucose concentrations could be introduced into the "anterior chamber" of the model eye. In one plot of V_o vs. glucose concentration over a range of zero to 3 grams/liter, the LMS linear fit to data had an $r^2 = 0.9989$, quite a good linear fit. These measurement were made using the full 6 mW output of the 512 nm diode laser.

In adapting this system to take accurate measurements from human eyes, the input light power will have to be seriously reduced, as discussed above. Also, the system will have to be calibrated for each user by taking several conventional finger-prick blood samples at different steady-state blood glucose levels along with V_o measurements. It will be a considerable challenge to develop a clinical and home version of this instrument.

15.7.5 DISCUSSION

In the preceding sections, we have described the prototype of a noninvasive, electro-optical system designed to enable diabetics to quickly, painlessly and frequently monitor their blood glucose concentration, and so adjust their intake of insulin or food and exercise to better achieve normoglycemia.

The present state of the art for home blood glucose monitoring requires taking a blood sample; no more than one or two drops of venous blood, using a small lancet or needle. Usually one of the finger tips or an earlobe is pierced. The blood drops are smeared on a chemically treated plastic strip, that, after about a 60-second reaction time, is read in a two-wavelength colorimeter, the output of which is the blood glucose concentration. This method strongly discourages frequent use by the patient, especially children, and has the following disadvantages:

1. The procedure is **invasive**. It provides a significant opportunity for infection in a population already predisposed to infections of the extremities.
2. The procedure is **painful**, especially when five or six pricks a day are required.
3. The procedure is **not accurate**. Accuracy can be off by as much as ± 20% relative to age and lot variations in the chemical strips, as well as changes in ambient temperature and non-adherence to a uniform testing procedure.
4. The procedure is **expensive**. While the monitors are generally inexpensive, as medical devices go, the manufacturers' profit is assured through the sale of the strips. A strip costs about 85 cents. Six strips a day times 365 days means that someone must pay about $1,862 per year for strips used in enhanced testing.

The overall objective of the research described has been to develop a prototype of an accurate noninvasive ocular polarimeter to estimate blood glucose concentration that will successfully replace the present finger prick-test-strip-colorimeter technology at a cost comparable to one year's supply of test strips. Any prototype instrument developed will have to undergo FDA approval before it can be marketed to help diabetics. To be marketable, it must have a reasonable cost, be easy to use, and have an accuracy better than the finger-prick method described above. A large market for the instrument exists — an estimated 16 million diabetics in the United

States alone, which is c. 6% of the population (NIDDK, 1999). Any accurate noninvasive glucose sensor would find an enormous potential market worldwide.

15.8 PULSE OXIMETRY

15.8.1 INTRODUCTION

Numerous medical procedures require a knowledge of the percent saturation of arterial blood hemoglobin with oxygen. Such procedures include childbirth (the baby), surgical anesthesia where the patient is artificially ventilated, any open-chest surgery where a heart-lung machine is used, treatment of obstructive lung diseases including pulmonary emphysema and acute asthma, the treatment of smoke inhalation and drowning, and general intensive care and surgical recovery.

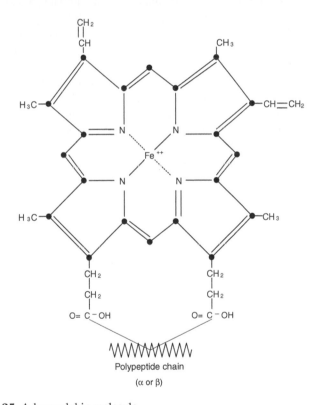

FIGURE 15.25 A hemoglobin molecule.

The molecular weight of hemoglobin (Hb) is c. 64,400 daltons. The hemoglobin molecule consists of four iron- (Fe^{++}) containing heme ring (shown in Figure 15.25) joined to two pairs of unlike polypeptide chains (the globins) to form a tetramer. The chains undergo conformational isomerization when the Hb molecule binds with oxygen. Initial binding of oxygen to Hb causes an *autocatalytic process* that facilitates the binding of oxygen to the three neighboring heme rings in a *heme–heme* interaction (West, 1985). About 15% of the blood by weight is hemoglobin contained inside the red blood cells (RBCs, aka erythrocytes). The total hemoglobin inside the RBCs (THb) can have one of four forms:

1. *Reduced (non-oxygenated) Hb* (HbR)
2. *Oxyhemoglobin* (HbO_2)
3. *Carboxyhemoglobin*, where Hb has combined with carbon monoxide (HbCO)
4. *Methemoglobin* in which the iron in the heme rings has oxidized to Fe^{+++} (metHb)

In the first three forms, iron is bound as Fe^{++}. Most of the THb is in the form of HbO_2 or HbR, the HbCO and metHb typically being < 1% of the THb. Pulse oximeters usually ignore the small amounts of metHb and HbCO and measure the concentration ratio between HbR and HbO_2 (Brown, 1980).

Hemoglobin in normal arterial blood is about 97% saturated with oxygen (97% HbO_2), and normal venous blood returning to the lungs contains about 75% HbO_2 (Guyton, 1991). Most pulse oximeters are ± 2% accurate in the normal physiological 70–100% oxygen saturation range. Pulse oximetry cannot distinguish between two pathological forms of hemoglobin: Carboxyhemoglobin (Hb combined with carbon monoxide), and methemoglobin. Pure carboxyhemoglobin (HbCO) reads 90% O_2 saturated Hb, and methemoglobin tends toward 90% O_2 saturation. A history and detailed analysis of optical blood oximetry can be found in the papers by Takatani and Ling (1994), de Kock and Tarassenko (1993), and Brown (1980).

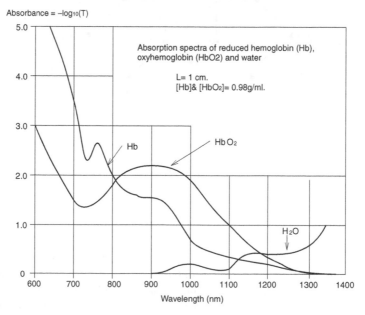

FIGURE 15.26 Optical absorbance of hemoglobin (reduced) and oxyhemoglobin (HbO_2) in the range from 600 to 1400 nm. Note the isobestic wavelength is at about 800 nm.

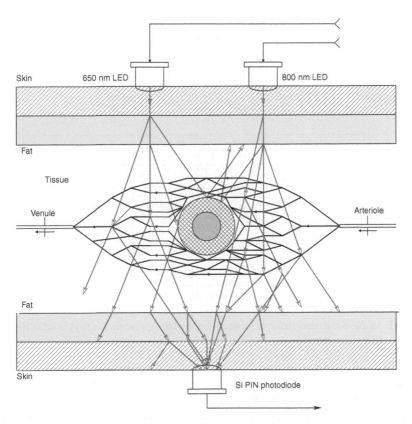

FIGURE 15.27 Schematic tissue cross-section showing representative rays in transmission pulse oximetry (TPOX). (The circular structure in the center can be a bone in a finger tip.)

15.8.2 PULSE OXIMETRY SYSTEMS

Transcutaneous *pulse oximetry* (TOX) is a noninvasive means used to estimate the percent O_2 saturation of peripheral blood hemoglobin using spectrophotometric techniques. Figure 15.26 illustrates the continuous optical absorbance (optical density) spectra of 100% O_2-saturated pure hemoglobin, reduced (deoxy-) hemoglobin (0% saturation), and water in a 1 cm cuvette vs. transmitted light wavelength. Note that, at a wavelength of about 800 nm, there is an *isobestic* point where the absorbance is the same regardless of the percent O_2 saturation of the hemoglobin molecules. The isobestic absorption depends only on the path length, L, and the Hb concentration, C. To spectrophotometrically measure PsO_2 of hemoglobin by TOX, it is not necessary to measure the entire absorbance spectrum. Generally, two light-emitting diodes (LEDs) are used, one in the NIR near the isobestic wavelength at 800 nm, and the other at c. 650 nm (red). In some oximetry applications, (red 650 nm) and IR on the long side (950 nm) if the isobestic wavelength have been used (de Kock et al., 1993).

While pure hemoglobin in a cuvette appears to obey the Beer-Lambert law governing optical absorption, hemoglobin in erythrocytes (RBCs) in whole blood

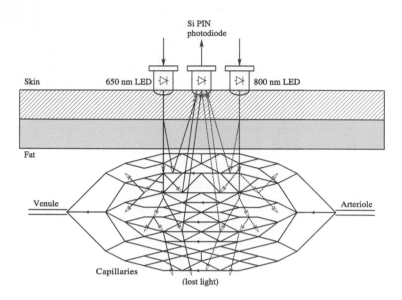

FIGURE 15.28 Schematic tissue cross-section showing representative rays in reflection pulse oximetry (RPOX).

does not (de Kock and Tarassenko, 1993), and nonlinear corrections must be made to obtain valid readings of the percent HbO_2 saturation (SpO_2). There is much scattering and reflection by the RBC membranes.

Two types of transcutaneous oximetry are possible: 1) The *transmission* or *forward-scattered* mode, in which light is passed through vascular tissue and collected at the other side with a photosensor. Tissues used for this application are the earlobe, finger tips, or toes. Figure 15.27 illustrates transmission pulse oximetry (TPOX) schematically. 2) The *reflection* or *backscattered* mode in which backscattered light is measured. This type of oximetry is used on cheeks, the forehead or the top of the head (infants during delivery). A schematic of reflectance pulse oximetry (RPOX) is shown in Figure 15.28. For either mode to work, the light must penetrate the skin, pass through layers of fat, connective tissue, muscle, capillary walls and erythrocyte (RBC) membranes at least twice. In addition, the light impinges on RBCs carrying hemoglobin at various degrees of SpO_2, depending on the capillary vascular anatomy, which can be variable among individuals, as is the blood flow rate through the capillaries. Thus, absorption is from an average of SpO_2 ranging from arterial inputs to venous outputs of the illuminated capillaries.

Most pulse oximeters are of the transmission type. As light propagates through the tissues, capillaries, and blood, it is attenuated and scattered. The useful information depends on the wavelength-dependent absorption by the mixture of Hb and HbO_2. Absorption is also dependent on the erythrocyte packing density in the blood (*hematocrit*) and the volume of blood in the capillaries. This latter factor gives pulse oximetry its name. At systole, peak blood pressure forces more blood (hence more RBCs) into the illuminated capillaries, thus absorbance varies in time, peaking at systole and reaching a minimum at diastole at the capillary bed. As well, at systole, RBCs carrying more HbO_2 enter the bed. Thus, in addition to a transient increase in absorber volume, there is a transient increase in HbO_2 at systole, and the voltage output wave-form from a pulse oximeter consists of a dc component plus a periodic wave that follows the systemic blood pressure with a slight lag due to propagation of the pressure wave through the arterial system. The components of optical absorption in tissues include:

1. Absorption due to skin, fat, bone and tissue
2. Absorption due to a fixed quantity of venous blood (c. 75% PsO_2)
3. A fixed component due to arterial blood (c. 97% PsO_2)
4. A variable, pulsatile, component due to arterial blood volume change

All but the first components are assumed to respond to Beer's law at the red (650 nm) wavelength, and have SpO_2-independent absorption at the 800 nm isobestic wavelength. Figure 15.29 illustrates how, with the concentration, C, and path length, L, being held constant, the absorbance of hemoglobin varies with SpO_2 at the red (650 nm) wave-length (i.e., essentially how the extinction coefficient, α_r, varies with SpO_2 at 650 nm. In the ideal case, it is a linear function of SpO_2 (dotted line), in practice, it probably is not (solid lines). To simplify the heuristic analysis below, we will assume that α_r varies linearly with PsO_2. That is:

$$\alpha_r = \alpha_{max} - m_r \overline{PsO_2}.\qquad\qquad 15.86$$

Where m_r is the magnitude of the slope of the linear approximation line, $\overline{SpO_2}$ is the average percent oxygen saturation of the illuminated, capillary blood, and α_{rmax} = α_{Hb}.

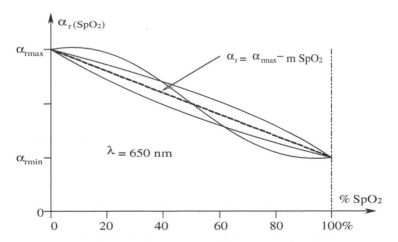

FIGURE 15.29 How the 650 nm extinction coefficient, α_{650}, of Hb varies with the SpO_2.

In most transmission-type pulse oximeters, two LEDs are used as nearly mono-chromatic photon sources; one is red (650 nm) and the other is at the near infrared isobestic wave-length (805 nm). The diodes are alternately pulsed in the sequence, red, NIR, dark. The dark interval is so that the oximeter can compensate for stray room light picked up by the photosensor. The photosensor is typically a silicon phototransistor or PIN photodiode, which has a peak sensitivity at about 770 nm. Sensitivity at 650 nm is about 0.9 the peak sensitivity in mA/mW.

To understand how an oximeter works, we first consider the case where there is no pulse, i.e., there is no time-variability of the absorbance due to pulsatile blood flow into the capillaries. First, let the red LED be on. The light that exits the earlobe or finger tip is attenuated by non-wavelength-dependent physical factors such as absorption by bone and tissues, as well as wavelength-dependent absorption by HbO_2 in the RBCs in the capillaries. The intensity of light exiting the earlobe can be approximated by Beer's law:

$$I_{or} = I_{inr} 10^{-(B_r + \alpha_r CL)} \qquad 15.87$$

Where α_r is the extinction coefficient for HbO_2 for red light (650 nm), C is the effective concentration of HbO_2, L is the mean path length, and B_r is the non-Hb absorption of tissues at 650 nm. The transmitted 650 nm light is collected by the PIN photodiode, converted to a proportional voltage, V_{ar}, by an op amp, and passed through a $\log_{10}(x)$ nonlinearity. These steps can be written:

$$V_{ar} = K_a I_{or} = K_a I_{inr} 10^{-(B_r + \alpha_r CL)} \qquad 15.88$$

$$V_{Lr} = K_L \log_{10}(K_a I_{or}) = K_L \log_{10}(K_a I_{inr}) - K_L (B_r + \alpha_r CL] \qquad 15.89$$

Now, let us substitute Equation 15.86 in Equation 5.89:

$$V_{Lr} = K_L \log_{10}\left(K_a I_{inr}\right) - K_L\left[B_r + CL\left(\alpha_{max} - m_r \overline{SpO_2}\right)\right] \qquad 15.90$$

Now the emerging light intensity from the 805 nm, LED is attenuated, but is independent of SpO_2. Its intensity can be written as:

$$I_{oi} = I_{ini} 10^{-B_i} \qquad 15.91$$

Now the NIR light is conditioned by a log amplifier as well. I_{inr} is made $= I_{ini}$.

$$V_{ai} = K_a I_{oi} \qquad 15.92$$

$$V_{Li} = K_L \log_{10}(K_a I_{oi}) = K_L \log_{10}(K_a I_{ini}) - K_L [B_i] \qquad 15.93$$

The oximeter's output is determined by subtracting V_{Li} from V_{Lr}:

$$V_o = (V_{Lr} - V_{Lr}) = K_L \log_{10}(K_a 1_{inr}) - K_L \left[B_r + CL(\alpha_{max} - m_r \overline{SpO_2}) \right]$$
$$- K_L \log_{10}(K_a 1_{ini}) + K_L (B_i)$$

15.94

Collecting terms, we have

$$V_o \cong (\overline{SpO_2})(K_L CL\, m_r) + K_L (B_i - B_r)$$

15.95

Equation 15.95 suggests that, if Beer's law were to hold, and the α_r extinction coefficient is a linear function of Hb SpO_2, then V_o will be a linear function of the average SpO_2 of hemoglobin in the capillary beds. In practice these ideal conditions do not occur, and V_o is a monotonically increasing, nonlinear function of $\overline{SpO_2}$. The actual $\overline{SpO_2}$ is found by a look-up table in the instrument.

A second complication of transmission pulse oximetry (TPOX) is the effect of the arterial pulse on V_o. At local systole at the capillary bed being studied, the rising blood pressure forces new, more oxygen-saturated RBCs into the capillaries, momentarily dilating them and raising the average SpO_2 in the illuminated volume. This action raises the effective concentration, C, of HbO_2, and the effective length, L, of the light path also increases slightly because the illuminated tissue swells with blood pressure. Hence, the output voltage from a typical pulse oximeter follows the peripheral blood pressure waveform. Thus, it can be used to measure heart rate and estimate blood pressure (after calibration), as well as estimate peripheral SpO_2.

Direct, accurate measurement of arterial SpO_2 appears to be impossible using TPOX in a clinical setting unless blood samples are taken to calibrate it. As we pointed out above, the effective SpO_2 in the illuminated capillary bed is an average of the levels of HbO_2 in the capillaries. This average is proportional to and lower than the arterial SpO_2. What can be relatively certain with a TPOX is that its sensitivity (i.e., output volts/SpO_2) is known and remains constant. The useful medical information obtained from a TPOX is that the $\overline{SpO_2}$ has dropped so many percentages from the initial (normal) value. Such a drop can be life-threatening, and generally signals the need for immediate corrective procedures.

Because the TPOX output is a periodic waveform that follows the brachial blood pressure wave-form (assuming a finger tip is used), several algorithms have been developed to read the average SpO_2. A common one is to sample the V_o waveform at some fixed threshold and do a running average of the samples. Another is to detect and sample the V_o peaks and average them. Still another is to sample the peaks and adjacent minima. A running average is calculated from the $(V_{opk} - V_{omin})/2$ series. As we pointed out above, the $V_o(t)$ waveform is due to volumetric and path length changes with BP, as well as SpO_2 varying with the cardiac cycle.

Reflection mode pulse oximetry (RPOX) has been used on body parts too thick for light transmission. Takatani and Ling (1994) described RPOX used to measure the mean SpO_2 of an infant's brain. RPOX has also been used to determine the SpO_2 in the blood vessels of the retina (de Kock et al., 1993).

Increased *hematocrit* (**H**) (the percent of blood volume that is RBCs) also has the effect of raising C in Beer's law (normal hematocrit is about 40%). Schmitt, Zhou and Miller (1992) developed a prototypical noninvasive *hematocrit measurement instrument* using two NIR isobestic wavelengths of Hb and HbO_2; 800 nm and 1300 nm. Its operation is very like a pulse oximeter. By measuring the optical density ratio, $\rho = OD_{800}/OD_{1300}$, of whole blood (*in vitro*), Schmitt et al. were able to plot a regression line: $\rho = 0.781 + 0.007389$ **H**, with a correlation coefficient r = 0.995 for $0 \leq \mathbf{H} \leq 100\%$. The fit was even better in the **H** range from 20 to 60%. Schmitt et al. tested their transmission-mode hemocritmeter on both a cuvette with whole blood and a more complex finger phantom. As in the use of pulse oximetry, their instrument was subject to uncertainties caused by skin pigmentation and other anatomical factors. Once this type of instrument is calibrated for a given individual, it would appear to be quite accurate.

15.8.3 Discussion

The modern pulse oximeter is a versatile noninvasive instrument. Often, an integrated oximeter front end containing the two LEDs, a silicon photodiode, and a connecting cable with connector is made disposable for clinical use. By adding a third LED emitting at 1300 nm, the oximeter can be adapted to measure not only SpO_2, but also hematocrit and pulse rate. We predict that the principle of measuring the absorbance of subcutaneous blood analytes at two or three wavelengths will eventually be extended to the transcutaneous measurement of analytes such as glucose, alcohol, heroin, etc., through the use of narrow-band laser diodes. Diode outputs can be conducted to the skin through fiber optic cables, and the transmitted or reflected light containing the information can also be collected and transmitted to a remote sensor by a fiber optic cable. The major problem with any transcutaneous optical system is individual variation in skin thickness and pigment, as well as variability in subcutaneous fat deposits and vasculature. This difficulty might be overcome if there were some blood analyte that is always fairly constant that could be used for normalization and calibration for an analyte — such as glucose.

At present, however, the state of the art is such that certain analytes can be measured transcutaneously with reasonable accuracy on a given individual, so long as the system is given a two-point "gold-standard" calibration using withdrawn blood samples (invasively taken). As soon as the measurement interface is moved or transferred to another patient, the system must be recalibrated.

15.9 NONINVASIVE MEASUREMENT OF CERTAIN BIOMOLECULES BY RAMAN SPECTROSCOPY

15.9.1 Introduction

Raman spectroscopy is based on the *Raman effect*, named for the Indian physicist C.V. Raman, who was awarded the 1930 Nobel prize for his discovery. In his seminal paper, published in the journal *Nature* in 1928, Raman observed that, when light interacted with matter, some small amount of its energy was scattered, and the frequency of the scattered light was shifted in a complex manner from that of the incident beam.

Since its discovery, the Raman effect has been developed into a sensitive analytical chemical tool with results that rival conventional spectroscopic techniques (UV, VIS, IR). The advent of monochromatic laser sources has expedited the rise of Raman spectroscopy as an analytical tool. In the past few years, Raman spectroscopy has been applied to various biomedical applications such as measuring various important analytes in blood and serum (Koo et al., 1999). Also, much attention has recently been given to developing noninvasive biomedical Raman systems (Hanlon et al., 2000).

Two kinds of Raman spectroscopy systems are currently in use: *conventional* and *stimulated*. Figure 15.30 illustrates a typical conventional *in vitro* Raman system. A high-power diode laser emitting in the NIR, typically at 830 or 850 nm, is used as the source. Its beam is chopped or otherwise amplitude-modulated to enable synchronous detection of the scattered light. NIR light is generally used to minimize any natural background fluorescence from a complex biological sample. (Recall that the shorter visible wavelengths and UV light excite fluorescence. See Section 15.3.) Most of the input light is elastically scattered (Rayleigh light) with no frequency shift by sample molecules. Inelastic (Raman) scattering in all directions occurs at about 10^{-8} times the intensity of the Rayleigh scattered light. Energy from the monochromatic input beam is absorbed in the process of exciting vibrations of the various interatomic bonds of the analyte. The Raman scattered (output) light thus has a complex spectrum depending on the chemical structure of the analyte(s). In general, the Raman shifts of the output spectrum are given by: $v_{in} - v_{scattered} = \Delta v_{Raman}$. Δv_{Raman} is also called the *Stokes shift*. The energy absorbed in the photon excitation of a particular interatomic bond resonance is proportional to the Δv_{Raman} of its spectral peak. That is, $E_{abs} = h \Delta v_{Raman}$.

To gather more of the weak Raman-scattered light, a parabolic mirror is often used near the sample. An *optical notch filter* is used to exclude light of frequency v_{in}. A holographic notch filter attenuates by c. 10^{-6} at the center of its stop band, and passes c. 90% of the input light at other wavelengths. The weak Raman light is passed through a dispersive spectrometer or monochromator that either projects the desired Raman spectrum on a linear CCD sensor array where the kth pixel intensity is proportional to Δv_{kRaman} , or light at a given Δv_{Raman} is directed onto a single photomultiplier sensor or some photodiode. For *in vitro* Raman spectroscopy, relatively large input intensities are used, typically in the hundreds of mW. Such high input power cannot be used for *in vivo* Raman measurements because of potential heat damage to tissues, including the retina.

Raman spectra are generally displayed in units of wave-number in cm^{-1}, which is proportional to the Hz frequency of the light. 1 cm^{-1} equals 3×10^{10} Hz, or 30 GHz. The frequency of 830 nm input light is $v_{in} = 3.61 \times 10^{14}$ Hz. Figure 15.31 shows the Raman spectrum of ethanol *in vitro*. Note the sharp signature peak at c. 800 cm^{-1}, and the two small peaks around 980 cm^{-1}. The conventional IR absorbance spectrum of a substance has the same peaks and peak spacing as does the Raman spectrum. Additional information is available from a Raman system in the form of the polarization of the scattered light. Peaks from non-polar chemical groups are

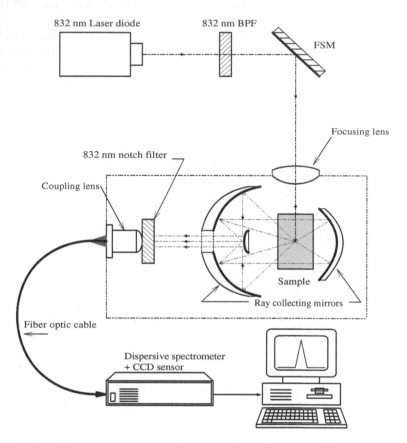

FIGURE 15.30 Schematic of an *in vitro* Raman spectrometer.

generally stronger in Raman spectroscopy, while the converse is true for conventional IR absorbance spectroscopy of the same analyte. Figure 15.32 illustrates both Raman and IR absorbance spectra from methanol. Notice that, in the two spectrograms, some congruent peaks are sharper and stronger than in the other spectrogram.

Stimulated Raman spectroscopy (SRS) is a technique that avoids the non-directional scattering of the frequency-shifted light emitted in conventional single-source Raman spectroscopy. In SRS, two lasers are used to excite the analyte — a pump laser and a tunable *probe laser*. The intersection of their beams defines an analyte volume. When the frequency (or wave-number) difference between the two lasers equals the $\Delta\nu_{Raman}$ of a Raman-active mode, there is an increase in the irradiance of the transmitted probe beam and a corresponding decrease of the irradiance of the transmitted pump beam. In one SRS system designed to sense D-glucose in biological samples, the $\Delta\nu$ between the pump and probe lasers is made to be the $\Delta\nu_{Raman}$ of a major glucose Raman peak, i.e., 518 cm^{-1} (Tarr and Steffes, 1993, 1998). (Recall that $\nu\lambda = c$, and the wave-number in cm^{-1} = 3.333×10^{-11} ν, ν in Hz.) The actual frequencies of the pump and probe lasers are not as important as the $\Delta\nu$ between

i

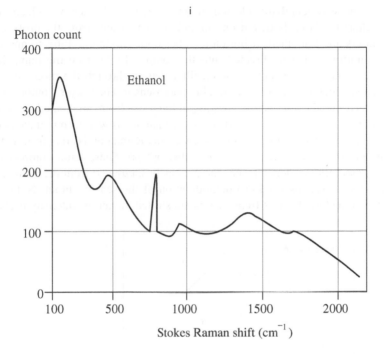

FIGURE 15.31 A sketch of the Raman spectrum of ethanol. (The actual curve has a ± 5 count noise added to it.)

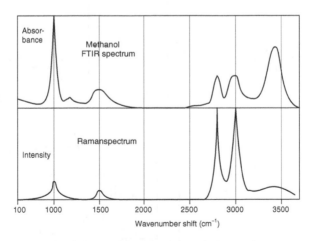

FIGURE 15.32 A sketch of the combined Raman emission and spectrometer absorbance spectra for methanol. Note wavenumber congruence in peak locations.

them. The pump frequency should be in the NIR, if possible, to avoid exciting intrinsic fluorescence of the specimen. The advantage of the SRS technique is that no expensive monochromator is used. As shown in Figure 15.33, the probe laser's output is both wavelength tunable and chopped, either mechanically or electronically, by switching the laser diode current on and off. The beams from the probe and the pump lasers are combined, using either fiber optic mixing or mirrors and a half-silvered mirror, and then directed into the sample. Light from the pump laser is greatly attenuated by an optical notch filter, letting through the modulated probe laser beam, which is directed to a suitable photosensor. The sensor's output contains a modulated signal component consisting of the probe beam attenuated as a function of the Raman-Stokes energy absorbed by the analyte, as well as modulated components from sample background fluorescence plus Raman emissions from the water solvent and from glass (cuvette, lenses, fiber optics). These latter components are artifacts with little Δv-dependence, and are easily subtracted from the desired signal following synchronous (lock-in) demodulation of the sensor output. Note that, in SRS, the probe laser beam's frequency is not shifted, rather, its intensity is changed.

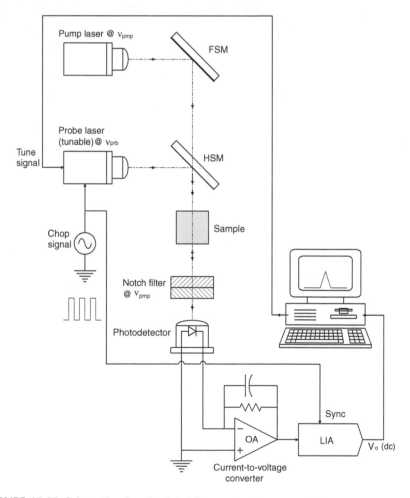

FIGURE 15.33 Schematic of a stimulated Raman spectroscopy system.

15.9.2 DIAGNOSTIC APPLICATIONS OF RAMAN SPECTROSCOPY

Most of the research and development to date on using Raman spectroscopy and SRS in noninvasive medical diagnosis has been in the form of *in vitro* studies on various biomolecules in solution, in blood and serum, and in excised non-living tissues. A comprehensive review of this active area of biomedical research can be found in the paper by Hanlon et al. (2000). For example, Salenius et al. (1998) did an *in vitro* study on the Raman spectra from the insides of samples of carotid and femoral arteries ranging from normal to those heavily affected by atherosclerosis. They looked for the Raman spectra from calcium deposits and cholesterol. Their results were well correlated with histological examination of the tissues, and demonstrated the feasibility of using the Raman approach *in vivo* as an invasive diagnostic procedure. Raman light would be conducted to the intravascular sites with a fiber optic catheter.

Because of its obvious importance in diabetes, the detection of glucose in blood, serum and in the aqueous humor of the eyes has been approached by a number of workers using Raman spectroscopy. In the 1993 U.S. patent of Tarr and Steffes, and in their 1998 paper, SRS is proposed to be used on the aqueous humor (AH) of the eye to sense glucose in the AH. It is known that the AH glucose concentration follows the blood glucose concentration with a lag and an attenuation factor. No one to date has done research on the dynamics relating AH glucose to blood glucose in humans, and how it may vary individually. What is assumed about this transfer function for humans has been deduced from animal data from the 1980s (Arnold and Klonoff, 1999). Thus, any measurement of AH glucose concentration, by whatever means, is an estimate of blood glucose based on a poorly known dynamic relation. Once the transfer function is known, then past AH glucose readings can be combined with the transfer function (assuming linearity, which I doubt) to more accurately find the present blood glucose concentration.

Tarr and Steffes' (1993, 1998) proposed SRS system to measure AH glucose concentration passed two coaxial SRS laser beams through the cornea from the side at an oblique angle so that they pass through the AH, across the front of the anterior chamber of the eye in front of the iris, and then exit obliquely. While not shown specifically in their patent and paper, the exit of the laser beams requires a coupling contact lens over the cornea with a refractive index greater than that of the cornea. Otherwise, the beams would remain trapped in the cornea because of the critical angle phenomenon (how fiber optic cables work to trap light in their cores). The need for the coupling contact lens was first appreciated by March (1977) and later by March, Rabinovitch and Adams (1982). The tangential anterior-chamber optical path may permit the use of higher optical power than ordinarily permitted for laser irradiation of the eye for diagnostic purposes, because only a small amount of Rayleigh- and Raman-scattered light would reach the sensitive retina over a large area. However, optical irradiation standards set by OSHA, FDA, etc., are set for any laser light entering the eye, regardless of path. Apparently, a practical approved *in vivo* SRS system using the aqueous humor will have to use about 1/00th the power of an *in vitro* system operating on blood or serum.

Another approach to the beam geometry problem is to use the reflection off the front surface of the lens as described by Browne (1998). Although the emergent beams will have net power on the order of 10s of nW, after filtering out the pump laser, the modulated probe beam can easily be measured with a photomultiplier sensor. Also, by chopping both the probe and pump laser beams, more peak input power can be used.

The simplicity of the SRS approach to glucose measurement in AH can be appreciated by the fact that glucose has a sharp peak in its stimulated Raman spectrum for a pump-probe laser wave-number difference of 512 cm^{-1} (Tarr and Steffes, 1993). Since only the AH glucose concentration is sought, the lasers do not need to be tunable.

Application of Raman spectroscopy to the measurement of glucose, cholesterol, triglyceri-des, urea (BUN), total protein and albumin in *in vitro* samples of human blood and serum (plasma) was reported by Berger et al. (1999). The excitation was a powerful 250 mW, 830 nm diode laser that was focused to a 50 μm diameter spot on the blood sample in a cuvette. The blood was stirred to reduce heating by the laser, but the samples were not cooled, nor were their temperatures measured. In spite of this casual attitude toward sample temperature, these authors obtained remarkably accurate results. One reason was that the Raman spectrum was dispersed into 1152 elements using a CCD array. The method of partial least squares was used to predict the concentration of each analyte. Further, they binned the CCD cells to form c. 8 cm^{-1} spectral resolution, and only the portion of the Raman spectrum between 565 and 1746 cm^{-1} was used. These authors' results on *in vitro* blood and serum samples showed that measurement of the six analytes listed above were more accurately done on serum than on whole blood. The signal-to-noise ratio of serum measurements was c. three times greater than for Raman spectrum measurements on whole blood. *In vitro* serum measurements were of acceptable accuracy for clinical use, however, a long 5 minutes was required to acquire and average the CCD pixel data to reduce noise in each of the six Raman spectra computed.

Hanlon et al. (2000) summarize various Raman studies done on the detection of breast cancer. They used principal component analysis in conjunction with logistic regression on spectra taken *in vitro* from biopsied breast tissue (normal and benign and malignant tumors). They found that out of 14 normal specimens, 14 benign and 33 malignant tumors, 31 malignant specimens were classified malignant, 2 malignant specimens were classified benign, 13 benign specimens were classified benign, 1 benign specimen was classified as normal and 14 normal tissue specimens were correctly classified as normal. Eventually, these workers propose to develop a fiber optic probe for invasive Raman breast tumor analysis.

Hanlon et al. also describe the application of Raman spectral analysis in the diagnosis of Alzheimer's disease (AD). In their own *in vitro* studies of AD by Raman spectroscopy, they found that, by subtracting an average normal Raman spectrum from one from a brain with AD, two characteristic peaks were seen at 940 and 1150 cm^{-1}. By using principal component analysis techniques, Hanlon and co-workers were able to discriminate 12 AD specimens from 5 normal spec-imens. They proposed developing a Raman instrument to detect AD in which a noninvasive fiber optic probe would be run up the nose c. 7 cm to the olfactory epithelium. IR laser light would penetrate the epithelium and the cribiform plate in the roof of the nasal cavity to illuminate the olfactory bulb (part of the CNS), where the spectrum would be formed.

15.9.3 DISCUSSION

We have seen that good *in vitro* results have been obtained measuring certain analytes in water, and blood plasma or serum. Mildly invasive procedures such as cystoscopy, broncoscopy and colonoscopy may provide a means to use Raman spectroscopy to examine lesions (candidate tumors) on the surface of the epithelium in these locations.

For noninvasive Raman spectroscopic diagnostic applications, the pump or excitation laser's energy must be introduced transdermally, and the very weak backscattered Raman shifted light must be collected and analyzed dispersively. Stimulated Raman spectroscopy could be used transdermally by shining the pump and probe lasers through a thin vascular tissue such as a finger web or an earlobe. A serious requirement in all forms of *in vivo* Raman analysis is to be able to do it at laser power levels that will not damage the biological tissues being irradiated (by heating).

15.10 SUMMARY

We have seen that there are many nonimaging applications of photon radiation in noninvasive medical diagnosis, at wavelengths ranging from infrared through visible, UV, and X-rays. Many of the techniques are used to quantify specific biomolecules whose concentrations are abnormal in disease states. In Section 15.2, we saw how X-ray energy at two different wavelengths is used to measure bone density and thus detect osteoporosis. Tissue fluorescence in response to short blue and UV light was introduced in Section 15.3. Many important biomolecules fluoresce, and have unique signature fluorescence emission spectra. Thus, fluorescence can be used to sense abnormally high concentrations of certain molecules associated with the higher metabolism of cancer cells, and thus localize the lesions. Any point on the skin, or part of the body reachable by an endoscope, can be probed for anomalous fluorescence.

Optical interferometric measurement of small displacements, covered in Section 15.4, is primarily a research tool looking for an application. Nanometer-sized vibrations on the skin surface and of a tympanic membrane have been measured. Interferometers are relatively delicate instruments and are sensitive to mechanical vibrations and optical path length modulations. If one is interested in measuring the peripheral blood circulation, laser Doppler velocimetry, covered in Section 15.5 is a preferred method. LDV is also a research tool looking for clinical application.

Transcutaneous IR spectroscopy, both dispersive and non-dispersive, have been shown to have promise for the measurement of molecules such as glucose, cholesterol, etc. Present problems with this type of spectroscopy, reviewed in Section 15.6, include repeatability and calibration. The reliable robust transcutaneous measurement of blood glucose by optical absorption at two or more discrete wavelengths still remains a pie in the sky.

Another physical technique for the measurement of blood glucose makes use of the fact that solutions of D-glucose exhibit optical rotation of linearly polarized light. An optically clear solution is required; the only one readily accessible by noninvasive means is the aqueous humor in the eye. Section 15.7 describes the attempts to measure the optical rotation of AH caused by glucose dissolved in it. This is a challenging instrumentation problem because the optical rotations are typically in the tens of millidegrees, the light intensity used is limited by safety reasons, only a very small fraction of the incident light intensity is reflected out of the eye, and the eyeball is continuously in motion (micronystagmus), even when staring at a fixation spot.

In Section 15.8, we examined pulse oximetry. This is a mature instrumentation technique that, happily, does have wide clinical employment. Pulse oximeters are simple low-cost devices that use a red and an NIR LED light source, and a common silicon photodiode to sense the backscattered light. They make use of the differential absorption of hemoglobin vs. oxyhemoglobin in the blood in the tissue under the device. Experimentally, the pulse oximetry principle has been modified to estimate blood hematocrit.

Finally, in Section 15.9, the principles of Raman spectroscopy are described. Raman spectroscopy has the ability to identify various biomolecules *in vitro* and transcutaneously. It has been used experimentally to measure dissolved glucose concentration *in vitro*, and it has been suggested that it may be suitable for measuring the glucose in aqueous humor. This may be another pipe dream, because exiting light reflected off the front surface of the lens is about 1/1000 the input intensity, and, of that, the actual Raman spectrum is c. 1 part in 10 million. There is no reason that Raman spectroscopy should not be effective on saliva samples, or even trans-cutaneously. In this case, the eye does not appear to be the chosen organ.

16 A Survey of Medical Imaging Systems

16.1 INTRODUCTION

Before the invention and application of simple X-ray shadow imaging in the early 20th century, the only noninvasive means of diagnosing diseases affecting internal organs was by palpation and visual observation of outward symptoms involving the skin, gums, eyes, tongue, teeth, breathing, urine, stool, etc. In the past 30 years, medical imaging systems have gained tremendous sophistication and effectiveness, largely due to the evolution of 2- and 3-D digital signal processing algorithms implemented on modern computers.

This chapter will examine the operating principles and key features of modern NI imaging systems. The mathematics of *tomography* and how it has been applied to various imaging modalities are described. Computer assisted (X-ray) tomography, the so-called CAT scanner, which has been around the longest of modern imaging systems, is certainly familiar to health care professionals and to most students in biomedical engineering. The principles of tomography have been adapted to other imaging modalities, namely *Ultrasound, Positron Emission Tomography* (PET), *Magnetic Resonance Imaging* (MRI), *Single Photon Emission Tomography* (SPECT), *Optical Coherence Tomography* (OCT), *Electrical Impedance Tomography,* and *Microwave Tomography.* The ability of a modern medical imaging computer to stack the tomographic "slices" to generate a 3-D image is now viewed as commonplace. Such 3-D views expedite diagnosis and aid in planning surgery. Three-dimensional reconstructions are particularly useful in diagnosing lung, brain and liver cancers.

Although noninvasive, the use of modern medical imaging techniques carry a small risk. X-rays, gamma rays, (and radioisotopes) are (or emit) ionizing radiations that have the potential to cause cell DNA damage and mutations. Ultrasound and microwaves generally do not carry risk in this form, but can damage cells and cell function by heating at high power levels. The small high-frequency currents used in electrical impedance tomography are probably the most innocuous of the modalities used to probe the body's inner 3-D structure. Only infrared imaging of body surface is completely without risk. Extremely small skin temperature differences that affect the body's blackbody radiation can be resolved. IR imaging is a completely passive means of detecting local "hot spots" that might be due to cancer growing near the skin surface, or cold spots indicative of circulatory anomalies. (IR imaging is not a tomographic technique.)

The first topics we consider below are the generation and detection of X-ray images.

16.2 X-RAYS

16.2.1 INTRODUCTION

X-rays are a broadband, short-wavelength, high-photon-energy electromagnetic radiation. They were discovered accidentally by German physicist Conrad Röntgen in November 1895. Röntgen was experimenting with cathode rays (electron beams) in a vacuum Crooke's tube, and noticed that fluorescence was produced on a screen far from the Crooke's tube, and correctly guessed that a new type of radiation was involved. He went on to show that these unknown "X-rays" had certain properties: they travel in straight lines, cast shadows of internal structures of opaque objects that they can penetrate, cause certain minerals to fluoresce, are not deflected by magnetic fields, and darken silver-halide photographic film. In fact, Röntgen made the first X-ray photograph of his wife's hand on 2 December 1895. He received the first Nobel prize in 1901 for his discovery and research.

16.2.2 SOURCES OF MEDICAL X-RAYS

The basic mechanism by which medical X-rays are produced has not changed since Röntgen's first discovery. In a vacuum, a focused beam of high-energy electrons from a tungsten filament cathode is directed to hit a solid anode. To gain their energy, the electrons are accelerated through a potential of anywhere from 15,000 to 150,000 volts from cathode to anode. There, the moving electrons interact with the metal atoms of the anode. Three forms of energy are produced: *X-rays, Auger electrons*, and a large amount of *heat*. The heat must be dissipated to prevent the temperature of the anode from rising to the anode metal's melting point. Various schemes are used to dissipate this thermal energy. One method is to keep the anode at ground potential, and liquid-cool it with circulating water or oil. Another common approach is to use a large motor-driven rotating anode so that the electron beam effectively has a larger target area, reducing the Watts/cm^2 on the anode. Anodes can rotate as high as 6,000 rpm, and are water cooled, as well. Figure 16.1 illustrates the design of a Coolidge-type X-ray tube with a fixed Cu anode, probably from the early 20th century. Many modern medical X-ray tubes have tungsten anodes; tungsten, also used for the cathode filament, has a high atomic number of $Z = 74$, and a high melting point (3,370° C). Molybdenum is also used as an anode metal.

An X-ray tube requires two power sources: a low-voltage, high-current, ac source to heat the tungsten filament, and a high-voltage, low-current, dc source to supply the electron beam. Figure 16.2 shows a two-phase high-voltage power supply. Note that the dc source does not have a filter capacitor to smooth the rectifier output. This is because the electron beam current is switched at the primary, and, if a filter capacitor were present, the beam current would not stop abruptly, but would decay exponentially, making it difficult to control the X-ray dose and wavelength. Note that the beam current varies in the form of a full-wave rectified sinusoid; peak X-ray energy occurs at the peak anode-cathode voltage, 40 kV, in the figure. For smoother, more monochromatic X-ray production, a three-phase ac supply and rectifier can be used. For really pure X-ray production, a dc beam current is required,

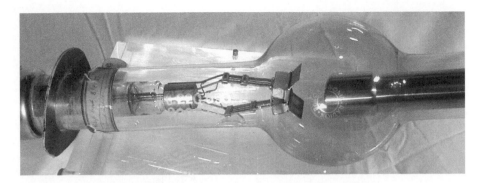

FIGURE 16.1 An early 20th-century X-ray tube with a massive copper anode. The electron gun is on the left. (With permission of Anders' X-ray Museum: wysiwyg://5/http://members.nbci.com/_XMCM/x-ray4you/ eng/x-ray_app.htm).

calling for a filter capacitor to smooth the rectifier pulses. In this case, an expensive high-voltage relay is required to switch the beam current.

Two mechanisms exist by which medical X-rays are produced. The first is called *bremsstrahlung radiation*. Bremsstrahlung is German for deceleration or slowing. The electrons striking the dense metal of the anode slow down abruptly, i.e., they decelerate. When a charged particle accelerates or decelerates, it radiates electromagnetic energy. The power radiated by a decelerating electron is given by (Liley, 1998):

$$P_x = \frac{q^2 \dot{v}^2}{6\pi\varepsilon_o c^3} \quad \text{Watts} \qquad\qquad 16.1$$

Where q is the electron charge, $\dot{v}$ is the deceleration, c is the speed of light, and ε_o the permittivity of free space. Because a single electron can collide with one or several anode atoms, and there are many electrons in the beam, bremsstrahlung radiation has a continuous energy spectrum similar to blackbody radiation. However, the peak energy is radiated in the range of wavelengths of tenths of an Å. In a one electron-one atom collision, the shortest X-ray wavelength that can be produced is given by:

$$\lambda_{min} = \frac{hc}{Vq} = \frac{6,624 \times 10^{-34} \times 3.0 \times 10^8}{V \times 1.603 \times 10^{-19}} \quad \text{meters} \qquad 16.2$$

Where h is Planck's constant, c is the speed of light, q is the coulomb electron charge, and V is the potential through which the electron is accelerated toward the anode. If V = 40 kV, then λ_{min} = 3.1 × 10⁻¹¹ m = 31 pm = 0.31 Å. Thus, there is a sharp cutoff of the bremsstrahlung spectrum for λs shorter than λ_{min}. However, the

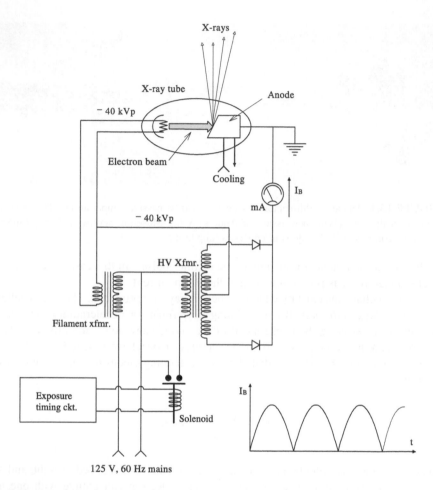

FIGURE 16.2 Schematic diagram of an unfiltered X-ray power supply. The applied cathode potential is a line-frequency full-wave rectified sine wave of −40 kV peak. Thus, the velocities of the electrons striking the anode range from near zero to $v_{max} = \sqrt{2}V_{pk}(q/m)$ m/s, producing a broad range of X-ray energies. Note that the anode is kept at ground potential to facilitate water cooling.

spectrum has a long tail over longer wavelengths. Only about 1% of the energy of the electron beam goes into making bremsstrahlung radiation; most of the beam energy is converted to heat.

The second source of X-radiation involves the interaction of the high-energy beam electrons with the deep shell electrons of the anode's metal. It is called the *characteristic radiation* of the anode metal. When the kinetic energy of the electron beam is above a threshold value called the *excitation potential*, electrons in the deep shells of the anode's atoms are knocked out, and outer shell, or loosely-bound conduction-band or valence electrons can fall into their place; in the process, X-ray photons are emitted having an energy equal to the energy difference between the displaced inner shell electron and the valence electron. Because these energy gaps are quantized, narrow peaks of X-ray energy occur at certain wavelengths above the continuous bremsstrahlung spectrum. These peaks are the X-ray "signatures" of the anode metal used. For example, molybdenum has *characteristic radiation peaks* at 70.93, 71.35, 71.07 and 63.23 pm; copper has peaks at 154.05, 154.43, 154.18 and 139.22 pm wavelength. Figure 16.3 illustrates a typical X-ray power spectrum, showing the bremsstrahlung and characteristic radiation peaks. Note that the dimensions of the spectrum are (Watts/cm²)/Å wavelength.

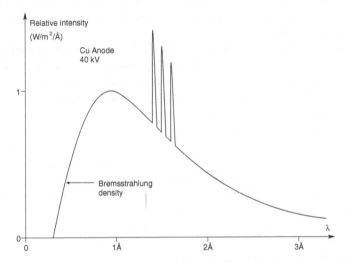

FIGURE 16.3 X-ray intensity spectrum for 40 kV electrons (constant). The broad bremsstrahlung curve occurs even with constant energy electrons striking the anode.

Many photons emitted in the characteristic radiation process interact with other atomic electrons in an *internal photoelectric* process. These electrons may gain sufficient energy to escape the metal surface as *Auger electrons*. When X-rays pass through free electrons (Auger or other electrons knocked loose by the beam), they experience the *Compton scattering effect* in which additional longer wavelength X-rays are generated.

X-ray beams emitted from an anode have an angular distribution of energy that is dependent on the shape of the incident electron beam. Quoting Powell (2001):

"The shape of the incident beam depends on the focal projection of the filament onto and from the anode material. X-ray beams that are parallel with wide projections of the filament have a focal shape of a *line*. X-ray beams that are parallel with the narrow projection of the filament have an approximate focal shape of a square, which is usually labelled as a *spot*. These two focal projections are necessarily about 90° apart in the plane normal to the filament-anode axis. The X-ray beams emitted from the anode travel in a variety of angular directions from the anode surface. As the angle from the anode surface is increased, the intensity of the beam increases, but the spot also becomes less focused. Thus, take-off angles are typically selected in the 3–6° range."

Also, as the angle of the X-ray departing from the anode increases, the peak of the bremsstrahlung spectum shifts to longer wavelengths. The beam leaving at the shallow angle (3°) has the least total energy, but its peak spectral wavelength is the shortest, hence its photons have the highest available energy (E = hc/λ eV).

Ideally, for imaging purposes, we would like monochromatic (single wavelength) X-rays focused in a tight pencil beam, or, equivalently, an X-ray laser. Unfortunately, there is no practical way to create a truly collimated monochromatic X-ray beam for medical purposes. (What is needed is a benchtop low-power CW X-ray laser; a device currently being sought by researchers.) Still, conventionally generated X-rays can be diffracted, filtered and focused to create narrow beams of limited wavelength range for imaging purposes.

The simplest collimator for stationary shadow X-ray imaging is a simple adjustable rectangular window or mask made of lead. The shadow of the collimator defines the active X-ray beam dimension. Other collimators are used to define narrow pencil beams used in certain tomographic applications. A narrow-beam collimator can be made from a small-diameter tube of an absorbing material such as lead. A second tube in line with the first is used to absorb and obliquely scatter X-rays from the first tube. In some tube collimators, lead glass capillaries are used. The diameter of these capillaries is c. 10 μm. These capillaries apparently act like wave guides to capture obliquely directed photons and aim them straight, increasing the intensity of the emerging collimated beam by a factor of 2 to 4 (Powell, 2001). Also reported is an X-ray collimator made from a bundle of small closely packed hexagonal tubes made of tantalum. The tantalum is 50 μm thick, and has an internal plating of tin 100 μm thick, over which is plated copper 50 μm thick. The plated sections are 4 cm in length (out of 20 cm tube lengths) beginning at the output end (Orlandini, 1994).

X-ray absorbing grids are often placed over the flat film case to block low-energy oblique X-rays scattered by interaction with atoms in the object. An X-ray grid resembles an open Venetian blind in structure. By blocking the oblique rays, the image is made sharper. Figure 16.4 illustrates the use of a grid in a conventional fixed X-ray system. First, the required area of the X-ray beam is defined by the collimator. Next, an aluminum plate is used to absorb low-energy X-ray photons that are less effective in imaging dense tissues. Their absorption reduces the overall dose of ionizing radiation to the patient. The lead grid is located between the patient and the film; as mentioned above, its function is to block low-energy oblique rays that would degrade the image. A stationary grid casts its shadow on the film, which can be distracting for the radiologist interpreting the picture. When the grid is moved back and forth during the X-ray exposure, it no longer leaves its shadow, but is still effective at blocking oblique rays; such a moving grid is called a *Bucky grid* (Jacobson and Webster, 1977). Pacific Northwest X-Ray Inc. markets a grid that has aluminum strips between the lead "slats." This design has dual functions; it blocks oblique low-energy rays and filters out the direct low-energy rays from the bremsstrahlung emission "tail."

16.2.3 X-Ray Detectors and Recording Media

The original X-ray recording medium was a flat plate of ordinary silver bromide photographic film kept in a light-tight cassette. Because the emulsion layer is thin

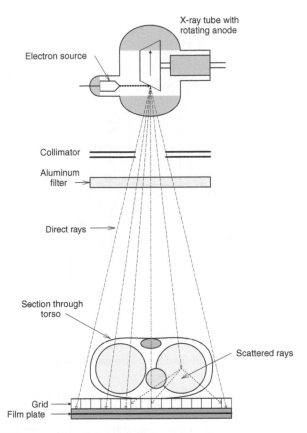

FIGURE 16.4 Schematic of an ordinary "shadow" X-ray system.

and AgBr is not a very efficient capturer of X-ray photons, a given degree of darkening on the developed film caused by photons interacting with the AgBr crystals requires a longer exposure than is required for two-emulsion film backed with scintillator plates. In this embodiment, the emulsions respond not only to direct X-rays, but also to visible photons emitted from the thin scintillation coatings pressed against the emulsions when X-rays excite the scintillator atoms. The scintillation is produced by high-atomic-weight (high-Z) molecules such as calcium tungstate ($CaWO_4$). Laminated scintillation film is from 20 to 100 times more sensitive than plain X-ray film, permitting the use of lower X-ray doses in a given application; obviously, it is also more expensive than plain film (Webster, 1992). An enlarged cross-section of laminated scintillation film is shown in Figure 16.5.

Direct fluoroscopy was an early means of visualizing internal organs in real time. In fluoroscopy, the radiologist stood behind a thin fluorescent screen in line with the X-rays emerging from the patient. This radiation caused visible photons to be emitted from the screen; the higher the ray intensity, the brighter the point on the screen. Conversion efficiency of transmitted X-rays to visible photons is small; only about 7% of the photon energy is converted to light. Thus, the radiologist had to view the dim green screen under low light conditions using dark-adapted eyes, which

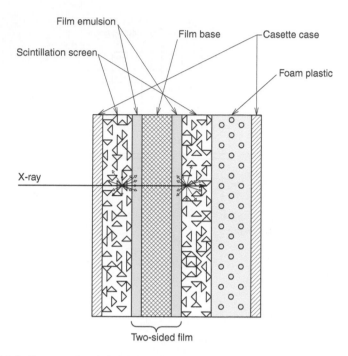

FIGURE 16.5 Cross-sectional detail through laminated, two-sided, scintillation X-ray film.

produce low visual resolution. The technique was used to visualize organs in motion, e.g., the heart and major blood vessels; often an iodine-contrast medium was injected to improve the contrast on heart valves, coronary vessels and aorta. Unfortunately, fluoroscopy resulted in high radiation doses for both the patient and the radiologist. It also took considerable skill and experience to read or interpret the tachistoscopically presented fluorescent images.

Modern fluoroscopic techniques have led to both reduced patient radiation dose and no dose for the radiologist. The *image intensifier tube* (IIT) improves the conversion efficiency for real-time fluoroscopy. A cross-sectional schematic of an IIT is shown in Figure 16.6. Its operating principle is very like the NIR night vision equipment used by the military. When an X-ray photon strikes the fluorescent screen, it emits photons. These stimulate an adjacent *photocathode* of the same size as the fluorescent screen to emit electrons, which are, in turn, accelerated by a c. 25 kV dc potential to strike a phosphor anode, similar to that of a conventional TV CRT. The phosphor anode re-emits bright visible photons as a result of impact by the accelerated photoelectrons. To recapitulate, X-ray photons cause fluorescent screen molecules to emit visible photons which, in turn, generate photoelectrons. The photoelectrons are accelerated and focused, striking a phosphor screen that emits high-intensity visible photons in the form of an X-ray shadow image. The IIT has a *brightness gain* that is the product of the *geometric gain* (ratio of the areas of the input fluorescent screen to the output phosphor screen) times the electronic gain (product of the accelerating potential, V, times the input fluorescent screen's quantum efficiency, η_i, the photo-cathode's efficiency, η_{pc}, and the output phosphor's efficiency, η_{op}). The intensified image on the phosphor can be viewed directly by eye using magnifying optics, or by analog or digital video camera. Thus, images can be stored, computer-enhanced, then played back in slow motion, etc. Direct view of the phosphor screen should make use of a 45° mirror and telescopic optics to place the observer out of the X-ray beam path. Note that one drawback of fluorescent screen imaging is that the visible photons released by collision with an energetic X-ray photon depart in all directions; some are scattered by adjacent phosphor particles and still emerge, degrading image quality.

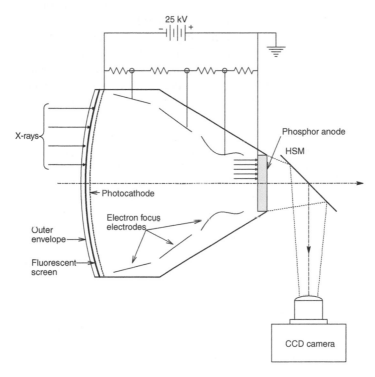

FIGURE 16.6 Cross-sectional schematic through an X-ray image intensifier tube (IIT) used for real-time fluoroscopy in applications such as angiography. HSM = half-silvered mirror beam splitter.

Recently, Industrial Quality, Inc., has developed a family of X-ray scintillating glasses under a U.S. Navy Phase III SBIR contract. IQI claims that the electronic images from their glass scintillators have less noise, and thus give a sharper picture. The glass can be made much thicker than conventional granular fluorescent screens, thus absorbing more X-rays and generating images that are less noisy and have a greater contrast range. There are no light-scattering problems from clear glass (Jones, 2001).

Research and development is currently under way on semiconductor sensor arrays that permit direct conversion of transmitted X-ray energy to electrical outputs in sub-millimeter sized pixel arrays. The problem here appears to be with the materials; an X-ray collision must liberate electrons in numbers proportional to the energy of the ray, and these electrons must be mobile and easily collected for charge-to-voltage conversion (Lachish, 2000). An experimental prototype, GaAs, a 92×100-pixel X-ray sensor array is being developed at the Physics Department of the University of Surrey, UK. The pixel pitch is 150 μm. The prototype chip is used with a prototype current integrator chip developed at Cornell University. The Surrey GaAs array has a dramatically higher detection efficiency for direct illumination with 40 keV X-rays than does one made of Silicon (Sellin, 2000). Besides GaAs, other materials are being investigated for solid-state X-ray-to-electron conversion at the pixel level; for example, cadmium-zinc-telluride crystals.

In summary, medical X-ray technology is heading toward filmless imaging, where eventually all X-ray image data will be captured digitally and stored magnetically or optically in DVD format. The ubiquitous CCD camera is playing a key role in this filmless technology in capturing images from scintillation plates. When perfected, large semiconductor X-ray imaging arrays promise to give better resolution by eliminating the noise and scattering inherent in phosphors. X-ray photons are directly converted to electrons in semiconductor arrays.

The contrast and spatial frequency resolution of X-ray images depend on many factors. Of great importance is the apparent size of the X-ray source spot. A large spot gives a fuzzy shadow of a sharp edge (density gradient) in the object. Image blurring is also caused by object motion (small motions from muscle tremor, heart action). Another source of fuzzy images comes from oblique scattered rays that get through the Bucky grid. Photon scattering in phosphor screens can also degrade spatial resolution.

A practical quantitative measure of the contrast and spatial frequency resolution of an entire X-ray imaging system or any component thereof is the *modulation transfer function* (MTF). Ideally, the MTF should be measured using an object having sinusoidal density for X-rays in one dimension. Because of the difficulty in constructing such a sinusoidal grid, the MTF is measured by using a lead spatial *square wave object* having a period of so many millimeters. In practice, to test an X-ray imaging system, it is better to use a series of grids, each with a progressively smaller spatial period. This is because the spatial frequency response of an image can be area- and orientation-dependent. For example, the highest spatial resolution might be at the center of the image and drop off at the edges. At very low spatial frequencies, the image of the grid is black (exposed) and clear (non-exposed) stripes. If film is the output medium, we can measure the *transmittance* of the clear and black areas. The *contrast* of the striped image is defined as:

$$C(u) \equiv \frac{T_{max} - T_{min}}{T_{max} + T_{min}} \qquad 16.3$$

Where u is the spatial frequency of the object (and image) in lines/mm, defined as $u = 1/\lambda$. T_{max} is the maximum transmittance of the film (in a clear area under a lead stripe), defined as $T_{max} = I_{outc}/I_{in}$. I_{outc} is the intensity of white light emerging from the film, given an input intensity of I_{in}. Similarly, in a dark area on the film (under a gap between lead stripes) $T_{min} = I_{outd}/I_{in}$. For very low u, C → 1.0.

As the spatial frequency of the striped lead object increases, the striped image becomes blurred at the edges of the stripes, and $T_{min} < 1.0$. For very high u, the image appears to be a fuzzy sinusoid, derived from the fundamental frequency in the Fourier series describing the square wave object; thus C(u) → MTF(u). In the limiting case, no periodicity is seen in the object; it is uniformly gray. The object's contrast is thus zero. Note that the spatial square wave object can be described by a Fourier series:

$$f(x) = f(x+\lambda) = F_o/2 + (2F_o/\pi) \sum_{k=1,odd}^{\infty} \sin(k2\pi x/\lambda)/k \qquad 16.4$$

In the limit, as $\lambda \to \lambda_{co}$, only the first harmonic creates an image, so the effective object is:

$$f(x) \cong F_o/2 + (2F_o/\pi)\sin(2\pi x/\lambda) \qquad 16.5$$

Note that F_o is the maximum X-ray density of the lead stripes, λ is their spatial wavelength in mm, x is the direction of the stripes periodicity in mm, and λ_{co} is the stripe period smaller than which, zero contrast is seen on the image.

Resolution of X-ray objects is complicated by the presence of noise in the image. Noise obscures the very small, high-spatial frequency, sinusoidal image of the grating. The noise appears as a fixed two-dimensional random pattern of low- and high-density areas on the film or intensifier screen. Thus, it is appropriate to talk about a *noise-limited bandwidth* for spatial objects.

Figure 16.7 illustrates typical MTFs for X-ray imaging by image intensifier and by film with fluorescent intensifier screens. In the latter case, the spatial cut-off frequency of the film with just the lead grid test object exceeds 10 cycles/mm. Noise from a living object overlying the lead grid gives a noise-limited bandwidth of about 3 cycles/mm, which can be considered to be the practical bandwidth of this system when X-raying humans (Jacobson and Webster, 1977).

Another factor in considering the MTF of film X-ray systems is the nonlinear optical density (OD) of exposed developed film vs. exposure (intensity × time). (OD is defined as $\log_{10}(1/T) = \log_{10}(I_{in}/I_{out})$.) Figure 16.8 illustrates a typical sigmoid curve for OD vs. relative exposure for X-ray film (Liley, 2001). Note that the center of the OD vs. relative exposure curve is fairly linear and can be approximated by:

$$OD \approx \gamma \log_{10}(E/E_o) \qquad 16.6$$

Where γ is the film's *gamma*, typically between 2 and 3, and E/E_o is the relative film exposure. Common sense tells us that if the X-ray exposure is too high, nearly all of the film will be black and very little spatial detail from the object will be visible. Similarly, if the film is underexposed, it will be too light, and a similar lack

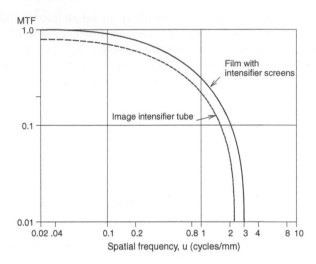

FIGURE 16.7 Typical modulation transfer function for an ordinary X-ray system using two-sided scintillation X-ray film (top curve), and for readout by an IIT. Note that the spatial frequency cutoff lies between 2 and 3 cycles/mm.

of contrast in the image will be present, ruining detail. In the figure, we see that the linear range is less than from $\log_{10}(E/E_o) = 1$ to 2. Thus, an object like a large bone (e.g., the femur) embedded in soft tissue (the leg muscles) may have the bone underexposed and lack detail, or the muscles over-exposed and too dark if the X-ray exposure is not matched to the absorbancy of the object. One way to avoid the problem of over- or underexposed film is to use a *dodger*, which is a shaped X-ray attenuator placed between the X-ray tube and the object to selectively reduce the exposure of soft tissue so that the entire film image is made in the linear gamma region, giving it maximum contrast and spatial frequency response (Jacobson and Webster, 1977).

It is expected that modern X-ray imaging systems such as a scintillation glass screen imaged by a 1024 × 1024-pixel CCD camera can easily exceed the 2.3 cycle/mm cut-off bandwidth of an image intensifier tube, as shown in Figure 16.7.

16.2.4 MAMMOGRAPHY

One of the great challenges in modern radiology is to be able to find lesions in soft tissues such as the breast, lung or liver. Subtle differences in X-ray absorption in soft tissues are more apparent when the X-rays are generated with a lower electron-accelerating voltage. Electron-accelerating voltages from 10 to 40 kV are used for mammography applications. At lower X-ray photon energies (e.g., from 10 to 20 keV), there are larger differences in the mass attenuation coefficients of soft tissues (fat, muscle, connective tissue, blood vessel, cyst, tumor. etc.), hence greater contrast in the X-ray images of soft tissues. By using a tube with a 25 kV accelerating potential and a molybdenum anode followed by a filter of 0.8 mm Be and 0.03 mm Mo, the emitted spectrum is attenuated sharply for X-ray energies above 20 keV, and there is a tall characteristic spike at c. 18 keV energy (VirtualMammo, 2000).

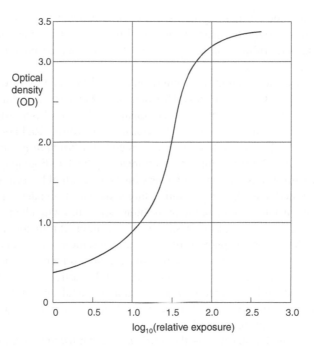

FIGURE 16.8 The sigmoid optical density vs. relative exposure for developed ordinary X-ray film.

Conventional X-ray mammography has not had outstanding results. In one Australian study (Howarth et al. 1999), researchers examined 155 women scheduled for breast cancer surgery. Multiple diagnostic modalities were used. Of 96 confirmed cancer cases, *scintimammography* correctly identified 81, while standard mammography correctly identified 61. On the other hand, scintimammography failed to detect 15 existing cancers while standard mammography missed 31. X-ray mammography indicated that 6 out of 19 cancer-free patients had cancer, while the number of false positives with scintimammography was only three out of 19. Scintimammography clearly appears to be a better noninvasive diagnostic technique for breast cancer than ordinary X-ray. Scintimammography makes use of the fact that cancer cells have higher metabolisms than other breast tissue, and will selectively take up a radioisotope-labeled metabolite; technetium-99m was the label. After a suitable time, any concentration of radioactivity in the breasts sensed with a gamma (scintillation) camera is suggestive of cancer, which can be verified by needle biopsy.

Digital mammography is another technique that offers an advantage over conventional X-ray film mammography. In this technique, the film is replaced with a digital camera in which X-rays are sensed by a high-resolution microchannel system, each pixel of which converts X-ray photons to electron charge. The gain of each microchannel photomultiplier is from 10^6 to 10^8 electrons/photon (Lochner, 2001). The charge from each pixel is integrated and converted to a voltage, thence to a digital signal. Digital mammograms taken with the GE Medical Systems' Senographe 2000D® digital mammography camera have better contrast and high spatial frequency detail, making it easier for the physician to interpret the image. Because the mammography image is in digital format, various linear and nonlinear spatial filtering algorithms can be applied to it to enhance suspicious areas of the primary image.

A new X-ray mammography technique is being developed by researchers at the University of North Carolina Chapel Hill School of Medicine in collaboration with the Brookhaven National Laboratory's National Synchrotron Light Source, the Illinois Institute of Technology, and the European Synchrotron Radiation Facility in Grenoble, France. The innovative technique is called *diffraction enhanced imaging* (DEI). (Fitzgerald, 2000); it may revolutionize medical radiography in the next decade. A synchrotron is the source of a very high-energy, highly collimated electron beam that is aimed at an X-ray-generating target such as molybdenum. The emitted X-rays have the usual broadband bremsstrahlung spectrum with characteristic emission spikes. They are directed to a silicon crystal monochromator, which has the property of reflecting X-ray photons of nearly all the same wavelength at a particular angle. These "monochromatic" X-ray photons are next directed to the object to be imaged. Because the synchrotron is a huge immobile particle accelerator, its beam geometry is fixed, and the target, monochromator, and analyzer crystal must remain fixed to function correctly. Thus, for the X-ray beam to scan the object, the object must be moved in relation to the beam.

The DEI method is sensitive to the *gradient of the refractive index* of the object. Recall that the simplest definition of refractive index is that it is the ratio of the speed of light *in vacuo* to the speed of light in a medium. Because of the complex internal tissue structures, medical X-ray objects have complex (vector) refractive indices that are functions of distance (x,y,z). In general, the refractive index can be given by: $\mathbf{n}(x,y,x) = 1 - \delta(x,y,z) - j\beta(x,y,z)$. The δ term incorporates refractive effects, and β is due to X-ray absorption (Fitzgerald, 2000). At typical mammography X-ray energies of 15–25 keV, δ is about 1000 time larger than β. Thus, it should be possible to sense phase contrast from within the object when absorption contrast (the basis of conventional shadow X-ray imaging) is undetectable. The DEI system is one means of visualizing object phase differences. Recall that the gradient of the scalar n(x,y,z) is a vector defined by:

$$\nabla \mathbf{n}(x, y, z) = \mathbf{i}\frac{\partial n}{\partial x} + \mathbf{j}\frac{\partial n}{\partial y} + \mathbf{k}\frac{\partial n}{\partial z} \qquad 16.7$$

Figure 16.9 shows the schematic of a DEI system. Insight into how the DEI system works can be found from the following quote from Fitzgerald (2000):

"[The] radiation that emerges from a monochromator [crystal] is essentially parallel. As the X-rays traverse a sample placed between the monochromator and the angular filter (termed the analyzer), they can be absorbed, scattered coherently or incoherently (by milliradians or more), or refracted through very small angles (microradians) due to the tiny variations in the refractive index. X-rays emerging from the sample and hitting the analyzer crystal will satisfy the conditions for Bragg diffraction only for a

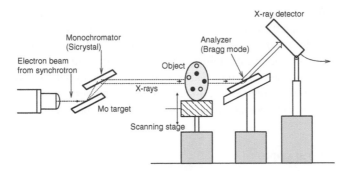

FIGURE 16.9 Schematic of a diffraction-enhanced (X-ray) imaging (DEI) system. Prototype DEI systems have exhibited phenomenal resolution of soft tissue details.

very narrow window of incident angles, typically on the order of a few μradians. X-rays that have been scattered in the sample will fall outside this window and won't be reflected at all. Refracted X-rays within the window will be reflected, but the reflectivity depends on the incident angle. This dependence [is] called the rocking curve....

" If the analyzer [crystal] is perfectly aligned with the monochromator, it will filter out any X-rays that are scattered or refracted by more than a few μrad. The resulting image at the X-ray detector will resemble a standard X-ray radiograph but with enhanced contrast due to scatter rejection.

"If, instead, the analyzer is oriented at a small angle with respect to the monochromator — say by the half-width at half-maximum of the rocking curve — then X-rays refracted by a smaller angle will be reflected less, and X-rays refracted by a larger angle will be reflected more. Contrast is therefore established by the small differences in refracted angle of X-rays leaving the sample."

Thus, the image can show changes in diffraction angles and highlights the edges of fine soft tissue structures in a breast. Preliminary studies have shown that the DEI technique has superior imaging properties; breast cancers are shown with detail increased by more than an order of magnitude over conventional mammograms. A present and major disadvantage of the DEI technique is that it requires a synchrotron particle accelerator to produce the monochromatic X-ray photons required. Clearly, what is needed is a low-cost portable source of collimated monochromatic X-rays, such as an X-ray laser.

If there is any lesson to be learned from mammography, it is that no one test modality is completely without error. The current gold standard would appear to be needle biopsy, but this is an invasive procedure generally used to confirm results. Available state-of-the-art NI tests that are more accurate than X-ray/film mammography include digital mammography, scintimammography, PET scan, and MRI. And, as you will see in Section 17.2, there may be biochemical tests on blood or urine that can sense breast cancer before it becomes evident on any imaging modality. Certainly a disease as important as breast cancer requires a multimodal approach to diagnosis to increase the detection probability.

In the future, we can expect to see DEI X-ray imaging be developed and used for almost all types of conventional shadow X-radiography. X-ray intereferometric imaging and phase-contrast radiography are also being investigated to exploit the high image resolution that can be obtained given a collimated monochromatic X-ray beam (Fitzgerald, 2000). Instead of labeling cancers with radioactive metabolites and using a gamma camera, the labels can be metabolites labeled with radio-dense elements such as iodine or barium that can be easily seen on DEI images. The DEI principle will also be extended to clinical computed tomographic imaging (Dilmanian et al., 2000). (A mathematical description of DEI can be found in the Dilmanian reference.)

16.3 TOMOGRAPHY

16.3.1 INTRODUCTION

The etymology of the word *tomography* comes from the Greek, *tomos,* a cut or slice, and *graphein*, to write. Tomography has been applied in a number of imaging modalities to reconstruct images of internal "slices" of body parts: the brain, lungs, intestines, skeletal structures, etc. In its simplest form, a tomogram is generated by computer calculations done on sensor outputs when the source sends radiation through the body to sensors on the opposite side. Of consideration in the computation is the radiation pattern of the source, the radiation absorption characteristics of body organs, the directional sensitivity function of the sensors, and the angle of the sources or sensors with respect to the body's axis. As you will see below, there are a number of possible geometric forms for scanning the object slice to obtain data to compute a tomographic image.

Tomographic reconstruction of the structure of inner body parts is done with many modalities. The first and foremost is X-ray *computed tomography* (CT), or computed axial tomography (CAT) developed in the early 1970s in England by G.N. Hounsfield and A. McCormack. We also have *positron emission tomography* (PET), *single photon emission computed tomography* (SPECT), *magnetic resonance imaging* (MRI), *ultrasound tomography* (UT), *electrical impedance tomography* (EIT), *microwave tomography,* and *optical coherence tomography* (OCT).

The first and simplest form of tomography is *X-ray motion tomography* (XMT), which is non-computed tomography. A single divergent-beam X-ray source is used, and an X-ray film plate is generally the sensor. The first type of XMT system uses linear parallel displacements of the X-ray source and films. As shown in Figure 16.10, the source and film are moved in a coordinated way so that when the source goes right by +x, the film plate moves left by a proportional amount, −kx. Because of the ray geometry, one plane in the object remains fixed in focus (the tomographic plane), while absorbers in other planes have their images blurred by (equivalent) spatial low pass filtering caused by the coordinated motions of source and film (Macovski, 1983, Ch. 7). In addition to linear motion, XMT can be carried out with radial and circular paths, depending on the application. In Figure 16.11, we see an XMT system devised by Ohno et al. (1976), in which the camera moves in an arc around the center of the tomographic plane, while the film is moved in a flat plane. A variable aperture limits the spread of the X-ray beam to the area of the object;

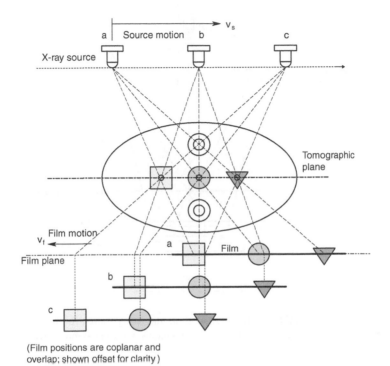

FIGURE 16.10 Schematic of a simple, X-ray motion tomography (XMT) system. Objects in the *tomographic plane* have the highest spatial frequency details. Objects out of the plane suffer lost high spatial frequency response. Note that transverse linear film motion is coordinated with transverse linear X-ray source motion in the opposite direction.

its aperture varies with the position of the source. Another type of XMT system is used to image the jaw and teeth to obtain detailed anatomical information relative to tooth implants. This dental system, the Veraviewepocs® XMT system by J. Morita Europe GmbH, rotates both the X-ray source and the film on circular sector paths. Figure 16.12 shows the geometry of the Veraviewepocs® XMT system.

However implemented, an XMT system can be used to image selected parts of the body inexpensively — for example, the spine, or the lungs without showing the ribs. The mathematical details of the projection geometry describing the resolution and spatial filtering of XMT systems can be found in Chapter 7 of Macovsky (1983).

Two disadvantages of XMT are cited by Macovsky. First, the radiation dose can be extensive if multiple planes are desired, because the whole volume of interest is irradiated for each XMT. Second, the quality of the XMT image is no better than a standard X-ray. No spatial frequency enhancement occurs for simple X-ray film.

To illustrate how computed tomographic data is acquired, let us first examine the evolution of the X-ray CAT scanner. The first practical X-ray CT scanner was developed in England by Dr. G.N. Hounsfield in the early 1970s.

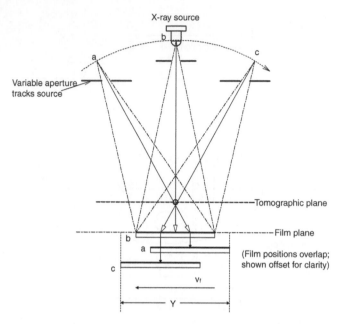

FIGURE 16.11 In the XMT system of Ohno et al., the X-ray source follows a curved path. The X-ray beam is directed through a collimating window, which also moves with the source.

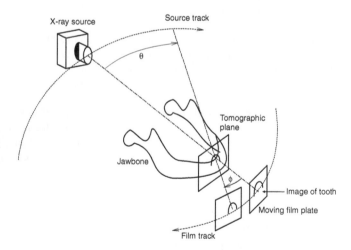

FIGURE 16.12 A dental XMT system in which both the source and the film move on curved paths.

1. This first-generation CT system used a single X-ray source emitting a highly collimated pencil beam and a single X-ray sensor opposite the source. Data was gathered by linearly translating the beam and sensor

across the patient and taking N intensity measurements (one every Δx cm) over a distance L spanning the patient. This data was digitized and stored in the 0° array. Next, the source and sensor were rotated some small angle, e.g., $\Delta\theta = 1°$, the linear scan of N points was repeated, and the digitized intensity data stored in the $1\Delta\theta$ array. This rotation by $\Delta\theta$ process was repeated a total of 179 times until an angle of $(180° - \Delta°)$ was reached, giving a total of 180 data arrays, each with N intensity values in it. The scanning took approximately 5 minutes, and it took the computer c. 20 minutes to reconstruct the data. This first-generation system used by Hounsfield was slow, and the patient was exposed to a relatively high dose of ionizing radiation. Still, it revealed for the first time the fine details in a tomographic slice of brain tissue.

2. The second-generation X-ray CT scanner used a single source emitting a uniform-intensity fan beam of X-rays. Multiple sensors were arranged in a fixed linear array. The fan source and sensors were still translated linearly across the object, then rotated $\Delta\theta$, which, in this case, could be larger, resulting in a c. 30-second total scan time, giving the patient shorter exposure to ionizing radiation. The image reconstruction algorithm was more complex than in the first generation because it had to deal with the angular fan beam geometry.

3. A third generation of scanning geometry was introduced in 1976 that eliminated the need for translation. A single fan beam source of X-rays was used along with an arc-shaped sensor array opposite the source. The whole assembly rotated around the center of the patient. Patient scan time was now reduced to c. 1 second.

4. In the fourth-generation scanner, a fixed sensor array of from 600 to 4,800 units (depending on the manufacturer) is arranged in a circle around the patient. A fan-beam X-ray source was rotated 360° around the patient. Again, scan time was c. 1 second.

5. In fifth-generation scanners, the X-ray exposure (scan) time has been reduced to c. 50 ms, fast enough to image a beating heart without excessive motion artifact. The fifth-generation system used a fixed semicircular sensor array and a special X-ray tube with a semicircular tungsten strip anode. A high-energy electron beam is electronically scanned around the anode, producing a moving fan-shaped beam of X-rays that rotates around the patient. There are no mechanical moving parts in the scanning process.

Other designs of X-ray CT scanners are evolving, being driven by three factors: reduce cost, minimize patient radiation dose, and improve resolution. Spiral (helically) scanned X-ray CT systems are being developed that will allow 3-D images to be acquired directly, instead of slice by slice.

In the following subsections, we introduce the reader to the complex mathematical processes required for CT image reconstruction.

16.3.2 Formation of Tomograms with the Algebraic Reconstruction Technique

We are all familiar with the simple stationary "shadow" X-ray picture on film, such as a doctor might order to visualize a broken bone. A conical beam of X-rays is directed at the body part of interest, directly under which is placed a film plate. The tissues in the body part, e.g., forearm, absorb X-ray photons according to Beer's law, thus the X-rays taken of the arm will have reduced intensities depending on the absorption coefficient of the type of tissue they pass through (e.g., bone, muscle, fat), and the path length they take through a particular type of tissue. Note that X-rays also can be scattered and emerge as secondary radiation, their photons traveling at an angle to the primary X-ray photons from the source. Often, a 2-D grid is placed over the film or scintillation detector to exclude these oblique secondary rays (see Figure 16.4). Thus, the tissue under study essentially casts a sharp X-ray shadow on the film; tissue like bone absorbs more energy, so the intensity of rays passing through bone are attenuated more than the rays emerging from soft tissue only. The more exposed an X-ray transparency plate is, the darker (more opaque) it is to light when developed. Thus, bones appear light on a conventional X-ray film, and a break in a bone shows up as a dark line.

Computed X-ray tomography allows us to see the fine structure of soft tissues that are normally hidden by bone in a conventional shadow X-ray, including the brain and spinal cord, as well as the lungs, etc. Because of its greater pixel resolution, CT can locate lesions in soft tissues such as the brain, liver, pancreas, or breast, that are not visible on conventional X-rays or XMTs. It is obvious that a real tissue is composed of a continuous mixture of absorbers, often arranged in layers or discrete geometries such as fat, blood vessels and bones. To explore the anatomical details of a real tissue, we examine it by imaging contiguous 2-D slices (tomograms). The absorbance details of the component tissues are measured on a discrete basis for instrumental and computational reasons. Each small area in a tomographic slice with the same computed absorbance is called a *pixel;* the smaller the pixels, the finer the resolution of the tissues. By processing the contiguous pixels in adjacent slices, we can define small isoabsorbance volume elements called *voxels.*

To introduce the algebraic reconstruction technique to form tomograms, consider a 2-D model X-ray absorber, shown in Figure 16.13. Four regions (pixels), each having a different absorbance, are shown. We assume that Beer's law holds: i.e., the transmittance along the jth ray path is:

$$T_j = 1_{jout}/1_{in} = \exp\left[-\sum_{k=1}^{2} \mu_k\right] \qquad 16.8$$

where μ_k is the *absorbance* of the kth pixel. When an X-ray beam passes through two pixels, the net absorbance is the sum of the two pixel's absorbances. Hence, the intensity of emerging beam 2 is $I_{2out} = I_{in} \exp(-(\mu_1 + \mu_2))$, and the intensity of the diagonal beam 3 is $I_{3out} = I_{in} \exp(-(\mu_1 + \mu_4))$, etc. The problem is to compute

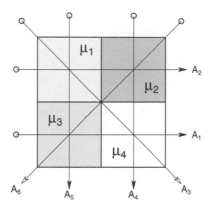

FIGURE 16.13 A 2-D four-element X-ray absorber used to demonstrate the linear algebraic reconstruction technique (ART) of finding a tomogram.

the $\{\mu_k\}$ from the intensities $I_{1out} \ldots I_{6out}$. By computing the natural logarithm of (I_{in}/I_{jout}), we have for example, the absorbance, $A_3 = \ln(I_{in}/I_{3out}) = \mu_1 + \mu_4$, etc. Note that A_j is in general, > 1. Since six beams can be passed through the four-pixel absorber in a unique manner, there are six equations available to solve for the four unknown $\{\mu_k\}$:

$$A_1 = \mu_3 + \mu_4$$

$$A_2 = \mu_1 + \mu_2$$

$$A_3 = \mu_1 + \mu_4$$

$$A_4 = \mu_2 + \mu_4$$

$$A_5 = \mu_1 + \mu_3$$

$$A_6 = \mu_2 + \mu_3$$

With six equations and four unknowns, it appears that the system is over-determined (four equations should be required to solve for four unknowns). However, solution for $\{\mu_k\}$ by using Cramer's rule to solve linear algebraic equations is impossible because the system determinant, $\Delta \equiv 0$. Macovski (1983) shows that the $\{\mu_k\}$ can be estimated by an iterative linear *algebraic reconstruction technique* (ART), illustrated below:

$$^{q+1}\mu_k = {}^{q}\mu_k + \left[A_j - \sum_{k=1}^{N} {}^{q}\mu_k \right] \Big/ N \qquad\qquad 16.9$$

Where q is the iteration number, $^{q+1}\mu_k$ is the estimated absorbance of the kth pixel in the jth ray path after the qth iteration, N is the number of pixels in the jth ray path, $\sum_{k=1}^{N} {}^q\mu_k$ is the sum of the estimated absorbances for the pixels in the jth ray

path, and A_j is the measured absorbance over the jth ray path.

Let us do a numerical example, following the procedure described in Tomovski (1983): Let: $\mu_1 = 2$, $\mu_2 = 8$, $\mu_3 = 5$, $\mu_4 = 1$. Thus $A_1 = 6$, $A_2 = 10$, $A_3 = 3$, $A_4 = 9$, $A_5 = 7$, $A_6 = 13$. To obtain the q = 1 estimates, Tomovski sets all the (initial) q = 0, $\{\mu_k\}$ estimates to zero, and considers the two vertical rays. For A_5:

$$^1\mu_1 = {}^1\mu_3 = 0 + (7 - 0)/2 = 3.5$$

For A_4:

$$^1\mu_2 = {}^1\mu_4 = 0 + (9 - 0)/2 = 4.5$$

Thus the q = 1 pixel estimates are: 3.5 4.5
                                       3.5 4.5

In the next (q = 2) iteration, the two horizontal rays are used. For A_2:

$$^2\mu_1 = 3.5 + (10 - 8)/2 = 4.5$$

$$^2\mu_2 = 4.5 + (10 - 8)/2 = 5.5$$

For A_1:

$$^2\mu_3 = 3.5 + (6 - 8)/2 = 2.5$$

$$^2\mu_4 = 4.5 + (6 - 8)/2 = 3.5$$

Now the trial absorbance values are: 4.5 5.5
                                     2.5 3.5

For the third iteration, Macovski uses the diagonals: For A_3:

$$^3\mu_1 = 4.5 + (3 - 8)/2 = 2$$

$$^3\mu_4 = 3.5 + (3 - 8)/2 = 1$$

For A_6:

$$^3\mu_2 = 5.5 + (13 - 8)/2 = 8$$

$$^3\mu_3 = 2.5 + (13 - 8)/2 = 5$$

Thus, we see that in only 3 iterations for this simple example, the exact $\{\mu_k\}$ values are obtained. When j, N and k are very large, convergence on the exact $\{\mu_k\}$ values can be very slow. Convergence can be tested by examining the magnitude of the normalized error for the jth path at the qth iteration.

$$\varepsilon_j = \left| \left[A_j - \sum_{k=1}^{N} {}^q\mu_k \right] \middle/ A_j \right|$$

16.10

The linear ART process can be halted when the largest ε_j reaches a preset minimum. Note that other nonlinear estimation techniques for the $\{\mu_k\}$ exist based on criteria such as the least MS error, etc., however, their description is beyond the scope of this chapter.

Current practice for finding the $\{\mu_k\}$ describing tomographic slices makes use of the *Radon transform,* rather than an ART.

16.3.3 USE OF THE RADON TRANSFORM IN TOMOGRAPHY

Figure 16.14 illustrates the geometry of a first-generation CT scanner. The pencil beam is linearly translated incrementally, then rotated some small $\Delta\theta$, and the process repeated until $k\Delta\theta = 180°$. Figure 16.15 illustrates the geometry of a third-generation CT system. In both cases, a family of plots of slice absorbance, $m(\theta, \rho)$ or $m(\theta, k\Delta\phi)$, is made, shown as continuous functions in the figures. This absorbance data is used to reconstruct the absorbance or X-ray density of the object in discrete pixels. A summary of the mathematics of tomographic reconstruction follows.

The *Radon transform* on Euclidean space was devised in 1917 by Johann Radon. Like many significant mathematical and physical discoveries, there was a substantial lag between its inception and a practical application. Not until the 1970s, following the development of the X-ray CAT scanner by EMI Ltd., was the Radon transform (RT) found useful in computing the absorbancies of the pixels in a tomogram. Although the discrete RT is used in modern CT applications, it is easier to describe the significance of the RT using the continuous form. Thus, we can write the net absorbance seen by an X-ray beam passing through an object at an angle θ to the y axis as the superposition of the differential absorbance elements in the ray path :

$$m(\rho, \theta) = \int_{(\rho,\theta \, \text{line})} \mu(x, y) \, d\sigma = \ln\left(I_{\text{in}} / I_{\text{out}}\right)$$

16.11

Where σ is the distance along the ray path in the object. Equation 16.11 can also be written using the Radon transform of a *projection slice* through the object of absorbance, $\mu(x,y)$, using the delta function to define the path of integration:

$$m(\rho, \theta) = \int_{-\infty}^{\infty} \int_{-\infty}^{\infty} \mu(x, y) \delta(\rho - x \cos\theta - y \sin\theta) \, dx \, dy$$

16.12

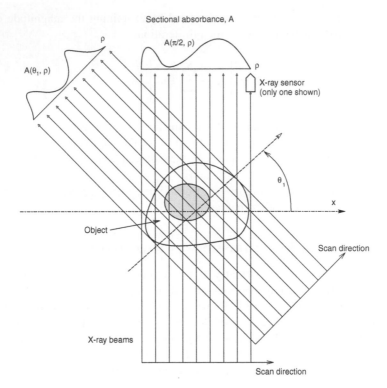

FIGURE 16.14 The parallel scanning geometry used in the first-generation CT scanners.

The delta function exists only for zero argument, and is zero for non-zero arguments. Its argument is the equation of a straight line in polar coordinates in the plane of $\mu(x, y)$, $\rho = x \cos\theta + y \sin\theta$. ρ is the perpendicular distance from the chosen line of integration to the x,y origin, and θ is the angle formed between the line over which the integration is done and the y axis. Figure 16.16 illustrates this geometry.

Some properties of the Radon transform (RT) are:

1. A $\mu(x, y)$ containing a straight line (not to be confused with the line of integration) or a line segment has a RT that exhibits an impulse or narrow peak at the RT coordinates ρ_o and θ_o, which correspond to the parameters of the polar equation of the straight line (along which the segment possibly lies).

2. A $\mu(x, y)$ function that has a single point at (x_o, y_o) has an RT which is non-zero along a sinusoidal curve in Radon space of equation: $\rho = x_o \cos\theta + y_o \sin\theta$.

3. The RT satisfies: *superposition:* $R[\mu_1(x, y) + \mu_2(x, y)) = R_{\mu 1}(\rho, \theta) + R_{\mu 2}(\rho, \theta)$
   linearity: $R[a\,\mu(x, y)) = a\,R_\mu(\rho, \theta)$
   scaling: $R[\mu(x/a, y/b)) = |a|\,R_\mu(\rho a/b, \theta/b)$
   rotation
   shifting

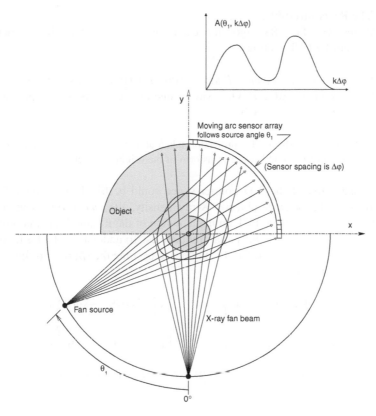

FIGURE 16.15 Fan beam scanning used in third-generation CT scanners.

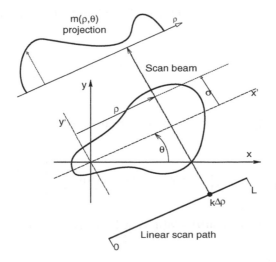

FIGURE 16.16 Scanning geometry relative to application of the Radon transform.

4. The RT is invertible.
5. A discrete, fast, RT algorithm exists, implementable in the frequency domain by FFT routines.

Computation of the *inverse Radon transform* (IRT) is used to estimate the original density image, $\mu(x, y)$. One way of finding the IRT is by by application of the *Fourier slice theorem* (FST):

> The 1-D Fourier transform of a projection taken at angle θ equals the central radial slice at angle θ of the 2-D Fourier transform of the original object.

The FST states that if the 2-D Fourier space could be filled, the inverse 2-D FT would recover the original object's X-ray density, $\mu(x, y)$. Filling can only be approximated using discrete FFT implementation of the RT and FST. Interpolations are required, especially at high spatial frequencies. To understand the FST, consider a rotation of the (x, y) coordinates by angle θ to become the (ρ, σ) coordinates. The rotation can be described by:

$$\begin{bmatrix} \rho \\ \sigma \end{bmatrix} = \begin{bmatrix} \cos\theta & \sin\theta \\ -\sin\theta & \cos\theta \end{bmatrix} \begin{bmatrix} x \\ y \end{bmatrix} \quad \text{and} \quad \begin{bmatrix} x \\ y \end{bmatrix} = \begin{bmatrix} \cos\theta & -\sin\theta \\ \sin\theta & \cos\theta \end{bmatrix} \begin{bmatrix} \rho \\ \sigma \end{bmatrix} \qquad 16.13$$

So $x = \rho\cos\theta - \sigma\sin\theta$, and $y = \rho\sin\theta + \sigma\cos\theta$, and the RT of $\mu(x, y)$ can also be written as:

$$m(\rho, \theta) = \int_{-\infty}^{\infty} \mu(\rho\cos\theta - \alpha\sin\theta, \rho\sin\theta + \sigma\cos\theta)\,d\sigma \qquad 16.14$$

Using Equation 16.14, the 1-D FT of $m(\rho, \theta)$ with respect to ρ is (at constant θ):

$$K\{m(\rho, \theta)\} = M(\omega, \theta) = \int_{-\infty}^{\infty} m(\rho, \theta)\exp[-j2\pi\omega\rho]\,d\rho$$

$$= \int_{-\infty}^{\infty}\int_{-\infty}^{\infty} \mu(\rho\cos\theta - \sigma\sin\theta, \rho\sin\theta + \sigma\cos\theta)\exp[-j2\pi\omega\rho]\,d\rho\,d\sigma \qquad 16.15$$

$$= \int_{-\infty}^{\infty}\int_{-\infty}^{\infty} \mu(x, y)\exp[-j2\pi\omega(x\cos\theta + y\sin\theta)]\begin{vmatrix} \partial\rho/\partial x & \partial\sigma/\partial x \\ \partial\rho/\partial y & \partial\sigma/\partial y \end{vmatrix}\,dx\,dy$$

$$= M(\omega\cos\theta, \ \omega\sin\theta) = M(u, v) \text{ in 2-D, spatial frequency space.}$$

Where $u \equiv \omega \cos\theta$, and $v \equiv \omega \sin\theta$, and the determinant is the Jacobean involved in changing from rectangular to polar coordinates.

Now the inverse 2-D FT is expressed in the polar coordinates, ω and θ in the (u,v) frequency space. Note that $du\ dv = \omega\ d\omega\ d\theta$.

$$\mu(x, y) = F_2^{-1}\{M(u, v)\} = \int_{-\infty}^{\infty}\int_{-\infty}^{\infty} M(u, v)\exp\left[j2\pi(xu + yv)\right] du\ dv$$

$$= \int_{0}^{2\pi}\int_{-\infty}^{\infty} M(\omega\cos\theta, \omega\sin\theta)\exp\left[j2\pi\omega(x\cos\theta + y\sin\theta)\right] \qquad 16.16$$

$$\begin{vmatrix} \partial u/\partial w & \partial v/\partial w \\ \partial u/\partial \theta & \partial v/\partial \theta \end{vmatrix} d\omega\ d\theta$$

The angle integral above can be split into two integrals; one from 0 to π, and the other from π to 2π. We then get:

$$\mu(x, y) = \int_{0}^{\pi}\int_{0}^{\infty} M(\omega, \theta)\exp\left[+j2\pi\omega(x\cos\theta + y\sin\theta)\right]\omega\ d\omega\ d\theta +$$

$$\qquad\qquad\qquad\qquad\qquad\qquad\qquad\qquad\qquad\qquad\qquad\qquad 16.17$$

$$\int_{\pi}^{2\pi}\int_{0}^{\infty} M(\omega, \theta + \pi)\exp\left[+j2\pi\omega(x\cos(\theta + \pi) + y\sin(\theta + \pi))\right]\omega\ d\omega\ d\theta$$

But is known from FT theory that if $\mu(x, y)$ is real, then $M(\omega, \theta + \pi) = M(-\omega, \theta)$. This identity is used in Equation 16.17 to write (Rao, Kriz et al. 1995):

$$\mu(x, y) = \int_{0}^{\pi}\left[\int_{-\infty}^{\infty} |\omega| M(\omega, \theta)\exp\left[j2\pi\omega\left(x\cos\theta \overset{(\rho)}{+} y\sin\theta\right)\right]d\omega\right]d\theta \qquad 16.18$$

In Equation 16.18, the inner integral operates to filter each projection profile in frequency space. Now we define the 1-D, inverse FT of the filtered kernel, Λ:

$$\Lambda(\rho, \theta) \equiv \int_{-\infty}^{\infty} M(\omega, \theta)|\omega|\exp\left[j2\pi\omega\rho\right]d\omega \qquad 16.19$$

Finally, we have the back-projection by the real integration:

$$\mathbf{B}\{\Lambda(\rho, \theta)\} = \int_{0}^{\pi} \Lambda(x \cos \theta + y \sin \theta, \theta)\, d\theta \cong \mu(x, y) \qquad 16.20$$

Multiplication by $|\omega|$ under the integral (in the frequency domain) serves as a high-pass filter applied to each projection profile in frequency space. Note that high-pass filtering accentuates noise, even if done over a finite ω range. Other band-pass filter functions can be used to minimize the effects of noise, and that filtering can also be done as real convolution in the spatial domain. The filtered profile, Λ, is summed along the ray paths in the image space.

Implementation of continuous *filtered back-projection* (FBP) requires infinite data to exactly reconstruct $\mu(x, y)$ of the object. The steps are (Rao, Kriz et al., 1995):

1. Find the 1-D FTs of the projections.
2. Perform the filtering operation on the projections in the frequency domain, then do inverse FTs.
3. Find the back-projections using Equation 16.20.

In practice, finite data are spatially sampled by the finite positions of the X-ray sensor array, and spatial anti-aliasing filtering is done to eliminate the effects of noise and high spatial frequencies in the object's $\mu(x, y)$. FFT and IFFT algorithms must be used. A noisy, discrete estimate of $\mu(x, y)$ is found, and interpolation and smoothing is then used to estimate the X-ray densities of the discrete pixels of $\mu(p\Delta x, q\Delta y)$ in the tomogram. To minimize the effect of spatial noise in the FBP process, it is common to multiply the $|\omega|$ function inside the integrals of Equation 16.18 and 16.19 with a common Hamming or Hanning windowing function used with discrete data. The development of the mathematics for FBP applied to angularly scanned objects follows a similar course as above, but is too complex to examine in detail here. The reader interested in the mathematical details of discrete RT and FBP computation can consult the paper by Rao, Kriz et al., 1995.

In summary, the reconstruction of the X-ray densities in each pixel of the tomographic image is a mathematically complex process. Many algorithms have been developed to interpolate and estimate $\mathbf{B}\{\mu(x, y)\}$. Modern parallel multiprocessor "supercomputers" can generate FBP density images in about 2–3 seconds (Rao et al., 1995).

16.4 POSITRON EMISSION TOMOGRAPHY (PET)

16.4.1 Introduction

Positron emission tomography (PET) is an imaging technique made possible by an amazing coincidence in nature. A PET image is basically a density map of radioactivity in a slice of tissue or organ viewed in two dimensions. The radioactivity, which comes from manmade isotopes, is used to tag and identify certain types of living tissue, such as cancers, or to investigate tissue metabolism, such as in heart muscle and the brain.

When certain kinds of unstable artificial radioisotopes return to a lower energy level, one of their protons emits a *positron* (a particle with + electron charge and electron mass) and a n*utrino,* and thus becomes a *neutron* in the isotope's nucleus. The positron travels a short distance to where it collides with an electron; the two annihilate each other in a matter–antimatter process that releases two energetic γ photons, each having an energy of 511 keV. The amazing coincidence is that the two photons originate at the same time and travel in opposite directions on nearly the same linear path (the *coincidence line*, or *line of response* (LOR)). The two photons exit the body and travel to two opposite sensors that are part of a multisensor ring array that defines the tomographic plane. Other photons leave the body out of the plane of the sensor ring and are not detected; obviously, only photons with paths in the tomographic plane contribute to the calculation of radio-density regions in the plane.

Because a variety of metabolites, drugs and hormones can be labeled with positron-emitting isotopes, the chemical affinities of these tracer compounds to membrane receptors, cancer cells, specific gland tissues, myocardial infarction sites, etc. can be determined in the PET process. Some of the more common positron-emitting radioisotopes used in PET include: ^{11}C (20.4 m, 4 mm), ^{13}N (9.97 m, 5.4 mm), ^{15}O (2.04 m, 8.2 mm), ^{18}F (110 m, 2.5 mm), ^{120}I (81 m, NA). The first number in each parenthesis is the half-life of the isotope in minutes, the second number is the mean range of the positron in water. (The longer the range, the higher the initial positron energy.) The short-lived isotopes are produced in pure form in a cyclotron by high-energy bombardment with protons or deuterons. Then the isotopes must be incorporated into the tracer molecules by chemical reactions, and promptly transported to the PET scanner site, where they are injected into the patient. Thus, a requirement for a PET scanner is a nearby cyclotron and radiochemistry lab.

An ^{15}O isotope is attached to tracer molecules such as carbon dioxide, molecular oxygen, and water. Ammonia is made with ^{15}N ($^{15}NH_3$). ^{11}C is used in acetate ($H_3C\text{-}^{11}COO^-$); Carfentanil, cocaine, diprenyl, N-methylspiperone, raclopride are all tagged with $-^{11}CH_3$; methionine and leucine are tagged with $-^{11}COOH$). $^{18}F-$ is used with: haloperidol, fluorodeoxyglucose, fluorodopa, fluorouracil, and fluoroethylspiperone (Strommer, 1996).

The isotopically labeled compound is injected (usually IV) and within a few heartbeats is uniformly distributed in the blood. The concentration of the isotope in the blood then slowly decreases as it is 1) taken up by target tissues and organs, 2) excreted, and 3) decays by positron emission. The isotope concentration rises to a peak in the target organ, then decreases to zero as it is metabolically destroyed, is removed from the site, and decays radioactively.

Sometimes, two different positron-emitting tracer compounds are given at once. For example, $^{15}NH_3$ and ^{18}fluorodeoxyglucose are used to view myocardial perfusion and infarcted heart muscle in the same PET scan.

16.4.2 THE PET PROCESS

Let us examine what happens to the two 511 keV photons emitted in the tomographic plane on a *line of response* (LOR). The two high-energy photons can interact with molecules in the body and undergo *Compton scatter* and *photoelectric absorption.* In Compton scatter, the photon interacts with an electron; the photon's direction is changed, the kinetic energy (KE) of the electron is increased, and the energy of the photon is decreased according to the formula:

$$E' = \frac{E_o}{1 + \left[E / \left(m_o c^2 \right) \right] (1 - \cos \theta)} \qquad 16.21$$

Where E and E′ are the photon's energy before and after the scattering collision, respectively, m_o is the rest mass of an electron, c is the speed of light, and θ is the scattering angle. In photoelectric absorption (PA), a photon is absorbed by an atom and, in the process, an electron is ejected from one of its bound shells. The probability of PA increases rapidly with increasing atomic number, Z, of the absorber atom. It also decreases rapidly with increasing photon energy. In water, the probability of photoelectric absorption decreases with approximately the third power of the photon's energy; it is negligible at 511 keV (Johns and Cunningham, 1983).

The reduction of PET data begins with coincidence detection of the two photons travelling on the LOR. There are four categories of *coincidence events* caused by two photons arriving at two scintillation sensors in the sensor ring within the time window that defines a coincidence event (CE). Figure 16.17A illustrates a true CE. Two PE photons traveling straight on the LOR arrive at sensors within the event time window that defines the LOR. Exact coincidence is very improbable, because of path length differences and tissue interactions with the two 511 keV photons. Generally, the two photons arrive within several ns of one another, however.

In Figure 16.17B, we see how random coincidences can define a false LOR and thus contribute to a noisy PET scan. Two independent positron emissions release four photons, two of which strike sensors within the coincidence time window. The rate of random CEs is roughly proportional to the square of the concentration(s) of positron-emitting isotope(s) in the slice viewed by the sensors. The phenomenon of scattered coincidence is shown in Figure 16.17C. Here, a false CE is caused by Compton scattering deflecting one or both photons emitted by a single positron–electron collision event. Scattered coincidence defines a false LOR that ultimately adds noise to the PET scan and also decreases its contrast. *Multiple coincidences* occur when two photons from two different positron–electron collision events strike the same sensor, while the other two photons strike a second and third sensor within the coincidence resolving time. Multiple coincidence events define two ambiguous LORs, and thus are rejected by the PET system; they are shown in Figure 16.17D.

The basic high-energy photon detection sensor in a PET system is a fast photomultiplier tube (PMT) that is optically coupled to a scintillation crystal. Many such sensors are arranged in a ring surrounding the patient; the plane of the ring defines the tomographic slice that is imaged. The scintillation event is produced

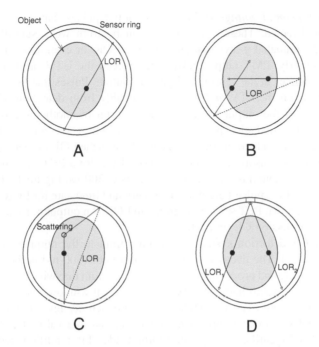

FIGURE 16.17 (A) A true PET event in the tomographic plane. (B) A coincidence event defining a false LOR. (C) A false LOR caused by scattering of one photon of the pair. (D) Two valid LORs from two coincident events are rejected by the counting system.

when an emitted high-energy γ photon strikes the scintillator crystal and causes the emission of a high-energy electron, either by Compton scatter or photoelectric absorption. The high-energy electron passes through the crystal, exciting other electrons, which lose energy in the form of radiated photons as they decay to their ground state energy.

A good scintillation crystal should have a high value of effective atomic number, Z. It should also generate a large number of scintillation photons when struck by a high-energy γ-ray photon. The crystal should have a low self-absorption factor for scintillation photons, and should have a refractive index close to that of the glass of the PMT to couple the scintillation light to the PMT's photocathode most efficiently. Many materials are suitable for scintillation detection; the scintillator of choice for PET sensors is *bismuth germanate* (BGO, or $Bi_3Ge_4O_{12}$), which has $Z = 74$, a linear attenuation coefficient (for scintillation photons) of 0.92 cm^{-1}, and a refractive index of 2.15. BGO emits 480 nm photons with a decay constant of 300 ns. Cerium-doped lutetium oxy-orthosilicate (LSO) is another material that promises to be effective for PET sensors. LSO's $Z = 66$, its linear attenuation coefficient is 0.87 cm^{-1}, and its refractive index $= 1.82$. LSO emits at 420 nm and has a decay constant of 40 ns, giving an improved coincidence detection and maximum counting rate (Daghigian et al., 1993).

Pulses from each sensor's PMT are conditioned by a fast *pulse-height window* circuit that has two adjustable threshold voltages; an *upper threshold voltage* (UTV) and a *lower threshold voltage* (LTV). PMT output pulses that do not exceed the LTV are not detected. These small pulses can be from weak scintillations from scattered and attenuated γ-rays that are not on a LOR, or even stray environmental radiation. Similarly, PMT output pulses that exceed the UTV originate from two photon coincidences at the sensor, and give no output. Pulses that lie in the voltage "window" between the LTV and UTV are probably from detection of a 511 keV emitted photon. If the output from a window circuit of another sensor across the diameter from the first also produces a pulse within τ seconds of the first, the coincidence circuit produces an output that establishes the LOR of that event between the two responding sensors. τ is typically about 12 ns for a PET system using BGO scintillators, even though the BGO decay time is c. 300 ns. Figure 16.18 illustrates a block diagram of the pulse-height discriminator and time gate for LOR coincidence detection between two PET sensors defining an LOR. An output pulse at V_o indicates a one-positron emission CE on LOR_{1k}.

The PET CE detection system has a finite limit to the number of CEs it can process per second. The decay time of the scintillator (300 ns) is the rate-limiting factor in identifying and processing LORs. The maximum rate with BGO scintillators is about 10^6/second/scintillator. The PMT, pulse-height window, and logic can effectively function at well over 100 MHz. If the radioactivity level is too high in the object, some CEs can occur separated by so small an interval that they cannot be discriminated and identified as separate LORs. Under this condition, certain CEs do not get processed, and their LORs do not go into the tomogram computation. The missed LORs are known as *dead-time losses* (Badawi, 1999).

Realization of the locations (or equivalently, the density) of the positron-emitting radioisotopes in the tomographic slice is accomplished by computing the intersections of the LOR vectors.

The finite angle of acceptance of each sensor, $\delta\theta$, leads to ambiguity in the calculation of the density of PE events in a tissue. The intersection of two separate LORs in the sensor ring plane originating from two isotope molecules only nm apart do not necessarily define a point on the tomogram. Instead, there is an uncertainty area where the two atoms are located defined by the geometry shown in Figure 16.19. Also contributing to the uncertainty area is the fact that an emitted positron from a radioactive tracer molecule can travel in the tissue as much as 4 to 5 mm in any direction before the positron is annihilated by an electron, and the two γ-ray photons are produced. The uncertainty area is on the order of 1 cm^2 in a 2-D PET tomogram.

In computing a PET tomogram, the collected LORs are arranged in sets of parallel lines, each set at some angle θ with the y-axis (the geometry is similar to the parallel beam approach to X-ray CT scanning). θ is varied in small increments over 0 to 180° − $\Delta\theta$. Just as in CT, a plot is made of the number of CEs on a given LOR path, $n(\theta, \rho)$ (see Figure 16.20). Unfortunately, as we have seen above, there are several sources of noise and error in gathering $n(\theta, \rho)$. Some of these have to do with the random (Poisson) nature of radioactive decay, others have to do with the geometrical fact that the horizontal pacing between LOR lines becomes smaller going from the center of the ring towards its edges, and the fact that the sensors spatially sample the CE lines due to their finite number and spacing around the circle.

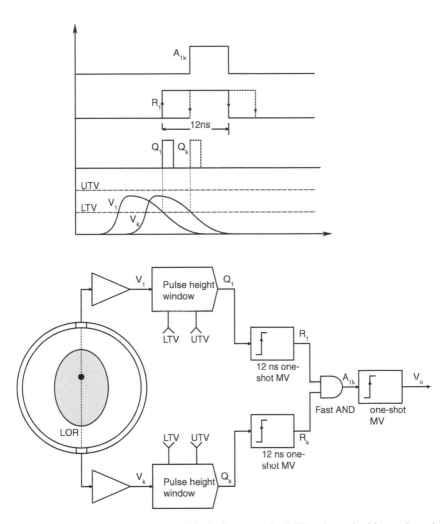

FIGURE 16.18 Timing diagram and block diagram of a PET pulse coincidence detection system.

PET images are calculated using the Radon transform and filtered back-projection as described in Section 16.3.3. Special attention has to be taken in the filtering to cut off high spatial frequencies in the data resulting from noise. An active research area in PET imaging is the application of statistical data reconstruction techniques to improve image detail (increase its MTF cutoff frequency).

16.5 MAGNETIC RESONANCE IMAGING (MRI)

16.5.1 INTRODUCTION

Magnetic resonance imaging is also called *magnetic resonance tomography* (MRT) because one of the display modes is tomographic slices. An MRI scanner is basically

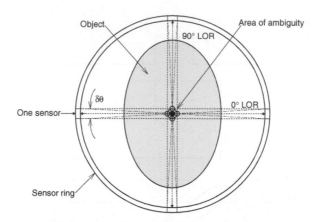

FIGURE 16.19 Ambiguity area defined by the finite acceptance angles of the photon counters when two events from the same point emit two intersecting LORs.

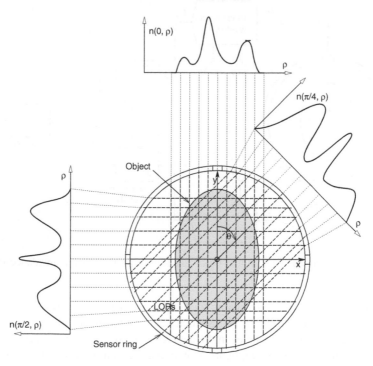

FIGURE 16.20 Representative photon counts for three different LOR angle arrays. There is a "hot spot" in the center of the slice.

a very large magnet with a hole in its center into which the patient is placed. Before describing the physical details of how MRI works, let us examine some of the pros and cons of this noninvasive imaging method. MRI advantages include:

- MRI is totally noninvasive and essentially risk-free. Unlike PET and CAT methods, there are no ionizing radiations from within or without.
- MRI gives excellent contrast for soft tissues including the brain, breasts, lungs and liver.
- MRI images blood vessels with high contrast because of the high water content of blood. This feature enables the detection of aneurisms, stenoses, areas of high perfusion in parts of the brain during specific tasks, and the vascularization accompanying tumors.

Some disadvantages of MRI are:

- An MRI scan takes a long time; c. 30 minutes, during which the patient must remain motionless to avoid blurring.
- MRI does not image bone well; tissue calcification is not easily seen.
- MRI is acoustically noisy. The gradient magnets are switched on and off, producing loud thunks from magnetostriction. In some cases, this noise can reach 95 dB. A patient should wear earplugs to prevent possible hearing loss.
- Because of the very high magnetic fields involved, patients wearing pacemakers or cochlear implants, or having implanted metal joints cannot undergo MRI. MRI is also avoided during the first trimester of pregnancy, although there have been no reported harmful effects to the fetus. An MRT has pixel resolution between 0.5 and 1 mm (HealthSystems, 2000).

16.5.2 MRI PHYSICS

First, let us define the orthogonal axes relevant to MRI. The z-axis is the center axis of the main electromagnet, and also runs the length of the body, feet to head. The y-axis runs perpendicular to the z-axis, from the back to the front (chest) of the patient. The x-axis is perpendicular to the z- and y-axes, and runs from left to right.

MRI exploits the magnetic and electromagnetic properties of certain atoms in a very strong magnetic field. The main, z-axis, magnetic field used in MRI is called B_z., which is typically on the order of 0.3 to 1.5 Tessla (1 Tessla = 1 Weber/m^2 = 10^4 Gauss). (By way of contrast, the earth's magnetic field is on the order of 0.5 Gauss.) A superconducting solenoidal magnet is generally used to generate B_z. The magnet has niobium-titanium alloy windings, and is chilled with liquid helium to make it superconducting, making it easy to maintain the desired high dc current without generating heat. The patient is placed in the center of the magnet's coil where the field strength is maximum. It can be shown that the field strength in the center of the coil is (Sears, 1953):

$$B_z = \frac{\mu_o NI}{L_c} \text{ Tessla} \qquad 16.22$$

Where μ_0 is the permeability of vacuum ($4\pi \times 10^{-7}$ N sec^2/Cb^2), N is the number of turns in the magnet coil, I is the coil current, and L_c is the coil's length in meters. At the ends of the coil, the magnetic field strength is about one-half that at the center.

It is known that atoms with an odd number of protons or neutrons possess a *nuclear spin angular momentum* vector, **M**, and thus exhibit the magnetic resonance phenomenon. Some of the atoms that are MR active include: ^{1}H (42.575, 1.000), ^{13}C (10.705, 0.016), ^{19}F (40.054, 0.830), ^{23}Na (11.262, 0.093), and ^{31}P (17.235, 0.066). The first number in parentheses is the (normalized) *Larmor frequency*, $f_L = \Gamma/2\pi$, in MHz/Tessla. The second number is the relative sensitivity vs. hydrogen (^{1}H).

Figure 16.21 illustrates the vector relationships when a charged particle (proton) moves in a circular path at constant tangential velocity, **v**, at radius r. The *orbital magnetic moment vector*, **M**, is given by the vector cross-product: $\mathbf{M} = \frac{1}{2}q\,(\mathbf{r} \times \mathbf{v})$, where **r** is the radius vector, and the angular momentum of the rotating particle, **L**, is defined by: $\mathbf{L} = m(\mathbf{r} \times \mathbf{v})$. Clearly, **M** and **L** are perpendicular to the plane of rotation of the proton.

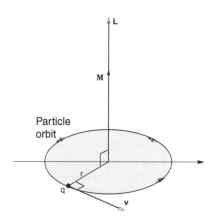

FIGURE 16.21 Vector magnetic moment, **M**, produced as the result of an orbiting proton.

When an atom's spinning proton interacts with an external magnetic field in the z-direction $\mathbf{B}_z$, a torque is experienced that causes its angular momentum axis to align with and precess about $\mathbf{B}_z$. (The z direction is defined as perpendicular to the plane of proton rotation.) The tip of the momentum vector describes a circle around $\mathbf{B}_z$. When $\mathbf{B}_z$ is first applied, it takes a finite *spin lattice relaxation time* for all the proton **M**s to respond. This response is characterized by an exponential equation of the form, $(1 - \exp(-t/T_1))$, where T_1 is the *spin lattice relaxation time constant*. ($T_1 = 2$ sec for urine, and 100–200 ms for fat.)

The steady-state frequency that the momentum vector revolves around $\mathbf{B}_z$ is the *Larmor frequency,* given by:

$$f_L = \Gamma\,|\,\mathbf{B}_z\,|\,/2\pi \text{ Hz} \qquad\qquad 16.23$$

Γ is the *gyromagnetic ratio,* given by the magnitude of the ratio of the orbital magnetic moment of the atom, **M**, to the *angular momentum* of the rotating proton, **L**. Γ can be shown to be equal to q/2m, where q is the proton charge, and m is its mass (Liley, 2001). Refer to Figure 16.22 for a description of the vectors.

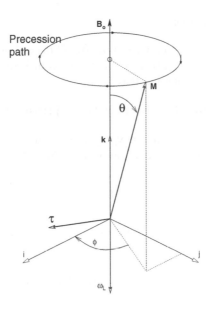

FIGURE 16.22 Vectors associated with a spinning proton interacting with an external magnetic field. The tip of **M** precesses around **B**$_o$ on the dotted line at the Larmor frequency.

It can be shown (Liley, 2001) that the vector differential equation of motion for one isolated magnetic moment subjected to **B**$_z$ is:

$$\dot{\mathbf{M}} = \Gamma\, \mathbf{M} \times \mathbf{B}_z \qquad\qquad 16.24$$

In an ensemble of many individual precessing **M**s, **M**$_e$ is the vector sum of the component **M**s.

In a static applied B field, **B**$_z$, the phases of an ensemble of many precessing magnetic moments are random. That is, each individual precessing **M** has a random position in its orbit (the dashed ellipse in Figure 16.22) induced by **B**$_z$. Because of this randomness, all of the x, y (or **i, j**) components of the individual **M**s cancel out. Thus the net macroscopic magnetic moment of the magnetized ensemble is aligned with **B**$_z$, even though individual protons are precessing around **B**$_z$ at the Larmor frequency. Thus, the static net **M**$_e$ = **M**$_z$, and $\dot{\mathbf{M}}_e$ = 0.

The crux of detecting the number of molecules contributing to **M**$_e$, hence the proton density in a volume element, is to perturb the individual **M**s by transiently changing the applied **B** vector's angle away from the z-axis (**k** unit vector). Because of the time-dependent motion of the x,y components of the tilted **M**s, and due to

Faraday's induction law, an ac voltage at the Larmor frequency is induced in a suitably placed pick-up coil. For a step change in the direction of $\mathbf{B_z}$, $\mathbf{M_{xy}}$ does not persist; it decays exponentially to zero with a characteristic time constant called the *effective spin relaxation time constant*, T_2^*. T_2^* is about 100 μs for protons. Thus, the induced Larmor EMF also decays in amplitude.

16.5.3 How MRI Works

So where does the resonance in MRI come from? Instead of a stepwise applied dc x-y component of $\mathbf{B}$, let us apply an x-y component of $\mathbf{B}$ that rotates at the Larmor frequency. That is, the net applied $\mathbf{B}$ is:

$$\mathbf{B} = \mathbf{B_z} + \mathbf{B_a}\,(\mathbf{i}\,\cos(\omega_L t) - \mathbf{j}\,\sin(\omega_L t)) \qquad 16.25$$

This $\mathbf{B_a}$ rotates with angular frequency, ω_L, in the same sense as the individual $\mathbf{M}$ vectors precess around $\mathbf{B_z}$. The equation of individual $\mathbf{M}$ vector motion is now:

$$\dot{\mathbf{M}} = \Gamma\,\mathbf{M} \times \left(\mathbf{B_z} + \mathbf{B_a}\right) \qquad 16.26$$

When we substitute Equation 16.25 into Equation 16.26, the following two ODEs result:

$$\dot{\phi} = \Gamma\left[B_a \cot(\theta)\cos\left(\omega_L t + \phi\right) - B_z\right] \qquad 16.27$$

$$\dot{\theta} = -\Gamma B_a \sin\left(\omega_L t + \phi\right) \qquad 16.28$$

When $\omega_L = \Gamma B_z$ is substituted in Equation 16.27, we find the solution:

$$\phi = -\Gamma\,B_z t - \pi/2 \qquad 16.29$$

and from Equation 16.28, $\dot{\theta}$ will be maximal and is given by $\dot{\theta} = \Gamma B_a$. Thus, a circularly polarized magnetic flux density rotating at the Larmor frequency determined by B_z will maximize the rate of nutation. However, it is easier to generate a *plane-polarized* $\mathbf{B_a}$ than the circularly polarized one described above. The plane-polarized flux density can be written:

$$\mathbf{B_a} = \mathbf{i}\,B_a \cos\left(\omega_L t\right) = \tfrac{1}{2}B_a\left\{\left[\mathbf{i}\cos\left(\omega_L t\right) - \mathbf{j}\sin\left(\omega_L t\right)\right] + \left[\mathbf{i}\cos\left(\omega_L t\right) + \mathbf{j}\sin\left(\omega_L t\right)\right]\right\} \;\; 16.30$$

The plane-polarized $\mathbf{B_a}$ is decomposed into right- and left-hand rotating components; the second term rotates opposite to the direction of precession and has negligible effect on nutation. It can be shown that when $\mathbf{B_a}$ rotates synchronously with the precessing magnetization vectors, a condition of *phase coherence* is induced in which the individual proton Ms are all nutated coherently and thus have the same fixed relationship around precessional orbits.

When the sinusoidal current producing $\mathbf{B_a}$ is gated on for about a microsecond, a peak *nutation angle* of c. 90° is produced in proton (^{1}H) MRI. (The nutation angle is the angle $\mathbf{L}$ makes with the z-axis.) The amplitude of the RF pulse from this angle-shifted $\mathbf{M_e}$ decays exponentially with a *transverse relaxation time constant,* T_2 ($20 < T_2 < 300$ ms). T_2 is basically the phase memory time constant of the spin. T_2 is shorter in inflamed, edematous or malignant tissues, and longer in fatty tissues. Note that $T_1 > T_2$ and T_2*, implying that different physical mechanisms are involved between the initial response to $\mathbf{B_a}$ on, and $\mathbf{B_a}$ off. Many complex interatomic magnetic reactions occur as the system goes from coherent spins to random phasing of the $\mathbf{M}$ rotations around $\mathbf{B_z}$. Note that the peak $|\mathbf{B_a}|/|\mathbf{B_z}|$ is typically ca. 0.005, a very small perturbation of $\mathbf{B_z}$. Control of the duration, period, and polarity of the $\mathbf{B_a}$ pulses and applied gradients are what give MRI images their exquisite contrast sensitivity. It can be shown that:

$$1/T_2^* = 1/T_2 + \Gamma|\Delta B_z|/2 \qquad\qquad 16.31$$

whereas before, T_2* is the effective spin–spin relaxation time constant, T_2 is the actual spin–spin relaxation time, and ΔB_z is the variation of the static magnetic field over the sample (Liley 2001).

Three major types of pulse sequences are used in MRI: Spin echo, inversion recovery, and gradient recalled echo. T_E is the time from the 90° $\mathbf{B_a}$ pulse to the receipt of the spin echo. Following the 90° pulse, the body's $\mathbf{M_e}$ is tilted in a transverse direction. If the 90° pulse is followed with a stronger 180° pulse, the individual $\mathbf{M}$s swing back so that initially, the slowest precessing protons now lead the change, and the faster-changing $\mathbf{M}$s are at the back of the group. The faster-responding ones catch up to the slow ones, so that they are back in phase; this causes the emitted signals to momentarily increase in amplitude. The fast and the slow responding $\mathbf{M}$s then go out of phase again and the RF signal again decreases. This increase in signal following the 180° pulse is called the *spin echo.* The timing of the 180° pulse following the 90° pulse is critical; it must be optimized to differentiate tissues on the basis of their T_2 values, so-called T_2-*weighted images* (Dawson, 2001).

MRI offers the option of being able to magnetically and electronically select the plane of the slice. If the main dc field is given a gradient, $\mathbf{B} = \mathbf{B_z} + G_x\, x$, where the field still points in the z-direction, but its amplitude varies in the x-direction (G_x is just dB_z/dx), the Larmor frequency is a function of x: $\omega_L(x) = \Gamma(B_z + G_x\, x)$. Now, if $\mathbf{B_a}$ with the excitation frequency $\omega = \Gamma B_z$ is applied, the slice x = 0 is selected. Spins in the y,z plane are tipped and emit RF signals, while other planes are not affected. The slice thickness, Δx, is controlled by the bandwidth of the bandpass filter acting on the RF signal from the pickup coil; a narrow filter bandwith gives a thin slice. Use of a $\mathbf{B_a}$ frequency of $\omega = \Gamma(B_z + G_x\, x_o)$ allows the y,z plane of interest to be shifted along the x axis to x_o. If a gradient, $\mathbf{B_z} + G_y\, y$, is used, the x,z plane is selected and the slice thickness is Δy. Oblique planes of constant Larmor frequency can be generated by making the main flux density a function of x, y, and z (Health-Systems, 2000).

Information from the amplitude and timing (T_1 and T_2) of the received RF transients taken along with the pickup coil position and the $\mathbf{B}_z$ gradient-defined slice allow the Radon transform and filtered back-projection to be used to form an MR image. As you can see, the process is much more complex than in forming a PET image. In PET we have discrete, all-or-nothing, coincidence events. In MRI, analog RF voltage wave-shapes and timing, taken along with the magnetic conditions that produced them, are factored into the image.

16.6 SINGLE PHOTON EMISSION TOMOGRAPHY (SPECT)

16.6.1 INTRODUCTION

The prototype *emission computed tomography* (ECT) device was developed by Kuhl and Edwards (1963). The first commercial SPECT device used a 32-channel gamma (Anger) camera called the Tomomatic-32 (Jaszczak, 1988). Since their inception, SPECT systems have steadily evolved; better, more highly collimated gamma cameras and improved DSP algorithms have improved image resolution (now c. 3.5 mm) and turned the SPECT system into a valuable diagnostic tool. An important application of SPECT is the identification of tissues with low blood flow, specifically, the brain following a stroke, and the heart with coronary artery disease. Liver, kidneys and other tissues are studied with SPECT, as well. A very important and promising application of SPECT is scintimammography —the detection of breast cancer by isoptopic labeling.

Like PET, SPECT also involves the administration to the patient of a short-lived radioisotope incorporated into a drug, hormone or metabolite with the object of measuring its density at target tissues relative to other tissues. However, the γ-ray emissions in SPECT occur as single random events, (at random times and directions) rather than in the synchronous pairs of photons that define the lines of response in PET. The path of a γ-ray in the SPECT process must be estimated from the ray collimation properties and the relative position of the gamma camera used to count the γ emissions. In the SPECT process, the camera is slowly rotated around the target tissue (e.g., the head) a full 360°. It stops every Δθ and accumulates counts in its N channels. The information gathered is the number of counts originating along each of the N parallel rays defined by the collimator. Similar to PET, the raw data are K data sets, n(jΔρ, kΔθ). K is the number of Δθ increments required to go from θ = 0° to 360°, and n is the number of discriminated radioactive events recorded in a given channel at a given camera angle. The K data sets, n(jΔρ, kΔθ) are discrete Radon transformed, then filtered back-projection is used to reconstruct the density of radioactivity in the tissue being scanned. Figure 16.23 illustrates a schematic top view of a human head being scanned by a SPECT system. Note that the lead tube collimator accepts only those γ photons that have paths that lie inside a certain acceptance angle, φ. Oblique rays striking the camera at angles greater than ± φ/2 to the normal to the camera plane are absorbed by the lead sides of the collimator tubes and are not counted. All the gamma cameras used in SPECT use collimators of one style or another. A collimated gamma camera is called an *Anger camera,* after its inventor, Hal Anger, who developed it at the Lawrence Berkeley Laboratory in the 1950s (Anger, 1964). Anger's original camera used a 1/2-in.-thick, 11-inch-diameter disk of NaI crystal as the scintillator, backed with 19 photomultiplier tubes (PMTs) (Blazek et al., 1995). A lead tube collimator was used in front of the crystal. A spatial resolution of c. 7 mm was claimed.

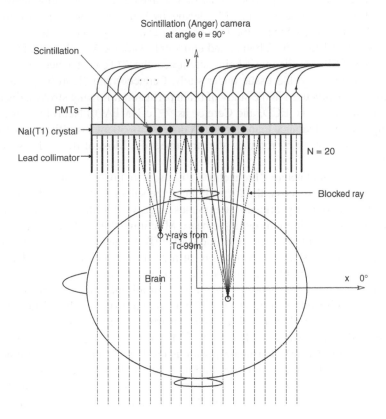

FIGURE 16.23 Schematic of a detector array picking up γ photons from ^{99m}Tc in the brain. Only those photons that enter a detector at less than its acceptance angle can be counted.

SPECT has a relatively poor resolution, partially due to the stochastic nature of the signals being counted, and partially due to the relatively large acceptance angles of the camera collimator tubes. However the cost of a SPECT procedure is about $1000, vs. $5000 for PET. A SPECT system is technically simpler than a PET scanner. All it requires is a high-resolution Anger camera, a system to move it precisely, electronics to discriminate and count the camera's outputs, and a powerful workstation to compute the tomogram. A PET system requires a ring of photon counters, pulse-height discrimination circuitry, coincidence and detection electronics, and, of course, a computer to reduce the data.

As in PET, gathering the data sets, $n(j\Delta\rho, k\Delta\theta)$, takes more time than actually computing the tomogram by filtered back projection. The SPECT data gathering process is more efficient than for PET because an Anger can have a square array and gather data for a number of slices at one time.

16.6.2 RADIOCHEMICALS USED IN SPECT

The radionuclide Technetium-99m was introduced by Harper et al. (1965) as a labeling agent. It is the byproduct of the radioactive decay of the radionuclide ^{99}Mo, produced by neutron activation. ^{99}Mo decays by beta (electron) emission to Technetium-99m (^{99m}Tc), which is the isotope most commonly used for tissue labeling. ^{99m}Tc has a half-life of 6.02 hours, and emits only 140.5 keV γ photons. Depending on the type of SPECT diagnosis being attempted, the ^{99m}Tc is attached to a chemical that has an affinity to the tissue under study. Ceretec® and Neurolite® are ^{99m}Tc-labeled compounds used in the study of brain perfusion following strokes. (Neurolite is also known as ^{99m}Tc-ECD, and Ceretec as ^{99m}Tc-HMPAO.) Neurolite has a faster brain uptake and clearance than Ceretec. A dose of 30–30 mCi (milliCuries) is given; imaging is done 30 to 60 minutes after the injection. Most of the ^{99m}Tc is excreted in urine.

IV ^{99m}Tc-pertechnetate (Technelite®) is used to image such tissues as brain lesions, the gastric mucosa, the thyroid gland, the salivary glands, and blood. ^{99m}Tc can be bound to many organic compounds, e.g., Cardiolite®, which is used to investigate coronary blood flow in the heart. Miraluma™ is a ^{99m}Tc compound used in scintimammography. Other applications of ^{99m}Tc-tagged pharmaceuticals include the study of renovascular hypertension, urinary tract infections, testicular cancer, brain metabolism, cardiovascular tissue, hepatobilary imaging, gastroesophageal reflux, etc. In fact, ^{99m}Tc is used in about 90% of all nuclear medicine studies.

Another radioisotope used in SPECT bone imaging and cardiac studies is Thallium-201. ^{201}Tl is produced with a cyclotron from ^{203}Tl. ^{201}Tl decays by electron capture to Mercury-201, a stable isotope. ^{201}Tl emits gamma photons with energies of 135 keV and 167 keV. Fortunately, little is used, as Tl and Hg salts are poisons.

Radioactive decay is a Poisson random process. That is, if the initial number of undecayed radioactive nuclei in a volume is N_o, then, after t time units (e.g., seconds, minutes, hours, etc.), the number, N, of undecayed nuclei in the volume is given by:

$$N = N_o \exp(-\lambda t) \qquad 16.32$$

λ is the *disintegration rate constant* characteristic of the radioisotope; its reciprocal is the decay time constant. In fact, the rate of disintegration is simply:

$$\dot{N} = -\lambda N \quad \text{events/time unit} \qquad 16.33$$

and the *half-life* of a radioisotope is simply:

$$T_{\frac{1}{2}} = \frac{\ln(2)}{\lambda} \text{ time units.} \qquad 16.34$$

16.6.3 Scintillation Crystals Used in Nuclear Medicine

Table 16.6.1 gives the important properties of the most common scintillation crystals used for SPECT, PET and nuclear imaging. Note that the scintillation decay time constant determines the event count rate of a given material. A high effective atomic number, Z, material is more effective at trapping γ photons.

TABLE 16.6.1
Properties of Some Important Scintillation Materials Used in Nuclear Medical Imaging

Properties	NaI(Tl)	BGO	CsI:Na	CsI:Tl	YAP:Ce	LSO:Ce
Chemical formula	NaI	$Be_4Ge_3O_{12}$	CsI	CsI	$YAlO_3$	$Lu_2(SiO_4)O$
Density (g/cm³)	3.67	7.13	4.51	4.51	5.37	7.40
Hygroscopicity	Yes	No	Slight	Slight	No	No
Refractive index, n	1.85	2.15	1.84	1.80	1.93	1.82
Peak emitted λ, nm.	410	480	420	565	365	420
Photons/meV	41,000	9,000	42,000	56,000	18,000	23,000
% of NaI:Tl	100	10	85	45	40	75
Scint. decay time (ns)	250	300	630	1000	27	40
Atten. length (cm) @ 140 keV	0.408	0.086	0.277	0.277	0.697	0.107
Effective Z	50	83			36	

16.6.4 Gamma Cameras and Collimators

An essential component of modern gamma (Anger) cameras is a means to convert the 140 keV photons from ^{99m}Tc to electronic signals. Anger used a single flat plate crystal of sodium iodide (NaI) as a scintillation interface between the γ photons and an array of photomultiplier tubes (PMTs). The use of NaI has continued to the present. The NaI scintillator has the following properties: Effective atomic number, 50; linear attenuation coefficient, 2.2 cm⁻¹ for 150 keV photons; optical index of refraction, 1.85; peak scintillation emission wavelength, 410 nm (violet); decay constant, 230 ns; mechanical, NaI is fragile and deliquescent. The latter property means that NaI crystals must be hermetically sealed, either in a vacuum or dry inert gas. Modern thallium-activated NaI crystals, such as those made and sold by Bicron Co., have been as large as a 17-in.-diameter disk, or a rectangular plate with a 38.5-in. diagonal. Bicron also manufactures curved NaI crystals to conform more closely to the curvature of the human body (Bicron, 1999). A typical thallium-activated NaI crystal used in SPECT is about 1 cm thick (Bertolucci, 1998).

When a 140 keV γ photon from ^{99m}Tc decay penetrates the collimator and strikes the NaI crystal, its energy is absorbed and converted to 410 nm photons that propagate in various directions through the crystal. In classical Anger camera design, a closely packed array of glass-enveloped PMTs sits on the back of the single NaI crystal. The PMTs generally have hexagonal end profiles to permit close packing (such as the Hammamatsu R3336 and R1537) to better capture the emitted scintillation photons.

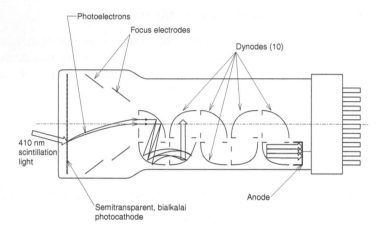

FIGURE 16.24 Cross-section of a photomultiplier tube with 10 dynodes.

Because light is reflected and refracted at interfaces, some energy from the 410 nm scintillation is lost in going from the NaI through the coupling medium to the PMT's glass envelope. In addition, absorption and attenuation of the oblique rays of 410 nm light occur in the crystal. In fact, some 410 nm light cannot leave the crystal because of *critical angle reflection*. If a 410 nm ray strikes the interface between the crystal and the coupling medium at more than the angle φ_c to the normal to the crystal surface, it will be totally reflected back into the crystal, where its energy will eventually be completely absorbed. From elementary optics, $\varphi_c = \sin^{-1}(n_1/n_2)$, where n_2 is the index of refraction of NaI at 410 nm (1.85), and n_1 is the index of refraction of the material outside the crystal but in intimate contact with it. The latter material can be a material such as microscope immersion oil with $n_1 = 1.515$, used to couple the scintillation light more efficiently to the PMT. With this n_1, $\varphi_c = 55°$, if air ($n_1 = 1$) is outside the NaI, then φ_c is only $32.7°$.

When a burst of 410 nm light strikes the PMT's photocathode, electrons are released and travel through the electric fields of a series of dynode electrodes where they gain kinetic energy in a stepwise manner. The electron pulse grows in size as it approaches the anode, because, as each bunch of electrons strikes a dynode, its kinetic energy dislodges even more electrons, etc. The more dynodes, the higher the PMT's current gain, but the longer it takes the initial photoelectron event to appear as a current pulse at the anode. A 10-dynode hexagonal PMT used in Anger cameras, such as the Hammamatsu R3336, has an electron transit time of 47 ns and a rise time of 6 ns. On the other hand, the microchannel plate R5916U series PMTs by Hammamatsu have a typical output pulse rise time of 188 ps (picoseconds) and a pulse fall-time of 610 ps. The half-height pulse width is 345 ps. This speed would be wasted counting scintillations in an NaI crystal, however, because of its 230 ns pulse decay time for scintillation events. Figure 16.24 illustrates a cross-sectional schematic of a PMT with 10 dynodes.

As remarked above, good γ-ray collimation is a necessary condition for a high-resolution SPECT image. Collimators are generally an array of tubes through a lead plate located over the front surface on the scintillation crystal. Taken as a whole, the collimator comprises a 2-D spatial sampling array, not unlike the facets of an insect's compound eye. And, like a compound eye, resolution is linked mathematically to the field of view of each tube in the array. Each tube defines an acceptance angle, φ, for incident γ rays. Rays incident at angles greater than $\varphi/2$ strike lead and are absorbed. The geometry of this collimation is shown in Figure 16.23, and in more detail for one tube in Figure 16.25A. From the geometry in the latter figure, it is easy to show that the total acceptance angle, $\varphi = 2 \tan^{-1}(w/L)$, where w is the tube diameter, and L its length. The smaller φ, the more directional the collimator, and the higher the image resolution. In fact, we can describe a *directional sensitivity function*, $f(\theta)$, for the tube based on the total intensity at the bottom of the tube (at the scintillation crystal's surface) as the function of angle θ made by an ideal continuous point source of radiation with the center line. $f(\theta) \equiv I(\theta)/I_{max}$, where $I(\theta)$ is the radiation intensity striking the bottom of the hole, i.e., the scintillator plate), and I_{max} is the maximum intensity. It can be shown that $f(\theta)$ is the normalized 1-D *spatial impulse response* of the tube (Northrop, 2001). Obviously, the intensity at the bottom of the tube is maximum when the point source is directly on-axis ($\theta = 0°$), and must be zero for $|\theta| \geq \varphi/2$. For $0° < |\theta| \leq \varphi/2$, there is a crescent "shadow" formed by the wall of the tube on the bottom, as shown in Figure 16.25B. The 1-D spatial frequency response of the tube collimator is proportional to the Fourier transform of $f(\theta)$, $F(u)$. $F(u)$ is real and even in the spatial frequency, u, because $f(\theta)$ is real and even. Note that the narrower $f(\theta)$, the broader the collimator's spatial frequency response. However, there is a trade-off between a high-frequency response (small w/L ratio) and system sensitivity. With a small w/L, few of the γ photons will be counted in a given interval; most will strike the sides of the lead tubes and be absorbed. Thus, to obtain high-definition SPECT plots, a longer counting time is needed at each camera angle. (The $f(\theta)$ illustrated in Figure 16.25C is "typical," no mathematical function was derived to describe it.)

A traditional Anger camera uses a flat collimator on a large flat NaI scintillation crystal backed with an array of PMTs. Because the object being imaged is generally oval or rounded in form, this means that the inherent ray geometry causes the image resolution at the edges of the camera to become degraded and distorted from that at the center. Center resolution is c. 3.5 mm (Balzek et al., 1995).

16.6.5 FUTURE TRENDS IN NUCLEAR MEDICAL IMAGING

To reduce the cost and complexity of the traditional flat-plate Anger camera design, and to improve on its imaging resolution, several new design strategies for gamma cameras for SPECT are being explored. In one approach being developed at the Karolinska Hospital in Stockholm, a cylindrical NaI scintillation crystal is used to better fit human anatomy; the head or body part is placed in the center of the cylinder. γ photons from ^{99m}Tc are coupled to the cylindrical scintillator through four lead collimators. 410 nm scintillation photons from the crystal are coupled to a radially oriented array of hexagonal PMTs, arranged in four rows and 18 columns, giving a total of 72 channels. U.S. Patent No. 5,783,829 (Sealock et al., 1998) describe another gamma camera made with separate curved sections of CsI scintillation crystals designed to better match the patient's geometry.

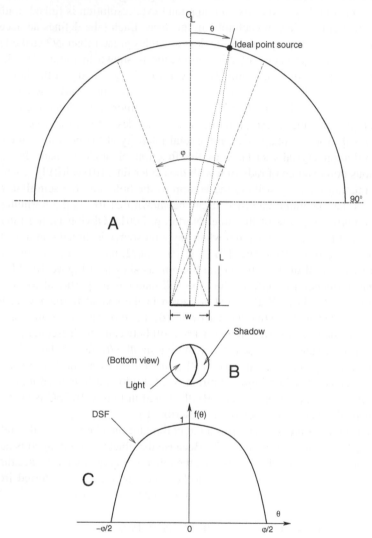

FIGURE 16.25 (A) Geometry of a system defining the acceptance angle of a γ photon collimator. Direct rays at angles $> |\varphi/2|$ do not strike the counter scintillator at the bottom of the tube; they are absorbed by the tube walls. (B) A crescent shadow is formed at the bottom of the collimator tube by a parallel ray bundle striking the tube mouth from an angle to the right, as shown in A. (The reader can verify this by shining a flashlight on a cardboard tube.) (C) A typical directional sensitivity function for a tube collimator. In an array of such collimators, the narrower the DSF, the higher the spatial frequency resolution of the array.

Scientists at the Instituto Nazionale di Fisica Nucleare in Rome (INFN-Roma), group on High Resolution Single Photon Emission Tomography (HIRESPET) are taking two innovative approaches to improving image quality in SPECT. One approach has been based on the innovative Hammamatsu *position sensitive photo-*

multiplier tube (PSPMT). The single PSPMT replaces dozens of conventional PMTs as scintillation photon detectors. Photoelectrons are emitted from various positions of the large area photocathode, depending on the distribution of input photons from the scintillators. A proximity mesh dynode structure produces electron multiplication and keeps the initial spatial distribution of the emission from the photocathode. Hammamatsu makes several models of PSPMTs; the R2486 series has a 76 mm (3-in.) diameter, disk photocathode; the R2487 series has a 3×3-in. square photocathode, and the R3292 series has a 5-in. diameter, 12-stage, bialkalai photocathode.

In the large R3292 PSPMT, the anode is formed by an orthogonal grid of 56 non-touching wires, i.e., 28 wires in the x-direction and 28 wires in the y-direction. In the square R2487 PSPMTs, the anode grid is 18×18 wires, and, in the round, R2486 PSPMTs, the anode grid is 16×16 wires. The anode grids have a square area, whether the shape of the photocathode is round or square. In the large R3292 PSPMT, the grid measures 53.34 mm (2.1 in.) on a side. Between each pair of wires on a side of the grid is a series of 1 k resistors, as shown in Figure 16.26. To understand how the PSPMT works, let us first consider the y-axis wires. The gray dot represents a beam of multiplied photoelectrons striking the grid; it behaves like a current source, $i_s(n,t)$, where it strikes the nth y-grid wire. The op amps are current-to-voltage converters. For example, i_{yb} flows into the op amp's summing junction, a virtual ground, and $V_{yb} = -i_{yb} R$. At the nth wire (n = 5 in this example), the voltage, V_{yn} can be shown to be:

$$V_{yn} = \frac{i_s R n(K-n)}{K}, \quad (0 \le n \le K) \qquad 16.35$$

And by Ohm's law, the current i_{ya} is:

$$i_{ya} = \frac{i_s R n(K-n)/K}{nR} = i_s(1 - n/K) \qquad 16.36$$

And i_{yb} is:

$$i_{yb} = \frac{i_s R n(K-n)/K}{(K-n)R} = i_s n/K \qquad 16.37$$

Thus, $V_{ya} = -i_s(1 - n/K)R$, $V_{yb} = -i_s(n/K)R$, and $(V_{ya} + V_{yb}) = -i_s R$; i.e., the sum signal gives the amplitude of $i_s(n,t)$. The difference, $(V_{ya} - V_{yb}) = -i_s R(1 - 2n/K)$. Thus, the four output voltages are sampled, and the ratio

$$\frac{\left(V_{ya} - V_{yb}\right)}{\left(V_{ya} + V_{yb}\right)} = 1 - 2n/K \qquad 16.38$$

is calculated. Note that the ratio is a linear function of the wire position in the y-grid. A similar relation can be developed for the x-grid. Thus, a transient amplified

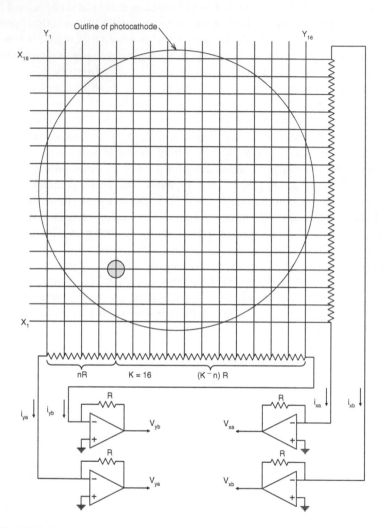

FIGURE 16.26 Schematic of the anode wires and analog readout electronics of a position-sensitive photomultiplier tube.

photocurrent pulse, i_s (x, y, t) can be located in terms of the wire numbers in the x, y grid of the PSPMT by simple signal processing.

Blazek et al. (1995) described a prototype high-resolution gamma camera. To take advantage of the PSPMT's high spatial resolution, they used individual small scintillator crystals, optically isolated from one another. Yttrium aluminum perovskit doped with cerium (YAlO$_3$:Ce, or YAP:Ce) was formed into thin square rods, $0.6 \times 0.6 \times 18$ mm. An array of 11×22 of these YAP:Ce "needles" was used with an R2486 PSPMT. The prototype camera was tested with various ^{99m}Tc phantoms;

it showed a resolution of c. 0.7 mm, a decided improvement over state-of-the-art collimated single-crystal Anger cameras.

Recently, (1999) a California start-up company, Gamma Medica marketed their LumaGem® gamma camera based on the same design strategy described in the paragraph above. The LumaGem uses a 5 × 5-in.-square array of 5625 individual "needle" scintillation crystals made from cesium iodide. The ends of the individual crystals are about 1.69 mm square. The crystals are coupled to a high-resolution PSPMT. Because of its small size, the LumaGem camera is ideally suited for scintimmamography and thyroid studies, as well as eventual application for brain SPECT. The manufacturer claims a spatial resolution of 1.75 mm for the camera in imaging tissue.

In the future, there will be continuing development of smaller high-resolution gamma cameras. Researchers at CERN (Geneva) and HIRESPET are developing an Imaging Silicon Pixel Array (ISPA) tube. The first version of this prototype device had geometry based on the venerable IR image intensifier tube. (See Figure 16.27.) Instead of IR photons striking a photocathode and generating photoelectrons, the UV photons from a scintillator crystal hit the ISPA tube photocathode, which emits photoelectrons. They are accelerated in straight lines, *in vacuo,* 20 to 50 mm by an electric field generated by a 20 to 25 kV potential. These high-energy, photoelectrons strike a chip with a 16 × 64 (1024) matrix of biased diode sensors on it. The active chip area is 4.8 × 8 mm. Each diode in the array has a 75 × 500 μm area. Diode reverse current is proportional to the electron current striking it. In the basic system, no external lead collimator was used in front of the single-plate YAP:Ce scintillator. 365 nm YAP:Ce scintillation photons were coupled to the ISPA tube's UV-sensitive photocathode through a quartz fiber optic (FO) coupler. Resolution was tested using a lead plate collimator source with two 350 μm holes drilled in it 1.2 mm apart. The ISPA tube prototype with the FO window could resolve objects at c. 700 μm. In another version, YAP:Ce needles with 600 × 600 μm end areas were used to convert γ photons to 365 nm scintillation photons. The YAP needles are optically isolated from each other and together act like a collimator. Resolution with the YAP needle ISPA tube was 310 μm (Puertolas et al., 1997).

A second-generation ISPA tube, shown schematically in Figure 16.28, uses an electric field lens to gather photoelectrons from a large photocathode (40 mm active diameter) and focus them on a smaller electron sensor chip. The demagnifying ratio of the prototype tube was 1/4.45 (D'Ambrosio et al., 1998, 1999). This cross-focusing (CF) ISPA tube will be studied using individual 1 × 1 mm column YAP:Ce crystals instead of the single YAP plate. I would predict the resolution to be c. 1 mm, suitable for scintimammography imaging and perhaps SPECT.

In summary, the ISPA tube approach detects photoelectrons arising from scintillations by a matrix of biased pn junctions. The PSPMT approach uses the crossed wire matrix of the PSPMT to sense the photoelectron current directly. The photomultiplier offers more photoelectron current gain, however, and probably will be more expensive.

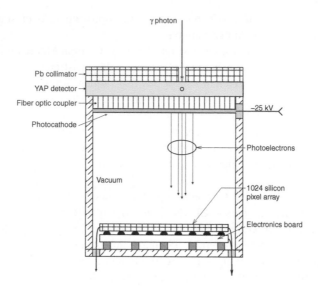

FIGURE 16.27 A first-generation imaging silicon pixel array (ISPA) tube.

16.7 OPTICAL COHERENCE TOMOGRAPHY (OCT)

16.71 INTRODUCTION

Optical coherence tomography is a new laser-based noninvasive non-contact imaging technique that can image tissue structures to a depth of 2 to 3 mm, *in vivo*, with a resolution of 5 to 15 µm (vs. 110 µm for high-frequency ultrasound). OCT was first developed in 1991 at MIT's Research Laboratory for Electronics (RLE) by James Fujimoto (Fujimoto et al. 1995).

OCT has been used with endoscopes to examine cancers and lesions on the surfaces of human mucosa, including that of the esophagus, larynx, stomach, colon, urinary bladder, and the uterine cervix (Sergeev et al., 1997; Feldchtein et al., 1998). OCT has also been used in the study and characterization of skin melanomas, and it also has application in the study of wound healing, e.g., for skin grafts in treating burns. Another important application of OCT is in ophthalmology. The anatomical layers of the retina can be displayed, both radially and tangentially, and its thickness measured. OCT has been found valuable in diagnosing diabetic retinopathy, macular holes, fluid accumulation, retinal detachments, etc. (Puliafito et al., 1996). The study of the fine structure of tooth enamel, dentin, caries and gums has also been made possible by OCT (Wang et al., 1999; Everett, 1998).

An OCT image from Boppart, S. et al. (*Nature Medicine*, 4(7): 1998) shows cells imaged by OCT on the left, and the same cells in a photomicrograph from a conventional histological (fixed) preparation are shown in Figure 16.29. Figure 16.30 from the same source illustrates a cross-section through frog abdominal skin. Note the capillaries. A radial (depth) slice OCT image of a normal retinal fovea is shown in Figure 16.31. (This image, originally in color, was on the NY Eye and Ear Infirmary website.)

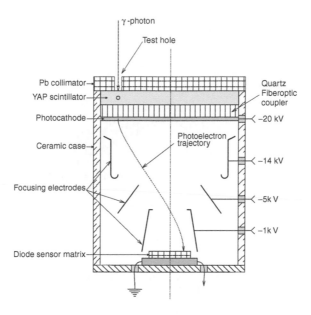

FIGURE 16.28 A second-generation ISPA tube using a larger photocathode and focusing electrodes to direct photoelectrons from the photocathode of area A_p to the smaller diode detector array of area A_d.

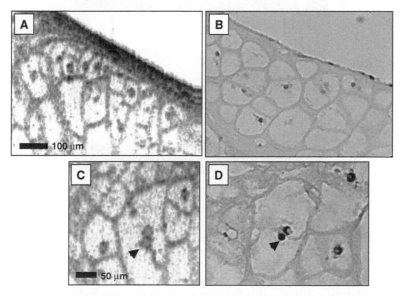

FIGURE 16.29 A comparison of cells imaged by optical coherence tomography (left) with conventional light microscopy (right) at the same magnification. (Used with permission of Dr. Stephen A. Boppart and *Nature Medicine*.)

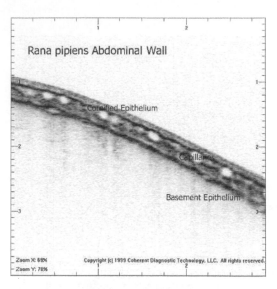

FIGURE 16.30 Transverse section through frog abdominal skin using OCT. (Used with permission of LightLab™ Imaging, LLC.)

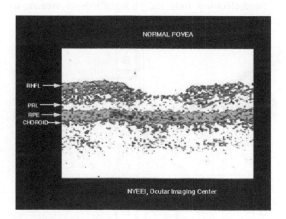

FIGURE 16.31 OCT image of the retinal fovea (original image in pseudocolor). Note the neural layers. (With permission of the New York Eye and Ear Infirmary.)

16.7.2 How Optical Coherence Tomography Works

The light source in OCT is generally a near-IR superluminescent light-emitting diode (SLD or SLED) with a narrow bandwidth (e.g., 17 nm half-intensity around an 812 nm peak). *Optical coherence length* is purposely short compared with a laser diode, only about 30 nm. SLDs are multilayer devices; in the 800 nm region they are fabricated from GaAS and AlGaAS. In the 1300–1500 nm range, they are made from InGaAsP and InP (Integrated, 1998). Near-IR is used in medical OCT for better tissue penetration.

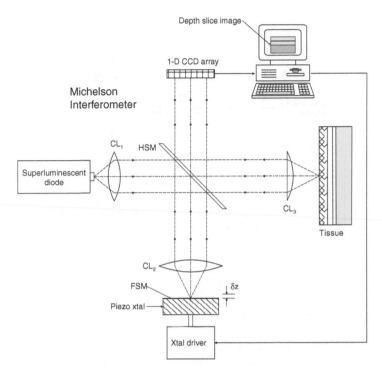

FIGURE 16.32 Schematic of an OCT system using a scanning Michelson interferometer. A short-coherence-length superluminescent diode (SLD) is used instead of a laser light source. The SLD is used to limit the thickness of the OCT image.

The SLD beam is directed to a *Michelson interferometer* (see Figure 16.32). The beam emerging from the interferometer is collimated into a small spot or a narrow line (in the y-direction) that is mechanically scanned over the tissue under study; in x and y for the spot and x for the line. The reflected light is collected and directed back through the interferometer. The amount and phase of the reflected light depend on the refractive index of the microscopic anatomical components of the tissue under study, as well as their absorption in x, y, and z.

With the low-coherence SLD source, interference fringes are generated only if the absolute path distance between the two arms is very small (less than half the coherence length). The δz modulation effectively scans the object in the depth (z) direction, once the coarse mirror position has been adjusted to balance the interferometer with the object. There is no fringe ambiguity problem such as would be caused with a highly coherent laser source. If the scanning mirror moves out of range of the SLD's coherence, the image vanishes. Thus, the OCT operator knows exactly the depth at which the scanning is taking place.

The backscatter intensity output of the interferometer is a function of depth (z) and position (x,y) over the target. By adjusting the interferometer to keep z constant, a 2-D, x,y slice of tissue structure can be displayed. Or x can be held constant and a 2-D depth slice image in z and y can be generated (most common for retinal scans).

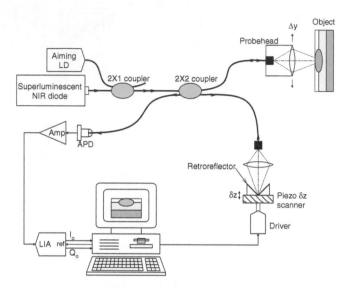

FIGURE 16.33 A fiber optic Michelson interferometer used with an SLD for OCT.

The intensity output from the interferometer is directed to a single photosensor for the spot probe, and a CCD line-scan sensor for the line probe.

16.7.3 Applications of OCT

A commercial OCT system for ophthalmological scanning has been marketed by Humphrey Instruments. The Humphrey OCT system can reproducibly quantify retinal and nerve fiber layer thickness to better than 11 µm. Roche Diagnostics Co. in Germany developed an OCT system using a chromium fosterite 1310 nm laser projecting a 4.5 µm spot. A single-mode optical fiber Michelson interferometer was used to condition the reflected radiation. Most OCT systems to date are experimental, because the technology in the field is evolving so rapidly. The trend today is away from the classical straight-beam Michelson interferometer to the use of single-mode optical fiber Michelson interferometers, such as illustrated in Figure 16.33. Note that a visible LED is used for targeting. The probe in this configuration produces a single, small spot.

An important enhancement of OCT being developed is Doppler optical coherence tomography (DOCT). DOCT is based on coherence gating. It combines laser Doppler flowmetry (LDF) (see Section 15.5 of this text) with OCT. Heterodyne mixing of the superimposed source light with the Doppler-shifted backscattered light at a photodiode surface yields a lower (RF) side-band whose frequency, f_D, is proportional to the velocity of moving scatterers parallel to the incident collimated beam. Because of the small beam diameter and low coherence of the source, A Doppler frequency can be determined for all of the moving reflectors in an OCT image pixel. Colors can be assigned by the imaging computer to give qualitative velocity information on pixels containing moving scatterers. The frequency of the detected Doppler shift was shown in Section 15.5 of this text to be:

$$f_D \equiv (v_s - v_r) = (2\ v_s/c')\ |\mathbf{v}|\cos(\theta) = (2/\lambda_s)\ |\mathbf{v}|\cos(\theta)\ \text{Hz} \qquad 16.39$$

Where $\mathbf{v}$ is the velocity vector of the moving scatterer, c' is the speed of light in the medium containing the moving scatterer, v_s is the frequency of the incident light of wavelength λ_s, v_b is the frequency of the backscattered light, and θ is the angle between $\mathbf{v}$ and the line between the scatterer and the source/pickup

Yazdanfar et al. (1997) studied DOCT on living *Xenopus laevis* tadpoles, and were able to observe the structure of and blood velocity in the tadpole's beating heart in real time. They found that the majority of Doppler shifts came from the motion of the ventricle itself; blood velocity was harder to measure because of turbulence in the ventricle. (Recall that the Doppler shift is caused by the reflector particles' velocity components parallel to the incident light.) The reader should consult Yazdanfar's paper for details of how they acquired and processed images. It appears that DOCT is well suited for experimental studies on microcirculation in tumors, the retina, the heart, healing wounds, and burns, etc.

Another variation on basic OCT exploits the *birefringence* in the tissue being scanned. That is, how the polarization vector of incident polarized light is changed by certain tissues at scattering. These changes provide additional information on the optical fine structure of the object's tissues, including refractive index and absorbance. Polarization-sensitive optical coherence tomography (PSOCT) has been carried out by several means. Figure 16.34 illustrates an air-path Michelson interferometer adapted to measure the polarization state of the selected OCT voxel (de Boer et al., 1999). de Boer et al. used an 856 nm, 0.8 mW superluminescent diode with a spectral half-peak intensity bandwidth (FWHM) of 25 nm. The beam from the SLD was linearly polarized horizontally by passing it first through a Glan-Thompson polarizer before the spectrophotometer. The beam was then split into two equal-intensity arms by a polarization-preserving beam splitter (PPBS). In the upper (reference) arm, the light was passed through a zero-order quarter-wave plate (QWP) oriented at 22.5° to the incident polarization, reflected off a moving 45° mirror and reflected from a retroreflector reference mirror. The reflected light was again directed to the moving mirror and again passed through the QWP, gaining a total E-vector rotation of 45° with respect to the horizontal. The moving mirror modulated the length of the reference channel path length by 20 μm to generate a carrier frequency. A neutral density filter (NDF) was used to reduce the intensity noise in the image by a factor of 50 (the OD was not given). Light in the sample arm passed through a second QWP oriented at 45° to the incident horizontal linear polarization; this produces circularly polarized light that is incident on the sample. The backscattered light passed again through the focusing lens, and again, the QWP. This light had an arbitrary (elliptical) polarization due to interaction with the sample. This light was recombined with the 45° polarized light in the reference arm and directed to a polarizing beam-splitting prism that separated the mixed beams into orthogonal polarization components that were directed to photodetectors. The optical theory that describes the detection process is too complex to pursue in detail here. The

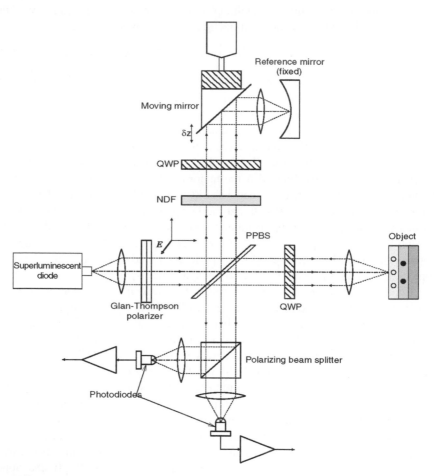

FIGURE 16.34 A Michelson interferometer adapted to measure the polarization state of the object in generating an OCT image. (System similar to that described by deBoer et al., 1999.)

interested reader should refer to the papers by de Boer et al., 1999, and Saxer et al., 2000 for details. Results in these papers showed that the OCT images made with polarization sensitivity had greatly increased contrast and detail. Pixel sizes in the range of 5 to 10μm square were demonstrated in the Saxer et al. paper.

Still another version of the OCT system was described by Sticker et al., 2000. These workers developed a variation on the birefringence-measuring OCT system described above, called *differential phase contrast OCT* (DPC-OCT). Their system was evaluated using a non-living optical test sample, and was shown to be responsive to the optical phase changes in the light returned from the object. It could display images based on very small optical path differences that were invisible in conventional intensity-based OCT imaging. Such path differences can be due to refractive index fluctuations or geometrical path variations.

A fiber optic Michelson interferometer version of the polarization-sensing OCT has special problems, because the optical fibers themselves exhibit birefringence when moved or subjected to mechanical strain. It is possible to compensate for these problems, but at the expense of some optical and signal processing complexity.

Perhaps in the future, polarization and Doppler enhancements can be combined in the same fiber optic OCT system.

16.8 ULTRASOUND IMAGING

16.8.1 INTRODUCTION

Ultrasonic imaging is a popular, widely used, form of noninvasive medical imaging that carries negligible risk to the patient. No ionizing radiations are used, nor are ultra-strong magnetic fields required; the sound pressure levels in medical ultrasound are too low to cause cell damage by heating or cavitation. Ultrasonic imaging is used on all major internal tissues, including the brain, eyes, heart, liver, intestines, breasts, uterus, testes, the fetus, placenta, etc. Pixel resolution in ultrasound imaging depends on, among other factors, the sound wavelength used. As with electromagnetic radiation (e.g., light), the wavelength, $\lambda = f/c$, where the sound frequency applied to the tissue is f, and c is the speed of sound in the tissue (typically 1540 m/sec in "soft tissue"). Medical ultrasound frequencies range from c. 1 to 50 MHz. Thus, λ for 10 MHz ultrasound (*in vivo*) is 154 μm, and for 50 MHz ophthalmological ultrasound, λ is 30.8 μm. While pixel resolution increases with increasing frequency, so does energy absorption by the biological tissue ensonified.

By combining Doppler ultrasound with imaging, it is possible to view major blood vessels in the body and quantitatively measure their blood velocity at the same time the image is made. Doppler ultrasonic imaging is invaluable in diagnosing kidney failure, coronary stenoses, pulmonary embolisms, and strokes.

Obstetric ultrasonic imaging is useful in determining such things as the number of fetuses, the sex of a fetus, critical fetal dimensions indicating normal growth and fetal age, possible birth defects, and, before delivery, how the fetus is lying, the head size (is a cesarian section indicated?), the placental location, the amount of amniotic fluid, and whether the umbilical cord is lying normally.

When it is impossible to view the retina of the eye through the cornea because of trauma (e.g., to the cornea, or blood in the eyeball), ophthalmological ultrasound can be used to diagnose a detached retina, or locate embedded foreign objects. True, OCT gives at least an order of magnitude better resolution of the retina and its pathologies than does ultrasound, but there must be a clear, undistorted optical path to enable its use.

16.8.2 The Physics of Ultrasound Propagation in Solids and Liquids

Ultrasound is basically sound of frequencies exceeding 20 kHz, up to 100s of MHz. In biological systems, sound propagation is generally in solids and liquids (e.g., blood, CSF, urine), and sometimes in air (in the lungs). The sonic energy is introduced into the body by a transmitting transducer in intimate contact with the skin so that its vibrational dispacements introduce sound waves through the skin into the body. Ultrasound propagates in the body by *longitudinal pressure waves* in which tissue elasticity allows a "particle" fixed in the volume to move back and forth longitudinally around a common center. Its motion is in the z-direction (direction of propagation of an acoustic plane wave). To describe the particle motion mathematically, consider that it has a differential element of mass, $dm = \rho\, A\, dz$. The acceleration of dm is $a = d^2\xi/dt^2$, where ξ is the particle displacement in the z direction. A Taylor's series can be used to find the differential force on dm:

$$F(z+dz) - F(z) = \left[F(z) + \frac{dF(z)}{dz}dz + \ldots \right] - F(z) = \frac{dF(z)}{dz}dz \qquad 16.40$$

So finally, by Newton's second law,

$$\frac{dF(z)}{dz}dz = \rho\, A\, dz \frac{d^2\xi(z)}{dt^2} \qquad 16.41$$

Equation 16.41 reduces to

$$\frac{dp}{dz} = \rho \frac{du}{dt} \qquad 16.42$$

Where in the above equations, $p = F/A$ in Newtons/meter^2 (Pascals), $u = \dot{\xi}$ the particle velocity in the z direction in m/sec, and ρ is the medium density in kg/meter^3.

The *specific acoustic impedance* of the medium is defined as $Z_s = p/u$. The fundamental dimensions of Z_s are $ML^{-2}T^{-1}$, and its units are *Rayls*. (For example, the Z_s of muscle is about 1.70×10^6 kg m^{-2} s^{-1}, or 1.70 M Rayls.) Another version of acoustic impedance is used in describing the properties of wind instruments. This definition is more analogous to Ohm's law for electricity. Here, $Z_{ac} = p/\dot{q}$. That is, Z_{ac} is equal to the pressure in Pascals at a point divided by the volume flow rate in m^3/sec It is easy to show that the fundamental dimensions of Z_{ac} are $ML^{-4}T^{-1}$; its units are often given as Pa sec/m^3 (Wolfe, 2000).

The following is a heuristic development of the *wave equation* for longitudinal particle motion in one dimension (z) in a non-lossy, elastic medium. Assume that a plane acoustic wave is propagating in the +z direction in a tube of area A. The medium has a uniform equilibrium density, ρ_o, kg/m^3. (Note that, in reality, ρ_o is a function of position in the ensonified object, i.e., ρ_o (x, y, z)).

Now the mass of a small slice of medium is: $\Delta m = \rho_0 \, A \, \Delta z$. Consider a particle displacement from z to $z + \Delta z$. The acceleration of this point at $z + \Delta z/2$ can be approximated by:

$$a \cong \frac{\partial^2}{\partial t^2}\left[\frac{\xi(z)+\xi(z+\Delta z)}{2}\right]$$

16.43

Thus, by Newton's second law of motion:

$$A\left(\Delta P_{12} - \Delta P_2\right) \cong \Delta m \frac{\partial^2}{\partial t^2}\left[\frac{\xi(z)+\xi(z+\Delta z)}{2}\right]$$

16.44

The left-hand term has the dimensions of force. ΔP_1 is the pressure change in the volume elements between $z - \Delta z$ and z; ΔP_2 is the pressure change in the volume elements between $z + \Delta z$ and $z + 2\Delta z$ due to medium deformation. These ΔPs follow from the definition of the *adiabatic bulk modulus of elasticity* of the medium, B:

$$\Delta P_1 \cong -B\left[\frac{\xi(z)-\xi(z-\Delta z)}{\Delta z}\right]$$

16.45

$$\Delta P_2 \cong -B\left[\frac{\xi(z+2\Delta z)-\xi(z+\Delta z)}{\Delta z}\right]$$

16.46

Substituting the relations above for the ΔPs we can write:

$$B\left\{\frac{\xi(z+2\Delta z)-\xi(z+\Delta z)}{\Delta z}-\frac{\xi(z)-\xi(z-\Delta z)}{\Delta z}\right\}\cong \rho_0$$
$$A \, \Delta z \frac{\partial^2}{\partial t^2}\left[\frac{\xi(z)+\xi(z+\Delta z)}{2}\right]$$

16.47

Now take the limit as $\Delta z \to 0$. The result is the one-dimensional wave equation:

$$\frac{\partial^2 \xi(z,\,t)}{\partial z^2} = \left(\rho_0/B\right)\frac{\partial^2 \xi(z,\,t)}{\partial t^2}$$

16.48

In three dimensions, the wave equation has the more general form:

$$\nabla^2 \xi(x,\,y,\,z,\,t) = \frac{1}{c^2}\frac{\partial^2 \xi(x,\,y,\,z,\,t)}{\partial t^2}$$

16.49

Where ∇^2 is the (scalar) Laplacian operator; and c is the wave velocity; c = $\sqrt{B/\rho_o}$ m/sec

$$\nabla^2(*) = \frac{\partial^2(*)}{\partial x^2} + \frac{\partial^2(*)}{\partial y^2} + \frac{\partial^2(*)}{\partial z^2} \qquad 16.50$$

Note that the wave equation can also be written in terms of the *instantaneous excess pressure*, p(x,y,z,t):

$$\nabla^2 p(x, y, z, t) = \frac{1}{c^2} \frac{\partial^2 p(x, y, z, t)}{\partial t^2} \qquad 16.51$$

The *characteristic acoustic impedance*, a property intrinsic to the medium, is defined as:

$$Z_c \equiv \rho_o c = \sqrt{B\rho_o} \ kg/m^2 \ sec \qquad 16.52$$

When an acoustic plane wave (with wavelength much smaller than the interface dimensions) strikes the interface between two media having different characteristic acoustic impedances, two things happen analogous to a light ray striking the boundary between two media with different refractive indices (see Figure 16.35):

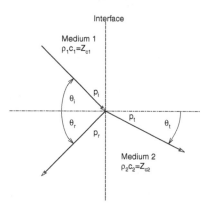

FIGURE 16.35 Vectors showing the reflection and refraction when acoustic plane waves strike a plane interface between two media having different characteristic acoustic impedances.

1. *Reflection.* If the propagation axis is at an angle θ_i with the normal to the interface, a portion of the incident wave is reflected at an angle $\theta_r = \theta_i$.
2. Transmission with *refraction* follows Snell's law: $\theta_t = \sin^{-1}((c_2/c_1) \sin(\theta_i))$. From boundary conditions, it can be shown that at the interface, the reflected wave has an intensity given by: $p_r = R \ p_i$, where:

$$R = \frac{\rho_2 c_2 \cos(\theta_i) - \rho_1 c_1 \cos(\theta_t)}{\rho_2 c_2 \cos(\theta_i) + \rho_1 c_1 \cos(\theta_t)} = \frac{Z_{c2} \cos(\theta_i) - Z_{c1} \cos(\theta_t)}{Z_{c2} \cos(\theta_i) + Z_{c1} \cos(\theta_t)} \qquad 16.53$$

Similarly, the pressure of the transmitted wave-front is given by: $p_t = T\, p_i$, where, for normal incidence:

$$T = 1 + R = \frac{2 Z_{c2}}{Z_{c1} + Z_{c2}} \qquad 16.54$$

R is typically ≤ 0.01 for soft tissue interfaces, thus, very little of the transmitted ultrasound energy is reflected back in pulse-echo imaging.

The intensity of an acoustic wave, I, is defined as the energy per unit time (power) that flows across a unit area perpendicular to wave propagation. Its units are Joules/sec m^2 or Watts/m^2, or, in cgs units, ergs/cm^2 sec. For the simple case of an infinite one-dimensional plane wave, it can be shown that:

$$I = 2\pi^2 f^2 (\rho_o\, c)\, \xi^2 = \omega^2 Z_c\, \xi^{2/}\ 2\ \text{Watts/m}^2 \qquad 16.55$$

All of the foregoing mathematical descriptions are based on the assumption that the propagating medium is perfectly elastic, that is, energy put into particle displacements is recovered, none is lost. In reality, all real propagation media are lossy; they are viscoelastic. Some of the acoustic energy put into particle displacement is lost as heat. Thus, an acoustic wave loses energy as it propagates; its pressure and particle velocity decrease with propagation distance.

Assuming that a sinusoidal plane wave is propagating in the +z direction, the excess pressure can be written as:

$$p(z, t) = P_o \exp(-\alpha z) \exp[-j(kz - \omega t)) \qquad 16.56$$

Where α is the absorption coefficient (actually, $\alpha(x,y,z)$), and the intensity as a function of p is given by:

$$I = \frac{|p|^2}{\rho_o c}\ \text{Watts/m}^2 \qquad 16.57$$

The intensity is attenuated with distance according to:

$$I(z) = I_o \exp(-2\alpha z) \qquad 16.58$$

$\mu \equiv 2\alpha$ is defined as the *intensity absorption coefficient*. In general, μ has an approximately linearly increasing function of frequency, i.e., $\mu(f) = \mu_o + \beta f$, so the cost of using higher frequency ultrasound to get better resolution is that its useful penetration depth is limited (Liley, 2001). This is not a problem, for example, for 50 MHz ophthalmic ultrasound, which only needs to penetrate to the depth of the eyeball to resolve retinal structure. To image deep tissues such as the liver, 3–10 MHz ultrasound is used.

16.8.3 ULTRASOUND TRANSDUCERS

Recall from Chapter 14 that a piezolectric material possesses the dual properties of generating a voltage (or equivalent internal charge displacement) if it is physically strained (compressed, twisted, bent, sheared, etc.), or, if a voltage is impressed across it producing an internal electric field, the transducer will exhibit a strain (ΔL/L). An important descriptor of piezotransducer behavior is the *short-circuit charge sensitivity to applied stress*, or *d parameter*, which has the dimensions of (coulombs/m^2)/(Newton/m^2) = Cb/N. d is also called the *piezoelectric strain constant* (Shung and Zipparo, 1996), or the *piezoelectric charge coefficient*. An alternate and dimensionally consistent interpretation of d when the transducer is used as a motor is (strain developed)/ (applied, internal E-field) (Germano, 1961).

A given transducer has three or more d parameters, d_{jk}. j and k refer to the orthogonal axes in which the transducer lies. The 3-D is the same as the z-axis along which the stress is developed (or stress is applied). The two- and three-dimensions are the same as the x- and y-axes. Thus, the *direct charge coefficient*, d_{33}, describes the charge/m^2 displaced along the z-axis of a *thickness-expander* transducer when the stress (N/m^2 = Pascals) is also applied along the z-axis. (The $_k$ parameter in d_{jk} is the direction in which the stress is applied.) d_{31} describes the behavior of a *length-expander* transducer which produces displaced charge density in the z-direction when the stress is in the x-direction. d_{33} is an important d parameter in that it gives the number of picocoulombs of charge, q, effectively separated in the transducer in the direction the stress is applied. The separated charge produces a voltage across the electrodes of an open-circuited transducer given by V_o = q/C, where C is the capacitance of the transducer. For a simple disk or plate transducer, C = $\kappa \varepsilon_o$A/L, where ε_o is the permittivity of space, κ is the piezoelectric material's dielectric constant, A is the area of the electrodes, and L is the distance separating the electrodes (the transducer thickness). The charge separated by a constant stress gradually leaks back to its equilibrium distribution in the transducer, allowing $V_o \rightarrow 0$.

There is also a *piezoelectric voltage coefficient* set, g_{jk}, that gives the strain (ΔL/L) produced by a mechanically unloaded transducer "motor" as the result of an applied charge density in Cb/m^2. Alternately, when a transducer is acting as a generator, it is useful to describe g units as the (open circuit E-field produced)/ (applied stress in N/m^2 or Pascals). In general, the g_{jk} parameters are related to the d_{jk} parameters by: g_{jk} = $d_{jk}/(\kappa_j \varepsilon_o)$ (strain developed)/ (applied charge density). κ_j is the dielectric constant of the transducer material in the j-direction.

Note that the d and g relationships for transducer behavior described above apply only for electrical and mechanical frequencies below the natural *mechanical resonant frequency* of the transducer. At and near mechanical resonance, the transducer's behavior can be modeled by a complex R,L,C, transformer equivalent circuit, the behavior of which will not be considered here.

Early piezoelectric transducers were naturally occurring materials such as used in World War II sonar systems, such as quartz, rochelle salt (NaKC$_4$H$_4$O$_6 \cdot$ 4H$_2$O, sodium potassium tartrate), or ammonium dihydrogen phosphate ($NH_4H_2PO_4$, ADP). The first synthetic piezoceramic material was barium titanate ($BaTiO_3$). Synthetic *ferroelectric* piezoceramics are not naturally piezoelectric; they must be *poled* by exposing them to a very strong internal electric field (c. 20 kV/cm) as they cure. Many different piezoceramics now exist; for example, many formulations of lead zirconate titanate (PZT, $Pb(Zr, Ti)O_3$), lead zirconate, lithium metaniobate ($LiNbO_3$) and lead metaniobate ($PbNb_2O_6$). One advantage to the use of piezoceramics is that they can be made in any desired shape to suit the application (disks, rods, bars, hollow cylinders, half-cylinders, hollow spheres, hemispheres, etc.).

An important consideration in the design of ultrasound transducer systems is that all transducer materials, with the exception of PVDF, exhibit mechanical resonance at frequency $f_n = \omega_n/2\pi$ Hz. This means that the efficiency of the ultrasound output (and input) is greatest when the ac driving frequency is at f_n, or when the acoustic wave impinging on the transducer is near f_n. In pulsed ultrasound, the transducer can be excited by a short burst of ac at f_n. The rate that the transducer oscillations' buildup and decay is governed not only by the ac pulse envelope, but the internal mechanical damping, ξ, of the loaded transducer. Decay is generally governed by an envelope of the form, $\exp(-\xi\omega_n t)$. If a transducer is excited by a single narrow dc pulse, the sound pressure produced at the transducer surface will be of the general shape of a damped sinusoid:

$$p(t) = P_o \exp(-\xi\omega_n t)\sin\left[\omega_n\left(\sqrt{1-\xi^2}\right)t + \varphi\right] \qquad 16.59$$

The Q or quality factor of a second-order damped resonant system can be shown to be: $Q = 1/(2\xi)$.

The electrical equivalent circuit of an ultrasound transducer near and at resonance is complex; its R,L,C transformer parameters depend not only on the mechanical properties of the transducer itself, but also upon its front- and rear-face acoustical loading. The rear face can be loaded with a material that will lower the overall Q of the transducer, and the front (driving) surface must be acoustic-impedance-matched to the tissue load for efficient energy transfer. Reflections occur at the interfaces of the matching media and the tissue. The tissue also absorbs far more sound energy than it reflects. In general, the loaded transducer at resonance presents a series or parallel R-C circuit to the driving power amplifier (Shung and Zipparo, 1996).

To measure the voltage generated by the piezotransducer or apply an internal electric field to cause it to move, thin metal electrodes are vapor-deposited on its active surfaces. Silver, gold or aluminum are generally used. Wires making contact with the thin electrodes are generally attached with silver-filled epoxy; the heat from soldering can damage the coating or the transducer. Contacts are also made with thin spring electrodes that press on the metalized transducer faces.

Because modern ultrasound imaging systems generally work in the pulsed mode, it is important that the transducer be adequately mechanically damped to prevent excess "ringing" when excited by a pulse of RF excitation. Damping is implemented by backing the transducer with a high-frequency, energy-absorbing material, or can be an intrinsic property of the transducer material. Lead metaniobate has a mechanical Q of 15, compared with LZT transducers where the Q is typically in the 100s. The Curie temperature (above which the material loses its piezoelectric properties) for lead metaniobate is $550°$ C, vs. a typical maximum operating temperature for LZTs of $150°$ C.

An unusual piezoelectric material is the plastic, polyvinylidene fluoride (PVDF). PVDF is a polymer composed of long molecular chains having the repeat unit, $-CH_2-CF_2-$. When the polymer is poled with a strong electric field, the polymer chains line up in parallel. Unlike a vitreous piezomaterial, PVDF has an extremely low Q. In fact, its frequency response runs from 0.005 Hz to a GHz. The basic half-wavelength thickness of a 28 μm-thick PVDF transducer is c. 40 MHz. PVDF has been successfully used at 50 Mz for ophthalmological investigations (Lockwood et al., 1996). As a consequence of its high internal damping, PVDF cannot handle high average radiated sound intensities without heating. Unfortunately, PVDF has a low maximum operating temperature of $100°$ C. PVDF is flexible and can adhere to body contours; it also has a low Z_c of 3.9×10^6 kg/m²sec (3.9 M Rayls), close to the Z_c of water (1.48 M Rayls) and of soft tissue (c. 1.63 M Rayls). Thus, it is easier to couple acoustic energy from PVDF to the body than from a hard piezoceramic like PZT, which has a Z_c c. 24×10^6 kg/m²sec.

Let us consider the case of a single cylindrical piston radiator launching ultrasonic vibrations into a uniform medium such as water. It can be shown (Liley, 2001) that the excess pressure magnitude varies along the z-axis according to:

$$|p| = (2\pi A/k) \left\{ 2 - 2\cos\left[k\left(\sqrt{r^2 + z^2}\right) - z \right] \right\}^{\frac{1}{2}}$$

        16.60

Where $k = 2\pi/\lambda$, A is a constant of proportionality related to the source pressure at the transducer face, and r is the transducer's radius. For P off the z-axis at some angle ϕ in the near field, the expression for $|p|$ is sufficiently complex to not be considered here. The typical behavior of $|p|$ on-axis is shown in Figure 16.36A. The z-value where the last peak occurs in the $|p|$ vs. z plot marks the boundary between *near-field* and *far-field* radiation behavior. z_b is given by: $z_b = r^2/\lambda - \lambda/4$. In the far-field, the excess pressure off axis can be modeled by:

$$|p| = \frac{A\pi r^2}{\rho} \left\{ \frac{2J_1[k\, r\sin(\phi)]}{k\, r\sin(\phi)} \right\}, \quad \rho > z_b$$

        16.61

Where $J_1(*)$ is a Bessel function of the first kind, and r, ρ, ϕ, A, k have been defined. Figure 16.36B illustrates a typical polar plot of *far-field* $|p|$ vs. ϕ. It can be shown that the angle at which $|p|$ first becomes zero is: $\phi_o = \sin^{-1}(0.61\, \lambda/r)$ (Shung and Zipparo, 1996). Side lobes are undesirable in ultrasonic imaging because they produce spurious return signals that decrease image resolution. Good transducer design requires a narrow main lobe and a large ϕ_o with weak side lobes. Also, it is often desirable to have a the focal point of the transducer closer than would be normally

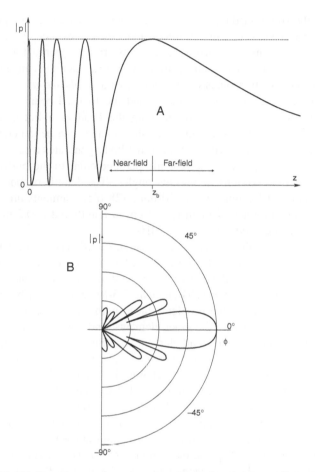

FIGURE 16.36 (A) On-axis sound pressure magnitude for a piston radiator showing near-field ($0 < z \leq z_b$) and far-field ($z > z_b$) behavior. (B) A typical constant intensity contour for a piston radiator in its far-field as a function of angle away from the z axis. Note the complex side lobes.

set by z_b. One answer to this design problem is to use an *acoustic lens* between the transducer and the tissue being scanned. An acoustic lens basically brings the radiated beam to a sharp focus at a $z_b' < z_b$ at the expense of a rapidly expanding beam beyond z_b'. Acoustic lenses must have dimensions larger than λ to be effective refractors. Some materials used for acoustic lenses are silicone rubber (Sylgard™), polyurethane and plexiglas.

The trend with modern ultrasound transducers is to use *multi-element arrays*. Such arrays allow the beam to be focused and steered electronically by varying the phases and amplitudes of the excitation signals to the individual array elements. A transducer array can be made in the shape of concentric annular piezoelectric rings, spaced with an appropriate inert material to acoustically isolate the transducers. This type of array produces a beam with circular symmetry; its focal point (point of maximum intensity and minimum cross section in z) can be set by adjusting the excitation to the ring transducers. Still another design, used in such applications as fetal imaging to image slices, uses a *linear array* of narrow rectangular transducers laid in parallel, separated by narrow *kerfs* of absorbing material for electrical and acoustic isolation. The sound beam from a linear array can be scanned laterally by exciting subgroups of transducers in sequence, or as a *phased array* where all the piezoelements are excited simultaneously, and the focused beam is steered at an angle ϕ from the array's center. By moving the head of a linear array slowly, perpendicular to its long axis, a "book" of slice images can be generated. Holding the array fixed and tilting it with respect to the body generates a set of fan images, and, rotating around its vertical axis while perpendicular to the body, generates a set of perpendicular sections at various angles. The length of one linear array marketed by Parallel Design, Inc., is 50 mm; 128 piezoelements are used, spaced 0.390 mm on centers. Each element is c. 1 cm in length and c. 0.2 mm wide. The array elements' center frequency is c. 8 MHz.

Rectangular 2-D multi-element arrays also are used. They, too, can be focused and the beam steered in two angular dimensions, ϕ and θ. Transducers in the rectangular array are long rods or posts, the diameters or end dimensions of which are much less than their lengths. A $42 \times 42 = 1764$-element, 2.5-MHz array has been investigated at Duke University. Among the problems faced with such large arrays are making physical electrical contact with the inner elements, and low signal-to-noise ratio due to poor acoustical isolation and small element size (Shung and Zipparo, 1996; Smith et al., 1996). Parallel Design, Inc. describes an experimental $11 \times 11 = 121$-element square array. Kerfs are 25 µm wide and each transducer face is 75×75 µm. The whole array measures a tiny 1.075×1.075 mm (Parallel Design, 1999).

It is mathematically difficult to calculate the spatial distribution of the sound pressure magnitude, $|p|$, at some point P at a radial distance, ρ, from the center of an array (O) and at an angle ϕ with the z-axis, and angle θ with the X-axis by a projection of ρ into the X-Y plane (see Figure 16.37). The calculation involves the superposition of the $|p|$s from each element of the array at P. Such design predictions are generally left to computer modeling.

16.8.4 DOPPLER ULTRASOUND IMAGING

Doppler ultrasound imaging combines traditional ultrasound imaging with Doppler velocity detection of moving scatterers. The scatterers are red cells in blood, or moving tissues such as heart valves or aneurisms. Recall from Chapter 14 that the Doppler frequency shift in reflected CW ultrasound is $f_D = 2|\mathbf{v}|f_T \cos(\theta)/c$ Hz, where f_T is the transmitted frequency, $\mathbf{v}$ is the scatterer velocity, θ is the angle a line from the transducer to the scatterer makes with $\mathbf{v}$, and c is the speed of sound in the medium surrounding the scatterer. Thus, the returning waves from the moving scatterers will have frequency $f_r = f_T \pm f_D$. (+ for scatterers approaching the transducer.),

Because modern Doppler imaging systems work in the pulsed mode, the Doppler effect can also be expressed in the time domain. The velocity $\mathbf{v}$ can be estimated from δt, the time difference in signal return from successive pulses. See Figure 16.38 for a description of the geometry. The ultrasound pulse repetition interval (PRI) is the reciprocal of the pulse repetition rate (PRR). (Note that the PRR is not f_n.) In

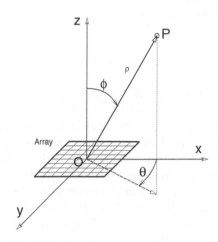

FIGURE 16.37 Spherical coordinates above a transducer array relevant to calculating its radiation pattern.

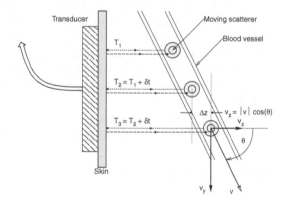

FIGURE 16.38 Diagram illustrating how a pulsed Doppler array can be used to find object velocity. At each successive pulse, the time for the return echo increases by an amount, δt, given by Equation 16.62 in the text. δt is then used to find $|\mathbf{v}|\cos(\theta)$.

the time interval PRI, the moving reflecting object moves away from the transducer by Δz. That is, $\Delta z = (\text{PRI})|\mathbf{v}|\cos(\theta)$, which means that the next ultrasound pulse must travel double this extra distance, taking an extra time, δt. Clearly,

$$\delta t = 2\,(\text{PRI})|\mathbf{v}|\cos(\theta)/c \qquad\qquad 16.62$$

Thus

$$|\mathbf{v}|\cos(\theta) = (c\,\delta t)/(2(\text{PRI})), \qquad\qquad 16.63$$

where c is the average sound velocity in the tissue between the transducer and the moving object. One can also think of the fractional time shift in terms of phase, that is, there will be a phase lag between successive returning pulses, φ, given by φ = 2π δt/(PRI) radians. If this relation is solved for PRI and substituted into Equation 16.63, we find:

$$|\mathbf{v}|\cos(\theta) = c \; \varphi/(4\pi) \; \text{m/s} \qquad\qquad 16.64$$

The moving objects are generally red blood cells (RBCs); there are c. 5×10^6 RBCs in a cubic mm of blood. Each RBC is a flattened disc of c.7.5 μm diameter and c.1.9 μm thick on the edge and c. 1 μm thick in the center. Thus, RBC dimensions are << λ of the ultrasound, which means they are much too small to present images. Also, in blood vessels with laminar flow, the blood velocity has a parabolic profile; maximum at the center and zero at the vessel walls. In the great arteries and in the chambers of the heart, flow can be turbulent over parts of the cardiac cycle. Thus, the reflected Doppler signals from blood are a superposition of many, many small scattered signals from moving RBCs with different cross-sections and velocities. In general, the intensity of the Doppler-shifted backscatter from moving RBCs is c. 40 dB less than that from surrounding tissues (Routh, 1996).

Doppler information is generally presented in ultrasound slice images of organs such as the heart, kidneys, aorta, carotid arteries, etc., as colors. For example, starting at +30 cm/sec velocity, yellow to orange to red to black at 0 velocity, then violet through blue to green as the velocity reaches −30 cm/sec. Doppler information is more qualitative than quantitative in this mode of display. Still, if there is a heart valve problem such as mitral regurgitation, it will show up well on the Doppler image, and can be correlated with another modality such as sonocardiography (see Section 3.3) (Routh 1996).

The processes whereby the Doppler information is inserted into the slice image are complex in terms of both hardware and software, and will not be covered here.

16.9 OTHER IMAGING MODALITIES

16.9.1 INTRODUCTION

In this survey of medical imaging methods, it is appropriate to briefly describe some of the less frequently encountered imaging methods and evaluate them for medical diagnostic utility or research potential. As we have seen, not every modality is without risk. Every imaging modality carries a cost–benefit ratio. The cost includes the dollar cost to the patient as well as risk of harm from radiation, contrast agent, anxiety, etc. The benefit of an imaging system lies in its resolution and its ability to diagnose specific important diseases such as various types of cancer, atherosclerosis, heart valve damage, etc.

Those imaging modalities involving ionizing radiations such as X-ray, X-ray CT, PET, and SPECT certainly carry more risk than MRI, ultrasound, impedance tomography and microwave tomography. In the sections below, we briefly describe long-wave infrared thermal imaging, microwave tomography and impedance tomography. Only LIR thermal imaging is risk-free; it is non-contact, noninvasive, and puts no energy or radioactivity into the body. However, it is pretty much limited to detecting circulatory defects, soft-tissue injuries, and breast cancer.

16.9.2 LIR THERMAL IMAGING OF BODY SURFACES

We know from Figure 6.2 in Section 6.32 that the IR blackbody radiation curve at 310 K peaks at 9.34 μm wavelength. Thus, sensors used to map and image surface IR radiation from human skin should cover from c. 2 to over 100 μm. Because of practical considerations, including infrared imaging optics, most IR cameras for body temperature imaging cover from 2 to 14 μm of source wavelength. The optics for IR thermographic imaging generally make use of materials that are opaque in visible wavelengths. Diamond-turned lenses of ZnSe (aka *Irtran-4*) are effective from 0.6 to 16 μm. The other Irtran materials are Irtran-1 (MgF$_2$, passes 1–9 μm); Irtran-2 (ZnS, passes 0.9–20 μm); Irtran-3 (CaF, passes <0.3–8 μm). Germanium passes from 2–14 μm, silicon passes from 1.2–8 μm, and KRS-5 passes from 0.6–50 μm. Mirrors (plane and spherical) are generally gold-coated. LIR Camera imaging optics can also be done entirely with mirrors to eliminate the need for exotic lenses, but such designs are generally bulky.

Two general classes of LIR detectors exist: *thermal* and *photon*. Thermal detectors work by blackbody absorption of LIR radiation causing a minute increase in the sensor's temperature, ΔT. Thermal detectors include *thermopiles, bolometers* and *pyroelectric sensors*. Thermopiles are arrays of miniature thermocouples that output microvolt-level signals.

The resistance of a bolometer increases with a slight rise in temperature; the ΔR is generally sensed with a bridge. Pyroelectric materials are special piezoelectric materials that generate voltages in response to thermally induced surface strain. Pyroelectric sensors must be used with a chopper. (See Section 6.3 for a detailed description of pyroelectric IR detection.) Thermopiles, bolometers and pyroelectic sensors are broadband in their IR wavelength responses (exclusive of limitations placed by the focusing optics). Photon detector sensors include *photodiodes* and *photoconductors* that work by incident LIR photons generating electron-hole pairs that cause increased current to flow. The longest wavelength detectable by a photon detector is given approximately by:

$$\lambda_{max} = 1.24/E_G \ \mu m \qquad 16.65$$

where E_G is the material's bandgap energy in eV. An advantage of photodiodes over photoconductors is that they can be operated at zero bias as photocurrent generators, also, they have no appreciable dark current, unlike voltage-biased photoconductors.

As might be expected when trying to measure small differences in Kelvin surface temperature around 300° K, thermal (Johnson) noise (and shot noise for photodiodes) is a problem. One way of reducing noise and enhancing thermal sensitivity is to operate the sensor array at reduced temperature. Heat extraction by boiling liquid nitrogen (LN$_2$), or liquid argon (LA) is often used to cool IR sensor arrays. (LN$_2$ boils at 77.35° K, and LA boils at 87.45° K.) Ricor, Ltd. offers miniature Stirling cycle coolers for LIR camera cooling. These compact devices will cool the detector array from 300° to 80° K in less than 8 minutes, and have steady-state cooling capacities of 0.25 to 0.5 W at 80° K. Typical input power for a 0.5 W cooler is 35 W @ 24 Vdc. Carting around several small rechargeable gelcell lead-acid batteries is considered less cumbersome than a Dewar of LN_2, and having to fill the camera's cryo-chamber every hour or so.

Recently, IR imaging cameras that operate at room temperature have come on the market, eliminating the need for cumbersome cryogenic enclosures and an expensive LN_2 supply.

Some materials for photodiodes include mercury cadmium telluride (MCT) and mercury manganese telluride (MMT); the latter material is useful from about 2 to 12 μm (Brimrose, 1992). Other materials used in photon-capture thermal imaging include indium antimonide (IA), $Pb_{1-x}Sn_xTe(In)$, and gallium arsenide.

Modern gallium arsenide IR cameras that run at 77° K can resolve temperature differences on human skin of ± 0.001° C in a 5 mm² patch of skin. Furthermore, 10 to 50 mK modulation of skin temperature can be followed at up to 10 Hz, enabling observation of skin temperature variations during the cardiac cycle, a good indicator of hemodynamics (Anbar 1998).

The Cincinnati Electronics Corp. makes a state-of-the-art portable LIR thermography focal plane array camera (model IRRIS-256ST) with a 256 × 256 InSb photodiode array operated at 80° K by a Sterling cooler. The camera operates over a 2.2–4.6 μm spectral range. It gives temperature-to-color image coding as well as a gray image of up to 256 levels, and typically can resolve surface temperature differences of 0.025° C. A full line of accessory lenses is available ranging from 13 to 250 mm focal length; all lenses are $f/2.3$. The camera is normally used with a color video image processor for medical applications.

Another commercial LIR thermography focal plane array camera is made by Sierra Pacific Infrared (SPI). Its Radiance 1™ camera also uses an 320 × 240-pixel InSb photodiode array. It uses a Dewar, so the array can be cooled to 77° K with LN_2. The SPI camera is responsive over 3.0 to 5.0 μm, and has a noise-equivalent temperature difference (NETD) of 20 mK. This camera also has a 12-bit digital output and a gray or pseudocolor display.

Equi-Thermal Imaging markets a hand-held thermal imaging camera that has application in veterinary medicine in spotting local hot spots due to strains and sprains in race- and show-horses. The company's Heat Seeker-2000™ IR camera is responsive over an 8–12 μm spectral band, using a 20 mm $f/0.7$ germanium lens. It uses an uncooled 120 × 120-pixel Honeywell thermopile (thermoelectric) array. A 2 Mbyte memory allows it to store up to 144 images. Image scan time is < 1.5 seconds, and the camera has a NETD of < 0.35° C at 30° C. This is not an exceptional thermal resolution, but is evidently adequate for veterinary applications. In general, thermal LIR sensors are too slow for TV-type imaging in real time, and, at present, are too noisy at room temperature. Chilled photon detector arrays are fast enough to permit a 30-frame/sec TV image rate, and offer NETDs one tenth that of room temperature thermal arrays.

An uncooled broadband bolometer LIR imaging array was described by White et al. (1998) at Lockheed Martin IR Imaging Systems in Lexington, Massachusetts.

A bolometer is a thermal detector heated by incident absorbed IR radiation, which undergoes a temperature rise that causes its resistance to increase. The array contains 327×245 micromachined bolometer elements, each about 46 μm square.

"Each microbolometer detector consists of a silicon nitride microbridge that lies above a CMOS silicon substrate and is supported by two silicon nitride legs. A vanadium oxide (VOx) film, which has an approximately 2% temperature coefficient of resistance at ambient temperatures, is deposited on the bridge to form the bolometer resistor. Each of the microbolometer detectors is connected to an underlying unit cell in the silicon CMOS readout integrated circuit (ROIC) substrate via two holes in the passivation layer on the top of the integrated circuit."

The detector's thermal time constant was 14 ms, and the detector resistance was 15–30 k. The array was put into the LTC500 camera, which had a spectral response of 7.5 to 14 μm, a frame update rate of 60 Hz, and an NEDT $< 0.1°$ K. Again, we see a tradeoff between the convenience of room temperature operation and lower thermal resolution because of noise.

Because the main source of heat exchange from the body's core to the skin is the peripheral circulation, the spatio-temporal distribution of skin temperature is closely associated with the behavior of the vascular system, including the cardiac cycle and the functioning of the autonomic nervous system, which controls vasodilation and contraction, and regulates the blood flow in veins and arteries. "Hot spots" on the skin indicate either increased blood flow to the region, for example, caused by local inflammation due to arthritis, infection or Paget's bone disease. Increased local blood flow can also be due to a highly vascular cancer near the skin surface (e.g., breast cancer). The neuromodulator, *nitric oxide* (NO) is a potent relaxer of vascular smooth muscle, causing vasodilation and increased blood flow. NO is known to be produced by a number of immune system cells involved in inflammatory reactions, as well as chondrocytes, osteocytes and different lines of cancer cells, including breast cancer, melanomas, squamous cell carcinoma and colorectal cancer. NO is also produced by the vascular epithelium in response to nervous stimulation. Cancer-induced NO may enhance angiogenesis in the cancer, and NO-induced regional vasodilation may also lead to metastasis (Anbar, 1998). Thus, the detection of a hot region on one breast not seen on the other indicates a high probability that a cancer may be present, and other more definitive tests should be done (e.g., scintimammography, biopsy, etc.). *Deep venous thrombosis* (DVT) in a leg can also cause anomalous heating on the back of that leg. Normally, the temperature of the back of the legs has a smooth gradient of about 3° from the upper thighs to the lower calves. If DVT is present, the temperature of the calf will be significantly raised. Thermographic diagnostic sensitivity to DVT is 97 to 100%, but thermography cannot localize the site of the thrombosis (Harding, 1998), and other means must be used to locate it.

"Cold spots" indicate anomalous reduced vascular perfusion of an area. This can have a nervous origin (extreme vasoconstriction signaled by sympathetic nerves that release norepinephrine, which causes the vascular smooth muscle to contract (Guyton, 1991). Local reduced perfusion can also have a mechanical cause such as injury, phlebitis, arteritis, or arteriosclerosis. If a thermogram of the face shows an asymmetric cold side, this can be due to reduced flow in the common or external carotid artery on that side. Such a hypothesis can be verified by Doppler ultrasound, or, more invasively, by X-ray angiography.

As medical imaging systems go, thermography is one of the safest and least expensive. Its major uses appear to be in the detection of breast cancer and other skin cancers, arthritis, infections (inflammation), and circulatory system dysfunction. As camera designs are perfected, expect to see larger arrays and lower NETDs.

16.9.3 MICROWAVE IMAGING

We normally think of microwaves in conjunction with radar and microwave ovens for cooking. However, microwaves penetrate living tissue, and, like other electromagnetic radiation, experience absorption, reflection, scattering and refraction as they interact with various tissue components. As in the case of ultrasound, if the intensity is kept low, heating is negligible, and there are no known long-term adverse effects to medical microwave exposure, and there is a trade-off between short wavelength (high resolution) and increasing absorption as wavelength decreases. Microwaves are not ionizing radiations. One property that makes microwave imaging attractive is that microwave absorption is a function of the (complex) dielectric constant of tissues. At a frequency of 2.5 GHz, dielectric permittivity varies from about 5 for fat to 56 for normal myocardium at body temperature. By comparison, the contrast range for soft tissue for X-rays is c. 2%, and is less than 10% for ultrasound (Semenov et al., 1996). In air, a 10 GHz source has a 3 cm wavelength; in the body, this falls to c. 3.4 mm because of the much slower speed of microwave radiation's being proportional *in vivo* to the reciprocal of the square root of the dielectric constant. The effective speed of EM radiation in tissue is $v = (0.34/3) \times 3 \times 10^8 = 4.4 \times 10^7$ m/sec.

Microwave imaging has great potential for the detection of breast cancer because of the greater contrast caused by the high dielectric constant of the cancer due to its higher water content. Several university laboratories are working to develop prototype microwave imaging and tomographic systems for mammography. An experimental microwave tomography system being studied in Russia at the Kurchatov Institute uses a power density of no more than 0.1 mW/cm². The Russian system and several in the United States use a tank of distilled water or other liquid into which the transmitting and receiving antennas are immersed along with the specimen. The water serves the same purpose as ultrasound coupling gel, i.e., impedance matching, to maximize energy transmission into the specimen.

Semenov et al. (1996) state:

"In microwave tomography there are extremely difficult mathematical problems connected with image reconstruction. The linear optics approximation which is used for X-ray tomographic image reconstruction cannot be used in the case of microwave tomography. For microwave tomographic image reconstruction it is necessary to solve the Maxwell equations or their scalar approximations. In the past few years this problem has been extensively investigated."

State-of-the-art resolution in experimental microwave medical imaging systems is c. 1 cm. This in itself is not exceptional, and, at this point, one could argue why bother? Certainly, other imaging modalities have better resolution. However, as we have indicated above, the strength of the method may lie in its ability to pick up, as high-contrast images, structures that have large gradients in dielectric constant compared with surrounding tissue, e.g., breast cancers.

Much of the future development of effective medical microwave imaging systems will be focused on perfecting the design of antennas and their radiation patterns. Semenov et al. (1996) suggest that at least 128 transmitting antennas and 128 receiving antennas will be required for accurate scattered field detection. Higher transmitted frequencies will be able to be used for microwave mammography because the overall transmission path is shorter and a greater absorption rate can be tolerated. Thus, resolution can be higher.

16.9.4 ELECTRICAL IMPEDANCE TOMOGRAPHY

One can think of electrical impedance tomography (EIT) as the ultimate problem in multiport circuit analysis. The object of the analysis is to describe the electrical parameters of a circuit distributed in a 2-D space, or tomographic slice. The circuit is a "black-box," and electrical access is by a finite number of electrode pairs distributed around its periphery, Γ. Furthermore, the circuit is continuous, rather than being composed of discrete *conductances* and capacitive *susceptances*. That is, there is an internal distribution of *admittivity*, $\gamma(x,y,z) = \sigma + j\beta$ Sicmens/m. The conductivity, σ, is a function of (x,y,z), and β is a function of the applied radian frequency, ω, and also is a function of the spatial distribution of the *permittivity*, $\varepsilon(x,y,z)$ in the tissue. The central problem is how to estimate the vector $\gamma(x,y,z)$ from a finite number of voltage measurements, given an ac current injected at each electrode in turn, and how to relate the estimated $\gamma(x,y,z)$ to medically important factors in the electrified volume, such as edema, lack of blood, swollen and inflamed organs, etc.

Because EIT uses innocuous levels of high frequency sinusoidal currents, and does not involve ionizing radiation, it is safe. Compared with other imaging modalities, it is also inexpensive; requiring only electrodes, signal sources, voltage-controlled current amplifiers, voltage preamplifiers, phase-sensitive rectifiers, multiplexors, A/D boards, and a computer.

Much of the ongoing research today on EIT is on algorithms to permit rapid and accurate estimation and mapping of $\gamma(x,y,z)$. Early EIT systems using the finite element approach assumed a circular boundary for the object being investigated. The EIT system of Edic et al. (1995), used 32 electrodes to apply 31 different 28.8 kHz current patterns to the body (torso) (one electrode was always the current return or ground). Thirty-two electrodes were used to measure the in-phase and quadrature voltages resulting from each current applied. A 496-element "Joshua tree" finite-element model (FEM) was used to model the admittance of the body. Edic et al. used a fast implementation of Newton's one-step error reconstructor (FNOSER) to calculate static, absolute, conductivity and permittivity distributions in the finite elements. Their study demonstrated the efficacy of their mathematical approach, but, in this writer's opinion, gave no results on which to base a diagnosis. Clearly, more electrodes are needed to improve resolution.

Better results were obtained in an EIT modeling study by Jain et al. (1997). They used a 6017-node mesh FEM with 512 boundary nodes to solve the *forward problem*, in which the voltages on the boundary nodes of the object are calculated given the interior admittance distribution and currents applied to the boundary. The governing continuous equations for the potential distribution in the object, $\phi(x,y,z)$, given $\gamma(x,y,z)$, are the Laplace equation for the area, Ω:

$$\nabla \bullet (\gamma \nabla \phi) = 0 \qquad\qquad 16.66$$

and the boundary equation for points x,y,z on the boundary, Γ, of Ω.

$$\gamma(x, y, z)\frac{\partial \phi}{\partial \eta} = \mathbf{J} \qquad\qquad 16.67$$

Where the partial derivative is the vector *directional derivative* of the potential on Γ, and $\mathbf{J}$ is the current density applied to the surface. We are after an estimate of $\gamma(x,y,z)$. Jain et al. also used the *boundary element method* (BEM) to generate the voltage data for inhomogenous conductivity distributions inside object areas with noncircular (e.g., elliptical) boundaries with success. Phantoms with controlled distribution of σ and β were used in their study.

The future success in EIT as an NI diagnostic imaging modality will depend on the development of better algorithms to estimate $\gamma(x,y,z)$, and also on the ability to cram more electrodes into a finite circumference. It should be possible to place 250 electrodes in a 1-meter circumference, and use two at a time for ac current injection, and the other 249 to record the voltage at points on the periphery. At present, EIT needs further refinement before it can compete effectively with any of the established imaging modalities in a particular diagnostic mode.

16.10 SUMMARY

As you have seen from this introductory chapter on medical imaging, a number of imaging modalities allow visualization of internal organs and their pathologies. Imaging had its beginning with the invention of the stationary shadow X-ray, evolved to simple motion tomography, and thence to various forms of computed tomography. X-ray imaging relies on differences in the X-ray photon absorbancy tissues, differences that can be very small in soft tissues such as the breast. Contrast agents can be injected into blood vessels for X-ray angiography to detect conditions such as coronary artery blockage or carotid artery stenosis.

Along with the inception of X-ray CT imaging, the mathematics of tomographic reconstruction has evolved, making use of the Radon transfer, filtered back-projection, and other image reconstruction algorithms. Imaging modalities such as MRI, PET, SPECT, etc., all use variations of these techniques.

Magnetic resonance imaging has developed into a high-resolution imaging modality that is primarily sensitive to the water density in tissue, and can be used to locate tumors with greater resolution than X-ray CT.

The use of radioisotopes and radionuclides attached to molecules that have affinity to particular tissues has enabled positron emission tomography (PET) and single photon emission tomography (SPECT) to locate tissues such as cancers. The high-energy, γ-photons in PET and SPECT are generally detected using collimators with scintillation sensors.

Ultrasound is the major noninvasive non-ionizing imaging modality. The amplitude, phase time or delay, and frequency of reflected and backscattered sound waves are used to construct tomographic images of internal organs and resolve details of fetuses *in utero*. This chapter has also considered elecrical impedance tomography, IR thermographic imaging (of the body surface), and microwave imaging.

A promising very high-resolution imaging modality currently under development is X-ray diffraction imaging. A beam of highly coherent monochromatic X-rays, which are generated with the aid of a synchrotron, is required. An invention that would really revolutionize medical imaging would be a compact low-powered X-ray laser.

17 Future Trends in NI Instrumentation and Measurements

17.1 INTRODUCTION

Cancers are generally detected in the body after they have reached a critical size where they can be seen on an imaging system (ca. 1 cm diameter in the case of breast cancer), palpated, disrupt some normal physiological process, or cause pain, discomfort or bleeding. The *latency period* of a cancer is the interval between initiation and clinical detection. For some slow-growing cancers, the latent period can be 5 years or more. A major objective in oncology is to minimize the latency period because it is easier to fight an identified small cancer than a large one, perhaps before it has had a chance to spread (turn metastatic).

For some types of cancer, when the body's immune system recognizes the tumor as foreign tissue because of damaged or mutated cancer cell surface proteins, it mounts an attack on the tumor cells. The attack may prove ineffectual because the tumor grows faster than the immune system can fight it, or the tumor cells may secrete substances that suppress the immune system's actions. Still, there will be circulating antibodies in the blood against signature tumor surface proteins. The problem is to detect these antibodies and use them as a sign that a particular type of cancer is growing in an otherwise asymptomatic body. The mitochondrial DNA of cancer cells may also be mutated, and can serve as a basis for cancer detection. The use of mitochondrial DNA to identify cancers in the normal latency period is described below.

Cancers growing in the body also produce shifts in the normal concentrations of certain biochemical components of saliva, sputum, urine and blood. Detection of these concentration shifts also holds promise for early NI (asymptomatic) cancer detection, and is discussed in the sections below.

Certain hereditary diseases can also be identified by DNA analysis; either there is a DNA base sequence that codes an abnormal (enzyme) protein, or the coding for an enzyme is missing. Other hereditary diseases involve DNA coding for bad or missing cell membrane receptor proteins. Again, DNA analysis can point to such diseases.

Fluorescence analysis is another growing field that combines immunology, molecular biology, and biophotonics. Fluoresecent molecular "probes," made by attaching fluorescent molecules (a *fluorophore*) to a specific antigen (or antibody) can be used to physically locate specific proteins on cell surfaces or circulating molecules (including antibodies) in the blood. *Fluorescent* in situ *hybridization* (FISH) is rapidly becoming an important technique for genetic analysis and cancer detection and characterization. FISH works in the following manner: a DNA double-stranded helix in the nucleus (nDNA) or in mitochondria (mtDNA) is enzymatically cleaved into single (complementary) strands exposing many nucleic acids. A DNA probe molecule is prepared with a desired base sequence that is complementary to and will mate up with the bases of one of the cleaved single DNA strands. The probe is tagged throughout its length with fluorescent molecules bound to its deoxyribose-phosphate side. Thus, a specific chromosome target can be tagged and made uniquely visible under short-wavelength general illumination. Shorter specific gene regions that code for specfic proteins can also be selected and marked. FISH is not at the present an NI or *in vivo* technique. It requires histological techniques in which a cell of interest is fixed and mounted on a microscope slide; its DNA is then cleaved by heating with formamide at 70° C. The fluorescent probe molecules are then introduced by a micropipette, and the preparation is covered with a cover glass and incubated for several hours at 37° C. After incubation, the excess probe molecules are washed away and all of the cell's DNA can be highlighted with a general stain fluorescing at a wavelength different from the probe's. The fluorochrome molecules used emit at characteristic wavelengths that are selected by a band-pass filter or monochromator attached to the viewing microscope (Miklos, 1999; Katzir et al., 1998).

Five different fluorochrome probes, each fluorescing at a different wavelength (one green, two red, two IR) can be used at the same time for complex human chromosomal (24) analysis by FISH (Speicher et al., 1996). A SpectraCube® system (described below) is used to perform the m-FISH analysis. Note that mitochondrial DNA (mtDNA), RNA (messenger RNA and retroviral RNA) can also be marked with complementary fluorescent probes.

Spectral karyotyping (SKY) is a powerful research tool enabling researchers to follow chromosomal rearrangements in mouse cancer cell lines. SKY is a variation of FISH. *Spectral pathology* (SPY) is a spectral imaging technique used with bright-field microscopy. Typically, chromogenic dyes such as hematoxylin and eosin are used to stain the tissue slices. By spectrally decomposing the image with a system like SpectraCube®, the information can be used to identify and characterize cancers (Miklos, 1999).

This chapter will also describe the *DNA Biochip*, an integrated circuit approach to chemical sensing in which sections of genetically engineered complementary strands of DNA "probe" molecules are bound to test cell sites on a silicon or glass substrate. When the sought-after single-strand DNA analytes appear in the test solution, they bind with the specific complementary DNA bases in the test cells. In one type of biochip, the binding of analyte to probe molecules causes an electrical current to flow for that cell that is proportional to the number of analyte molecules bound; this dc current is amplified and displayed. The DNA biochip principle is not limited to DNA and RNA analysis; antigen and antibody binding can also be used to gate current.

Finally, we will describe the innovative SpectraCube® system, and show some of its applications in diagnosis.

17.2 NONINVASIVE CHEMICAL TESTS FOR CANCER NOT INVOLVING DNA

With the rise of new methods in analytical biochemistry, and cost- and health-driven goals for the early detection of cancer, researchers have found a number of substances in blood, urine, saliva and sputum (other than DNA) that are well correlated with the diagnosed presence of various cancers. Many of these substances may be present as the result of the increased metabolism of cancer cells, or may be the result of substances secreted by cancer cells as they grow. Changes in some immune system proteins can also occur as cancers grow.

One of the earliest reports was by Faraj et al., (1981). These workers observed significantly elevated concentrations of *L-dopa, dopamine,* and *3-o-methyldopamine* in the urine of patients who had diagnosed malignant melanoma. An enzyme-radioimmunoassay was used to quantify the concentrations of these substances. There was no significant rise in the concentrations in normal patients, and the elevated concentrations in melanoma patients decreased after surgery to remove the melanomas.

Melatonin (MEL) is a hormone secreted by the pineal gland in the brain. Control of pineal secretion of MEL is from nerve stimulation that has origin in the body's biological clock (zeitgeber) located in the suprachiasmatic nucleus. The secretion rate of MEL follows a circadian rhythm, being higher at night during the period of sleep and lower in the daytime. Figure 17.1 illustrates its structural formula. Melatonin is a pleiotropic hormone, i.e., it has multiple effects on different target organs in the body. Melatonin is known to influence nearly all glandular secretions of the endocrine system (Bartsch et al., 1992; Goldman, 1999). It has become popular to take exogenous MEL at night to promote deep sleep, and to aid recovery from jet lag. MEL has also been found to have an antioxidant effect similar to vitamin C. That is, it destroys free radicals before they can cause cell damage and possible cancer. Exogenous MEL has also been used in high doses with interleukin-2 (IL-2) to treat cancers; in some cases it has been found effective (NTP, 1996).

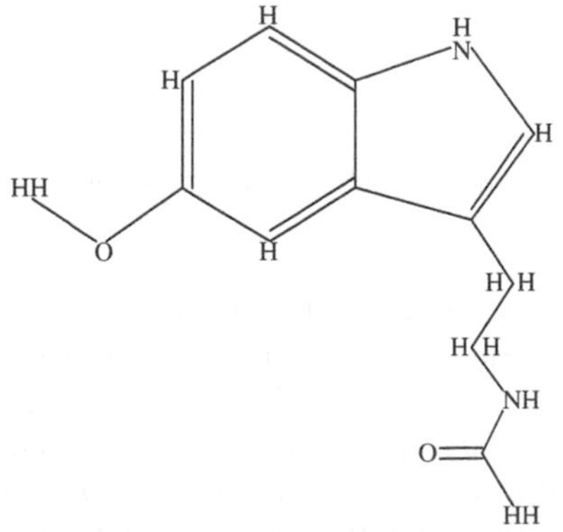

FIGURE 17.1 A melatonin molecule.

Our interest here is how cancers growing in the body affect the MEL concentration in urine and plasma. Following extensive clinical studies, Bartsch et al., (1992) reported that initial growth of the cancer (breast cancers with estrogen receptors, and prostate cancers) is associated with an increased nocturnal secretion rate of MEL; as the tumor grows, nocturnal MEL secretion is markedly suppressed. Nocturnal MEL secretion rate returns to normal when the cancer metastasizes or when the patient is treated with antiestrogen therapy with tamoxifen. Although the relationship between cancer growth and nocturnal MEL secretion rate seems well established, apparently no work has been done to see how sensitive the MEL test is in detecting occult breast or prostate cancers.

It is known that certain cancer cells produce an excess of a class of molecule known as pteridines. Figure 17.2 illustrates the structural formulas of some common pteridines (pteridine, pterin and biopterin). Pteridines are a class of bicyclic heterocyclic molecules, the more important of which are folic acid, biopterin and their derivatives. Biopterin in its tetrahydro form participates in the enzymatic conversion of the amino acids phenylalanine, tyrosine, and tryptophan by various hydroxylation reactions to different members of the catecholamine family, important neurotransmitters. Tetrahydrobiopterin (THBP) is also an essential factor in the three forms of nitric oxide (NO) synthase. NO is an important cell signaling substance.

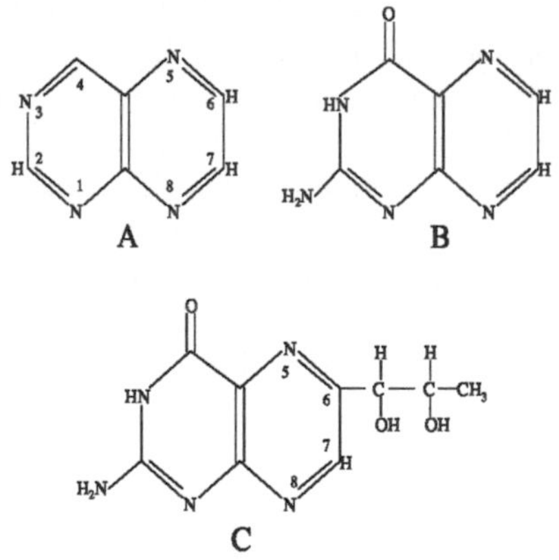

FIGURE 17.2 (A) The pteridine molecule. (B) The pterin molecule. (C) The biopterin molecule.

Capillary electrophoresis was used to separate the pteridines in urine. Concentrations of the various pteridine components were measured by counting photons from laser-induced fluorescence as the various electrophoretic components migrated past the laser beam. Preliminary studies have shown that there is a significant increase in certain pteridines in the urine of cancer patients. Future research may show that "signatures" based on the concentrations of the various pteridine components have a potential to detect cancers in their latency period, and possibly discriminate among different kinds of cancer (Han et al., 1999).

Yet another potential cancer screening modality may make use of the ratio between two different subgroups of immunoglobulins in blood associated with the IgG class of antibodies. Research by Schauenstein and Schauenstein (1998) on the subgroups of the IgG class of antibodies showed that the ratio of concentration of the subgroups, $(IgG_1)/(IgG_2)$, was found to decrease in patients with various cancers. These authors stated:

"Originally based on a biochemical assay to detect a reactive inter-heavy chain disulphide group (SS*) in the hinge region of IgG_1, it turned out accidentally that the majority of human sera derived from patients suffering from cancer of various organ systems exhibited significantly decreased values of SS*, indicating a selective decrease in the percentage of IgG_1 as compared with the total IgG fraction, whereas the percentage of IgG_2, containing the only accessible free SH group of IgG, tended to increase. Later, these initial findings were substantiated with larger numbers of patients afflicted with malignant diseases of selected tissues, such as the female breast, the female genital tract, and the prostate gland. These first studies revealed that benign proliferative or inflammatory diseases of the same organs did not exhibit a similar phenomenon. With breast cancer, it was shown that the decrease of SS*, that is, the percentage of IgG_1, occurs very early and becomes highly significant at tumor stages where conventional serological markers, such as CEA, CA 15-3, and TPA are largely still in the normal range. Furthermore, as shown for the first time for gynecological malignancies, the drop in the percentage of IgG1 turned out to be useful in the postoperative monitoring of tumor patients. The mechanism(s) of this tumor-mediated dysregulation of $(IgG_1)/(IgG_2)$ is (are) still undetermined."

The authors go on to state that clinical trials are being done to evaluate the effectiveness of this serological marker as a sensitive diagnostic tool for cancer screening. Time will reveal its effectiveness.

Transferrin is an 80 kDa glycoprotein found in the blood plasma. Transferrin has the role of transporting iron in the ferric form (Fe^{3+}) from the gut, and from its storage form bound to ferritin in liver cells to red blood cells (RBCs), where the transferrin binds with RBC membrane receptors in the process of transfering the iron into the cell where it is incorporated into hemoglobin. At any given time, about 0.1% of the total iron in the body is bound to tranferrin, 66% is in hemoglobin, 3% is in myoglobin, 30% is stored intracellularly in ferritin, 1% is chelated, and 0.1% is in heme enzymes (Re: Transferrin, 1997).

Baker (2000) reported on the *Transferrin Receptor Red Cell Assay,* (also called the E-Tr test) developed by Dr. Joseph Gong at the University of Buffalo. Gong's test reveals the extent of cumulative bone marrow stem cell damage from X-ray exposure, other ionizing radiation, and from certain chemicals that mimic ionizing radiation exposure. Gong said:

"All cancers develop from a pool of mutated cells that are 'turned on' by one or more triggers. The larger the pool of mutated cells, the greater the risk. Cancer can take years to develop, depending on the type. This test provides a way to measure the (radiation) damage before the first sign of cancer appears. It can also determine if cell mutations from ionizing radiation are increasing over time. If so, the individual can take steps to stop the increase, perhaps through a change in job, diet or environment. It gives people more control over their health."

Gong and co-workers found that the number of RBCs with transferrin receptors increases monotonically with ionizing radiation exposure. Thus, the simple bioassay for the RBC ferritin receptors in a drop of blood can give an accurate physiological indication of a person's radiation exposure and cell damage. The E-Tr test is functionally better than the conventional fogged film badge or electrometer dosimeter, which merely measure radiation, per se. Gong's test is covered by U.S. Patent #5,691,157 (Gong and Glomski, 1997). Fluorescent labeled antibodies are used to bind with those RBCs with a radiation-induced increase in transferrin receptors. In the patent, Gong and Glomski show a very linear increase in RBCs with transferrin receptors vs. radiation dose over a range of 0 to c. 2 Gy (Gray; 1 Gy = 100 rad).

We have seen that cancers perturb the biochemical milieu around them in subtle ways, perhaps leading to the development of NI screening tests based on the changes in certain biochemical constituents in blood, urine, saliva or sputum. Growing cancers also have altered metabolic needs, generally because they are growing faster than the tissues surrounding them. This property also makes them vulnerable to NI diagnosis. Researchers at the Mayo Clinic and at the University of Minnesota have recently developed a technique for diagnosing latency-period breast cancer that uses radioisotope-labeled vitamin B12 (cobolamin). Vitamin B12 is preferentially taken up by breast cancer cells, and also by lung cancer in patients with metastases; the cancer's radioactivity is above the body's background radioactivity and is detected with a gamma camera. Vitamin B12 is involved in the production of genetic material in dividing cells, and also is essential for the metabolism of certain amino acids, and fats. It is also required for the conversion of inactive folate to active form (FYCCO 2000; Gustafson, 1999).

The amino acid *homocysteine* is formed by the demethylation of the natural amino acid methionine (See Figure 17.3). A number of workers (Chao et al., 1999; Boushey et al., 1995; Perry et al., 1995; Verhoef et al., 1996; Bronstrup et al., 1998) have found that a high level of homocysteine in the blood is a potent risk factor for cardiovascular disease (atherosclerosis), heart attack and stroke. It may also be associated with kidney disease, psoriasis, breast cancer and acute lymphoblastic leukemia (Moghadasian et al., 1997; Follest-Strobl et al., 1997). The exact cause for elevated homocysteine concentration is not clear; it may be related to disease-caused stress, and it undoubtedly has a complex biochemical explanation. The administration of vitamins B12 and B6 brings the level of homocysteine down, presumably reducing the risks. Thus, it appears that measurement of elevated blood homocysteine concentration does not have specific predictive diagnostic value, but is indicative of a spectrum of possible future or ongoing health problems.

17.3 FLUORESCENCE TESTS FOR BIOMOLECULES; FISH AND SKY

In Section 15.3, we described the use of fluorescence to detect cancers and other lesions noninvasively, that is, using endoscopes to directly examine the fluorescent

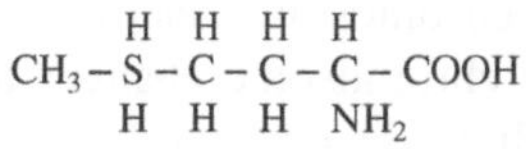

H H H H
CH₃ – S – C – C – C – COOH
H H H NH₂

A

H H H
HS – C – C – C – COOH
H H NH₂

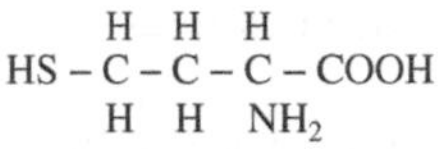

B

FIGURE 17.3 (A) The amino acid methionine. (B) The amino acid homocysteine.

properties of the cells in the surface of a lesion. In this section, we further explore this topic, including how the use of fluorescent dyes bonded to probe molecules can reveal chromosomal, gene, and oligonucleotide structures. The ability to probe the structure of DNA and RNA sequences is currently an extremely active research topic in oncology and genetic medicine. Cancer cells not only exhibit mutations in their nuclear DNA (nDNA), but also in their mitochondrial DNA (mtDNA), providing possible early tests for cancers and aiding researchers to understand the causes of various types of cancer.

Generally, fluorescent tests on DNA can be done on prepared cancer cells taken by biopsy (an invasive procedure) using fluorescent nucleic acid labeling techniques and confocal fluorescence microscopy. Alternately, the cells and mtDNA to be analyzed can be found in specimens of urine, saliva and sputum (NI procedures). DNA fragments (oligonucleotides) can be "amplified" or reproduced enzymatically by the *polymerase chain reaction* (PCR) technique, so more identical molecules are available to study.

Fluorescent *in situ* hybridization (FISH) is a molecular labeling technique used to detect the chromosomal location (and presence) of a specific genomic target. FISH was invented at the Lawrence Livermore National Laboratory in the mid-1980s by J.W. Gray and D. Pinkel. The FISH technique involves the selective binding of one or more probe molecules, each labeled with a separate unique fluorescent dye (fluorochrome) to target single strands of DNA or RNA. The single-strand labeled DNA (or RNA) probe molecules are synthesized in lengths dependent on the application. Multiple complementary probes can be synthesized from all of the fragments from a single long strand of DNA of a particular chromosome. These probes can label the total target chromosome. Alternately, chromophore-labeled probes can be made for a single gene, or be a relatively short oligonucleotide composed of as few as eight nucleotides. Short oligonucleotide probes can be used to find and label the complementary target sequences in any single-strand chromosomal DNA.

FISH can be used to distinguish all of the chromosomes; five or more unique fluorescent markers (fluors) must be used in various combinations to effect unique marking of all 23 chromosomes. The use of multiple fluors is called M-FISH. A sixth fluor can be used to give banding patterns. M-FISH has great potential for cancer research for the diagnosis and evaluation of treatments, particularly for various leukemias, where the chromosomes can be "jumbled." M-FISH will aid in the identification of recurrent chromosome changes and rearrangements. Speicher et al., (1996) developed epifluorescence wavelength filter sets and software that allows the detection and discrimination of 27 different DNA probes hybridized simultaneously to human chromosomes. The perfection of this technology led to the development of *spectral karyotyping* (SKY), which enables the simultaneous differentiation of all 24 human chromosomes in 24 colors. To quote Miklos (1999):

> "SKY takes advantage of the fact that Spectral Bio Imaging, in contrast to traditional filter systems, is not influenced by intensity variations which often impair the results of FISH experiments or make them simply not analyzable. ... The analysis of multi-color FISH experiments by (Applied) Spectral Imaging (Ltd.) provides a high number of measurement points along the spectral axis for each point (pixel) of the image which yields an extremely high signal to noise ratio.
>
> "For Spectral Karyotyping, all 24 flow-sorted human chromosome painting probes are combinatorially labeled with a set of 5 different fluorochromes (1 x green, 2 x red, 2 x infrared). Each chromosome is assigned a unique combination of fluorochromes and thereby a highly characteristic emission spectrum, which is used for definite chromosome recognition. Image acquisition is achieved with the SpectraCube® system (cf. Section 17.5 below), a combination of an interferometer (used as a Fourier spectrometer) and a CCD camera, which can be mounted on nearly every existing fluorescence microscope via a C-mount without the need for sophisticated microscope automation. ..."

Mitochondria are cell organelles that are responsible for the synthesis of adenosine triphosphate (ATP) (largely from oxygen and glucose) in a complex series of enzymatically controlled chemical reactions. ATP is a ubiquitous molecule, used by the body's cells as a common energy currency; it drives many of the chemical reactions in the body including various *ion pumps* used by neurons, muscle cells, kidney tubule cells, etc., as well as powering the synthesis of glucose from lactic acid, the synthesis of fatty acids from acetyl coenzyme A (acetyl Co-A), the synthesis of cholesterol, phospholipids, hormones and many other substances. Mitochondria are unique because they have a double-walled membrane isolating them from the cytosol, and they have their own circular 16.5-kilobase DNA chromosome that codes for 13 proteins and several regulating enzymes. There are about 10 copies of the genome in each mitochondrion, and up to 10^4 mitochondria in a cell. Damage to mtDNA (e.g., from ionizing radiation) is more common than to nDNA; mutations occur most frequently in the NADH dehydrogenase subunit 4 gene and in the displacement loop region (Hochhauser, 2000). About 90% of mitochondrial proteins are coded by genes from DNA in the cell nucleus (nDNA), however, suggesting that, in the process of evolution, genes have been lost from the mtDNA. mtDNA is inherited from the unfertilized ovum, hence everyone's mtDNA comes from their mother.

When a cancer cell dies (undergoes apoptosis or is attacked by the immune system's natural killer cells), cell fragments and mtDNA enter the surrounding medium (urine, saliva, etc.). In a key pilot study, Fliss et al., (2000) found that mtDNA isolated from the urine of patients having bladder cancer showed mutations.

The same mtDNA mutations were found by direct examination of biopsied cells from the cancer. Similar results were found for head, neck and lung cancers using saliva and lung lavage samples from the respective patients. Mutations were also found in cancer cells' nDNA, as might be expected, but the mtDNA mutation tests are many times more sensitive because a cancer cell has only one nucleus with nDNA and thousands of mitochondria, each with up to 10 copies of its mtDNA. Lung, neck and bladder cancers strike over 260,000 persons per year, as well as kill an estimated 180,000 victims. Thus, the screening of fluids obtained noninvasively (urine, saliva, sputum) for mutations in mtDNA using FISH, SKY, spectral imaging techniques or a DNA biochip, hold promise for rapid and inexpensive cancer screening in the future.

17.4 THE SPECTRACUBE® SYSTEM

The SpectraCube® system, a product developed and patented by Applied Spectral Imaging Co. in Israel, is a unique imaging system that allows the detailed wavelength (spectral) information associated with each pixel of an illuminated object to be determined and displayed. The object can be a length of fluorescently tagged DNA in a cell nucleus, a tissue probed with a Raman laser, an autofluorescent tissue such as a growing cancer viewed by an endoscope, or varieties of DNA tagged with fluorescent oligonucleotide probes bound to a DNA biochip. (The SpectraCube system can also be used in geological and natural resource image analysis (remote sensing); it is not limited to medical diagnosis.) U.S. Patent No. 5,539,517 (Cabib et al., 1996) Method for Simultaneously Measuring the Spectral Intensity as a Function of Wavelength of All the Pixels of a Two Dimensional Scene, describes the optical technology used in the SpectraCube system. U.S. Patent No. 5,995,645 (Soenksen et al., 1999) Method of Cancer Cell Detection, illustrates how the SpectraCube system can be used to find cancerous cells. Suspect cells from a biopsy are stained with two dyes, one of which binds preferentially to cancer cells. Spectral imaging is used to detect those cells imaged in certain pixels that are cancerous. The SpectraCube system not only gives intensity information for every pixel, but also measures the spectrum of each pixel in a predetermined range.

The heart of the SpectraCube system is an *interferometer* that allows computation of the spectrum of the light reflected or emitted from each object pixel using the *Fourier transform (FT) spectrogram method* (described in detail in Section 8.2.2 of this text). Note that the use of an interferometer and the FT method replaces the need for a monochromator or many narrow-band band-pass filters for spectral decomposition. Cabib et al. (1996) show that several different kinds of interferometer can be used to derive the spectrum of the light from each object pixel. They show that both interferometers with moving mirrors to vary the optical path distance (OPD), and also interferometers with fixed mirrors (where the OPD is varied by the angle of incidence of rays from object pixels) can be used. For illustrative purposes, they illustrate embodiments of their invention with internally modulated Fabry-Perot and Michelson, and fixed Michelson and Sagnac interferometers.

Figure 17.4 is a block diagram of the SpectraCube® system covered by U.S. Patent No. 5,539,517 (Cabib et al., 1996). An optical schematic diagram of a

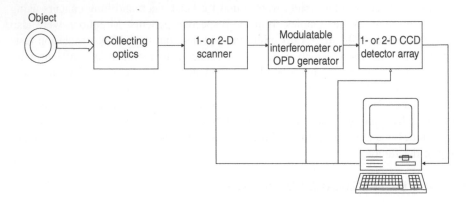

FIGURE 17.4 Block diagram of the SpectraCube® system.

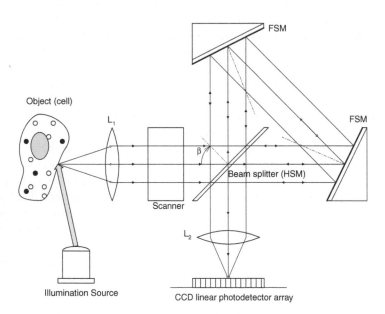

FIGURE 17.5 Schematic of a SpectraCube® system in which the interferometer is a Sagnac type with fixed mirrors.

typical SpectraCube configuration is shown in Figure 17.5. Note that, in this embodiment, a *Sagnac interferometer* with fixed mirrors is used. The OPD required to form an interferogram is inherent in the angle of incidence, β, of the incoming rays. It is shown in Cabib et al. (1996) that the OPD in the Sagnac interfero-meter is proportional to β. Figure 17.6 illustrates a Michelson interferometer with an OPD varied by a mirror mounted on a piezoelectric crystal transducer. Horizontal scanning is not required in this embodiment because a square CCD photosensor array is used, rather than the CCD linear array seen in Figure 17.5. To quote Cabib et aet al., l. (1996):

"In all the embodiments of the invention described below [in the Patent text], all the required optical phase differences are scanned simultaneously with the spatial scanning of the field of view in order to obtain all the information required to reconstruct the spectrum, so that the spectral information is collected simultaneously with the imaging information.

"A method and apparatus according to the present invention may be practiced in a large variety of configurations. Specifically, the interferometer used may be of either the moving (mirror) or the non-moving type and the detector array may, independently of the type of interferometer, be one- or two-dimensional. When the interferometer is of the moving type and the detector array is two-dimensional, no scanning (of the object) is required, except for movement of the interferometer which is an OPD scan. When the interferometer is of the moving type and the detector array is one-dimensional, spatial scanning (of the object) in one dimension is required. When the interferometer is of the non-moving type and the detector array is two-dimensional, OPD scanning in one dimension is required (to vary β, hence the OPD). When the interferometer is of the non-moving type, and the detector array is one-dimensional, scanning in two-dimensions is required, with one dimension relating to a spatial scan while the other relates to an OPD (β) scan."

In the internally modulated Michelson interferometer of Figure 17.6, the output is directed to a 2-D CCD photodetector array. Note that no external scanning is required. Once the image and the spectra of its pixels have been computed, the information can be used to screen tissue samples (generally obtained by biopsy) for cancer cells. The affinities for various fluorescent dye molecules of cancer cells differ from normal cells', and the pattern recognition software used with a SpectraCube system can be programmed to "recognize" cancer cells by their spectral signatures. The same technique can be used in DNA analysis using multiple fluorescent tags on probe oligonucleotides, either on chromosomes on a prepared microscope slide, or on a DNA biochip, as described in the next section. SpectraCube systems are enabling efficient, rapid and accurate SKY to be done, where genetic aberrations in both nDNA and mtDNA can be located and characterized. SKY is useful in research on genetic diseases and on the causes of cancer.

Another application of the SpectraCube system is in ophthalmology. The ophthalmic applied spectral imaging system (OASIS) has been developed by the Applied Spectral Imaging Co. The OASIS system is a sophisticated fundus camera that allows resolution of chemical as well as structural details in the retina. For example, the processor can be programmed to map regions of low oxygen saturation (see Section 15.8 on Pulse Oximetry) in the retina, a condition relating to vascular disease caused, for example, by diabetes (i.e., diabetic retinopathy). OASIS can also detect drusen by their spectral characteristics. (Drusen can be present in retinas affected by age-related macular degeneration; see Section 2.2.1.) The OASIS system uses a modified and cooled Hamamatsu C4880-81 CCD camera with 640×480-pixel resolution. The interferometer used in the OASIS system has fixed mirrors; the OPD length is

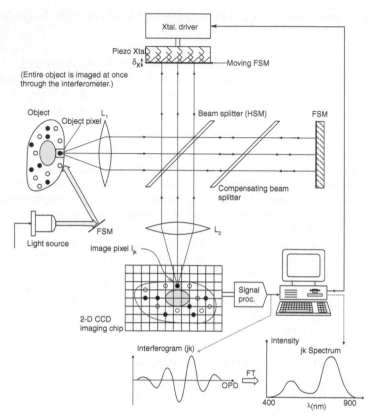

FIGURE 17.6 Schematic of a SpectraCube® system in which an OPD-modulated Michelson interferometer is used to find the spectrum of each pixel using Fourier transform calculations.

modulated by parallax angle to get c.100 data points in the interferogram for each pixel. Each pixel's interferogram is FFTd to give a corresponding spectrogram. The system's computer is programmed to analyze each spectrogram and assign a (pseudo)color to each pixel, depending on how it matches the property sought (i.e., oxyhemoglobin) (Curran, 2000).

17.5 THE DNA MICROARRAY

DNA microarrays, aka DNA biochips, come in many embodiments; they are actively being developed by many corporations and university laboratories around the world. There are several forces driving their invention; one is the economy resulting from the speed of analysis they permit, which effectively makes use of molecular parallel processing. They require fewer personnel than do conventional analytical techniques, and they offer high analytic accuracy. DNA microarrays are used to determine the molecular structure of chromosomes, genes and other oligonucleotides (oligos). They also can be used to analyze proteins, including antigens, antibodies and receptors on cell surfaces. They have many applications in the fields of genetic medicine, cancer diagnostics, and pharmaceutical development. For example, they provide genetic analysis of bacterial strains, showing how mutations can lead to drug resistance.

A microarray is composed of a rectangular grid of open compartments or "cells" formed on a flat substrate such as silicon or glass. The cell dimensions on DNA microarrays are on the order of 10s to100s of μm, at least two orders of magnitude larger than features on a typical electronic microcircuit. Much art and ingenious surface chemistry have been invested in attaching probe molecules to an array's cells. In one scheme, developed at Rockefeller University in New York, Shivashankar and Libchaber (1997) used an atomic force microscope and laser "tweezers" to graft a single strand of DNA to a 3-μm-diameter latex bead and then bond this complex into a microarray cell so the DNA could be probed with fluorophore-labeled oligos in solution. Another approach has used an electric field applied to the target cell to attract charged probe molecules to that cell; the process is repeated until all the cells are filled with different probes. The company Affymetrix has adapted a photolithographic process to assemble various fluorescent probes in the array's cells. Experimental microarrays with over 96,000 cells containing different oligonucleotides have been built as gene probes (CMGS, 1998). Note that probe molecules generally have known base sequences and are labeled with fluorescent molecules; probes can be in solution, or be tethered to substrate molecules in the cells. The target molecules are the analytes; their base sequence is unknown and to be determined. If the probe molecules are tethered, the target analytes are in solution, and vice versa.

There are three basic detection or readout schemes that are currently used with DNA microarrays:

1. The most common method is based on fluorescent labeling of probe molecules that bind with target molecules in the microarray's "cells." Fluorescence can be read out by interrogating each cell sequentially with a collimated laser beam that excites the fluorescence in a particular cell, if any. Bandpass filters are used to read each type of fluorescence. Alternatively, the entire microarray can be illuminated with the UV-exciting light, and a SpectraCube® system can be used to analyze all the fluorescent signatures of the cells, all at once.

2. Radioactive labeling of probe molecules in solution is a second means of detecting probe-target ligands. The target molecules are bound to cells in the array. Autoradiography with film is used to detect bound complexes on the array; a more qualitative than quantitative approach.

3. The third type of readout is electrical. Clinical MicroSensors, a subsidiary of Motorola, Inc., has developed a charge-based method in which various oligonucleotide probes are bound to array cells. When a target complementary DNA section binds to an oligo probe on a cell, a third molecular probe carrying iron can bind to the ligated probe and DNA. The presence of the iron is sensed electronically by the altered E field around the cell, and a current flows for that cell proportional to the amount of third probe molecule attached in the cell. Thus, a dc current readout is possible from each cell, the magnitude of which is indicative of the amount of target DNA bound to a given cell's probe oligo.

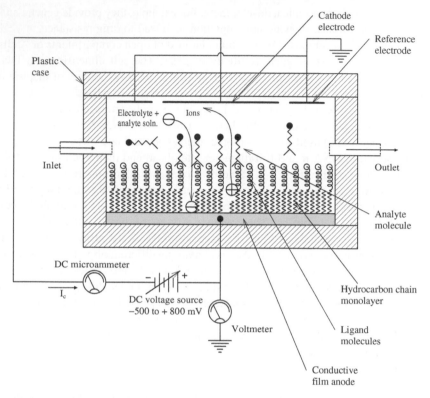

FIGURE 17.7 The Lennox 2000 biosensor system. When an analyte molecule binds with the target site on a ligand molecule, the underlying dense hydrocarbon monolayer parts and allows ions to flow. DC cell current is proportional to the bound analyte concentration.

Another electronic detection means for detecting probe-target binding is described by Lennox (2000), in U.S. Patent No. 6,107,180, Biosensor Device and Method. Lennox's invention uses conductivity-based phenomena as well as a field effect. Figure 17.7 illustrates a cross section through the simplified array cell of Lennox's system. In one embodiment of his biosensor, a monolayer of 8 to 22 carbon-saturated hydrocarbon (SHC) chains are bound to the conductive substrate by sulfhydryl linkages. The chain density is 3–5 per nm^2. Ligand (probe) molecules are then attached to the distal ends of a small fraction of the chains. In the absence of target analyte molecules, the dense, ordered packing of the SHC chains forms an effective, high-resistance barrier to electron flow through the cell. When a target molecule forms chemical bonds with a probe molecule, the ordered geometry of the SHC chains is perturbed, allowing certain ions from the bathing solution capable of undergoing a redox reaction to react at a noble metal electrode surface. A typical redox ion could be $Fe(CN)_4^-$, or $Fe^{+++} \rightarrow Fe^{++}$ (reduction). Lennox claims that only one binding event (probe to analyte) triggers 10^2 to 10^6 redox events and electrons to flow per second, thus is highly multiplicative. A cell's electron current is proportional to the number of reacted probe molecules in the cell. To quote Lennox:

"By analogy to a (field effect) transistor, the redox solution serves as the 'source,' the monolayer as the 'gate,' and the underlying electrode as the 'drain.' Current flow in a transistor is initiated by applying a threshold voltage to the gate. In the *biosensor* of the invention, current flow is initiated by a stimulus — in this case, a ligand receptor binding event — to the monolayer 'gate.'"

Of course, a suitable dc potential must be maintained to support the redox reaction used.

Electrical readout of DNA microarrays is especially attractive because no expensive lasers and fluorescence imaging CCD cameras are required; only N current-to-voltage converters, an analog multiplexer, and an analog-to-digital converter to interface with the computer used to manage data. The N cells on a biosensor "chip" require noble metal electrodes (gold or platinum) for the redox reactions. A drawback of the electrical DNA microarray is that this type of system has very high temperature sensitivity; the electrical conductivity of ionic solutions, and redox reactions have very high positive tempcos. This means that the temperature environment of an electrical DNA biosensor must be strictly regulated.

A future readout system for microarrays can make use of *surface plasmon resonance* (SPR) (see Section 8.2.4). A rectangular matrix of probe molecules, each having an affinity to a particular target molecule, will be deposited in cells on the surface of an SPR grating or prism. When the probe molecule in any one cell binds to its target molecule, the dielectric constant and refractive index change in the chemical layer, affecting surface plasmon generation. We have seen in Section 8.2.4 that the binding reaction affects the absorption of input photon energy and its conversion into plasmons. One way this binding can be detected is by shining a beam of monochromatic, linearly polarized light on the metal film on the grating directly under the cell in question. The intensity of the reflected beam is monitored. Binding causes a shift in the light beam angle at which maximum absorption (minimum reflection) occurs, as shown in Figure 8.14.

In an alternate readout approach, the light beam is kept at a fixed angle and a wavelength is chosen that will give minimum intensity of the reflected light beam shone on the unreacted cell in question. When target molecules bind to the probe molecules in the cell, the wavelength for maximum absorption (minimum reflection intensity) will shift. This alternate readout approach requires a monochromator to vary the λ of the input beam at constant intensity and angle. Figure 8.15 illustrates this wavelength-dependent absorption shift at constant incidence angle as binding occurs.

If the *variable angle method* is used, a simple diode laser can be used to test for probe binding with a single photomultiplier detector. The mechanical design in this case is more complex; for N cells, the laser and detector must be moved to systematically cover each cell, and also scanned in angle. Using the *fixed angle method,* the entire SPR cell array can be illuminated with one beam at a fixed angle and λ. Detection can be by a square-array CCD camera, also at a fixed angle with respect to the SPR microarray. The wavelength of the illuminating beam can be repetitively swept over the λ range of interest, and each of the CCD ouputs averaged to improve SNR and to measure binding dynamics. The λ of the input beam can be varied continuously with a monochromator, or discretely with a bank of narrow band-pass filters acting on a white light source. I believe the latter method will be simpler and less expensive because nothing moves (except the gratings in the mono-chromator or the filters).

Applications of molecular biosensors are growing with the number of designs available. As we have described above, cancer screening through genetic mutation detection of nDNA and mtDNA is very important. The DNA microarray is also finding application in drug design. As various kinds of bacteria become resistant to older antibiotics, it is possible to track the mutations leading to changes in internal enzymes, etc., that confer this resistance. Thus, new antibiotics can be designed to exploit weaknesses in the more stable parts of a bacterium's genome. The DNA microarray is not limited to DNA. RNA from retroviruses such as HIV can be analyzed for mutations as well.

Simple cells with bound *protein antigens* can be designed to test for particular antibodies in the blood or other body fluids; conversely, monoclonal antibodies can be bound as probes to detect a particular bacterial antigen such as on *E. coli,* streptococcus, pneumococcus, etc., and even read out the subtype to facilitate anti-biotic selection. They can facilitate detection of *PLA2*, a protein produced by prostate cancers cells and *melastatin,* a protein produced by melanoma cancer cells.

17.6 SUMMARY

The two disciplines that will contribute most to the next generation of noninvasive diagnostic instrumentation are photonics and biochemistry. We have seen how pho-tonics in the embodiment of Fourier transform spectroscopy, as in the SpectraCube® system, can analyze the spectral absorption of biological surfaces at the pixel level. Such analysis will make the detection of skin cancer more reliable.

The use of fluorophore-tagged molecules with affinities for various antigens, antibodies, biomolecules and nucleic acid fragments has opened up another growing group of modalities for noninvasive photon-based diagnosis, including FISH and SKY. DNA biochips are emerging as a potent diagnostic tool. In some designs, the readout is electric, in others, readout is by fluorescent taggants scanned by a blue laser.

We might also expect to see the development of reliable transcutaneous spec-trophotometric measurement of critical blood analytes, including glucose, certain hormones, opioids, drugs, etc. (At present, the percent oxyhemoglobin and hemat-ocrit can be measured transcutaneously by spectrophotometric analysis.)

Bibliography and References*

Adler, F.H. 1933. *Clinical Physiology of the Eye.* Macmillan, NY.

Advisory Committee on Human Radiation Experiments (ACHRE) — Final Report. Available as Stock # 061-000-00-848-9 from the Superintendent of Documents, the U.S. Government Printing Office, Washington, D.C. 20402. Available on-line at URL: http://tis.eh.doe.gov/ohre/roadmap/achre/intro.html

Affymetrix Technologies: Product Technology: GeneChip® Technology. URL accessed: www.affymetrix.com/products/tech_probe_content.html

Alenius, S. 1999. On Noise Reduction in Iterative Image Reconstruction Algorithms for Emission Tomography: Median Root Prior. (Web paper on noise reduction in PET and SPECT. At URL:) www.cs.tut.fi/~sakkeus/v/thesis.htm

Anbar, M. 1998. Clinical thermal imaging toaday. *IEEE Engrg. in Med, and Biol. Mag.* 17(4): 25–33.

Andersson, B., et al. 1998. Glucose concentration in parotid saliva after glucose/food intake in individuals with glucose intolerance and diabetes mellitus. *Eur. J. Oral Sci.* 106(5): 931–937.

Anger, H.O. 1964. Scintillation camera with multichannel collimators. *J. Nuc. Med.* 5: 515–531.

Arnold, M.A. and D.C. Klonoff. 1999. Noninvasive laser measurement of blood glucose in the eye: A bright idea or an optical illusion? Editorial in *Diabetes Technology and Theraputics.* 1(2): 117–119.

Badawi, R. 1999. *Introduction to PET Physics.* (University of Washington, Div. of Nuclear Medicine. URL: http://nucmed.rad.washington.edu/web/teaching/physics_intro/toc.html

Bains, S. 1998. DNA molecules grafted on silicon with optical tweezers. *OE Reports.* 171: March 1998. SPIE Web. www.spie.org/web/oer/march/mar98/ltconstr.html

Baker, L. 2000. Blood test measures radiation damage. *The University of Buffalo Reporter.* 31(18): URL: www.buffalo.edu/reporter/vol31/vol31n18/n8.html

Barnes Engineering Co. 1983. *Handbook of Infrared Radiation Measurement.* Barnes Engineering Co., Stamford, CT.

Barro, S., M. Fernández-Delgado, J.A. Villa-Sobrino, C.V. Regueiro and E. Sánchez. 1998. Classifying multichannel ECG patterns with an adaptive neural network. *IEEE Engrg. Med. and Biol. Mag.* 17(1): 45–55.

Bartsch, C., H. Bartsch and T.H. Lippert. 1992. The pineal gland and cancer: facts, hypotheses and perspectives. *Cancer J.* 5(4): 10p. URL: www.infobiogen.fr/agora/journals/cancer/articles/5-4/bart.htm

Bastiaans, M.J. 1997. Application of the Wigner distribution function in optics. In *The Wigner Distribution–Theory and Applications in Signal Processing.* Mecklenbräuker, W. and F. Hlawatsch, Eds. Elsevier Science. 375–426.

Belcaro, G.V., U. Hoffmann, A. Bollinger and A.N. Nicolaides, Eds. 1994. *Laser Doppler.* Med-Orion Pub. Co.

Berger, A.J., T-W. Koo, I. Itzkan, G. Horowitz and M.S. Feld. 1999. Multicomponent blood analysis by near-infrared Raman spectroscopy. *Applied Optics.* 38(13): 2916–2926.

---

* All URL's were accessed successfully in the period from 6/2000 to 3/2001.

Berger, A.J., J.F. Brennan III, R.R. Dasari, M.S. Feld, I. Itzkan, K. Tanaka and Y. Wang. 1997. *Apparatus and Methods of Raman Spectroscopy for Analysis of Blood Gases and Analytes.* U.S. Patent No. 5,615,673. 1 April 1997.

Bertolucci, E. 1998. *Medical Imaging with Ionizing Radiation.* Tutorial paper at URL: www.wirescript.com/cgibin/HyperNews/get.cgi/bb9901.html

Best, M., T.A. Kelly and M.A. Galin. 1970. The ocular pulse–technical features. *Acta Ophthalmologica.* 48: 357–367.

Best, M, G. Plechaty, L. Harris and M.A. Galin. 1971. Ophthalmodynamometry and ocular pulse studies in carotid occlusion. *Arch. Ophthal.* 85: 334–338.

Best, M. and R. Rogers. 1974. Techniques of ocular pulse analysis in carotid stenosis. *Arch. Ophthal.* 92: 54–58.

Bicron. 1999. Curved Scintillator Plates Advance PET Technology for Better Diagnosis. (Bicron Corp. white paper, at URL:) www.bicron.com/bicronmed/snm2.htm

Blank, T.B., T.L. Ruchti, S.F. Malin and S.L. Monfre. 1999. The use of near infrared diffuse reflectance for the noninvasive prediction of blood glucose. LEOS paper at URL: www.ieee.org/organizations/Newsletters/leos/oct99/article6.htm

Blazek, K., F. De Notaristefani, et al. 1995. YAP multi-crystal gamma camera prototype. *IEEE Trans. Nucl. Sci.* 42(5): 1474–1482.

Bonnick, S.L. 1998. *Bone Densitometry in Clinical Practice: Application and Interpretation.* Humana Press.

Boushey, C.J., et al. 1995. A quantitative assessment of plasma homocysteine as a risk factor for vascular disease. *JAMA.* 274(13): 1049–1057.

Braig, J.R., D.S. Goldberger and S.B. Bernhard. 1997. Self-Emission Noninvasive Infrared Spectrophotometer with Body Temperature Compensation. U.S. Patent No. 5,615,672. 1 April 1997.

Breindel, B. 1998. C-140R Trends in Noninvasive and Minimally Invasive Diagnostic Equipment. URL: http://buscom.com/health/C140R.html

Brimrose, 1992. Infrared Products brochure. Brimrose Corp. of America. Baltimore, MD, 21236.

Bronstrup, A., et al. 1998. Effects of folic acid and combinations of folic acid and vitamin B12 on plasma homocysteine concentrations in healthy young women. *Am. J. Clin. Nutrition.* 68: 1104–1110.

Brookner, C.K., et al. 2000. Autofluorescence patterns in short-term cultures of normal cervical tissue. *Photochemistry and Photobiology.* 71(6): 730– .URL: www.aspjournal.com/premium/vol71/iss6/html/v71i6p730.htm

Brown, L.J. 1980. A new instrument for the simultaneous measurement of total hemoglobin, percent oxyhemoglobin, percent carboxyhemoglobin, percent methemoglobin, and oxygen content in whole blood. *IEEE Trans. Biomed. Engrg.* 27(3): 132–138.

Browne, A.F., T.R. Nelson and R.B. Northrop. 1997. Microdegree polarimetric measurement of glucose concentrations for biotechnology applications. *Proc. 23rd Ann. New England Bioengineering Conf.* IEEE Press, NY. 9–10.

Browne, A.F. 1998. A New Approach to Monitoring Glucose Concentrations Based on Reflection of Polarized Light from a Liquid/Lens Interface and Detection by an Improved Closed-Loop Optical Polarimeter. Ph.D. dissertation, The University of Connecticut. Area: BioMedical Engineering. (R.B. Northrop, advisor.)

Burmeister, J.J., M.A. Arnold and G.W. Small. 1998. Spectroscopic considerations for noninvasive blood glucose measurements with near infrared spectroscopy. LEOS paper at URL: www.ieee.org/organizations/Newsletters/leos/apr98/infrared.htm

Cabib, D., et al. 1996. Method for Simultaneously Measuring the Spectral Intensity as a Function of Wavelength of All the Pixels of a Two Dimensional Scene. U.S. Patent No. 5,539,517. July 23, 1996.

Cabib, D., et al. 1998. Spectral Bio-Imaging Methods for Biological Research, Medical Diagnosis and Therapy. U.S. Patent No. 5,784,162. July 21, 1998.

Cavallerano, A.A., et al. 1997. Optometric Clinical Practice Guideline: Care of the Patient with Macular Degeneration. American Optometric Association web publication. At URL: www.aoanet.org/cpg-6-armd.html

CES. 1999. CES Medical Applications in Cardiology. White paper on MCG. At URL: http://ces-squid-systems.com/medical.html

Chao, C-L, et al. 1999. Effect of short-term vitamin (folic acid, vitamins B6 and B12) administration on endothelial function induced by post-methionine load hyperhomocysteinemia. *Am. J. Cardiol.* 84: 1359–1361.

Chin, T.J. and M. McGrath. 1998. Diagnoses of deep vein thromboses. *Austr. Prescr.* 21: 6pp. URL: www.australianprescriber.com/vol21no3/diagnosis_thrombosis.htm

Clayton, R.H., R.W.F. Campbell and A. Murray. 1998. Characteristics of multichannel ECG recordings during human ventricular tachyarrhythmias. *IEEE Engrg. Med. and Biol. Mag.* 17(1):. 39–44.

CMGS (Clinical Molecular Genetics Society). 1998. Mutation detection using DNA chip technology. At URL: www.ich.ucl.ac.uk/cmgs/chips98.htm

Collins, R.D. 1968. *Illustrated Manual of Laboratory Diagnosis.* J.B. Lippincott Co., Philadelphia.

Cornwall, M. 1999. Diagnostic Electromyography. Web notes for class PT580 at Northern Arizona Univ. URL: http://jan.ucc.nau edu/~cornwall/pt580/class/EDX/EMGassign2 -4-1.html

Coté, G.L., M.D. Fox and R.B. Northrop. Optical Glucose Sensor Apparatus and Method. U.S. Pat. # 5,209,231. 11 May 1993.

Curran, L.J. 2000. Imaging system equips ophthalmologists with noninvasive detection method. *Vision Systems Design.* August. 30–32.

Daghigian, F., et al. 1993. Evaluation of a cerium doped lutetium orthosilicate (LSO) scintillation crystal for PET. *IEEE Trans. Nucl. Sci.* 40(4): 1045–1047.

Dähne, C. and D. Gross. 1987. Spectrophotometric Method and Apparatus for the Non-Invasive [sic]. U.S. Patent No.4,655,225. 7 April 1987. (NIR transcutaneous measurement of glucose.)

D'Ambrosio, C., et al. 1998. The ISPA-tube and the HPMT, two examples of a new class of photodetectors: the hybrid photo detectors. *Nucl. Physics B* (Proc. Suppl.) 61B: 638–643.

D'Ambrosio, C., et al. 1999. Further developments on an ISPA-camera for γ-rays in nuclear medicine. *Nucl. Physics B* (Proc. Suppl.) 78: 598–603.

Daskalov, I.K., I.A. Dotinsky and I.I. Christov. 1998. Developments in ECG acquisition, preprocessing, parameter measurement and recording. *IEEE Engrg. Med. and Biol. Mag.* 17(2): 50–58.

Dawson, P. 2001. MRI Theory Made Child's Play. AroSoft, Ltd. active server page web site. URL: www.image-publishing.com/chapt.asp?vol=1&chapt=14

de Berardinis, E., O. Tieri, A. Polzella and N. Iuglio. 1965. The chemical composition of the human aqueous humor in normal and pathological conditions. *Exp. Eye Rsch.* 4: 179–186.

de Boer, J.F., et al. 1997. Two-dimensional birefringence imaging in biological tissue by polarization-sensitive optical coherence tomography. *Optics Letters.* 22(12): 934–936.

de Boer, J.F., et al. 1999. Polarization effects in optical coherence tomography of various biological tissues. *IEEE J. Sel. Top. in Quantum Electronics.* 5(4): 1200–1204.

de Kock, J.P. and L. Tarassenko. 1993. Pulse oximetry: theoretical and experimental models. *Med. and Bio. Engrg. and Computing.* 31: 291–300.

de Kock, J.P., et al. 1993. Reflectance pulse oximetry measurements from the retinal fundus. *IEEE Trans. Biomed. Engrg.* 40(8): 817–823.

Dilmanian, F.A., et al. 2000. Computed tomography of X-ray index of refraction using the diffraction enhanced imaging method. *Phys. Med. Biol.* 45: 933–936.

Ding, M., et al. 2000. Short-window spectral analysis of cortical event-related potentials by adaptive multivariate autoregressive modeling: data preprocessing, model validation, and variability assessment. *Biological Cybernetics.* 83: 35–45.

Di Palma, J.A. 2000. Lactose hydrogen breath test methods. In *Online J. Digestive Hlth.* URL: www.gastronews.com/digestive.dir/physio.dir/physio.html

Drake, A.D. and D.C. Leiner. 1984. A fiber Fizeau interferometer for measuring minute biological displacements. *IEEE Trans. Biomed. Engrg.* 31(7): 507–511.

Duteil, L., J.C. Bernengo and W. Schalla. 1985. A double wavelength laser Doppler system to investigate skin microcirculation. *IEEE Trans. Biomed. Engrg.* 32(6): 439–447.

Edic, P.M., G.J. Saulnier, J.C. Newell and D. Isaacson. 1995. A real-time electrical impedance tomograph. *IEEE Trans. Biomed. Engrg.* 42(9): 849–859.

Ercal, F. A., Chawla, W.V., Stoecker, H-C Lee, and R.H. Moss. 1994. Neural network diagnosis of malignant melanoma from color images. *IEEE Trans. BioMed. Engrg.* 41(9): 837–845.

Everett, M. 1998. Optical coherence tomography for dental applications. (LLNL Medical Technology Program review article. At URL:) http://lasers.llnl.gov/lasers/mtp/oct.html

Faraj, B.A., et al. 1981. Melanoma detection by enzyme-radioimmunoassay of L-dopa, dopamine, and 3-o-methyldopamine in urine. *Clin. Chem.* 27(1): 108–112.

Feke, G.T., D.G. Goger, H. Tagawa and F.C. Delori. 1987. Laser Doppler technique for absolute measurement of blood speed in retinal vessels. *IEEE Trans. Biomed. Engrg.* 34(9): 673–680.

Fellows, K.R. 1997. The Design of a Non-Dispersive Spectrophotometer to Measure Oxyhemoglobin. MS dissertation in Biomedical Engineering. The University of Connecticut, Storrs. (R.B. Northrop, major advisor.)

Feldchtein, F.I., et al. 1998. Endoscopis applications of optical coherence tomography. *Optics Express.* 3(6): 257–270.

Ferraro, J.A. and R.P. Tibbils. 1999. SP/AP area ratio in the diagnosis of Ménière's disease. *Am. J. Audiology.* 8(1): URL: http://journals.asha.org/1059-0089/v8n1/ferraro.html

Fitzgerald, R. 2000. Phase sensitive X-ray imaging. *Physics Today Online.* July, 2000. URL: www.aip.org/pt/vol-53/iss-7/p23.html

Fliss, M., et al. 2000. Facile detection of mitochondrial DNA mutations in tumors and bodily [sic] fluids. *Science.* 287(5460): 2017 –2019.

Follest-Strobl, P.C., et al. 1997. Homocysteine: a new risk factor for atherosclerosis. *Am. Fam. Physician.* 56: 1607–1612.

Forbat, L.N., R.E. Collins, G.K. Maskell and P.H. Sonksen. 1981. Glucose concentrations in parotid fluid and venous blood of patients attending a diabetic clinic. *J. Royal Soc. Med.* 74: 725–728.

Forbes, M., P. Guillermo, Jr., and B. Grolman. 1974. A noncontact applanation tonometer. *Arch. Ophthal.* 91(2): 134–140.

Fox, M.D. 1978. Multiple crossed-beam ultrasound Doppler velocimetry. *IEEE Trans. Sonics and Ultrason.* 25(5): 281–286.

Fox, M.F. and J.F. Donnelly. 1978. Simplified method for determining piezoelectric constants for thickness mode transducers. *J. Acoust. Soc. Am.* 64(5): 1261–1265.

Fox, M.D. and W.M. Gardiner. 1988. Three-dimensional Doppler velocimetry of flow jets. *IEEE Trans. Biomed. Engrg.* 35(10): 834–841.

Fraden, J. 10 Jan. 1989a. Infrared electronic thermometer and method for measuring temperature. U.S. Pat. #4,797,840.

_____. 8 Aug. 1989b. Radiation thermometer and method for measuring temperature. U.S. Pat. #4,845,730.

_____. 7 July 1992. Apparatus and method for temperature measurement by radiation. U.S. Pat. #5,127, 742.

_____. 12 Jan. 1993a. Balanced infrared thermometer and method for measuring temperature. U.S. Pat. # 5,178,464.

_____. 1993b. *AIP Handbook of Modern Sensors.* American Institute of Physics, NY.

_____. 15 Nov. 1994. Infrared electronic thermometer and method for measuring temperature. U.S. Pat. #RE34,789.

Friedman, R.J., et al. 1985. Early detection of malignant melanoma: The role of physician examination and self-examination of the skin. *Ca–A Cancer Journal for Clinicians.* 35(3): 130–151.

Fujimoto, J.G., et al. 1995. Optical biopsy and imaging using optical coherence tomography. *Nature Medicine.* 1: 970.

FYCCO. 2000. Radioactive B12 diagnosis? URL: www.earlier.org/radioactive_b12_ diagnosis.html

Fye, W.B. 1998. Profiles in Cardiology: Rudolf Albert von Koelliker. On-line in *Clinical Cardiology.* 22: 376–377. URL: www.clinical-cardiology.org/briefs/9905briefs/22-376.html

Galin, G.A, M. Best, et al. 1972. The ocular pulse. *Trans. Am. Acad. Ophthal. and Otolaryngol.* 76: (Nov.–Dec.) 1535–1541.

Germano, C.P. 1961. On the Meaning of "g" and "d" Constant as Applied to Simple Piezoelectric Modes of Vibration. Technical Paper TP-222. Gould, Inc., Piezoelectric Division, Bedford, OH.

Gerster, J., et al. 1998. Non-magnetic low noise pulse tube cryocooler for cooling high-T_c DC-SQUID gradiometers. URL: www.physik.uni-jena.de/~tief/itk98/2-98.html

Gilham, E.J. 1957. A high-precision photoelectric polarimeter. *J. Sci. Instrum.* 34: 435–439.

Glass, L., et al. 1997. *Virtual Stethoscope.* McGill University's website of downloadable heart, lung and breath sounds and their T-F spectrograms. URL: www.music.mcgill.ca/ausculation/ausculation.html

Goldman, Z.Z. 1987. *Human Auditory and Visual Continuous Evoked Potentials.* Ph.D. Dissertation in Biomedical Engineering. The University of Connecticut. (R.B. Northrop, major advisor.)

Goldmann, H. 1957. Applanation tonometry. In *Glaucoma: Trans. of Second Conf., Dec. 3,4,5, 1956. Princeton, NJ.* F.W. Newell, ed. Madison Printing Co. 167–220.

Graylab. 1998. *The On-Line Medical Dictionary.* URL: www.graylab.ac.uk/omd/index.html

Grin, C.M., et al. 1990. Accuracy in the clinical diagnosis of malignant melanoma. *Arch. Dermatol.* 126: 763–766.

Gustafson, C. 1999. New procedure assists in cancer detection. *The Minnesota Daily Online.* Sept. 27. URL: www.mndaily.com/daily/1999/09/27/news/paten/ [sic]

Guyton, A.C. 1991. *Textbook of Medical Physiology,* 8th ed. W.B. Saunders Co., Philadelphia.

Hahn, C.E.W. 1998. Electrochemical analysis of clinical blood gases, gases and vapors. *The Analyst.* 123: 57R–86R.

Hall, G., F. Petak, N. Dore, M.J. Hayden, Z. Hantos and P.D. Sly. 1988. Respiratory mechanics in normal infants using low-frequency forced oscillations. *Proc. Thoracic. Soc. Australia and New Zealand.* Adelaide, 15–18 March.

Han, F., et al. 1999. Pteridine analysis in urine by capillary electrophoresis using laser-induced fluorescence detection. *Analyt. Chem.* 71: 1265–1269.

Hanlon, E.B., R. Manoharan, T-W Koo, K.E. Shafer, J.T. Motz, M. Fitzmaurice, J.R. Kramer, I. Itzkan, R.R. Dasari and M.S. Feld. 2000. Prospects for *in vivo* Raman spectroscopy. *Phys. Med. Biol.* 45(2): R1–R59.

Hannaford, B. and S. Lehman. 1986. Short time Fourier analysis of the electromyogram: fast movements and constant contraction. *IEEE Trans. Bio-Med. Engrg.* 33(12): 1173–1181.

Harding, J.R. 1998. Investigating deep vein thrombosis with infrared imaging. *IEEE Engrg. Med. and Biol. Mag..* 17(4): 43–46.

HealthGate. 1999. *Single Fiber Electromyography.* On-line description of diagnostic procedure. URL: wysiwyg://19/http://www.healthgate.co.uk/dp/dph.0217.shtml

HealthSystems. 2000. *Magnetic Resonance Imaging.* Teaching Files, 26 pp. URL: www.healthsystems.com/MRI/mri01.htm

Hecht, E. 1987. *Optics.* 2nd ed. Addison-Wesley, Reading, MA.

Heintzelmann, D.L., R. Lotan and R.R. Richards-Kortum. 2000. Characterization of the autofluorescence of polymorphonuclear leucocytes, mononuclear leucocytes, and cervical epithelial cancer cells for improved spectroscopic discrimination of inflammation from dyplasia. *Photochemistry and Photobiology.* 71(3): 327–332. URL: www.aspjournal.com/premium/vol71/iss3/html

Heise, H.M., L. Küpper and R. Marbach. 1999. Limitations of infrared spectroscopy for noninvasive metabolite monitoring using the attenuated total reflection technique. LEOS paper. URL: www.ieee.org/organizations/Newsletters/leos/oct99/article6.htm

Herscovici, H. and D.H. Roller. 1986. Noninvasive determination of central blood pressure by impedance plethysmography. *IEEE Trans. Biomed. Engrg.* 33(6): 617–625.

History of SQUID Technology in the United States and Japan. (1996). URL: www.itri.loyola.edu/sce196/06-02.htm

Hochhauser, D. 2000. Relevance of mitochondrial DNA in cancer. (A commentary and review article at the *Lancet* web site.) URL: www.findarticles.com/m0833/9255_356/63566598/p1/article.jhtml

Hong, H-D. and R.B. Northrop. 1991. Ultrasonic phase-shift oxygen measuring system. *Proc. 17th Ann. Northeast Bioengineering Conf.* IEEE Press, NY. 53–55.

Hong, H-D. and M.D. Fox. 1993. Detection of skin displacement and capillary flow using an optical stethoscope. *Proc. 19th Ann. Northeast Bioengineering Conf.* IEEE Press, NY. 189–190.

Hong, H.D. 1994. Optical Interferometric Measurement of Skin Vibration for the Diagnosis of Cardiovascular Disease. Ph.D. Dissertation on Biomedical Engineering. The University of Connecticut, Storrs. (M.D. Fox, advisor.)

Hørven, I. and H. Nornes. 1971. Crest time evaluation of corneal indentation pulse. *Arch. Ophthal.* 86: 5–11.

Hørven, I. 1973. Dynamic tonometry. *Acta Ophthalomogica.* 51: 353–366.

Hørven, I. and H. Gjønnaess. 1974. Corneal indentation pulse and intraocular pressure in pregnancy. *Acta Ophthalomogica.* 91: 92–98.

Howarth, D., et al. 1999. Scintimammography: An adjunctive test for the detection of breast cancer. *Med. J. Aust.* 170: 588 -591.

Hutchinson, J. 1846. On the capacity of the lungs, and on the respiratory functions, with a view of establishing a precise and easy method of detecting disease by the spirometer. *Med. Chir. Trans.* (London) 29: 137–.

Imaginis Corp. 2000. *Medical Procedures: Endoscopy.* URL: www.imaginis.com/endoscopy/index.asp?mode=1.

Inaguma, M. and K. Hashimoto. 2000. Porphyrin-like fluorescence in oral cancer: *In vivo* fluorescence spectral characterization of lesions by use of a near-ultraviolet excited autofluoresnce diagnosis system and separation of fluorescent extracts by capillary electrophoresis. *Mouth Cancer.* URL: www.oncolink.upenn.edu/cancernet/00/feb/702275.html

Integrated Publishing. 1998. *Light-Emitting Diodes.* URL: wysiwyg.://102/http://www.tpub.com/neets/tm/110-4.htm

ISCEV* Standards for clinical electroretinography (1999 update). *International Society for Clinical Electrophysiology of Vision. URL: http://sun11.ukl.uni-freiburg.de/aug/iscev/standards/erg1999.html

ISCEV Standards for Clinical Electro-oculography. 2000. URL: http://sun11.ukl.uni-freiburg.de/aug/iscev/standards/eog.html

ISCEV Guidelines for Calibration of Stimulus and Recording Parameters Used in Clinical Electrophysiology of Vision. 2000. URL: http://sun11.ukl.uni-freiburg.de/aug/iscev/standards/cal.html

ISCEV Visual Electrodiagnostics. 2000. URL: http://sun11.ukl.uni-freiburg.de/aug/iscev/standards/proceduresguide.html

ITRI. 1998. History of SQUID Technology in the United States and Japan. URL: www.itri.loyola.edu/scel96/06_02.htm

Jacobson, B. and J.G. Webster. 1977. *Medicine and Clinical Engineering.* Prentice-Hall, NY.

Jain, H., D. Isaacson, P.M. Edic and J.C. Newell. 1997. Electrical impedance tomography of complex conductivity distributions with noncircular boundary. *IEEE Trans. Biomed. Engrg.* 44(11): 1051–1060.

Jaszczak, R.J., P.H. Murphy, D. Huard and J.A. Burdine. 1977. Radionuclide emission computed tomography of the head with Tc-99m and a scintillation camera. *J.Nuc. Med. Inst. Phys.* 18(4): 373–.

Jaszczak, R.J. 1988. Tomographic radiopharmaceutical imaging. *Proc. IEEE.* 76(9): 1079–1094.

Jenkins, D. 1997. ECG Library: A Brief History of Electrocardiography. URL: http://homepages.enterprise.net/djenkins/ecghist.html

Johns, H.E. and J.R. Cunningham. 1983. *The Physics of Radiology,* 4th ed. C.C. Thomas, IL.

Jones, T. 2001. Scintillating Glass Provides High Quality X-Ray Imaging. URL: www.navysbir.brtc.com/SuccessStories/IndustrialQualityInc.htm

Jory, M.J., G.W. Bradberry, P.S. Cann and J.R. Sambles. 1995. A surface-plasmon-based optical sensor using acousto-optics. *Meas. Sci. Technol.* 6: 1193–1200.

Jossinet, J, P. Castello and F. Risacher. 1995. Multichannel impedance plethysmography discriminates leg arteries. Paper 1.2.6.19. EMBC95. URL: http://funsan.biomed.mcgill.ca/~funnell/embc95_cd/texts/217.htm

Kaiser, N. 1979. Laser absorption spectroscopy with an ATR prism. *IEEE Trans. Biomed. Engrg.* 26(10): 597–600.

Kandel, et al. 1991. *Principles of Neural Science*, 3rd ed. Appleton and Lange, Norwalk, CT. (McGraw-Hill).

Katz, B. 1966. *Nerve, Muscle and Synapse.* McGraw-Hill, NY.

Katzir, N., et al. 1998. Method for Classification of Pixels into Groups According to their Spectra Using a Plurality of Wide Band Filters and Hardwire [sic] Therefore. U.S. Patent #5,834,203. Nov. 10, 1998.

Kelly, R.G. and A.E. Owen. 1991. Microelectronic ion sensors: A critical survey. In *Microsensors*. R.S. Muller, R.T. Howe, S.D. Senturia, R.L. Smith and R.M. White. IEEE Press, NY.

Kelley, L.M., et al. 1997. Scanning laser ophthalmoscope imaging of age related macular degeneration and neoplasms. *J. Ophthal. Photog*, URL: http://webeye.ophth.uiowa.edu/ops/journal/97/dec/jour1.htm

Kemp, D.T. 1978. Stimulated acoustic emissions from within the human auditory system. *J. Acoust. Soc. Am.* 64: 1386–1391.

Klonoff, D.C., Braig, J., et al. 1998. Mid-infrared spectroscopy for noninvasive blood glucose monitoring. IEEE/LEOS Newsletter. URL: www.ieee.org/organizations/Newsletters/leos/apr98/midinfrared.htm

König, F., D. Schnorr, S.A. Loening, R. Paul, L. Pfeifer, A. Lehmann, A. Scheer and F. Fink. 1994. Laser-induced autofluorecence of prostate- and bladder tissue. *Proc. of OE/LASE '94,* Los Angeles, USA: SPIE-Vol 2134, Laser Tissue Interaction V.

Koo, T-W., A.J. Berger, I. Itzkan, G. Horowitz and M.S. Feld. 1999. Reagentless blood analysis by near infrared Raman spectroscopy. *Diabetes Technology and Theraputics.* 1(2): 153–157.

Korean Research Institute of Standards and Science, Superconductivity Group. URL: http://krissol.kriss.re.kr/quantum/supercon/k360.html

Korhonen, P.S. Lukkarinen, R. Sepponen, J. Backman, J. Ruotoistenmäki, K., Rajala. Frequency response measurements on commercially available stethoscopes. URL: www.hut.fi/Yksikot/Electron...jects/Audioscope/NBC-96/indec.html

Kraus, R., Jr. 1999. First phantom and human evoked response measurements for a whole-head super-conducting imaging surface MEG system. (Poster # 160, *5th Intl. Conf. on Functional Mapping of the Human Brain.* URL: www.apnet.com/hbm99/2637.html

Kronfeld, P.C. 1943. *The Human Eye in Anatomical Transparencies.* Bausch and Lomb Press, Rochester, NY.

Kuhl, D.E. and R.Q. Edwards.1963. Image separation radioisotope scanning. *Radiology.* 80: 653–662.

Lachish, U. 2000. The Role of Semiconductors in Digital X-Ray Medical Imaging. URL: wysiwyg://6/http://urila.tripod.com/xray.htm

Lacourse, J.R. and D.A. Sekel. 1986. A contact method of ocular pulse detection for studies of carotid occlusions. *IEEE Trans. Biomed. Engrg.* 33(4): 381–385.

Lambert, J., M. Storrie-Lombardi and M. Borchert. 1998. Measurement of physiological glucose levels using Raman spectroscopy in a rabbit aqueous humor model. URL: www.ieee.org/organizations/Newsletters/leos/apr98/aqueoushumor.htm

Le, H.V. 1999. Image Processing and Analysis for Melanoma Detection. MS dissertation in computer science at Cal. State Univ. at Pomona. Lee, advisor. URL: http://members.nbci.com/_XMCM/hvle/thesis/contents.html

Leach, W.M., Jr. 1996. A two-port analogous circuit and SPICE model for Salmon's family of acoustical horns. *J. Acoust. Soc. Am.* 99(3): 1459–1464.

Lee, Y.W. 1960. *Statistical Theory of Communication.* John Wiley and Sons., NY.

Lee, P.S., R.F. Majowski and T.A. Perry. 1991. Tunable diode laser spectroscopy for isotope analysis – Detection of isotopic carbon dioxide in exhaled breath. *IEEE Trans. Biomed. Engrg.* 38(10): 966–973.

Lei, H., Z. Chongxun, H. Ying and C. Qun. 1997. Detecting myocardial ischemia with 2-D spectrum analysis of VCG signals. *IEEE Engrg. Med. and Biol. Mag.* 16(4): 33–40.

Lennox, R.B. 2000. Biosensor Device and Method. U.S. Patent #6,107,180. Aug. 22, 2000.

Leonard, G., J. Smurzynski, M.D. Jung and D. Kim. 1990. Evaluation of distortion product otoacoustic emissions as a basis for the objective clinical assessment of cochlear function. *Advances in Audiology.* 7: 139–148.

Leunig, A., K. Rick, H. Stepp, R. Gutmann, G. Alwin, R. Baumgartner and J. Feyh. 1996. Fluorescent imaging and spectroscopy of 5-aminolevulinic acid induced protoporphyrin IX for the detection of neoplastic lesions in the oral cavity. *Am. J. Surg.* 172(6): 674–677.

Leunig, A., C.S. Betz, R. Baumgartner, G. Grevers and W.J. Issing. 2000. Initial experience in the treatment of oral leukoplakia with high-dose vitamin A and follow-up 5-aminolevulinic acid induced protoporphyrin IX fluorescence. *Eur. Arch. Otorhinolaryngol.* 257: 327–331.

LightLab™ Imaging, LLC. 2000. Website with many OCT images. URL: wysiwyg://16/http://octimaging.com/

Liley, D.T.J. 2001. Course Notes for Medical Imaging, HET 408, at Swinburn University of Technology, Australia. Excellent on-line course notes on medical imaging modalities. URL: http://marr.bsee.swin.edu.au/~dtl/het408.html

Lochner, J. 2001. Microchannel Plates. URL: wysiwyg://29/http://imagine.gsfc.nasa/science/how_12/microchannels.html

Lockwood, G.R., D.H. Turnbull, D.A. Christopher and F.S. Foster. 1966. Beyond 30 MHz: Applications of high-frequency ultrasound imaging. *IEEE Engr. in Med. and Biol. Mag..* 15(6): 60–71.

Lum, E., MDand T. Gross, MD. 2000. Spirometry: Interpretation of Pulmonary Function Tests. Brochure from the University of Iowa Virtual Hospital. URL: http://www.vh.org/Providers/Simulations/Spirometry/SpirometryModule.html

Macovski, A. 1983. *Medical Imaging Systems.* Prentice-Hall, Inc. Englewood Cliffs, NJ.

Magnin, P.A. 1986. Doppler effect: History and theory. *Hewlett-Packard J,* June.

March, W.F. 29 March 1977. Non-Invasive Glucose Sensor System. U.S. Patent #4,014,321.

March, W.F., B. Rabinovitch and R.L. Adams. 1982. Noninvasive glucose monitoring in the aqueous humor of the eye. Part 2: Animal studies and the scleral lens. *Diabetes Care.* 5(3): 259–265.

March, W.F. 1984. Ocular glucose sensor. *Proc. 1984 IEEE/NSF Symp. on Biosensors.* IEEE Press. 79-81.

Marelius, J. 1995. Autofluorescence Imaging of Living Cells. MSc thesis at the University of Zurich. URL: www.student.ibg.uu.se/~john/autofl/1st.htm

Maron, S.H. and C.F. Prutton. 1958. *Principles of Physical Chemistry.* MacMillan Co., NY.

McKusick, V.A., S.A. Talbot and G.N. Webb. 1959. Spectral phonocardiography: Problems and prospects in the application of the Bell spectrograph to phonocardiography. *Bull. Johns Hopkins Hosp.* 94: 187–198.

McDonald, B.M. 1992. Two-Phase Lock-In Amplifier with Phase-Locked Loop Vector Tracking. M.S. Dissertation, The University of Connecticut, Storrs. (R.B. Northrop, Major advisor.)

McDonald, B.M. and R.B. Northrop. 1993. Two-phase lock-in amplifier with phase-locked loop vector tracking. *Proc. Eur. Conf. Circuit Theory and Design.* Davos, Switzerland. 30 Aug.–3 Sept. 1993. 6 pp.

McGill University, Canada. Virtual Stethoscope: Cardiac Auscultation and Pulmonary Auscultation. URL: www.music.mcgill.ca/auscultation/auscultation.html

Mellors, R.C. 1995. Neoplasia. Tutorial paper. URL: http://edcenter.med.cornell.edu/CUMC_PathNotes/Neoplasia/Neoplasia.html

Mendelson, Y., A.C. Clermont, R.A. Peura and B-C. Lin. 1990. Blood glucose measurement by multiple attenuated total reflection and infrared absorption spectroscopy. *IEEE Trans. on Biomed. Engrg.* 37(5): 458–465.

Merk. 2000. *The Merk Manual of Diagnosis and Therapy.* Section 17. Genitourinary Disorders: Ch. 214. Clinical Evaluation of Genitourinary Disorders. The Merk Manual online. URL: www.merk.com/pubs/mmanual/section17/chapter214/214a.htm

Miklos, J. 1999. Chromosome painting, a powerful tool for chromosomal analysis. Web review paper. URL: http://artsci.wustl.edu/~jstader/miklos.html

MJA. 1998. Otoacoustic Emissions. Comments on OE testing in on-line *Australian Med. J.* URL: www.mja.com.au/public/issues/xmas98/lepage/lepage1.html

Moghadasian, M.H., et al. 1997. Homocysteine and coronary artery disease. *Arch. Internal. Med.* 157: 2299–2308.

Möller, K.D. 1988. *Optics.* University Science Books, Mill Valley, CA.

Montgomery, L.D., et al. 1997. Visual discrimination assessment using cortical energy analysis. Paper at 68th Ann. Scientific Mtg. Aerospace Med. Assoc. URL: http://msttp.arc.nasa.gov/eeg.html

Morris, M.D., Ed. 1999. Biomedical applications of Raman spectroscopy. *SPIE Proceedings.* 3608: 1–19. SPIE Web Publications Abstracts. URL: www.spie.org/web/abstacts/3600/3608.html

Moseley, P.T., J.O.W. Norris and D.E. Williams. 1991. *Techniques and Mechanisms in Gas Sensing.* Adam Hilger, NY.

Nanoptics, Inc., 1999. *Fiber Optics Tutorial.* URL: www.nanoptics.com/FiberopticTutorial.htm

Nave, R. 2000. *Blackbody Radiation.* (Web notes on BB radiation from the Georgia State University Hyperphysics web pages.) http://hyperphysics.phy-astr.gsu.edu/hbase/mod6.htm

Nelson, T.R. 1999. Development of a Type I Nonlinear Feedback System for Laser Velocimetry and Ranging. M.S. Dissertation in Biomedical Engineering. R.B. Northrop, advisor.

NIDDK. 1999. *Diabetes Statistics.* URL: www.niddk.nih.gov/diabetes/pubs/dmstats/dmstats.htm

Niemeyer, G. 1995. Selective rod- and cone-ERG responses in retinal degeneration. *Digital Journal of Ophthalmology.* URL: www.djo.harvard.edu/meei/OA/NIEMEYER/INDEX.html

Northrop, A.E.P. 1994. Comments on gas used for laparoscopy. *Personal communication, 9/94.*

Northrop, R.B. and S.S. Nilakhe. 1977. A no-touch ocular pulse measurement system for the diagnosis of carotid occlusions. *IEEE Trans. Biomed. Engrg.* 24(3): 139–148.

Northrop, R.B. and B.M. Decker. 1978. Assessment of cerebral hemodynamics by no-touch ocular pulse. *Proc. 6th New Engl. Bioengineering Conf.* Dov Jaron, Ed. (23–24 March, Univ. of Rhode Island, Kingston.) Pergamon Press. pp 105–108.

Northrop, R.B. 1990. *Analog Electronic Circuits.* Addison-Wesley Pub. Co., Reading, MA.

_____. 1997. *Introduction to Instrumentation and Measurements.* CRC Press. Boca Raton, FL.

_____. 2000. *Endogenous and Exogenous Regulation and Control of Physiological Systems.* CRC Press. Boca Raton, FL.

NTP Nomination History and Review. 3/96. *Melatonin.* CAS No. 73-31-4. URL: http://ntpserver.niehs.nih.gov/htdocs/Chem_Background/ExecSumm/Melatonin.html

Nunez, P.L. 1981a. A study of the origins of the time dependencies of the scalp EEG: I–Theoretical basis. *IEEE Trans. Biomed. Engrg.* 28(3): 271–280.

_____. 1981b. A study of the origins of the time dependencies of the scalp EEG: II–Experimental support of theory. *Ibid.* 281–288.

Ogata, K. 1970. *Modern Control Engineering.* Prentice-Hall, Englewood Cliffs, NJ.

Ohno, H. and Y. Hayashi. 1976. X-ray Tomography Apparatus. U.S. Patent #3,963,932. 15 June 1976.

Olson, H.F. 1940. *Elements of Acoustical Engineering.* D. Van Nostrand Co., Inc. NY.

Orlandini, M. 1994. [X-ray] *Collimators.* URL: www.tesre.bo.cnr.it/Research/SAX/sax_pds/node4.html)

Ornadel, D. 2000. How to Use a Stethoscope. Tutorial paper. Dept. of Chest Medicine, Whittington Hospital, London. URL: www.studentbmj.com/search/data/st09ed2.html

Pallas-Areny, R. and J.G. Webster. 1991. *Sensors and Signal Conditioning.* John Wiley and Sons, NY.

Papoulis, A. 1965. *Probability, Random Variables and Stochastic Processes.* McGraw-Hill Book Co., NY.

_____. 1977. *Signal Analysis.* McGraw-Hill Book Co., NY.

Parallel Design, Inc. 1999. Web pp. describing various linear (1-D) and rectangular (2-D) ultrasonic transducer arrays. URL: www.pardesign.com

Perkins, P. 1999. Gastroenterology Breath Tests. (White paper for Hotel Dieu Hospital, Kingston, Ontario. URL: www.hoteldieu.com/breath.htm

Perry, I.J., et al. 1995. Prospective study of serum total homocysteine concentration and risk of stroke in middle-aged British men. *The Lancet.* 346: 1395–1398.

Phan, H. 1999. Fundamental infrared spectroscopy. *TN-100.* The MIDAC Corp. URL: www.midac.com/applications.htm

Phan, H. 1999. FTIR sampling techniques. *TN-101.* The MIDAC Corp. URL: www.midac.com/applications.htm

Pharminfo. 1996. H. pylori *News*: Issue #1, May 1996. URL: www.pharminfo.com/disease/ulcers/hypnew1.html

Photon Technology International (PTI). 1999. About fluorescence. URL: www.ptinj.com/fluorescence_2.html

Pierce, R., MD and D.P. Johns. 1995. Spirometry: The Measurement and Interpretation of Ventilatory Function in Clinical Practice. The Thoracic Society of Australia and New Zealand, URL: http://hna.ffh.vic.gov.au/asthma/spiro/toc.html

Pimmel, R.L., R.A. Sunderland, D.J. Robinson, H.B. Williams, R.L. Hamlin and P.A. Bromberg. 1977. Instrumentation for measuring respiratory impedance by forced oscillations. *IEEE Trans. Biomed. Engrg.* 24(2): 89–93.

Pinto, L.H. and P.J. Dallos. 1968. An acoustic bridge for measuring the static and dynamic impedance of the eardrum. *IEEE Trans. Biomed. Engrg.* 15(1): 10–16.

Pohlmann, A., S. Sehati and D. Young. 1999. Towards acoustic imaging — influence of lung density on acoustic transmission in the respiratory system. *Trans. ESEM'99.* Barcelona, Spain.

Potter, J.B., J.B. Brown, J.F. Patrick and J.M. Schramp. 1975. A spectrophotometer for the direct determination of sample extinction by simultaneous measurement at multiple wavelengths and application of Allen's correction. *IEEE Trans. Biomed. Engrg.* 22(6): 528–532.

Powell, D.R. 2001. *X-Ray Generation.* U. Kansas Crystallography Home Page. URL: www.msg.ukans.edu/~xraylab/notes/xray.html

Proakis, J.G. and D.G. Manolakis. 1995. *Digital Signal Processing: Principles, Algorithms and Applications,* 3rd ed. Prentice-Hall, Englewood Cliffs, NJ.

Puertolas, D., et al. 1997. Biomedical applications of an imaging silicon pixel array (ISPA) tube. *Nucl. Instr. and Methods in Physics Res.* A. 387: 134–136.

Puliafito, C.A., M.R. Hee, J.S. Schuman, J.G. Fujimoto and N.J. Thorofare. 1996. Optical Coherence Tomography of Ocular Diseases. SLACK, Inc. 376 pp.

Qi, J-X. 1990. Determination of Cu, Zn, Fe, Ca, Mg, Na, and K in serum flame by atomic absorption spectroscopy. Varian AA Application Note AA-93.

Rabinovitch, B., W.F. March and R.L. Adams. 1982. Noninvasive glucose monitoring of the aqueous humor of the eye. Part 1: Measurements of very small optical rotations. *Diabetes Care.* 5(3): 254–258.

Rader, R.L. 1998. A White Noise Processing Approach in the Analysis of the Pulmonary System. M.S. Dissertation in Biomedical Engineering, The University of Connecticut, Storrs, CT. (R.B. Northrop, advisor.)

Raman, C.V. and K.S. Krishnan. 1928. A new type of secondary radiation. *Nature.* 121(3048): 501.

Rao, R.P.V., R.D. Kriz, et al. 1995. Parallel Implementation of the Filtered Back Projection Algorithm for Tomographic Imaging. Web paper. URL: www.sv.vt.edu/xray_ct/parallel/Parallel_CT.html

Rawlings, C.A. 1991. *Electrocardiography.* SpaceLabs, Inc., Redmond. WA.

Redhead, J.T. 1998. Otoacoustic Emissions and Recreational Hearing Loss. *.Med. J. Austral.* URL: www.mja.com.au/public/issues/xmas98/redhead/redhead.html

Reilley, C.N. and D.T. Sawyer. 1961. *Experiments for Instrumental Methods.* McGraw-Hill, NY.

Reisch, S., H. Steltner, J. Timmer, C. Renotte, and J. Guttmann. 1999. Early detection of upper airway obstructions by analysis of acoustical respiratory input impedance. *Biol. Cybernetics.* 81: 25–37.

Rice, D. 1983. Sound speed in pulmonary parenchyma. *J. Appl. Physiol.* 54: 304–308.

Rijpma, A.P., H.J.M. ter Brake, M.J. Peters and H. Rogalla. 1999. Design for a fetal heart monitor for clinical use. *4th Intl. Conf. on Neuroscience and Neuroimaging,* Friedrich Schiller Univ., Jena. 9/26/99.

Riley. 1996. Slit Lamp Illuminations and Slit Lamp Examination. URL: www.opt.indiana.edu/optlib/Riley/Rileyslit.html

Rosow, E., F. Beatrice and J. Adam. 1998. A virtual instrumentation system evaluates fiber-optic endoscopes. Paper with illustrations. URL: www.evaluationengineering.com/pctest/articles/e711med.htm

Routh, H.F. 1996. Doppler ultrasound. *IEEE Engrg. Med. and Biol. Mag.*15(6): 31–40.

Rowell, N.D. 2000. Gains made in macular degeneration treatment. *Photonics Spectra.* 34(12): 50–55.

Salenius, J.P., J.F. Brennan III, A. Miller, Y. Wang, T. Aretz, B. Sacks, R.R. Dasari and M.S. Feld. 1998. Biochemical composition of human peripheral arteries examined with near-infrared Raman spectroscopy. *J. Vasc. Surg.* 27(4): 710-9.

Saxer, C.E., J.F. de Boer, et al. 2000. High-speed fiber-based polarization-sensitive optical coherence tomography of *in vivo* human skin. *Optics Letters.* 25(18): 1355–1357.

Schauenstein, K. and E. Schauenstein. 1998. Diagnostic relevance of non-specific tumor associated immune dysfunctions. *Cancer J.* 11(3). URL: www.infobiogen.fr/agora/journals/cancer/articles/11-3/scha.htm

Schlager, K.J. 1989. Non-Invasive Near Infrared Measurement of Blood Analyte Concentrations. U.S. Patent #4,882,492. (Transcutaneous non-dispersive spectrophotometry used to sense blood glucose using 900–1800 nm light.)

Schrock, E., et al. 1996. Multicolor spectral karyotyping of human chromosomes. *Science.* 273(5274): 494–497.

Schmitt, J.M., G-X. Zhou and J. Miller. 1992. Measurement of blood hematocrit by dual-wavelength near-IR photoplethysmography. SPIE. 1641: 150–161.

Sellin, P. 2000. GaAS X-ray Imaging Detectors. URL: www.ph.surrey.ac.uk/rmm/imaging/gaas/

Semenov, S.Y., et al. 1996. Microwave tomography: Two-dimensional system for biological imaging. *IEEE Trans. Biomed. Engrg.* 43(9): 869–877.

Sergeev, A.M., et al. 1997. *In vivo* endoscopic OCT imaging of precancer and cancer states of human mucosa. *Optics Express.* 1(13): 432–440.

Sears, F.W. 1949. *Optics.* Addison-Wesley Press, Inc., Cambridge, MA. Ch. 14. "Color."

Sears, F.W. 1953. *Electricity and Magnetism.* Addison-Wesley Pub. Co., Cambridge, MA.

Sergeev, A.M., et al. 1997. *In vivo* endoscopic OCT imaging of precancer and cancer states of human mucosa. *Optics Express.* 1(13): 432 -440.

Shalhoub, G.M. 1996. Blackbody Radiation and Planck Distribution Law. (Web essay. URL: http://www.monmouth.edu/~tzielins/mathcad/GShalhoub/doc003.htm

Shepherd, A.P. and P.Å. Oberg, Eds. 1990. *Laser Doppler Blood Flowmetry.* Kluwer Academic Publishers.

Sherman, S.E. 2000. Hermann von Helmholtz and His Discovery of the Ophthalmoscope. (Web paper. The American Academy of Opththalmology. URL: www.eyenet.org/public/museum/Helmholtz.html

Shi, L. 2001. DNA Microarray (genome Chip)–Monitoring the Genome on a Chip. A review article on DNA microarrays and their applications; many hot-link references. URL: wysiwyg://22/http://www.gene-chips.com/

Shivashankar, G.V. and A. Libchaber. 1997. Single DNA molecule grafting and manipulation using a combined atomic force microscope and optical tweezers. *Appl. Physics Letters.* 71: 22 Dec.

Shung, K.K. and M. Zipparo. 1996. Ultrasonic transducers and arrays. *IEEE Engrg. in Med. and Biol. Mag.* 15(6): 20–30.

Signal Processing, S.A. 1999. Introducing DOP Ultrasonic Velocimeter. Tech. white paper. URL: www.signal-processing.com/tech/introducing_dop.htm

Simon, H.J. 8 Dec. 1998. Sensor Using Long Range Surface Plasmon Resonance with Diffraction Double Grating. U.S. Pat. # 5,846,843.

Sirohi, R.S. and M.P. Kothiyal. 1991. *Optical Components, Systems, and Measurement Techniques.* Marcel Dekker, Inc., NY.

Smith, S.W., R.E. Davidson and C.D. Emery. 1996. Update on 2-D array transducers for medical ultrasound. *1995 IEEE Ultrasonics Symp. Proc.* 1273.

Sodal, I. and G.D. Swanson. 1982. Making the mass spectrometer an efficient anesthetist's aide. *IEEE EMB Mag..* 1(1): 32–35.

Sodickson, L.A. and M.J. Block. 1994. Kromoscopic analysis: a possible alternative to spectroscopic analysis for noninvasive measurement of analytes *in vivo. Clin. Chem.* 40: 1838–1844.

_____. 1995. Non-Spectrophotometric Measurement of Analyte Concentrations and Optical Properties of Objects. U.S. Patent #5,434,412. 18 July 1996.

Soenksen, D.C., et al. 1999. Method of Cancer Cell Detection. U.S. Patent #5,995,645. Nov. 30, 1999.

Spalterholz, W. 1914. *Handatlas der Anatomie des Menschen,* Band 3. Verlag von S. Hirzel, Leipzig.

Spear, C. 1999. Controversies in glaucoma care. *Review of Optometry.* 7 pp. URL: www.revoptom.com/issue/ro07f7.htm

Speicher, M.R., B.S. Gwyn and D.C. Ward. 1996. Karyotyping human chromosomes by combinatorial multifluor FISH. *Nature Genetics.* 12(4): 368–375.

Srinavasan, R., D.M. Tucker and M. Murias. 1998. Estimating the spatial Nyquist of the human EEG. *Behavior Res. Meth, Instruments and Computers.* 30(1): 8–19.

Stanford Exploration Project. 1997. Time-Frequency Resolution. Web tutorial. URL: http://sepwww.stanford.edu/sep/prof/fgdp/c4/paper_html/node2.html

Stark, H., F.B. Tuteur and J.B. Anderson. 1988. *Modern Electrical Communications.* Prentice-Hall, Englewood Cliffs, NJ.

Steinke, J.M. and A.P. Shepherd. 1986. Role of light scattering in spectrophotometric measurements of arteriovenous oxygen difference. *IEEE Trans. Biomed. Engrg.* 33(8): 729–734.

Sticker, M., C.K. Hitzenberger and A.F. Fercher. 2000. Direct extraction of phase information in differential phase contrast OCT. Web paper, 6 pp. URL: http://optics.sgu.ru/SFM2000/report/Hitzenberger

Strommer, J. 1996. Let's Play PET. An extensive description of PET, at UCLA Molecular and Medical Pharmacology website. URL: http://laxmi.nuc.ucla.edu:8000/lpp/lpphome.html

Suki, B. and K.R. Lutchen. 1992. Pseudorandom signals to estimate apparent transfer and coherence functions of nonlinear systems: Applications to respiratory mechanics. *IEEE Trans. Biomed. Engrg.* 39(11): 1142–1150.

Swanson, E.A., J.G. Fujimoto, et al. 1993. *In vivo* retinal imaging by optical coherence tomography. *Opt. Lett.* 18(21): 1864–1866.

Takatani, S. and J. Ling. 1994. Optical oximetry sensors for whole blood and tissue. *IEEE Engrg in Med. and Biol. Mag..* June/July. 347–357.

Tarr, R.V. and P.G. Steffes. 1993. Noninvasive Blood Glucose Measurement System and Method Using Stimulated Raman Spectroscopy. U.S. Patent #5,243,983. 14 September 1993.

_____ . 1998. The noninvasive measure of d-glucose in the ocular aqueous humor using stimulated Raman spectroscopy. LEOS paper. URL: www.ieee.org/organizations/leos/apr98/dgloucose.htm [sic].

Tearney, G.J., J.G. Fujimoto, et al. 1996. Scanning single-mode fiber optic catheter-endoscope for optical coherence tomography. *Opt. Lett.* 21(7): 543–545.

Tech Transfer News. 11 Oct. 2000. Motorola's Clinical MicroSensors division receives five key US patents; coverage is central to com [sic]. (re: DNA Biochip technology. UVentures' URL: www.uventures.com/servlets/UVTechNews/1408

Tenenbaum, D. 1999. *A new urine test?* URL: http://whyfiles.org/shorties/urine_test.html

Thakor, N.V., J.M. Ferrero, Jr, J. Saiz, B.I. Gramatikov and J.M. Ferrero, Sr. 1998. Electrophysiological models of heart cells and cell networks. *IEEE Engrg. Med. and Biol. Mag.* 17(5): 73–83.

Thomas, S.W.H. and W.R. Preuhsner. 1995. Fetal Pulse Oximetry Sensor. U.S. Patent # 5,411,024. May 2, 1995. Assignee: Corometrics Medical Systems, Wallingford, CT.

Tian, Y., et al. 1999. Flip-chip-type high-T_c gradiometer for biomagnetic measurements in unshielded environment. Web paper. URL: www.chinainfo.gov.cn/periodicals/zgkx-e/kx-a2000/0001/000110.htm

Tilson-Chrysler, A. 2000. Understanding Heart Sounds, Part I. URL: www.chiroweb.com/archives/12/11/02.html

Tope, W.D., E.V. Ross, N. Kollias, A. Martin, R. Gillies and R.R. Anderson. 1998. Protoporphyrin IX fluorescence induced in basal cell carcinoma by oral 5-aminolevulinic acid. Photochemistry and Photobiology Abstract. 67: 249. URL: www.pol-us.net/PAPhome/Vol67/pap67249.html

Transferrin. 1997. Iron Transport and Cellular Uptake. Web paper, 11 pp with refs. URL: http://sickle.bwh.harvard.edu/iron_transport.html

Truax, B., Ed. 1999. Handbook for Acoustic Ecology. On-line reference text on acoustics and sound. Cambridge Street Publishing. URL: www.sfu.ca/sonic-studio/index.html

Turner Designs. 1998. An Introduction to Fluorescence Measurements. Web tutorial. URL: www.turnerdesigns.com/applications/998_0050/998_0050.htm

Tustison, C.J. 1999. Melanoma FAQ. URL: wysiwyg://53/http:/westbyserver.westby.mwt.net/ctustis/melfaq.html

Verdon, W., Director, Electrodiagnostic and Vision Functions Clinic. URL: http://spectacle.berkeley.edu/ucbso/vfc/

Verhoef, P., et al. 1996. Homocysteine metabolism and risk of myocardial infarction; relation with vitamins B6, B12 and folate. *Am. J. Epidemiol.* 143(9): 845–859.

Viera, P. c. 2000. Tomographic Reconstruction of the Retina Using the Confocal Scanning Laser Ophthalmoscope. Web paper. URL: www.biomed.abdn.ac.uk/abstracts /A03F00/ Virtual Mammo, 2000. *VirtualMammo User Manual.* URL: www.oxiva.com/doc/vmum/xmvPhysics.htm

Wallace, V.P, D.C. Crawford, P.S. Mortimer, R.J. Ott, and J.C. Bamber. 2000. Spectrophotometric assessment of pigmented skin lesions: methods and feature selection for evaluation of diagnostic performance. *Phys. Med. Biol.* 45: 735–751.

Wang, X-J., et al. 1999. Characterization of dentin and enamel by use of optical coherence tomography. *Applied Optics.* 38(10): 2092–2096.

Ward, J.W. 1977. Automatic Acoustic Impedance Meter. U.S. Patent #4,009,707. 1 March 1977.

Webster, J.G., ed. 1992. *Medical Instrumentation: Application and Design.* 2nd edition. Houghton-Mifflin Co., Boston.

_____. 1998. *Medical Instrumentation: Application and Design.* 3rd edition. John Wiley and Sons. NY.

Wesseling, G.J. 1999. Respiratory impedance measurement in clinical lung function testing. Thesis abstract. Univ. Maastricht, Netherlands. 23 Nov. URL: http://www2.uni-maas.nl/~pulmo/sum_wes.htm

West, J.B., Ed. 1985. *Best and Taylor's Physiological Basis of Medical Practice,* 11th ed. Williams and Wilkins, Baltimore.

Williams, C.S. 1986. *Designing Digital Filters.* Prentice-Hall, Inc. Englewood Cliffs, NJ.

Wodicka, G.B., K.N. Stevens, H.L. Golub, E.G. Cravalho and D.C. Shannon. 1989. A model of acoustic transmission in the respiratory system. *IEEE Trans. BioMed. Engrg. 36(9):* 925–934.

Wolfbeis, O.S., Ed. 1991. *Fiber Optic Sensors and Biosensors. Vol. 1.* CRC Press, Boca Raton, FL.

Wood, J.C., A.J. Buda and D.T. Barry. 1992. Time-frequency transforms: A new approach to first heart sound frequency dynamics. *IEEE Trans. Biomed. Engrg.* 39(7): 730–740.

Wood, J.C. and D.T. Barry. 1995. Time-frequency analysis of the first heart sound. *IEEE Engrg. in Med. and Biol. Mag.* March/April. 144–151.

Yamaguchi, M., M. Mitsumori and Y. Kano. 1998. Noninvasively measuring blood glucose using saliva. *IEEE Engrg. Med. and Biol. Mag.* 17(3): 59–63.

Yamashita, T., H. Ushida, et al. 1990. Development of a high resolution PET. *IEEE Trans. Nucl. Sci.* 37(2): 594–599.

Yazdanfar, S., M.D. Kulkarni and J.A. Izatt. 1997. High resolution imaging of *in vivo* cardiac dynamics using color Doppler optical coherence tomography. *Optics Express.* 1(13): 424–431.

Young, S.S., D. Tesarowskiá, L.Viel. 1996. Frequency dependence of forced oscillatory mechanics in horses with heaves. *APS Abstracts.* 3:0497A.

Young, P.R. 1996a. *Infrared Absorbances for Common Functional Groups.* Organic Chemistry OnLine. URL: http://chipo.chem.uic.edu/web1/ocol/spec/IRTable.htm

_____. 1996b. *Basic Mass Spectroscopy.* Organic Chemistry OnLIne. URL: http://chipo.chem.uic.edu/web1/ocol/spec/MS.htm

Index

---

* Pages with boldface numbers contain figures relating to keywords.